I0057334

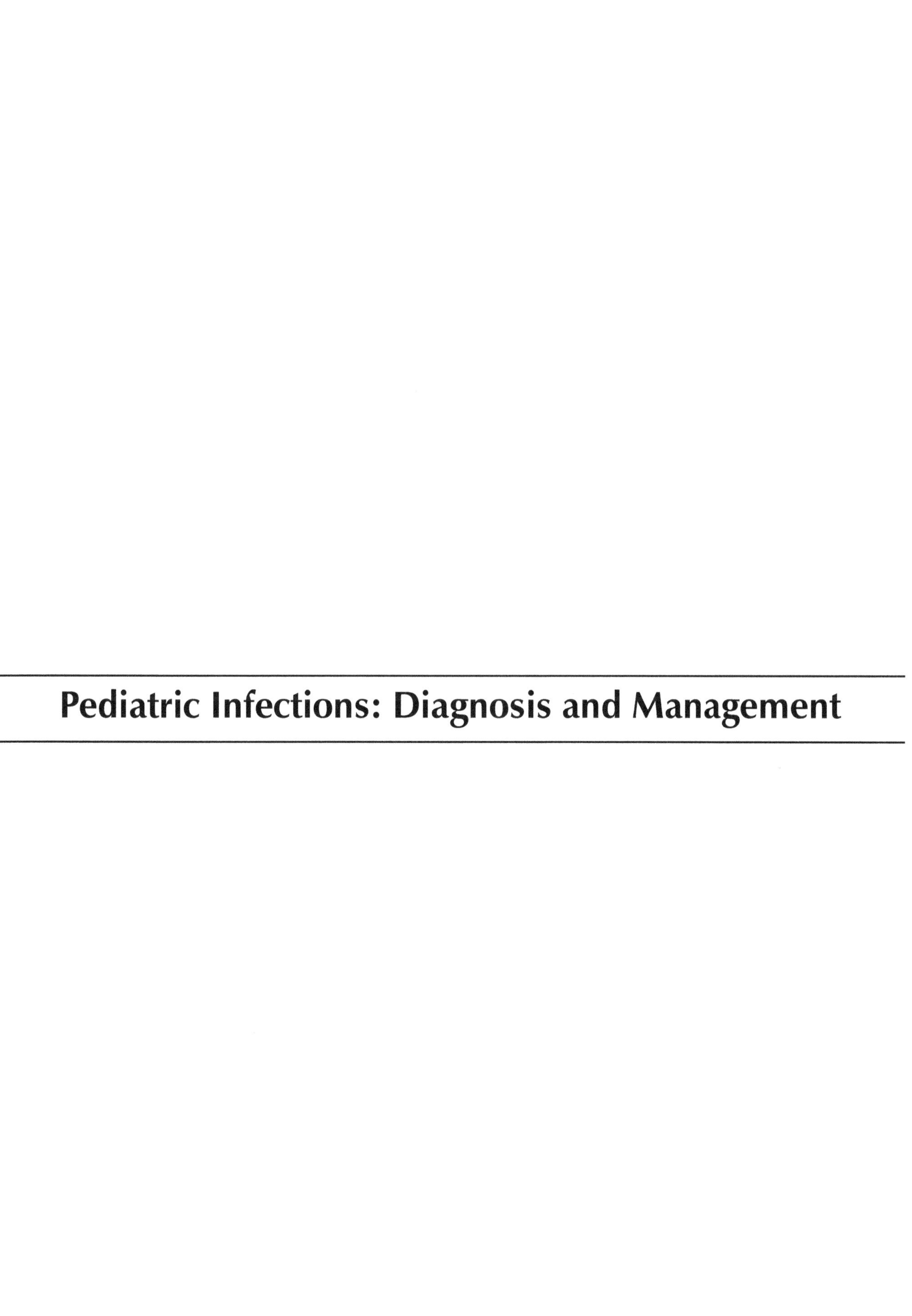

Pediatric Infections: Diagnosis and Management

Pediatric Infections: Diagnosis and Management

Editor: Caroline Francis

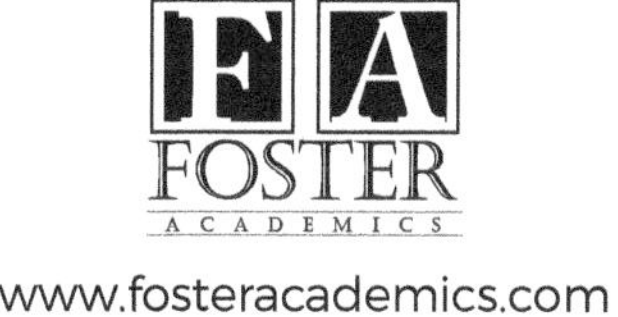

www.fosteracademics.com

www.fosteracademics.com

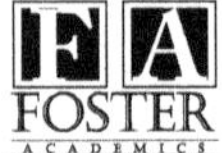

Cataloging-in-Publication Data

Pediatric infections : diagnosis and management / edited by Caroline Francis.
p. cm.
Includes bibliographical references and index.
ISBN 978-1-63242-779-3
1. Infection in children. 2. Children--Diseases--Diagnosis. 3. Children--Diseases--Treatment.
4. Bacterial diseases in children. 5. Pediatrics. 6. Infection. I. Francis, Caroline.
RJ401 .P43 2019
618.929--dc23

© Foster Academics, 2019

Foster Academics,
118-35 Queens Blvd., Suite 400,
Forest Hills, NY 11375, USA

ISBN 978-1-63242-779-3 (Hardback)

This book contains information obtained from authentic and highly regarded sources. Copyright for all individual chapters remain with the respective authors as indicated. All chapters are published with permission under the Creative Commons Attribution License or equivalent. A wide variety of references are listed. Permission and sources are indicated; for detailed attributions, please refer to the permissions page and list of contributors. Reasonable efforts have been made to publish reliable data and information, but the authors, editors and publisher cannot assume any responsibility for the validity of all materials or the consequences of their use.

Trademark Notice: Registered trademark of products or corporate names are used only for explanation and identification without intent to infringe.

Contents

Preface

Young children and infants can suffer from a wide range of immunologic and infectious diseases, caused by viral, bacterial, fungal and parasitic agents. These diseases can be complicated or common. Some of such diseases are meningitis, tuberculosis (TB), respiratory infections, hepatitis, bone and joint infections, acquired immunodeficiency syndrome (AIDS), etc. Physicians who specialize in pediatric infectious diseases study the causative pathogens and transmission pathways of such diseases. They also design the therapeutic and prevention techniques for each of these conditions. Many research domains are relevant to this field, such as antibiotic resistance, production of safe and effective vaccines, and emerging infections. The topics included in this book on pediatric infections are of utmost significance and bound to provide incredible insights to readers. It presents researches and studies performed by experts across the globe on the diagnosis and management interventions of pediatric infections. It will help new researchers by foregrounding their knowledge in this domain.

Significant researches are present in this book. Intensive efforts have been employed by authors to make this book an outstanding discourse. This book contains the enlightening chapters which have been written on the basis of significant researches done by the experts.

Finally, I would also like to thank all the members involved in this book for being a team and meeting all the deadlines for the submission of their respective works. I would also like to thank my friends and family for being supportive in my efforts.

Editor

Differences in Epidemiological and Molecular Characteristics of Nasal Colonization with *Staphylococcus aureus* (MSSA-MRSA) in Children from a University Hospital and Day Care Centers

Erika A. Rodríguez[1,2], Margarita M. Correa[1], Sigifredo Ospina[3], Santiago L. Atehortúa[3], J. Natalia Jiménez[1,2]*

1 Grupo de Microbiología Molecular, Escuela de Microbiología, Universidad de Antioquia, Medellín, Colombia, **2** Grupo de Investigación en Microbiología Básica y Aplicada - MICROBA, Escuela de Microbiología Universidad de Antioquia, Medellín, Colombia, **3** Hospital Universitario de San Vicente Fundación, Medellín, Colombia

Abstract

Background: Clinical significance of Staphylococcus aureus colonization has been demonstrated in hospital settings; however, studies in the community have shown contrasting results regarding the relevance of colonization in infection by community-associated MRSA (CA-MRSA). In Colombia there are few studies on *S. aureus* colonization. The aim of this study was to determine the molecular and epidemiological characteristics of nasal colonization by *S. aureus* (MSSA-MRSA) in children from a university hospital and day care centers (DCCs) of Medellin, Colombia.

Methods: An observational cross-sectional study was conducted in 400 children (200 in each setting), aged 0 months to 5 years, during 2011. Samples were collected from each nostril and epidemiological information was obtained from the parents. Genotypic analysis included *spa* typing, PFGE, MLST, SCC*mec* typing, detection of genes for virulence factors and *agr* groups.

Results: Frequency of *S. aureus* colonization was 39.8% ($n = 159$) (hospital 44.5% and DCCs 35.0%) and by MRSA, 5.3% ($n = 21$) (hospital 7.0% and DCCs 3.5%). Most *S. aureus* colonized children were older than two years ($p = 0.005$), the majority of them boys (59.1%), shared a bedroom with a large number of people ($p = 0.028$), with history of β-Lactamase inhibitors usage ($p = 0.020$). MSSA strains presented the greatest genotypic diversity with 15 clonal complexes (CC). MRSA isolates presented 6 CC, most of them (47.6%) belonged to CC8-SCC*mec* IVc and were genetically related to previously reported infectious MRSA strains.

Conclusion: Differences in epidemiological and molecular characteristics between populations may be useful for the understanding of *S. aureus* nasal colonization dynamics and for the design of strategies to prevent *S. aureus* infection and dissemination. The finding of colonizing MRSA with similar molecular characteristics of those causing infection demonstrates the dissemination capacity of *S. aureus* and the risk of infection among the child population.

Editor: Herminia de Lencastre, Rockefeller University, United States of America

Funding: This research was supported by the Comité para el Desarrollo de la Investigación - CODI, Universidad de Antioquia, Project: CIMB-032-11 and received support from Estrategia para la Sostenibilidad de Grupos 2011–2012, Code EO1624. The funders had no role in study design, data collection and analysis, decision to publish, or preparation of the manuscript.

Competing Interests: The authors have declared that no competing interests exist.

* Email: nataliajiudea@gmail.com

Introduction

Staphyloccocus aureus is one of the principal human pathogens, responsible for various types of important infections in the community and hospital settings [1]. This microorganism is characterized by its high capacity to adapt to antimicrobials by the acquisition of resistance mechanisms particularly against methicillin, further complicating the treatment of infections [1].

Besides its advantages as a pathogen and its capacity to develop resistance mechanisms, *S. aureus* presents a great ability to colonize humans, primarily their nose [2]. Colonization is an important factor in the pathogenesis and epidemiology of infections by *Staphyloccocus aureus* methicillin-sensitive (MSSA) and methicillin-resistant (MRSA) [2]. It is suggested that there is a greater risk for previously colonized individuals of developing infection or of invasive infection after colonization by MRSA [3]. Children are particularly susceptible to colonization by *S. aureus* with prevalences that vary from 7.6–53.8%, depending on the age group [4,5]. Furthermore, they generally present a pattern of persistent colonization and may act as vectors disseminating *S. aureus* throughout the community and in healthcare institutions [6].

The importance of colonization has been defined in more detail in hospital environments, while its significance in the community is

Table 1. Epidemiological characteristics of *S. aureus*-colonized children in the overall population and by institution (hospital - day care centers).

Characteristics				Hospital (n = 200)			DDCs (n = 200)		
	No. of *S. aureus*-colonized children (%)			No. of *S. aureus*-colonized children (%)			No. of *S. aureus*-colonized children (%)		
	Yes 159 (39.8)	No 241 (60.2)	P[a]	Yes 89 (44.5)	No 111(55.5)	P[a]	Yes 70 (35)	No 130 (65)	P[a]
Age:									
Median	3	2	**0.027**[d]	1	1	**0.006**[d]	3	2	0.207[d]
Range	(1–4)	(1–3)		(0–4)	(0–3)		(2–4)	(2–4)	
Age (years):									
>2	86 (54.1)	96 (39.8)	**0.005**	35 (39.3)	21 (18.9)	**0.001**	51 (72.9)	75 (57.7)	**0.034**
≤2	73 (45.9)	145 (60.2)		54 (60.7)	90 (81.1)		19 (27.1)	55 (42.3)	
Gender:									
Male	94 (59.1)	123 (51)	0.112	56 (62.9)	57 (51.4)	0.101	38 (54.3)	66 (50.8)	0.635
Female	65 (40.9)	118 (49)		33 (37.1)	54 (48.6)		32 (45.7)	64 (49.2)	
History of *S. aureus* in the previous year [e]	-	-	-	0	2 (1,8)	0.503[b]	-	-	.
History in the previous year of:									
Hospitalization	74 (46.5)	103 (42.7)	0.454	63 (70.8)	82 (73.9)	0.627	11 (15.7)	21 (16.2)	0.936
Surgery	27 (17)	38 (15.8)	0.747	22 (24.7)	28 (25.2)	0.935	5 (7.1)	10 (7.7)	0.888
Dialysis	1 (0.6)	0 (0)	0.397[b]	0	0	_	1 (1.4)	0	0.350[b]
Stay in ICU	25 (15.7)	36 (14.9)	0.831	24 (27)	34 (30.6)	0.570	1 (1.4)	2 (1.5)	0.99[b]
Antimicrobial use in the previous 6 months:	78 (49.1)	114 (47.9)	0.821	47(52.8)	60 (54.1)	0.861	31 (44.3)	54 (42.5)	0.811
Penicillin	51 (65.4)	83 (72.8)	0.271	21 (44.7)	37 (61.7)	0.080	30 (96.8)	46 (85.2)	0.146[b]
Macrolides	7 (9)	17 (14.9)	0.222	6 (12.8)	14 (23.3)	0.164	1 (3.2)	3 (5.6)	0.99[b]
β-Lactamase inhibitors	16 (20.5)	10 (8.8)	**0.020**	16 (34)	10 (16.7)	**0.038**	0	0	-
Co-morbidities:	78 (49.1)	120 (49.8)	0.885	54 (60.7)	77 (69.4)	0.199	24 (34.3)	43 (33.1)	0.863
Diabetes Mellitus	1 (0.6)	2 (0.8)	0.99[b]	1 (1.1)	2 (1.8)	0.99[b]	0	0	_
Atopy	46 (28.9)	80 (33.2)	0.369	25 (28.1)	39 (35.1)	0.288	21 (30)	41 (31.5)	0.822
Neoplasia	4 (2.5)	6 (2.5)	0.99[b]	4 (4.5)	6 (5.4)	0.99[b]	0	0	_
Immunosu- pression	12 (7.5)	15 (6.2)	0.606	12 (13.5)	14 (12.6)	0.856	0	1 (0.8)	0.99[b]
Chronic renal disease	0 (0)	2 (0.8)	0.520[b]	0	2 (1.8)	0.504	0	0	_
Cardiovascular disease	6 (3.8)	6 (2.5)	0.553[b]	6 (6.7)	6 (5.4)	0.693	0	0	_
Chronic lung disease	4 (2.5)	5(2.1)	0.745[b]	4 (4.5)	5 (4.5)	0.99[b]	0	0	_
Malnutrition	13 (8.2)	11 (4.6)	0.137	11 (12.4)	11 (9.9)	0.582	2 (2.9)	0	0.121[b]
Pneumococcal conjugate vaccination	47 (33.1)	90 (40.7)	0.144	22 (29.7)	45 (46.9)	**0.023**	25 (36.8)	45 (36)	0.916
Influenza vaccination	130 (84.4)	204 (88.3)	0.269	70 (82.4)	89 (85.6)	0.546	60 (87)	115(90.6)	0.437
Family and personal history of SSTI in the previous year	62 (39)	80 (33.2)	0.236	36 (40.4)	43 (38.7)	0.806	26 (37.1)	37 (28.5)	0.207
Hospitalization of a family member within the previous 3 months	31 (19.6)	31 (12.9)	0.071	21 (23.6)	18 (16.4)	0.201	10 (14.5)	13 (10)	0.345

Table 1. Cont.

Characteristics				Hospital (n = 200)			DDCs (n = 200)		
	No. of *S. aureus*-colonized children (%)			No. of *S. aureus*-colonized children (%)			No. of *S. aureus*-colonized children (%)		
	Yes 159 (39.8)	No 241 (60.2)	P^a	Yes 89 (44.5)	No 111(55.5)	P^a	Yes 70 (35)	No 130 (65)	P^a
Contact with healthcare workers	18 (11.4)	40 (16.6)	0.149	13 (14.6)	24 (21.6)	0.204	5 (7.2)	16 (12.3)	0,269
Type of housing:									
Lodging	2 (1.3)	6 (2.5)	0.341[c]	2 (2.2)	6 (5.4)	0.597[c]	0	0	0.96[c]
Apartment	33 (20.8)	55 (22.8)		20 (22.5)	22 (19.8)		13 (18.6)	33 (25.4)	
House	113(71.1)	171 (71)		62 (69.7)	77 (69.4)		51 (72.9)	94 (72.3)	
Tenement house	11 (6.9)	8 (3.3)		5 (5.6)	5 (4.5)		6 (8.6)	3 (2.3)	
No. of occupants in the dwelling:									
Median	5	5	0.531[d]	5	5	0.623[d]	5	5	0.209[d]
Range	(4–7)	(4–6)		(4–7)	(4–7)		(4–7)	(4–6)	
No. of occupants in the bedroom:									
Median	3	3	**0.028[d]**	3	3	0.151[d]	3	2	0.188[d]
Range	(2–4)	(2–3)		(2–4)	(2–3)		(2–3)	(2–3)	
No. of minors sharing the dwelling:									
No. of children younger than 10:									
Median	3	3	0.137[d]	1	1	0.415[d]	3	3	0.188[d]
Range	(2–4)	(2–3)		(1–2)	(1–2)		(1–2)	(1–2)	
No. of minors between 11–18:									
Median	1	1	0.431[d]	1	1	0.485[d]	3	3	0.678[d]
Range	(1–2)	(1–2)		(1–1)	(1–2)		(1–2)	(1–2)	
Shared personal items:	63 (39.9)	99 (41.1)	0.810	26 (29.2)	1 (0.9)	0. 627	37 (53.6)	70 (53.8)	0. 976
Shared soap	59 (93.7)	96 (97)	0.432[b]	24 (92.3)	28 (96.6)	0.598[b]	35 (94.6)	68 (97.1)	0.608[b]
Shared towels	30 (47.6)	40 (40.4)	0.366	16 (61.5)	8 (27.6)	**0.011**	14 (37.8)	32 (45.7)	0.434
Mother's school grade:									
Elementary	62 (39)	80 (33.2)	0.178[c]	35 (39.3)	47 (42.3)	0.262[c]	27 (38.6)	33 (25.4)	0.130[c]
High school	69 (43.4)	102 (42.3)		39 (43.8)	35 (31.5)		30 (42.9)	67 (51.5)	
Higher education	9 (5.7)	31 (12.9)		4 (4.5)	12 (10.8)		5 (7.1)	19 (14.6)	
Illiterate	17 (10.7)	25 (10.4)		9 (10.1)	15 (13.5)		8 (11.4)	10 (7.7)	
No data reported	2 (1.3)	3 (1.2)		2 (2.2)	2 (1.8)		0	1 (0.8)	
Using nasal spray or nasal wash	47 (32.4)	70 (34.8)	0.640	37 (48.1)	60 (63.8)	**0.038**	10 (14.7)	10 (9.3)	0.277
Passive smoking	64(40.5)	82 (34)	0.189	38 (42.7)	37 (33.3)	0.174	26 (37.7)	45 (34.6)	0.667
Household pets:	59 (37.3)	78 (32.4)	0.306	32 (36)	42 (37.8)	0.784	27 (39.1)	36 (27.7)	0.099
Dog	44 (74.6)	53 (67.9)	0.398	25 (78.1)	28 (66.7)	0.279	19 (70.4)	25 (69.4)	0.937
Cat	16 (27.1)	17 (21.8)	0.471	10 (31.2)	10 (23.8)	0.475	6 (22.2)	7 (19.4)	0.787

Table 1. Cont.

Characteristics				Hospital (n = 200)			DDCs (n = 200)		
	No. of *S. aureus*-colonized children (%)			No. of *S. aureus*-colonized children (%)			No. of *S. aureus*-colonized children (%)		
	Yes 159 (39.8)	No 241 (60.2)	P^a	Yes 89 (44.5)	No 111(55.5)	P^a	Yes 70 (35)	No 130 (65)	P^a
Rabbit	2 (3.4)	4 (5.1)	0.699[b]	0	2 (4.8)	0.502[b]	2 (7.4)	2 (5.6)	0.99[b]
Birds	17(28.8)	25 (32.1)	0.684	13 (40.6)	20 (47.6)	0.549	4 (14.8)	5 (13.9)	0.99[b]
Other pets	4 (6.8)	9 (11.5)	0.347	3 (9.4)	6 (14.3)	0.723[b]	1(3.7)	3 (8.3)	0.629[b]

Significant differences ($p<0.05$) are shown in bold. Chi-square test[a], Fisher's exact test[b], likelihood ratio test[c], Mann-Whitney U tests[d]. Variable evaluated only in hospitalized children[e].

still controversial. It is suggested that colonization has little relevance to pathogenesis and infection by community-associated MRSA (CA-MRSA) [7]. However, an increase in nasal colonization has been implicated as the principal risk factor in the emergence of MRSA infections, especially in healthy children [8,9]. In Colombia and particularly in Medellin, few studies have been carried out on *S. aureus* colonization in children or to describe the molecular characteristics of the colonizing strains. Considering that the epidemiology of *S. aureus* depends on the particular conditions of each population, the objective of this study was to determine the molecular and epidemiological characteristics of nasal colonization by *S. aureus* (MSSA-MRSA) in children from a university hospital and day care centers (DCCs) in the city of Medellin, Colombia.

Materials and Methods

Study Population

An observational cross-sectional study was conducted in children aged 0 months to 5 years admitted to the Pediatric Department of Hospital Universitario de San Vicente Fundación (HUSVF) and from eight DCCs of Medellin, the second largest city of Colombia, during 2011. The research and informed consent protocols for this study were approved by the Bioethics Committee for Human Research of the University Research Center, Universidad de Antioquia (CBEIH-SIU-UdeA) (approval No 10-041-277), as well as by the Research Ethics' Committee of HUSVF. Written informed consent to participate in the study was obtained from the children parents or guardians prior to sample collection. Hospital Universitario de San Vicente Fundación is a fourth-level care center with 648 beds, and its Pediatric Department has 186 beds. The children included in the study were randomly selected from the different services of the Pediatric Department and included, general hospitalization, nursing, oncology and nephrology. According to data from the HUSVF-Clinical Microbiology Service, during 2010 the prevalence of MRSA in all types of infections was 31.8%. The eight DCCs (A–H), are located in neighborhoods of low socio-economic status and belong to the "Buen comienzo" (Good Start) program sponsored by the municipality government. The number of children attending the DCCs varied, A ($n=100$), B ($n=55$), C ($n=90$), D ($n=75$), E ($n=150$), F ($n=75$), G ($n=100$) and H ($n=60$).

Sample size was estimated based on an expected rate of 0.5 *S. aureus* positive children, for a total sample of 400 children (200 from each setting, hospital and DCCs). Children with more than 48 h of hospitalization or more than 6 months of attendance to the DCCs were included in the study. Children taken antibiotics during the previous seven days to sampling were excluded.

Clinical and epidemiological data

Epidemiological information was obtained from the medical records and parents or guardians for each child. Information included demographic aspects, medical history, antimicrobial usage, history of previous hospitalization, comorbidities, number of family members, smokers in the household and other possible factors linked to colonization.

Collection of nasal swabs and microbiological procedures

Samples from each nostril were collected using sterile cotton swabs with sterile 0.9% saline solution, rotated two or three times in the vestibule of both anterior nares and immediately placed in Amies transport medium with charcoal, conserved at 4–8°C and transported to the microbiology laboratory within 4 h of collection

Table 2. Bivariate and multivariate analyses of risk factors associated with *S. aureus*- colonized children in the overall population.

Variable	Crude PR (95% confidence interval)	P	Adjusted PR (95% confidence interval)	P
Hospitalization	1.271 (0.995–1.623)	0.0659	1.458 (1.133–1.876)	0.003
Age (years) >2	1.411 (1.107–1.797)	0.0070	1.712 (1.384–2.118)	0.001
β-Lactamase inhibitors usage in the previous 6 months	1.647 (1.147–2.366)	0.0340	1.655 (1.348–2.032)	0.001
Passive smoking	1.179 (0.924–1.505)	0.2270	1.361 (1.106–1.674)	0.004

[10]. In the lab, samples were immediately inoculated onto mannitol-salt agar, incubated at 37°C, for 24–48 h. Colonies with mannitol-salt fermentation and morphology suggestive of *Staphylococcus* were subcultured onto blood agar plates. Gram staining, catalase and rabbit plasma coagulase tests were performed [11].

Molecular typing

Previous to molecular typing, confirmation of *S. aureus* and methicillin resistance was performed by amplification of species-specific *nuc* and *femA* genes, and of *mecA* gene encoding resistance to methicillin, as previously described [12,13].

Spa typing was performed on all MRSA and on fifty percent of MSSA strains randomly selected (69 isolates, 39 from hospital and 30 from DCCs) [14]. Amplification products were sequenced and *spa* types were determined using Ridom Staphtype software (version 1.4; Ridom, GmbH, Wurzburg, Germany [http://spa.ridom.of/inofx.shtml]).

MLST was performed on a subset of 10 isolates representing the more frequent *spa* types (11% of all *spa* typed isolates ($n = 90$) [15]. Allele numbers and sequence types (ST) were assigned using the database maintained at http://saureus.mlst.net/, while CC were inferred using eBURST analysis [16]. CC for the strains not processed by MLST were inferred by *spa* repeat pattern analysis [17,18] or by referring to the Ridom Spa Server website.

SCC*mec* types and subtypes for MRSA isolates were determined using a set of multiplex PCR reactions [19,20].

Pulsed-field gel electrophoresis (PFGE) was performed on a representative subset of 64 colonizing *S. aureus* isolates, corresponding to all MRSA ($n = 21$) and 43 MSSA isolates randomly selected, representative of both settings and in a similar number of the resistant strains (22 from the hospital and 21 from DCCs) [21]. Digestion was carried out with *SmaI* enzyme. DNA fragment patterns were normalized using *S. aureus* strain NCTC 8325. Band assignments were manually adjusted after automatic band detection and only bands ranging from 36 kb to 600 kb were included in the analysis. Cluster analysis was performed using the Dice coefficient in BioNumerics software version 6.0 (Applied Maths, Sint-Martens-Latem, Belgium). Dendrograms were generated by the unweighted pair group method using average linkages (UPGMA), with 1% tolerance and 0.5% optimization settings. Similarity cutoffs of 80% and 95% were used to define types and subtypes, respectively [21]. Representatives of the most common infectious MRSA clones described in Colombia [22] and clone USA300-0114 CA-MRSA were used as reference strains.

Detection of virulence factors and *agr* genes

All isolates were screened for the genes encoding staphylococcal enterotoxins (*sea, seb, sec, sed, see*), toxic shock syndrome toxin 1 (*tst*) and exfoliative toxins A and B (*eta, etb*), using the protocols and primers described by Mehrotra et al. [13] The identity of the *lukS/F-PV* genes enconding Panton-Valentine Leucocidine (PVL) was performed as previously reported [23]. Accessory gene regulator (*agr*) typing was amplified by Multiplex PCR to determine four types of *agr* [24]. The *arcA* gene coding for the arginine catabolic mobile element (ACME) was detected by PCR [23,25].

Statistical analyses

Comparisons of clinical, epidemiological and molecular characteristics were carried out between *S. aureus* colonized and non-colonized, and MSSA- and MRSA- colonized children. Categorical variables were compared using the Chi-square test or Fisher's exact test and Mann–Whitney U test for continuous variables. Values $p \leq 0.05$ were considered to be statistically significant. Multiple binomial regression analysis was applied to explore risk factors associated with *S. aureus* colonization in the overall population. Initially, a bivariate analysis was performed to estimate the prevalence ratios (PR) and the 95% confidence interval (CI). Variables that had a p-value <0.25 or that were epidemiologically important were included in the multivariate model, such as, institution, age, history of β-Lactamase inhibitors and passive smoking. Multiple binomial regression analysis of risk factors associated with colonization by MRSA was not performed due to lack of power as there were very few observations. Statistical analyses were carried out using the software package SPSS v20.0 (SPSS Inc., Chicago, USA) and Stata 11 (StataCorp, College Station, TX, USA).

Results and Discussion

In Colombia few studies have been conducted to evaluate nasal carriage of S. aureus, and most of them have been performed in hospital settings evaluating healthcare personnel, and only recently, colonization in the pediatric population has been evaluated [26,27]. This is the first study in Colombia, simultaneously characterizing, epidemiologically and molecularly, nasal colonization by *S. aureus* in two different pediatric populations, from the hospital and the community. The information provided is useful for the understanding of *S. aureus* nasal colonization dynamics in these populations and for the design of strategies to prevent *S. aureus* infection and dissemination.

Frequency of nasal colonization by *Staphylococcus aureus*

The frequency of nasal colonization by *S. aureus* among the 400 children was 39.8% ($n = 159$) and of MRSA, 5.3% ($n = 21$). This findings are similar to previous reports for other countries of colonization frequencies among pediatric population of different ages, that vary between 7.6–53.8% [4,5], and for MRSA between 0.3%–13.2% [28,29]. Colonization at the hospital was 44.5% ($n = 89$), while in DCCs was 35.0% ($n = 70$) ($p = 0.0659$). Notoriously, a higher MRSA colonization frequency was observed in hospitalized children compared to DCCs, 7.0% ($n = 14$) vs. 3.5% ($n = 7$), although, this difference was no significant ($p = 0.1786$).

Table 3. Epidemiological characteristics of children colonized by MRSA and MSSA.

Characteristics	Total Population (n=159) No. %			Hospital (n=89) No. %			Day care centers (n=70) No. %		
	MRSA positive No. (%) 21 (13.2)	MSSA positive No. (%) 138 (86.8)	p[a]	MRSA positive No. (%) 14 (15.7)	MSSA positive No. (%) 75 (84.3)	p[a]	MRSA positive No. (%) 7 (10)	MSSA positive No. (%) 63 (90)	p[a]
Gender									
Male	18 (85.7)	76 (55.1)	**0.008**	12 (85.7)	44 (58.7)	**0.054**	6 (85.7)	32 (50.8)	0.116[b]
Female	3 (14.6)	62 (44.9)		2 (14.3)	31(41.3)		1 (14.3)	31 (49.2)	
History in the previous year of:									
Hospitalization	14 (66.7)	60 (43.5)	**0.047**	13 (92.9)	50 (66.7)	**0.058[b]**	1 (14.3)	10 (15.9)	0.99[b]
Surgery	7 (33.3)	20 (14.5)	**0.055[b]**	7 (50)	15 (20)	**0.037[b]**	0	5 (7.9)	0.99[b]
Antimicrobial use in the previous 6 months:	13 (61.9)	65 (47.1)	0.206	12 (85.7)	35 (46.7)	**0.007**	1 (14.3)	30 (47.6)	0.123[b]
Co-morbidities:									
Immunosu-ppression	4 (19)	8 (5.8)	**0.055[b]**	4 (28.6)	8 (10.7)	0.091[b]	0	0	-
Malnutrition	4 (19)	9 (6.5)	0.073[b]	4 (28.6)	7 (9.3)	0.067[b]	0	2 (3.2)	0.99[b]
Contact with healthcare workers	5 (23.8)	13 (9.5)	0.068[b]	5 (35.7)	8 (10.7)	**0.029[b]**	0	5 (8.1)	0.99 [b]
No. of occupants in the bedroom:									
Median	3	3	0.056[c]	3	3	0.390[c]	4	3	0.072[c]
Range	(3–4)	(2–3)		(2–4)	(3–4)		(2–6)	(2–3)	
No. of children younger than 10 who share the dwelling:									
Median	2	1	0.085[c]	2	1	0.507 [c]	2	1	**0.0493[c]**
Range	(1–4)	(1–2)		(1–2)	(1–2)		(2–4)	(1–2)	
Shared personal items	13 (61.9)	50 (36.5)	**0.027[b]**	8 (57.1)	18 (24)	**0.022[b]**	5 (71.4)	32 (51.6)	0.437[b]
Passive smoking	11(52.4)	53 (38.7)	0.234	5 (35.7)	33 (44)	0.565	6 (85.7)	20 (32.3)	**0.010[b]**

Significant differences ($p<0.05$) are shown in bold. Chi-square test[a], Fisher's exact test[b], Mann–Whitney U tests[c].

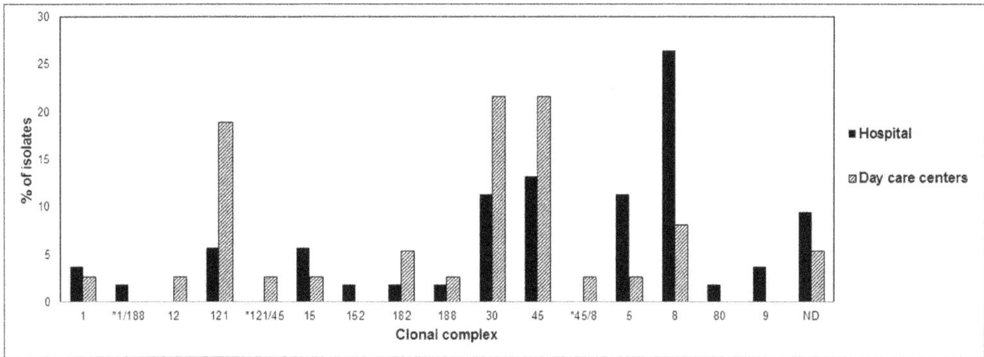

Figure 1. Clonal diversity of *Staphylococcus aureus* isolates among hospital and day care centers. The percent of isolates (Y-axis) is plotted against clonal complex type (X-axis). Abbreviations: ND: not determined. *Colonization with multiple *Staphylococcus aureus* strains with different clonal complexes.

These findings agree with other studies that have reported an increased frequency of MRSA colonization in healthy children [8,9], and also indicate that DCCs are reservoirs that favor MRSA transmission in the community [30].

In previous studies in Latin America including children from DCCs of similar age to the ones in this study, the frequency of MRSA colonization varies, for example in Mexico, 0.93% [31], Brazil, 1.2% [6], Cuba, 2.2% [32] and Argentina 4.4% [33]. In the present study, MRSA colonization in DCCs children (3.5%), is similar to the frequencies detected in these countries, but lower than previously reported in other Colombian cities, e.g. 4.8% in Cartagena [26] and 12.6% in Montería [27]. Variations in colonization frequencies have been attributed to differences in socio-demographic characteristics [34]. Children included in this study belonged to low socioeconomic status neighborhoods, and for the studies in other Colombian cities only the one reporting higher frequencies (12.6%) [27], indicated that the children were from low socioeconomic neighborhoods. Although, the economic factor may influence colonization frequencies, other factors may be involved, such as the geographic background [34] and the number of anatomical sites sampled, thus, detection of MRSA carriers can be enhanced by taking samples from other body parts such as throat, skin, perineum, armpits and rectum [35]. In contrast to this work, in the Monteria study samples were taken from throat and nostrils, which in addition to the socioeconomic background, may have increased colonization frequencies.

Epidemiological characteristics of the children colonized by *Staphylococcus aureus*

The epidemiological characteristics of children colonized by *S. aureus* in the overall population and by institution are described in Table 1. In general, children colonized by *S. aureus* were older than

Table 4. Molecular characteristics of MRSA isolates.

Clonal complex[a]	*spa* type[a]	SCC*mec*	*LukS/F-PV*	*arc*A	No (%)[b]	Population (No.)
1	t922	NT	-	-	1 (4.8)	D (1)
121	**t645**	NT	-	-	**2 (9.5)**	D (2)
182	t7862	NT	+	-	1 (4.8)	H (1)
45	New (X1-K1-A1-New-X2-B1-K1-B3-B3-A1-M1-B3)	IVa	+	–	1 (4.8)	H (1)
	t050	NT	+	–	1 (4.8)	H (1)
	t065	NT	+	–	1 (4.8)	D (1)
45/8	t065/t1635[c]	NT	+	–	1 (4.8)	D (1)
5	t002	IVa	–	–	1 (4.8)	H (1)
8	**t008**	IVc	+	–	**1 (4.8)**	H (2)
		NT	+	–	**1 (4.8)**	
	t024	IVc	+	–	**3 (14.3)**	H (3)
	t1610	IVc	+	–	**2 (9.5)**	H (1) D (1)
	t1635	IVa	+	–/+	**2 (9.5)**	H (2)
	t3308/t008[c]	IVc	+	–	1 (4.8)	H (1)
ND	New (Z1-B1-M1-E2-L1-J1-N1-N1-Q1-Q1)	NT	–	–	1 (4.8)	D (1)
	New (NEW-F1-G1-F1-M1-W2-W5)	IVa	+	–	1 (4.8)	H (1)

[a]The most prevalent clonal complexes and *spa* types are shown in boldface, defined by Ridom or e- genomics.
[b]Number and percentage of isolates with a specific clonal complex (CC), *spa* type and SCC*mec* type combination.
[c]Colonization with multiple *Staphylococcus aureus* strains with different *spa* type. NT: non-typeable, H: hospital, D: Day care centers.

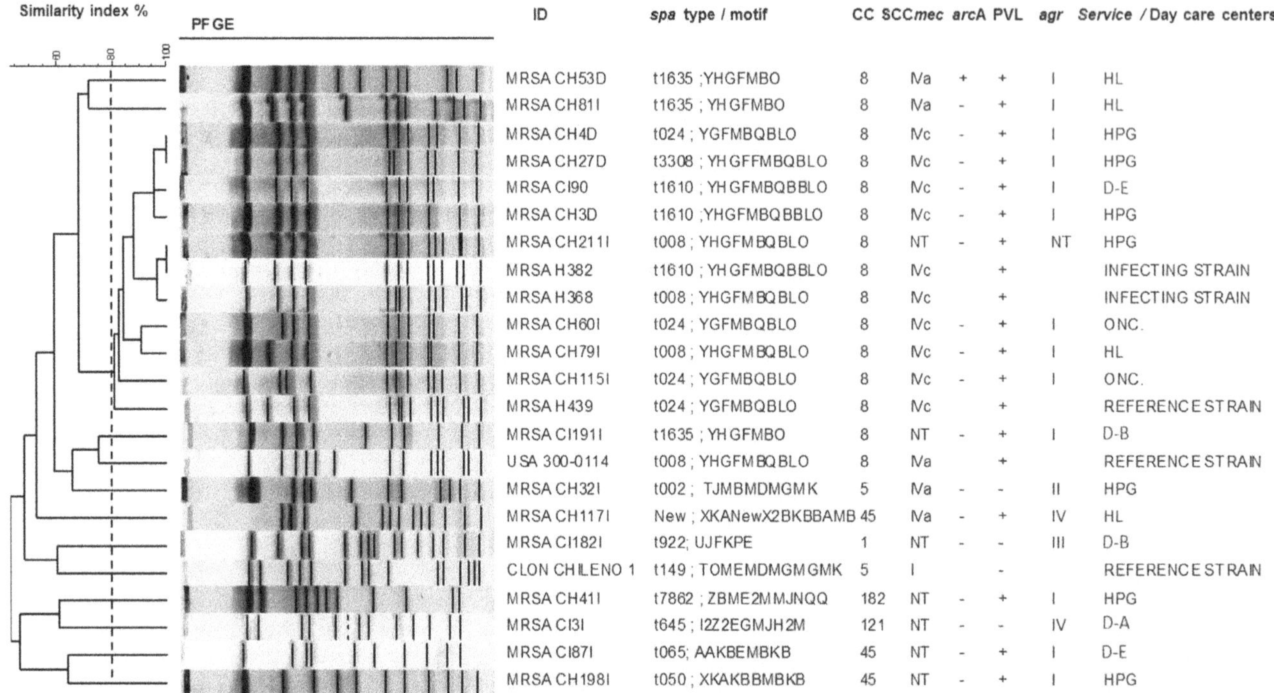

Similarity index %
PFGE
ID
spa type / motif
CC SCCmec arcA PVL agr Service / Day care centers
MRSA CH53D t1635 ;YHGFMBO 8 IVa + + I HL
MRSA CH81I t1635 ; YHGFMBO 8 IVa - + I HL
MRSA CH4D t024 ; YGFMBQBLO 8 IVc - + I HPG
MRSA CH27D t3308 ; YHGFFMBQBLO 8 IVc - + I HPG
MRSA CI90 t1610 ; YHGFMBQBBLO 8 IVc - + I D-E
MRSA CH3D t1610 ;YHGFMBQBBLO 8 IVc - + I HPG
MRSA CH211I t008 ; YHGFMBQBLO 8 NT - + NT HPG
MRSA H382 t1610 ; YHGFMBQBBLO 8 IVc + INFECTING STRAIN
MRSA H368 t008 ; YHGFMBQBLO 8 IVc + INFECTING STRAIN
MRSA CH60I t024 ; YGFMBQBLO 8 IVc - + I ONC.
MRSA CH79I t008 ; YHGFMBQBLO 8 IVc - + I HL
MRSA CH115I t024 ; YGFMBQBLO 8 IVc - + I ONC.
MRSA H439 t024 ; YGFMBQBLO 8 IVc + REFERENCE STRAIN
MRSA CI191I t1635 ; YHGFMBO 8 NT - + I D-B
USA 300-0114 t008 ; YHGFMBQBLO 8 IVa + REFERENCE STRAIN
MRSA CH32I t002 ; TJMBMDMGMK 5 IVa - - II HPG
MRSA CH117I New ; XKANewX2BKBBAMB 45 IVa - + IV HL
MRSA CI182I t922; UJFKPE 1 NT - - III D-B
CLON CHILENO 1 t149 ; TOMEMDMGMGMK 5 I - REFERENCE STRAIN
MRSA CH41I t7862 ; ZBME2MMJNQQ 182 NT - + I HPG
MRSA CI3I t645 ; I2Z2EGMJH2M 121 NT - - IV D-A
MRSA CI87I t065; AAKBEMBKB 45 NT - + I D-E
MRSA CH198I t050 ; XKAKBBMBKB 45 NT - + I HPG

Figure 2. Genetic relatedness among MRSA isolates. UPGMA dendrogram showing genetic relatedness among MRSA isolates as determined by PFGE with *SmaI*. The broken line corresponds to the cutoff level (80%) used to define related PFGE clones. Note that CC8 MRSA isolates form a separate cluster by PFGE and were genetically related to infectious MRSA strains previously reported in the city.

two years ($p = 0.005$), and the majority were boys (59.1%). In both populations, colonized children were more likely to share a bedroom with a large number of people ($p = 0.028$) and presented antecedents of β-Lactamase inhibitors usage ($p = 0.020$ for the general population, $p = 0.038$ for the hospital). Other characteristics such as sharing a towel ($p = 0.011$) were more frequently observed among the hospital children. Noteworthy, non-colonized, hospitalized children more likely used nasal sprays or washes ($p = 0.038$), or were vaccinated against *Streptococcus pneumoniae* (46.9%), as compared to colonized children ($p = 0.023$).

Multivariate analysis indicated that the variables that remained associated with an increased risk for *S. aureus* in the child population were, ages over two years (RP, 1.712; 95% CI, 1.384 to 2.118; $p = 0.001$), β-Lactamase inhibitors usage in the previous 6 months (RP, 1.655; 95% CI, 1.348 to 2.032; $p = 0.001$), exposure to cigarette smoke (RP, 1.361; 95% CI, 1.106 to 1.674; $p = 0.004$) and hospitalization (RP, 1.458; 95% CI, 1.133 to 1.876; $p = 0.003$) (Table 2). An additional factor that has often been correlated to *S. aureus* colonization frequencies is age. It has been reported that colonization decreases considerably during the first year of life, from 53,8% in the first month to 11,9% at 14 months [36]. In contrast, a gradual increase in colonization frequency is observed from two to five years of age [37], as observed in the present study. In addition, colonized children were exposed to cigarette smoke, which agrees with previous reports of an association of passive smoking with an increased risk of colonization in children [38]. Other epidemiological characteristics that have been correlated with *S. aureus* colonization and specifically MRSA are antibiotic usage in the previous 6 months and hospitalization [30]. Similarly, in this study, β-Lactamase inhibitors usage in the previous 6 months and hospitalization were also significant factors influencing colonization in the children population. These also constitute risk factors for *S. aureus* infection [3,39,40] and reinforces the importance of preventing *S. aureus* transmission in hospitalized children [41].

Epidemiological characteristics of the children colonized by MRSA

Comparison of the epidemiological characteristics between children colonized by MRSA and by MSSA (Table 3), demonstrated that MRSA was more common among boys ($p = 0.008$). In the general population variables such as prior history of hospitalization ($p = 0.047$) and immunosuppression ($p = 0.055$) were related to colonization by MRSA. Most MRSA carriers had antecedents of surgery ($p = 0.055$ general population and $p = 0.037$ in hospital) and of sharing personal items ($p = 0.027$), especially among hospitalized children. In addition, in hospitalized, MRSA-colonized children antecedents of antibiotic usage ($p = 0.007$) and contact with healthcare workers ($p = 0.029$) were significant; in contrast, for children at DCCs, previous exposure to cigarette smoke ($p = 0.010$) and sharing a dwelling with children younger than 10 years ($p = 0.0493$) were the most frequent characteristics detected. These findings coincide with previous reports that show that colonization by MRSA is associated to characteristics such as male gender [11], previous history of hospitalization and surgery [42], previous contact with healthcare workers [8,11], sharing personal objects [38] overcrowding conditions and high physical contact among children [37].

Molecular characteristics of colonizing *Staphylococcus aureus* strains

Results of the molecular characterization of *S. aureus* colonizing pediatric population constitute one of the most relevant aspects of this work. Genotypes of *S. aureus* from hospitalized and DDCs populations revealed the presence of *S. aureus* strains with different

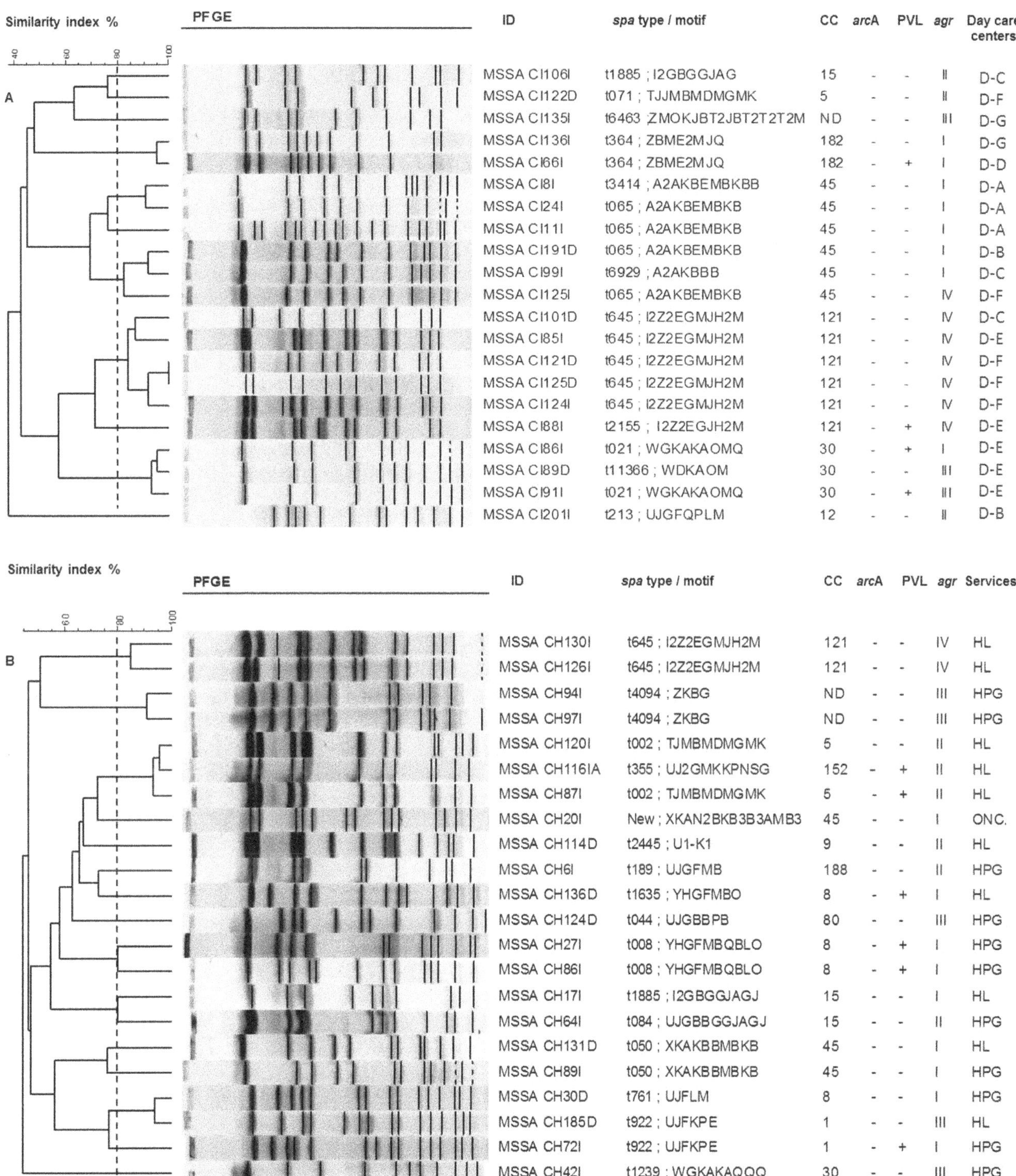

Similarity index %
PFGE
ID
spa type / motif
CC
arcA
PVL
agr
Day care centers
40
60
80
100
A
MSSA CI106I t1885 ; I2GBGGJAG 15 - - II D-C
MSSA CI122D t071 ; TJJMBMDMGMK 5 - - II D-F
MSSA CI135I t6463 ;ZMOKJBT2JBT2T2T2M ND - - III D-G
MSSA CI136I t364 ; ZBME2MJQ 182 - - I D-G
MSSA CI66I t364 ; ZBME2MJQ 182 - + I D-D
MSSA CI8I t3414 ; A2AKBEMBKBB 45 - - I D-A
MSSA CI24I t065 ; A2AKBEMBKB 45 - - I D-A
MSSA CI11I t065 ; A2AKBEMBKB 45 - - I D-A
MSSA CI191D t065 ; A2AKBEMBKB 45 - - I D-B
MSSA CI99I t6929 ; A2AKBBB 45 - - I D-C
MSSA CI125I t065 ; A2AKBEMBKB 45 - - IV D-F
MSSA CI101D t645 ; I2Z2EGMJH2M 121 - - IV D-C
MSSA CI85I t645 ; I2Z2EGMJH2M 121 - - IV D-E
MSSA CI121D t645 ; I2Z2EGMJH2M 121 - - IV D-F
MSSA CI125D t645 ; I2Z2EGMJH2M 121 - - IV D-F
MSSA CI124I t645 ; I2Z2EGMJH2M 121 - - IV D-F
MSSA CI88I t2155 ; I2Z2EGJH2M 121 - + IV D-E
MSSA CI86I t021 ; WGKAKAOMQ 30 - + I D-E
MSSA CI89D t11366 ; WDKAOM 30 - - III D-E
MSSA CI91I t021 ; WGKAKAOMQ 30 - + III D-E
MSSA CI201I t213 ; UJGFQPLM 12 - - II D-B
Similarity index %
PFGE
ID
spa type / motif
CC
arcA
PVL
agr
Services
60
80
100
B
MSSA CH130I t645 ; I2Z2EGMJH2M 121 - - IV HL
MSSA CH126I t645 ; I2Z2EGMJH2M 121 - - IV HL
MSSA CH94I t4094 ; ZKBG ND - - III HPG
MSSA CH97I t4094 ; ZKBG ND - - III HPG
MSSA CH120I t002 ; TJMBMDMGMK 5 - - II HL
MSSA CH116IA t355 ; UJ2GMKKPNSG 152 - + II HL
MSSA CH87I t002 ; TJMBMDMGMK 5 - + II HL
MSSA CH20I New ; XKAN2BKB3B3AMB3 45 - - I ONC.
MSSA CH114D t2445 ; U1-K1 9 - - II HL
MSSA CH6I t189 ; UJGFMB 188 - - II HPG
MSSA CH136D t1635 ; YHGFMBO 8 - + I HL
MSSA CH124D t044 ; UJGBBPB 80 - - III HPG
MSSA CH27I t008 ; YHGFMBQBLO 8 - + I HPG
MSSA CH86I t008 ; YHGFMBQBLO 8 - + I HPG
MSSA CH17I t1885 ; I2GBGGJAGJ 15 - - I HL
MSSA CH64I t084 ; UJGBBGGJAGJ 15 - - II HPG
MSSA CH131D t050 ; XKAKBBMBKB 45 - - I HL
MSSA CH89I t050 ; XKAKBBMBKB 45 - - I HPG
MSSA CH30D t761 ; UJFLM 8 - - I HPG
MSSA CH185D t922 ; UJFKPE 1 - - III HL
MSSA CH72I t922 ; UJFKPE 1 - + I HPG
MSSA CH42I t1239 ; WGKAKAQQQ 30 - - III HPG

Figure 3. Genetic relatedness among MSSA isolates from (A) day care centers and (B) hospital. UPGMA dendrogram showing genetic relatedness among MSSA isolates as determined by PFGE with *SmaI*. The broken line corresponds to the cut off level (80%) used to define related PFGE clones.

molecular characteristics circulating in both settings; one of the main differences being their frequency of presentation (Fig. 1). Thus, isolates belonging to clonal complex CC8, CC30, CC45 and CC5 were most frequent in the hospital population and CC30, CC45 and CC121, in children of DCCs. The presence of CC30 and CC45 in both populations agrees with previous reports that indicate that these clonal complexes are among the most prevalent and successful colonizing strains [43,44]. Further, isolates belonging to these clonal complexes have also been reported causing infection [45].

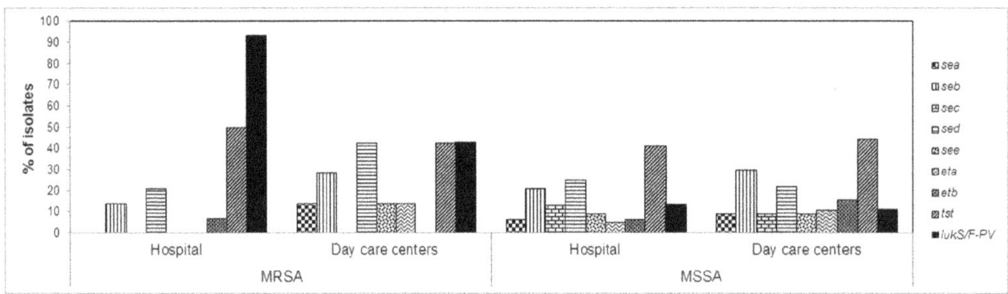

Figure 4. Frequency of distribution of virulence genes among MRSA and MSSA isolates according to institution. Abbreviations: *sea, seb, sec, sed* and *see*: staphylococcal enterotoxin genes A–E; *eta* and *etb*: exfo-liative toxin genes A and B; *tst*: toxic shock syndrome toxin 1 gene; *lukS/F-PVL*: Panton-Valentine Leucocidine.

Among MRSA isolates (Table 4), six clonal complexes were determined, with predominance of CC8 (47.6%), CC45 (14.3%) and CC121 (9.5%). Furthermore, eleven *spa* types were detected, the most common were t024 (14.3%), t1610 (9.5%), t645 (9.5%), t1635 (9.5%) and t008 (9.5%). SCC*mec* typing showed that 33.3% ($n=7$) of the MRSA strains carried SCC*mec* IVc, 23.8% ($n=5$) SCC*mec* IVa and 42.9% ($n=9$) were not typifiable.

PFGE analysis of all MRSA isolates showed a cluster of eight closely related isolates (coefficient of similarity 80–85%) (Fig. 2) that belonged to CC8, represented *spa* types t024, t008 and t1610 and SCC*mec* IVc, carried the PVL genes *lukS/F-PV* and *agrI*. Seven of these strains came from general hospitalization and oncology services, and one from a DCC (CC8-SCC*mec* IVc-t1610). Notoriously, these colonizing isolates were also closely related (coefficient of similarity 80–85%) to infectious isolates form a previous study, included in the PFGE assay as reference strains. Those strains represented the *spa* types t1610, t024 and t008, that were previously predominant in the hospitals, included the one evaluated here [22,46]. These findings suggest the circulation and acquisition of these MRSA strains in the hospital environment. In addition, the finding of an infectious genotype colonizing children in a DCC, albeit at a low frequency, demonstrates its circulation among the general public; an issue of importance in public health given the pathogenic capacity and ability to disseminate of these type of strains. In the DCC population, a few MRSA strains belonging to CC1 and CC45 were detected. This is similar to results of the previous study on infectious MRSA that found a small proportion of these genotypes [22,46]. Interestingly, two MRSA isolates belonging to CC121, not previously reported in Medellin were detected in DCCs. Notoriously, CC121 is uncommon among resistant isolates [45]. Finally, MRSA genotypes found in both populations differed from those detected at highest frequencies in colonized children of countries such as Brazil (CC8-ST239-SCC*mec* IVc-III) [6] and Argentina (CC5-ST5-SCC*mec* IV) [33]. Data that further evidences changes in the epidemiology of colonizing MRSA among different countries.

Greater genotypic diversity was detected in MSSA of both populations, as previously described [47,48]. In this work, MSSA isolates belonged to 15 clonal complexes, the most frequent being CC30 (20.3%), CC45 (17.4%) and CC121 (11.6%). The most common *spa* types were t645 and t021 (both 8.7%), t002 and t050 (both 5.8%) and t1635 (4.3%). PFGE analysis of MSSA isolates, carried out by institution confirmed the genotypic diversity of these isolates (Figs. 3A and B).

Detection of virulence factor genes and *agr* types

Detection of virulence factor genes in the 159 *S. aureus* isolates showed that 74.2% ($n=118$) carry at least one virulence factor gene (Fig. 4). In general, a higher proportion and diversity of virulence factors were detected among MSSA isolates. This finding is of importance because it has been suggested that the presence of virulence factor genes predicts, to a certain extent, the pathogenic capacity of colonizing isolates [23].

Genes *lukS/F-PV* were present in 14.3% (n = 1 0) and 25.8% (n = 23) of DCCs and hospital colonizing isolates, respectively. The frequency for these genes in DCCs is higher than previously

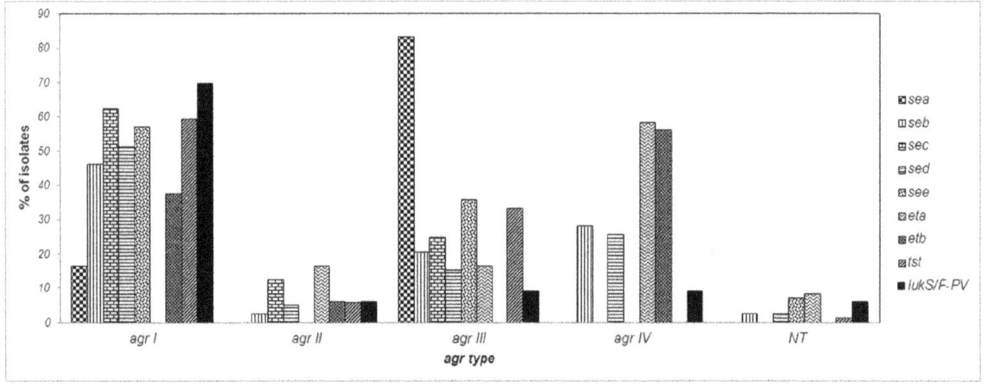

Figure 5. Percentage distribution of virulence genes according to *agr* type in *S. aureus* isolates. Abbreviations: *sea, seb, sec, sed* and *see*: staphylococcal enterotoxin genes A–E; *eta* and *etb*: exfo-liative toxin genes A and B; *tst*: toxic shock syndrome toxin 1 gene; *lukS/F-PVL*: Panton-Valentine Leucocidine genes.

reported in a similar study in Cartagena, Colombia (14.3% vs. 5.8%) [26], but it is lower than the one found among children of countries such as China (22.4%) [49]. PVL genes (*lukS/F-PV*) were detected in 76.2% (n = 16) of the MRSA isolates, 42.2% (n = 3) from DCCs and 92.9% (n = 13) from the hospital. The percentage of the PVL genes in hospital MRSA colonizing strains was similar to previously reported for infectious isolates from the child population of the same hospital, with 94.0% of the isolates carrying these genes [50]. The frequency of PVL genes among colonizing MSSA strains was 12.3%, higher than reported among Swiss children (1.6%) [51]. Recent studies have reported on an increase in their frequency in S. aureus (MRSA-MSSA), colonizing and clinical isolates [52]. A hospital MRSA isolate carried the arcA gene for ACME (CC8-SCCmec IVa-t1635), PVL (lukS/F-PV) and agrI. PFGE did not reveal any relationship with the rest of colonizing MRSA isolates or with a few infectious isolates form a previous study and strain USA300-0114 CA-MRSA (ST8-SCC*mec* IVa), included in the PFGE assay as reference strains. Presence of the ACME-*arcA* gene has been correlated with strains USA300 [53], but particularly, most isolates circulates in Colombia are ACME-*arcA* negative, known as the "Latin American variant" clone, USA300-LV [54]. Besides the finding of an ACME-*arcA* colonizing isolate, one infectious strain with this gene was recently reported from Bogotá, the capital city of Colombia [55]. This suggests the importance of a continued surveillance for this type of virulence factors; particularly, it has been suggested that ACME could provide *S. aureus* with an increased survival and colonization ability, conferring a selective advantage and improving its virulence capacity [56].

One of the principal regulatory genes of *S. aureus* is *agr*, which controls the temporal expression of most virulence factors [51]. The distribution of virulence factors within each *S. aureus agr* group is shown in Fig. 5. The *agrI* group contained 76.2% of MRSA and 58.0% of the MSSA isolates. Interestingly, these percentages are similar to reports for *agrI* in infectious MRSA isolates, e.g. 71% [57] and up to 96% [58] of. Presumably, there is a correlation between the type of *agr* with the presence of some virulence factor genes or with the genetic background of the strains [59]. Accordingly, in the present study, all the strains that belonged to CC30 were *agr*III, also of 17 CC8 isolates, 15 were *agr*I, and of 10 CC121 isolates, eight were *agr*IV.

In addition, a relationship between virulence factors and clonal complex was detected, thus of 17 CC8 isolates, 16 presented *lukS/F-PV* and 14 *tst* genes. Of 14 CC30 strains, 13 had *tst* and nine, *sea*. Of 10 CC121 isolates, seven carried *eta* and eight *etb*. The importance of this finding resides in that CC121 is known as the "impetigo clone" because of its association with impetigo affected patients, a very contagious condition affecting mostly children, and often related with *eta* and *etb* gene [48]. Most *S. aureus* CC121 isolates were detected in DCCs, results that should guide prevention measures.

Among the limitations of this work are, that as a cross-sectional study it was not possible to detect variations in colonization patterns, e.g. persistent carriers, intermittent carriers or non-carriers. Also, sampling only the nostrils without including other body parts may represent an underestimation of the frequency of MRSA [35], and finally, the inability to detect if colonization originated in the hospital or the community limits our ability to make generalizations about the results.

Nevertheless, our findings provide relevant information on *S. aureus* and MRSA colonization behaviors in the pediatric population at the local level. The finding of colonizing MRSA with similar molecular characteristics to infectious strains demonstrates the importance for public health of monitoring these populations, because of the risks of these strains disseminating and causing infection. Furthermore, the differences in epidemiological characteristics between the populations provide the baseline for the design of control and prevention strategies for colonizing and infectious *S. aureus*.

Author Contributions

Conceived and designed the experiments: EAR JNJ MMC SO SLA. Performed the experiments: EAR JNJ. Analyzed the data: EAR JNJ MMC SO. Contributed reagents/materials/analysis tools: EAR JNJ MMC SO SLA. Wrote the paper: EAR JNJ MMC SO.

References

1. Aires de Sousa M, de Lencastre H (2004) Bridges from hospitals to the laboratory: genetic portraits of methicillin-resistant *Staphylococcus aureus clones*. FEMS Immunol Med Microbiol 40: 101–111.
2. Kluytmans J, van Belkum A, Verbrugh H (1997) Nasal carriage of *Staphylococcus aureus*: epidemiology, underlying mechanisms, and associated risks. Clin Microbiol Rev 10: 505–520.
3. Safdar N, Bradley EA (2008) The risk of infection after nasal colonization with *Staphylococcus aureus*. Am J Med 121: 310–315.
4. Regev-Yochay G, Raz M, Carmeli Y, Shainberg B, Navon-Venezia S, et al. (2009) Parental *Staphylococcus aureus* carriage is associated with staphylococcal carriage in young children. Pediatr Infect Dis J 28: 960–965.
5. Lebon A, Labout JA, Verbrugh HA, Jaddoe VW, Hofman A, et al. (2010) Author's correction. Dynamics and determinants of *Staphylococcus aureus* carriage in infancy: the Generation R Study. J Clin Microbiol 48: 1995–1996.
6. Lamaro-Cardoso J, de Lencastre H, Kipnis A, Pimenta FC, Oliveira LS, et al. (2009) Molecular epidemiology and risk factors for nasal carriage of *Staphylococcus aureus* and methicillin-resistant *S. aureus* in infants attending day care centers in Brazil. J Clin Microbiol 47: 3991–3997.
7. Miller LG, Diep BA (2008) Clinical practice: colonization, fomites, and virulence: rethinking the pathogenesis of community-associated methicillin-resistant *Staphylococcus aureus* infection. Clin Infect Dis 46: 752–760.
8. Creech CB, 2nd, Kernodle DS, Alsentzer A, Wilson C, Edwards KM (2005) Increasing rates of nasal carriage of methicillin-resistant *Staphylococcus aureus* in healthy children. Pediatr Infect Dis J 24: 617–621.
9. Huang YC, Hwang KP, Chen PY, Chen CJ, Lin TY (2007) Prevalence of methicillin-resistant *Staphylococcus aureus* nasal colonization among Taiwanese children in 2005 and 2006. J Clin Microbiol 45: 3992–3995.
10. Pathak A, Marothi Y, Iyer RV, Singh B, Sharma M, et al. (2010) Nasal carriage and antimicrobial susceptibility of *Staphylococcus aureus* in healthy preschool children in Ujjain, India. BMC Pediatr 10: 100.
11. Halablab MA, Hijazi SM, Fawzi MA, Araj GF (2010) *Staphylococcus aureus* nasal carriage rate and associated risk factors in individuals in the community. Epidemiol Infect 138: 702–706.
12. Brakstad OG, Aasbakk K, Maeland JA (1992) Detection of *Staphylococcus aureus* by polymerase chain reaction amplification of the *nuc* gene. J Clin Microbiol 30: 1654–1660.
13. Mehrotra M, Wang G, Johnson WM (2000) Multiplex PCR for detection of genes for *Staphylococcus aureus* enterotoxins, exfoliative toxins, toxic shock syndrome toxin 1, and methicillin resistance. J Clin Microbiol 38: 1032–1035.
14. Shopsin B, Gomez M, Montgomery SO, Smith DH, Waddington M, et al. (1999) Evaluation of protein A gene polymorphic region DNA sequencing for typing of *Staphylococcus aureus* strains. J Clin Microbiol 37: 3556–3563.
15. Enright MC, Day NP, Davies CE, Peacock SJ, Spratt BG (2000) Multilocus sequence typing for characterization of methicillin-resistant and methicillin-susceptible clones of *Staphylococcus aureus*. J Clin Microbiol 38: 1008–1015.
16. Feil EJ, Li BC, Aanensen DM, Hanage WP, Spratt BG (2004) eBURST: inferring patterns of evolutionary descent among clusters of related bacterial genotypes from multilocus sequence typing data. J Bacteriol 186: 1518–1530.
17. Mathema B, Mediavilla J, Kreiswirth BN (2008) Sequence analysis of the variable number tandem repeat in *Staphylococcus aureus* protein A gene: *spa* typing. Methods Mol Biol 431: 285–305.
18. Strommenger B, Kettlitz C, Weniger T, Harmsen D, Friedrich AW, et al. (2006) Assignment of *Staphylococcus* isolates to groups by *spa* typing, *Sma*I macroreiction analysis, and multilocus sequence typing. J Clin Microbiol 44: 2533–2540.
19. Kondo Y, Ito T, Ma XX, Watanabe S, Kreiswirth BN, et al. (2007) Combination of multiplex PCRs for staphylococcal cassette chromosome *mec* type assignment: rapid identification system for *mec*, *ccr*, and major differences in junkyard regions. Antimicrob Agents Chemother 51: 264–274.
20. Milheirico C, Oliveira DC, de Lencastre H (2007) Multiplex PCR strategy for subtyping the staphylococcal cassette chromosome *mec* type IV in methicillin-

resistant *Staphylococcus aureus*: 'SCC*mec* IV multiplex'. J Antimicrob Chemother 60: 42–48.
21. Mulvey MR, Chui L, Ismail J, Louie L, Murphy C, et al. (2001) Development of a Canadian standardized protocol for subtyping methicillin-resistant *Staphylococcus aureus* using pulsed-field gel electrophoresis. J Clin Microbiol 39: 3481–3485.
22. Jimenez JN, Ocampo AM, Vanegas JM, Rodriguez EA, Mediavilla JR, et al. (2012) CC8 MRSA strains harboring SCC*mec* type IVc are predominant in Colombian hospitals. PLoS One 7: e38576.
23. McClure JA, Conly JM, Lau V, Elsayed S, Louie T, et al. (2006) Novel multiplex PCR assay for detection of the staphylococcal virulence marker Panton-Valentine leukocidin genes and simultaneous discrimination of methicillin-susceptible from -resistant staphylococci. J Clin Microbiol 44: 1141–1144.
24. Shopsin B, Mathema B, Alcabes P, Said-Salim B, Lina G, et al. (2003) Prevalence of *agr* specificity groups among *Staphylococcus aureus* strains colonizing children and their guardians. J Clin Microbiol 41: 456–459.
25. Diep BA, Gill SR, Chang RF, Phan TH, Chen JH, et al. (2006) Complete genome sequence of USA300, an epidemic clone of community-acquired meticillin-resistant *Staphylococcus aureus*. Lancet 367: 731–739.
26. Rebollo-Perez J, Ordonez-Tapia C, Herazo-Herazo C, Reyes-Ramos N (2011) Nasal carriage of Panton Valentine leukocidin-positive methicillin-resistant *Staphylococcus aureus* in healthy preschool children. Rev Salud Publica (Bogota) 13: 824–832.
27. Tovar C, Zubiria M, Brango D, Buelvas F, Ramos L, et al. (2011) Prevalencia y determinación de perfi les de susceptibilidad de *Staphylococcus aureus* resistente a meticilina (SARM) en niños de hogares infantiles de la ciudad de Montería. Rev Chil Infect 28 (Supl 2): S 60–S 67.
28. Ciftci IH, Koken R, Bukulmez A, Ozdemir M, Safak B, et al. (2007) Nasal carriage of *Staphylococcus aureus* in 4–6 age groups in healthy children in Afyonkarahisar, Turkey. Acta Paediatr 96: 1043–1046.
29. Lo WT, Lin WJ, Tseng MH, Lu JJ, Lee SY, et al. (2007) Nasal carriage of a single clone of community-acquired methicillin-resistant *Staphylococcus aureus* among kindergarten attendees in northern Taiwan. BMC Infect Dis 7: 51.
30. Lo WT, Wang CC, Lin WJ, Wang SR, Teng CS, et al. (2010) Changes in the nasal colonization with methicillin-resistant *Staphylococcus aureus* in children: 2004–2009. PLoS One 5: e15791.
31. Velazquez-Guadarrama N, Martinez-Aguilar G, Galindo JA, Zuniga G, Arbo-Sosa A (2009) Methicillin-resistant *S. aureus* colonization in Mexican children attending day care centres. Clin Invest Med 32: E57–63.
32. Torano G, Quinones D, Hernandez I, Hernandez T, Tamargo I, et al. (2001) [Nasal carriers of methicillin-resistant *Staphylococcus aureus* among cuban children attending day-care centers]. Enferm Infecc Microbiol Clin 19: 367–370.
33. Gardella N, Murzicato S, Di Gregorio S, Cuirolo A, Desse J, et al. (2011) Prevalence and characterization of methicillin-resistant *Staphylococcus aureus* among healthy children in a city of Argentina. Infect Genet Evol 11: 1066–1071.
34. Kuehnert MJ, Kruszon-Moran D, Hill HA, McQuillan G, McAllister SK, et al. (2006) Prevalence of *Staphylococcus aureus* nasal colonization in the United States, 2001–2002. J Infect Dis 193: 172–179.
35. Bitterman Y, Laor A, Itzhaki S, Weber G (2010) Characterization of the best anatomical sites in screening for methicillin-resistant *Staphylococcus aureus* colonization. Eur J Clin Microbiol Infect Dis 29: 391–397.
36. Lebon A, Labout JA, Verbrugh HA, Jaddoe VW, Hofman A, et al. (2008) Dynamics and determinants of *Staphylococcus aureus* carriage in infancy: the Generation R Study. J Clin Microbiol 46: 3517–3521.
37. Chen CJ, Hsu KH, Lin TY, Hwang KP, Chen PY, et al. (2011) Factors associated with nasal colonization of methicillin-resistant *Staphylococcus aureus* among healthy children in Taiwan. J Clin Microbiol 49: 131–137.
38. Bogaert D, van Belkum A, Sluijter M, Luijendijk A, de Groot R, et al. (2004) Colonisation by *Streptococcus pneumoniae* and *Staphylococcus aureus* in healthy children. Lancet 363: 1871–1872.
39. von Eiff C, Becker K, Machka K, Stammer H, Peters G (2001) Nasal carriage as a source of *Staphylococcus aureus* bacteremia. Study Group. N Engl J Med 344: 11–16.
40. Wertheim HF, Vos MC, Ott A, van Belkum A, Voss A, et al. (2004) Risk and outcome of nosocomial *Staphylococcus aureus* bacteraemia in nasal carriers versus non-carriers. Lancet 364: 703–705.
41. Milstone AM, Goldner BW, Ross T, Shepard JW, Carroll KC, et al. (2011) Methicillin-resistant *Staphylococcus aureus* colonization and risk of subsequent infection in critically ill children: importance of preventing nosocomial methicillin-resistant *Staphylococcus aureus* transmission. Clin Infect Dis 53: 853–859.
42. Horowitz IN, Baorto E, Cirillo T, Davis J (2012) Methicillin-resistant *Staphylococcus aureus* colonization in a pediatric intensive care unit: risk factors. Am J Infect Control 40: 118–122.
43. Argudin MA, Argumosa V, Mendoza MC, Guerra B, Rodicio MR (2013) Population structure and exotoxin gene content of methicillin-susceptible *Staphylococcus aureus* from Spanish healthy carriers. Microb Pathog 54: 26–33.
44. Sangvik M, Olsen RS, Olsen K, Simonsen GS, Furberg AS, et al. (2011) Age- and gender-associated *Staphylococcus aureus spa* types found among nasal carriers in a general population: the Tromso Staph and Skin Study. J Clin Microbiol 49: 4213–4218.
45. Monecke S, Coombs G, Shore AC, Coleman DC, Akpaka P, et al. (2011) A field guide to pandemic, epidemic and sporadic clones of methicillin-resistant *Staphylococcus aureus*. PLoS One 6: e17936.
46. Jimenez JN, Ocampo AM, Vanegas JM, Rodriguez EA, Mediavilla JR, et al. (2013) A comparison of methicillin-resistant and methicillin-susceptible *Staphylococcus aureus* reveals no clinical and epidemiological but molecular differences. Int J Med Microbiol 303: 76–83.
47. Ghasemzadeh-Moghaddam H, Ghaznavi-Rad E, Sekawi Z, Yun-Khoon L, Aziz MN, et al. (2011) Methicillin-susceptible *Staphylococcus aureus* from clinical and community sources are genetically diverse. Int J Med Microbiol 301: 347–353.
48. Blumental S, Deplano A, Jourdain S, De Mendonca R, Hallin M, et al. (2013) Dynamic pattern and genotypic diversity of *Staphylococcus aureus* nasopharyngeal carriage in healthy pre-school children. J Antimicrob Chemother 68: 1517–1523.
49. Fan J, Shu M, Zhang G, Zhou W, Jiang Y, et al. (2009) Biogeography and virulence of *Staphylococcus aureus*. PLoS One 4: e6216.
50. Jimenez JN, Ocampo AM, Vanegas JM, Rodriguez EA, Garces CG, et al. (2011) Characterisation of virulence genes in methicillin susceptible and resistant *Staphylococcus aureus* isolates from a paediatric population in a university hospital of Medellin, Colombia. Mem Inst Oswaldo Cruz 106: 980–985.
51. Megevand C, Gervaix A, Heininger U, Berger C, Aebi C, et al. (2010) Molecular epidemiology of the nasal colonization by methicillin-susceptible *Staphylococcus aureus* in Swiss children. Clin Microbiol Infect 16: 1414–1420.
52. Rolo J, Miragaia M, Turlej-Rogacka A, Empel J, Bouchami O, et al. (2012) High Genetic Diversity among Community-Associated *Staphylococcus aureus* in Europe: Results from a Multicenter Study. PLoS One 7: e34768.
53. Ellington MJ, Yearwood L, Ganner M, East C, Kearns AM (2008) Distribution of the ACME-*arc*A gene among methicillin-resistant *Staphylococcus aureus* from England and Wales. J Antimicrob Chemother 61: 73–77.
54. Arias CA, Rincon S, Chowdhury S, Martinez E, Coronell W, et al. (2008) MRSA USA300 clone and VREF–a U.S.-Colombian connection? N Engl J Med 359: 2177–2179.
55. Portillo BC, Pinilla G, Escobar J, Moreno JE, Gomez NV (2010) Estudio de la transcripción del elemento móvil para el catabolismo de la arginina en *Staphylococcus aureus* extrahospitalario. Infectio. pp. 73–74.
56. David MZ, Daum RS (2010) Community-associated methicillin-resistant *Staphylococcus aureus*: epidemiology and clinical consequences of an emerging epidemic. Clin Microbiol Rev 23: 616–687.
57. Liu Q, Han L, Li B, Sun J, Ni Y (2012) Virulence characteristic and MLST-*agr* genetic background of high-level mupirocin-resistant, MRSA isolates from Shanghai and Wenzhou, China. PLoS One 7: e37005.
58. Liu M, Liu J, Guo Y, Zhang Z (2010) Characterization of virulence factors and genetic background of *Staphylococcus aureus* isolated from Peking University People's Hospital between 2005 and 2009. Curr Microbiol 61: 435–443.
59. van Trijp MJ, Melles DC, Snijders SV, Wertheim HF, Verbrugh HA, et al. (2010) Genotypes, superantigen gene profiles, and presence of exfoliative toxin genes in clinical methicillin-susceptible *Staphylococcus aureus* isolates. Diagn Microbiol Infect Dis 66: 222–224.

2

A Population Based Study of Seasonality of Skin and Soft Tissue Infections: Implications for the Spread of CA-MRSA

Xiaoxia Wang[1]*, Sherry Towers[1], Sarada Panchanathan[2,3], Gerardo Chowell[1,4]

1 Mathematical, Computational and Modeling Sciences Center, School of Human Evolution and Social Change, Arizona State University, Tempe, Arizona, United States of America, **2** Department of Pediatrics, Maricopa Integrated Health System, Phoenix, Arizona, United States of America, **3** Department of Biomedical Informatics, Arizona State University, Tempe, Arizona, United States of America, **4** Division of Epidemiology and Population Studies, Fogarty International Center, National Institutes of Health, Bethesda, Maryland, United States of America

Abstract

Methicillin resistant *Staphylococcus aureus* (MRSA) is currently a major cause of skin and soft tissue infections (SSTI) in the United States. Seasonal variation of MRSA infections in hospital settings has been widely observed. However, systematic time-series analysis of incidence data is desirable to understand the seasonality of community acquired (CA)-MRSA infections at the population level. In this paper, using data on monthly SSTI incidence in children aged 0–19 years and enrolled in Medicaid in Maricopa County, Arizona, from January 2005 to December 2008, we carried out time-series and nonlinear regression analysis to determine the periodicity, trend, and peak timing in SSTI incidence in children at different age: 0–4 years, 5–9 years, 10–14 years, and 15–19 years. We also assessed the temporal correlation between SSTI incidence and meteorological variables including average temperature and humidity. Our analysis revealed a strong annual seasonal pattern of SSTI incidence with peak occurring in early September. This pattern was consistent across age groups. Moreover, SSTIs followed a significantly increasing trend over the 4-year study period with annual incidence increasing from 3.36% to 5.55% in our pediatric population of approximately 290,000. We also found a significant correlation between the temporal variation in SSTI incidence and mean temperature and specific humidity. Our findings could have potential implications on prevention and control efforts against CA-MRSA.

Editor: Michael Otto, National Institutes of Health, United States of America

Funding: This work was supported by the Arizona Biomedical Research Commission (http://azdhs.gov/biomedical/) with Commission Contract No.1216. The funders had no role in the study design, data collection and analysis, decision to publish, or preparation of the manuscript.

Competing Interests: The authors have declared that no competing interests exist.

* E-mail: xwang248@asu.edu

Introduction

Methicillin resistant *Staphylococcus aureus* (MRSA) is endemic in many US hospitals [1], long-term care facilities [2], and communities [3,4]. MRSA was estimated to be associated with 125,969 hospitalizations annually in the United States from 1999 to 2000 [5]. Moreover, estimates of MRSA-related hospitalizations more than doubled from 1999 through 2005 [1]. While the rates of health care associated (HA) -MRSA infections are declining in the US [6], community acquired (CA) -MRSA infections, predominantly skin and soft tissue infections (SSTI) [7,8], have increased markedly in the last decade in the United States [3,9]. Because CA-MRSA infections are often acquired in the community and treated in emergency rooms and offices [8,10], the effect of traditional transmission control measures in hospitals is limited [11]. Thus, improving our understanding of the temporal trend and seasonality patterns of CA-MRSA infections at the population level has the potential to inform surveillance and public health control strategies.

A short-term retrospective study of SSTIs diagnosed in the Pediatric Emergency Department of Johns Hopkins Hospital covering November 1, 2003 to October 31, 2005 suggested that MRSA infections could follow a seasonal pattern worth of close examination. That study reported the highest number of SSTIs during July-September [12]. Using MRSA isolates submitted to Rhode Island Hospital microbiology laboratory from January 2001 to March 2010 and the associated emergency department (ED) visits, Mermel et al. [13] reported higher CA-MRSA incidence during months July-December compared to months January-June. This pattern was more pronounced among pediatric patients. In another study, Frei et al [14] employed hospital discharge SSTIs records during 1996–2006 in the US and found peak CA-MRSA incidence in children (aged 0–19 years) occurring from May to December with variation across geographic regions in the USA. Leekha et al. [15] recently reviewed a number of epidemiological studies that have evaluated the seasonality in *S. aureus* colonization and infection and found that 31 out of 41 studies reported seasonal variation in *S. aureus*. In particular, all of the 10 studies on *S. aureus* –associated SSTIs noted its seasonal pattern with varying peak timing between summer and autumn. Also, it was pointed out that only a few of these studies have attempted to correlate seasonal patterns of *S. aureus* infections with climate-related factors such as temperature and humidity [16–19]. They also underscored the need to apply appropriate statistical methods (e.g., time-series analysis) to assess seasonality patterns based on incidence at the population level rather than absolute case counts. Thus, studies based on time-series analysis techniques and MRSA case counts in outpatient settings that cover a significant fraction of the population for several years are needed

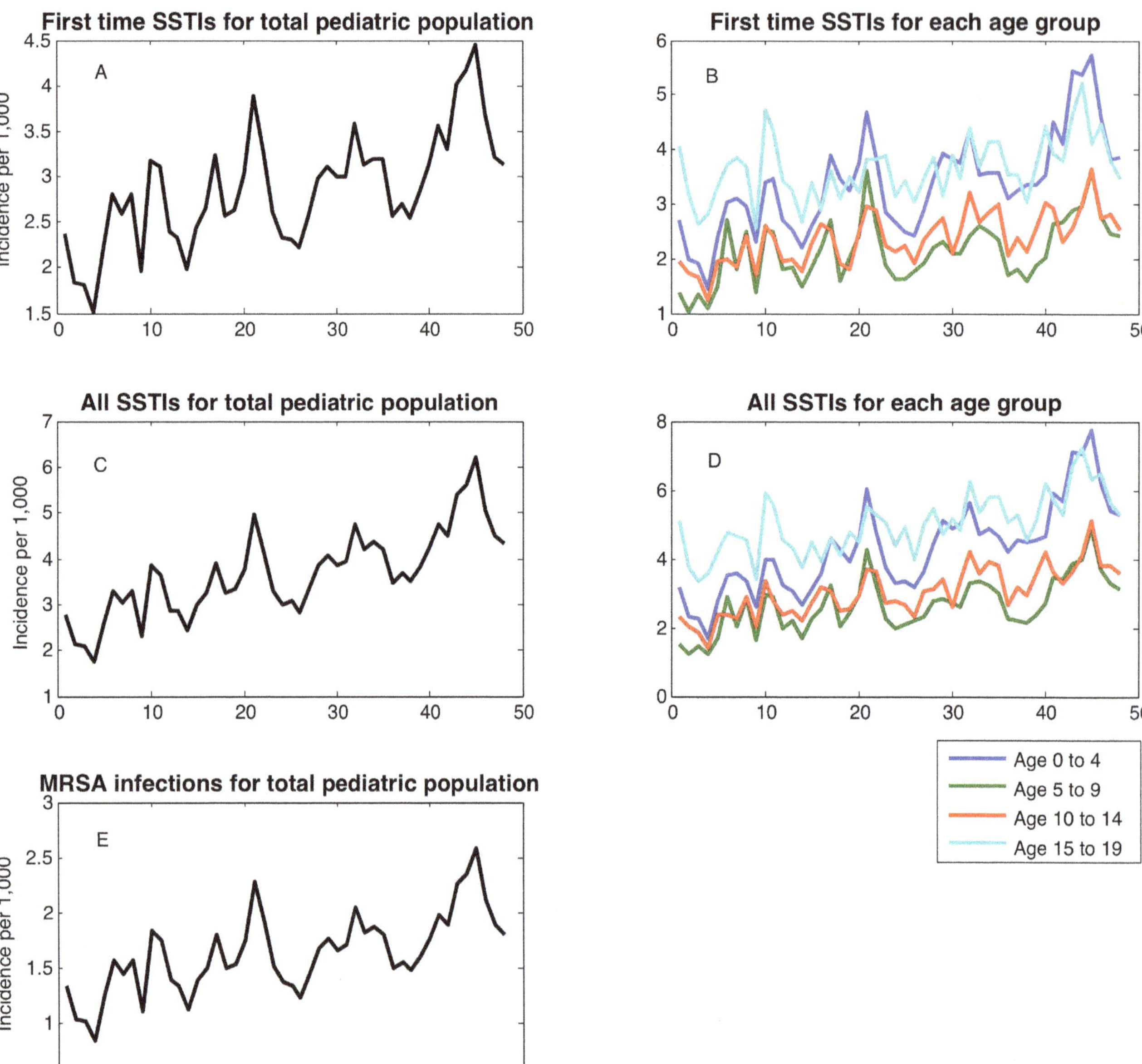

Figure 1. Time series of incidence of general SSTIs in total pediatric population and four pediatric age groups: first time (A and B); sum of first time and recurrent (C, D); incidence of first time and recurrent MRSA-related SSTIs in total pediatric population (E).

in order to comprehensively assess seasonality patterns and trends in MRSA infections.

In this paper, we use a population-based research data repository of SSTIs in children and youth aged 0–19 years covering the period from January 1, 2005 to December 31, 2008 to determine the temporal trend, seasonality pattern, and peak timing of MRSA infections in different age groups. We also examine the correlation between MRSA infections and potentially associated environmental factors such as average temperature and humidity.

Materials and Methods

Study location: Maricopa County, Arizona

Maricopa County is the third most populous local public health jurisdiction in the US, behind New York City and Los Angeles County, with a population of 3.8 million comprising 60% of Arizona's population.

Epidemiologic Data Collection

We obtained our study data from the Center for Health Information Research (CHIR). CHIR is a university-community partnership between ASU and several Arizona providers, insurers and employers. It maintains a research data repository that integrates Arizona-based administrative, clinical and public health data across a large number of sources permitting the conduct of

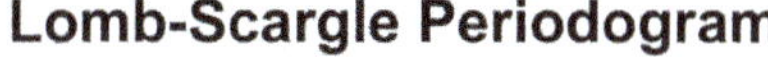

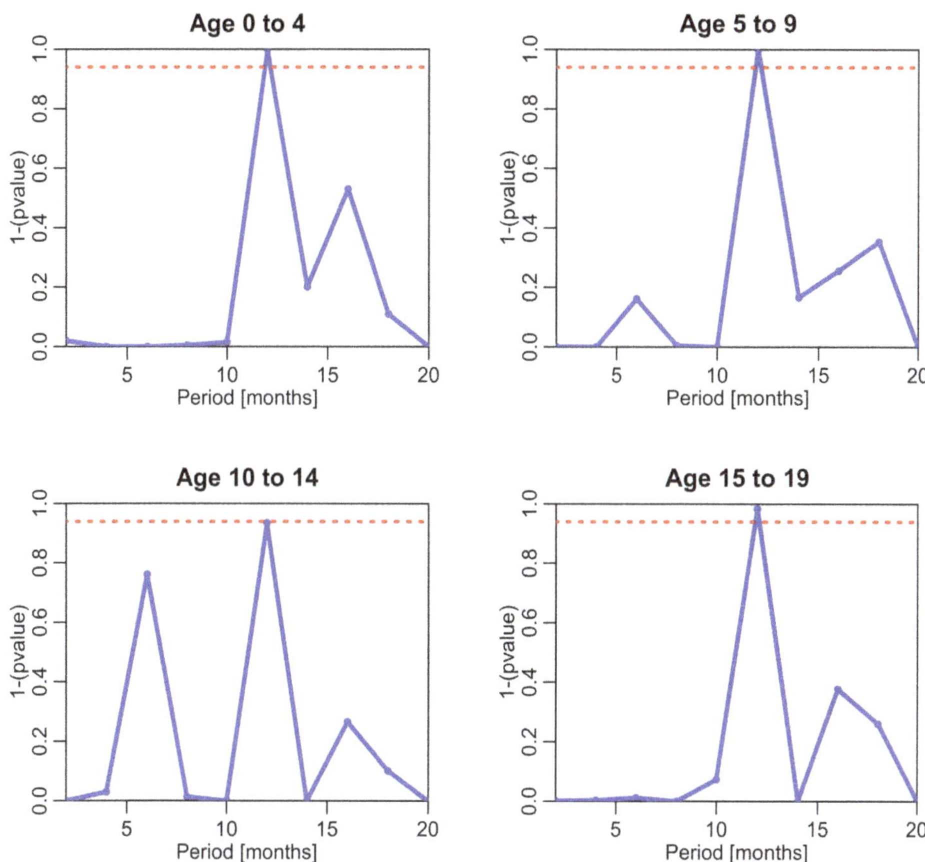

Figure 2. Lomb-Scargle periodograms testing the significance of cyclical patterns of periods between 2 and 20 months in the time series of incidence monthly SSTIs. Points above the red dotted line indicate the period is significant to $p<.05$.

population-based research on residents of Arizona [20]. Specifically, we obtained data on hospitalization and outpatients visits of children and youth (age< = 19 year) who were continuously enrolled for at least 6 months in the Arizona Health Care Cost Containment System (AHCCCS) program (Medicaid) during the period January 1, 2005 to December 31, 2008. The records of all encounters with individuals aged < = 19 years and diagnosed with skin or soft tissue infection based on ICD 9 codes (680.xx–682.9x) in Maricopa County were extracted. These codes correspond to cellulitis and abscesses, but do not include superficial skin infections such as impetigo. A recurrent infection was presumed to have happened if a second visit was greater than 30 days after an initial visit while visits occurring prior to that time were presumed to be follow-up visits. These were clinical case definitions since most often cellulitis is treated without any laboratory testing and test results for abscesses are often unavailable at the time of visit. Our data comprises 51,287 patient encounters including both first-time and recurrent infections during the 4-year period, with a stationary covered population, ranging from 287,091 to 293,550. Information regarding the prevalence of methicillin resistance in staphylococcal isolates in the community was obtained from statistics on wound cultures from 3 urban emergency departments representative of the Greater Phoenix area. The percentage of SSTIs caused by MRSA was 47.8%, 46%, 43.1%, and 41.8% respectively in the 4-year study period [20].

We stratified patients into 4 age groups: 0–4 years, 5–9 years, 10–14 years, and 15–19 years. Using the corresponding denominator population obtained from CHIR, we generated time series of monthly SSTI incidence per 1,000 people as shown in Figure 1. Of note, this incidence curve corresponds to SSTIs including MRSA. We then applied the percentage of MRSA in wound cultures for each year to derive incidence curves for MRSA infections.

Climate data

To assess the temporal correlation between SSTI incidence and climatological variables, we obtained daily time series of mean temperature, specific humidity, and relative humidity from the National Oceanic and Atmospheric Administration records, accessible from the Weather Underground website (http://www.wunderground.com/).

Statistical Methods

For the time-series of SSTI incidence for each age group, we used a well-known spectral analysis least-squares method known as the Lomb-Scargle periodogram [21–23] to determine the frequency spectrum (or period). The Lomb-Scargle method is similar to Fourier spectral analysis methods, except with the added benefit that bootstrapping methods are used to calculate the probability of false-alarm peaks in the spectrum (i.e., the bootstrapping methods determine the statistical significance of

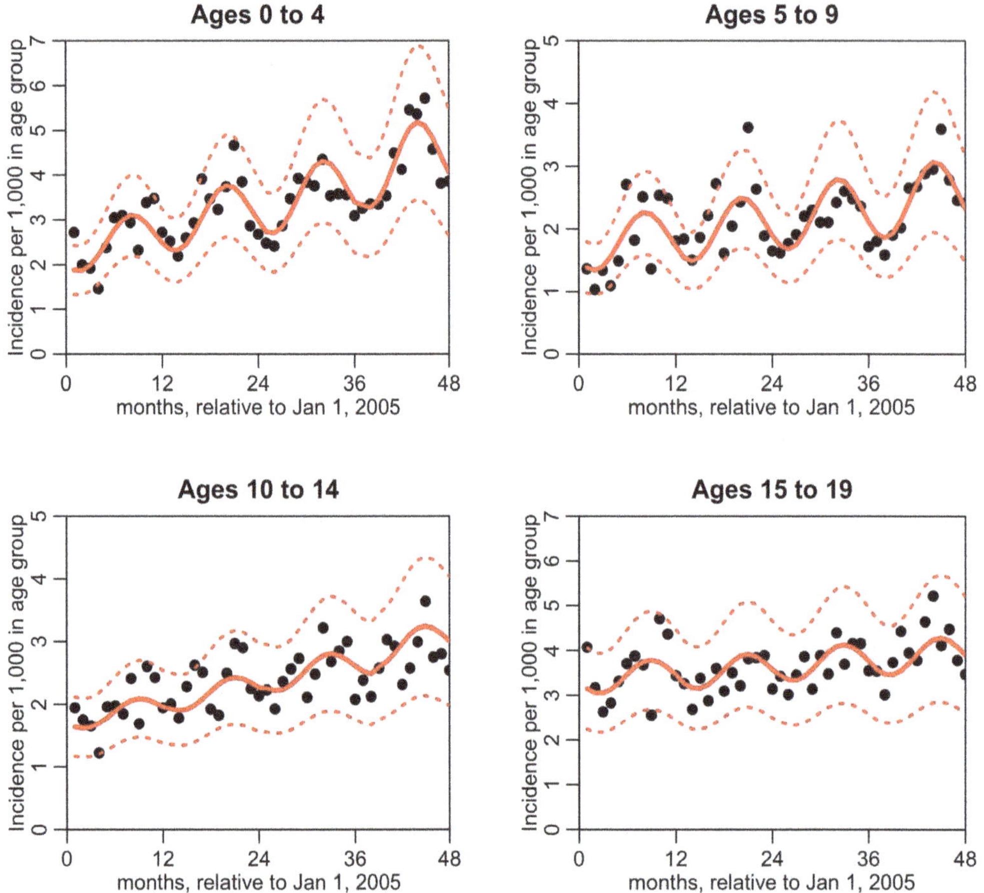

Figure 3. Time series of monthly SSTI incidence in four pediatric age groups (points), and the best fit of linear trend plus seasonality with period 12 months (red line). The dotted red lines indicate the 95% CI on the fit prediction.

observed peaks in the spectrum). It is implemented in R language and available from http://research.stowers-institute.org/efg/2005/LombScargle. After the period T being determined, in order to estimate the overall linear trend and peak of the seasonal pattern, we fitted the following nonlinear regression model (in R language)

$$y_i=(at_i+b)(1+\varepsilon\cos(\frac{2\pi(t_i-\phi)}{T})) \quad (1)$$

where (t_i,y_i) is the incidence data point, a and b parameterize the overall linear trend, ε is the degree of seasonality (or the strength of the seasonal forcing), ϕ is the phase in incidence which gives the month of the year when SSTI incidence is maximal.

Results

The monthly incidence of first time SSTIs showed an overall increasing trend with annual periodicity between January 1, 2005 and December 31, 2008 for the entire pediatric population (Figure 1A) and for each age group (Figure 1B). The overall incidence, when recurrent infections are included, shows a similar seasonality pattern and temporal trend (Figure 1C and Figure 1D). Moreover, the same pattern can be observed for monthly incidence of MRSA-related SSTIs, by applying the percentages of MRSA from wound cultures [20](Figure 1E). The overall yearly incidence of all SSTIs was 3.36%, 4.12%, 4.59% and 5.55% for the years 2005–2008 respectively.

Figure 2 shows the significance of the seasonal pattern using period lengths from 3 to 20 months across four age groups. In this analysis we consider seasonality with periods that are significant at the 95% level. We found a statistically significant ~12 month periodic cycle in incidence for all four age groups.

The best-fit models for the four age groups are shown in Table 1 and Figure 3. The 95% confidence intervals for ε (seasonality forcing) are greater than zero for all four age groups, indicating a significant annual seasonality pattern in all four age groups. The 95% confidence intervals forϕ (phase of the seasonality) of the four age groups overlap, and indicate that the month of September is

Table 1. Best-fit estimate and confidence interval for ε(seasonality forcing) and ϕ(phase of the seasonality, or where the peak of a period is).

Age group	ε	ϕ
0 - 4	0.19 [0.14,0.24]	7.9 [7.4,8.4]
5 - 9	0.22 [0.16,0.29]	8.1 [7.5,8.7]
10 - 14	0.09 [0.03,0.14]	8.6 [7.4,9.8]
15 - 19	0.10 [0.04,0.15]	8.7 [7.8,9.7]

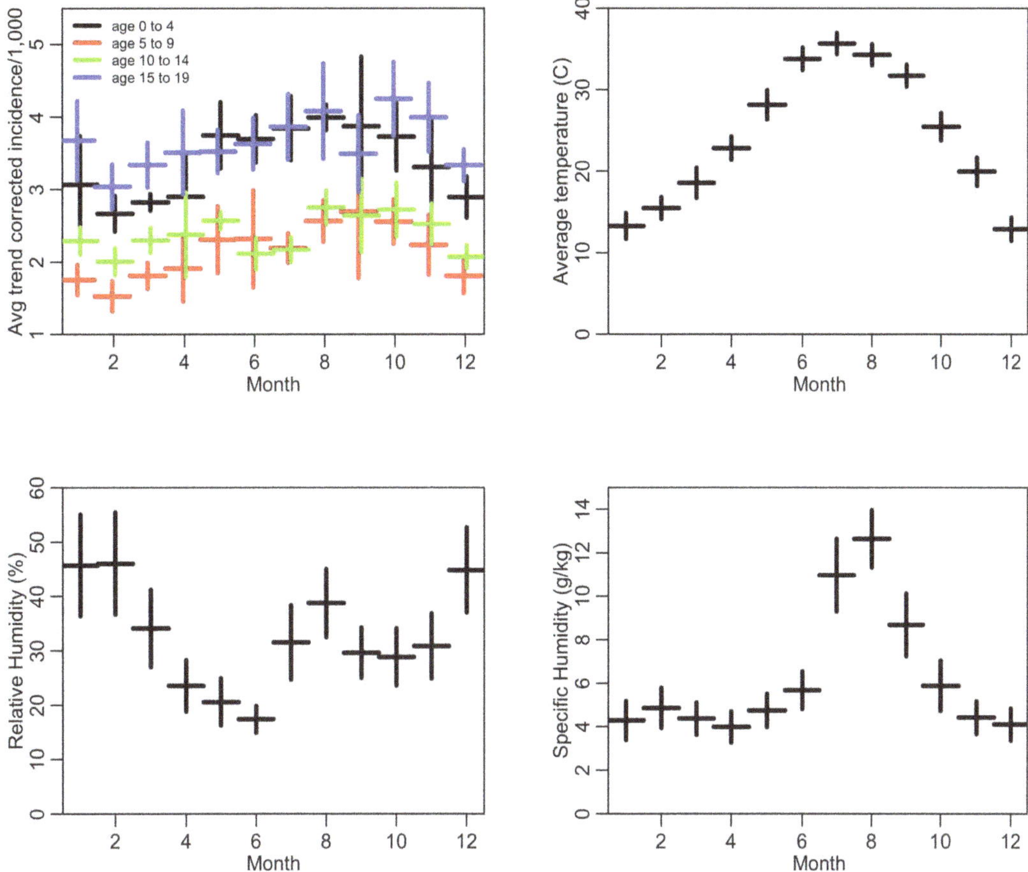

Figure 4. The first plot shows the within-month average of the trend-correlated incidence of SSTIs for each of the four pediatric age groups. The vertical error bars represent the one standard deviation error on the mean. The trend corrected incidence is the incidence minus the trend term in the regression model ($at+b$ in Equation (1)). The second to fourth plots show the within-month average of temperature, relative humidity, and specific humidity, respectively.

when SSTI incidence peaks for children of all ages. The p-value testing the hypothesis that all four values of ϕ are drawn from the same mean is $p=$ 0.14 (Pearson two-tailed).

All age groups show a significant upward incidence trend. Based on the model fit of the nonlinear regression model (Equation (1)), we estimate that in 5 years (year 2013) the incidence will be 1.6 to 1.9 times greater than in 2008 for the 0 to 4 age group (95% CI). Similar but smaller increases could also be expected for other age groups, with the confidence intervals being [1.3, 1.8], [1.2,1.7], and [1.0, 1.6] in the 5 to 9, 10 to 14, and 15 to 19 age groups respectively.

In Figure 4 we show the within-month average of temperature, relative humidity, and specific humidity between 2005 and 2008. In all four age groups, temperature is significantly correlated to SSTI incidence (one tailed $p<.05$). Specific humidity is also significantly correlated to incidence across all age groups except for those aged 10–14 years.

Discussion

We have carried out a time series analysis of age-specific SSTI infections in children and adolescents $<=19$ years who were enrolled in AHCCCS, the Medicaid program in Arizona. We found that the temporal trend of SSTIs follows strong annual seasonality with peak timing in incidence occurring approximately in early September. Further, all of the 4 pediatric groups in our data share this pattern. Our findings may be explained by the high correlation between skin infection and environmental factors such as temperature and specific humidity. The average temperature in Maricopa County in Arizona is as high as 38 °C in summer months (May – September), with peak average temperature in late July. Humidity in the skin from perspiration may facilitate SSTI development by increasing bacterial load on skin and making certain areas of the skin more vulnerable to bacterial infection. This may also explain regional variation in temporal peak of CA-MRSA infections as found in other studies (e.g., [14]). Another potential factor associated with this temporal pattern could be the start of school activities in early August (or early September in other parts of the country). CA-MRSA, like all strains of S *aureus*, is transmitted by direct contact with the index patient or carrier, usually by skin-to-skin contact with a colonized or infected individual. It is well documented that contact frequency among young children increases during school time compared to summer vacation period [24]. The delay of approximately one month from the start of school activities to the timing of the infection peak in early September could be explained by the intrinsic disease dynamics including the multiple stages of the MRSA infection cycle (contact-colonization-infection) and possible downward household transmission from school-aged children to their younger siblings. We also observed higher incidence in children in the age groups 0–4 year and 15–19 year. Other studies have reported similar results (e.g., [25–27]). The increased incidence in older adolescents could also be due to increased skin abrasions during contact sports while the increased incidence in children may be related to diaper use in this age group since a large number of MRSA abscesses start in broken skin in the diaper area.

Our study has limitations that should be noted. Our dataset captures only those cases coded as SSTI, and hence cannot directly capture the infections caused by CA-MRSA. Utilizing laboratory diagnosis of MRSA will not be accurate in a population based study including office visits, and is likely to underestimate the burden of infections caused by MRSA. Although incidence in our study is based on the total number of SSTIs, with the specific fraction caused by MRSA as determined from microbiology statistics, this represents true clinical practice at this time. That is, most cases of SSTIs were clinically diagnosed and specimens for microbiological testing were not collected. Future studies using clinical and laboratory data are warranted to corroborate our findings and pinpoint the correlation and contribution of MRSA to SSTIs.

Our study is one of the few where incidence in a population can be described, since the majority of SSTIs are treated in the offices of primary care physicians, rather than in hospitals. We chose to use only Medicaid data, since these data were the most complete in our data repository. It is important to note that patients under Medicaid coverage belong to a lower income population, where rates of infection have been described to be higher than in the general population [28,29]. Therefore our data are likely to overestimate the actual incidence in the overall population. However, the seasonality pattern described here is likely to be representative of the general population.

Another limitation is the retrospective nature of our study. We note that the percentage of MRSA in wound cultures decreased from 2005 to 2008. This could be explained by the change in antibiotic prescription practices as health care workers became more aware of CA-MRSA, but the specific antibiotics used for treatment of each SSTI were not examined.

A clear picture of the seasonality and trend of SSTIs, especially those MRSA-related, at the population level has implications for clinical treatment and public health interventions. With this information, potential factors affecting MRSA infection and transmission could be targeted. However, the exact interaction of age, length of contact, temperature, and other factors effecting MRSA infection and transmission remain to be elucidated. Also, further studies are needed to determine the cause of the September peak in incidence. However, peak incidence timing in September could inform prevention efforts and control interventions. Of note, current treatment and decolonization (e.g., with mupirocin [30]) strategies do not change throughout the year. However, our results suggest that enhanced decolonization efforts in the patient and his/her household contacts could be conducted during the summer months as a mitigation strategy. Conversely, a less aggressive approach during the remaining part of the year could decrease the probability of emergence of further antibiotic resistance to mupirocin in CA-MRSA strains [31]. However, prospective studies examining such strategies would be needed to determine their impact on incidence and the dynamics of antibiotic resistant infections.

Author Contributions

Conceived and designed the experiments: XW SP GC. Performed the experiments: XW ST SP GC. Analyzed the data: XW ST. Contributed reagents/materials/analysis tools: XW ST SP GC. Wrote the paper: XW SP GC.

References

1. Klein E, Smith DL, Laxminarayan R (2007) Hospitalizations and deaths caused by methicillin-resistant staphylococcus aureus, United States, 1999-2005. Emerg Infect Dis 13: 1840–1846.
2. Nicolle LE (2012) Antimicrobial resistance in long-term care facilities. Future Microbiol 7: 171–174.
3. Crum NF, Lee RU, Thornton SA, Stine OC, Wallace MR, et al. (2006) Fifteen-year study of the changing epidemiology of methicillin-resistant staphylococcus aureus. Am J Med 119: 943–951.
4. Lowy FD (1998) Staphylococcus aureus infections. N Engl J of Med 339: 520–532.
5. Kuehnert MJ (2005) Methicillin-resistant staphylococcus aureus hospitalizations, United States. Emerg Infect Dis 11: 468–872.
6. Kallen AJ, Mu Y, Bulens S, Reingold A, Petit S, et al. (2010) Health care-associated invasive MRSA infections, 2005–2008. JAMA 304: 641–648.
7. Frazee BW, Lynn J, Charlebois ED, Lambert L, Lowery D, et al. (2005) High prevalence of methicillin-resistant staphylococcus aureus in emergency department skin and soft tissue infections. Ann Emerg Med 45: 311–320.
8. Moran GJ, Krishnadasan A, Gorwitz RJ, Fosheim GE, McDougal LK, et al. (2006) Methicillin-resistant S. aureus infections among patients in the emergency department. N Engl J Med 355:666–674.
9. Creech CB 2nd, Kernodle DS, Alsentzer A, Wilson C, Edwards KM (2005) Increasing rates of nasal carriage of methicillin-resistant staphylococcus aureus in healthy children. Pediatr Infect Dis J 24: 617–621.
10. Pallin DJ, Egan DJ, Pelletier AJ, Espinola JA, Hooper DC, et al. (2008) Increased US emergency department visits for skin and soft tissue infections, and changes in antibiotic choices, during the emergence of community-associated methicillin-resistant staphylococcus aureus. Ann Emerg Med 51: 291–298.
11. Walraven CJ, Lingenfelter E, Rollo J, Madsen T, Alexander DP (2012) Diagnostic and therapeutic evaluation of community-acquired methicillin-resistant staphylococcus aureus (mrsa) skin and soft tissue infections in the emergency department. J Emerg Med 42: 392–399.
12. Szczesiul JM, Shermock KM, Murtaza UI, Siberry GK (2007) No decrease in clindamycin susceptibility despite increased use of clindamycin for pediatric community-associated methicillin-resistant staphylococcus aureus skin infections. Pediatr Infect Dis J 26: 852–854.
13. Mermel LA, Machan JT, Parenteau S (2011) Seasonality of MRSA infections. PLoS One 6: e17925.
14. Frei CR, Makos BR, Daniels KR, Oramasionwu CU (2010) Emergence of community-acquired methicillin-resistant staphylococcus aureus skin and soft tissue infections as a common cause of hospitalization in united states children. J Pediatr Surg 45:1967–1974.
15. Leekha S, Diekema DJ, Perencevich EN (2012) Seasonality of staphylococcal infections. Clin Microbiol Infect 18:927–933.
16. Eber MR, Shardell M, Schweizer ML, Laxminarayan R, Perencevich EN (2011) Seasonal and temperature-associated increases in gram-negative bacterial bloodstream infections among hospitalized patients. PLoS One 6:e25298.
17. Elegbe IA (1983) Influence of seasonal and weather variation on the incidence of coagulase positive staphylococci isolates among nigerians with boil infections. J R Soc Health 103:118–119.
18. Kaier K, Frank U, Conrad A, Meyer E (2010) Seasonal and ascending trends in the incidence of carriage of extended-spectrum ss-lactamase-producing escherichia coli and klebsiella species in 2 german hospitals. Infect Control Hosp Epidemiol 31:1154–1159.
19. Perencevich EN, McGregor JC, Shardell M, Furuno JP, Harris AD, et al. (2008) Summer peaks in the incidences of gram-negative bacterial infection among hospitalized patients. Infect Control Hosp Epidemiol 29:1124–1131.
20. Panchanathan SS, Petitti DB, Fridsma DB, Fridsma DB (2010) The development and validation of a simulation tool for health policy decision making. J Biomed Inform 43:602–607.
21. Lomb N (1976) Least-squares frequency analysis of unequally spaced data. Astrophys Space Sci 39: 447–462.
22. Scargle J (1982) Studies in astronomical time-series analysis.2. statistical aspects of spectral-analysis of unevenly spaced data. Astrophys J 263: 835–853.
23. Press W, Rybicki G (1989) Fast algorithm for spectral-analysis of unevenly sampled data. Astrophys J 338: 277–280.
24. Hens N, Ayele GM, Goeyvaerts N, Aerts M, Mossong J, et al. (2009) Estimating the impact of school closure on social mixing behaviour and the transmission of close contact infections in eight european countries. BMC Infect Dis 9:187.
25. Vaska VL, Nimmo GR, Jones M, Grimwood K, Paterson DL (2012) Increases in Australian cutaneous abscess hospitalisations: 1999–2008. Eur J Clin Microbiol Infect Dis 31:93–96.
26. Munckhof WJ, Nimmo GR, Carney J, Schooneveldt JM, Huygens F, et al. (2008) Methicillin-susceptible, non-multiresistant methicillin-resistant and multiresistant methicillin-resistant Staphylococcus aureus infections: a clinical, epidemiological and microbiological comparative study. Eur J Clin Microbiol Infect Dis 27:355–364.

27. Fridkin SK, Hageman JC, Morrison M, Sanza LT, Como-Sabetti K, et al. (2005) Methicillin-resistant Staphylococcus aureus disease in three communities. N Engl J Med 352:1436–1444.
28. Fritz SA, Garbutt J, Elward A, Shannon W, Storch GA (2008) Prevalence of and risk factors for community-acquired methicillin-resistant and methicillin-sensitive staphylococcus aureus colonization in children seen in a practice-based research network. Pediatrics 121: 1090–1098.
29. Bratu S, Landman D, Gupta J, Trehan M, Panwar M, et al. (2006) A population-based study examining the emergence of community-associated methicillin-resistant staphylococcus aureus USA300 in new york city. Ann Clin Microbiol Antimicrob 5:29.
30. Ammerlaan HS, Kluytmans JA, Wertheim HF, Nouwen JL, Bonten MJ (2009) Eradiction of methicillin-resistant staphylococcus aureus carriage: a systemtic review. Clin Infect Dis 48: 922–930.
31. Fritz SA, Hogan PG, Camins BC, Ainsworth AJ, Patrick C, et al. (2013) Mupirocin and chlorhexidine resistance in staphylococcus aureus in patients with community-onset skin and soft tissue infections. Antimicrob Agents Chemother 57:559–568.

3

Positive Attitudes to Pediatric HIV Testing: Findings from a Nationally Representative Survey from Zimbabwe

Raluca Buzdugan[1,2]*, Constancia Watadzaushe[3], Jeffrey Dirawo[3], Oscar Mundida[4], Lisa Langhaug[3], Nicola Willis[5], Karin Hatzold[6], Getrude Ncube[7], Owen Mugurungi[7], Clemens Benedikt[8], Andrew Copas[1], Frances M. Cowan[1,3]

1 University College London, Research Department of Infection & Population Health, London, United Kingdom, **2** University of California, Berkeley, School of Public Health, Berkeley, California, United States of America, **3** University of Zimbabwe, ZAPP-UZ, Community Medicine, Harare, Zimbabwe, **4** National AIDS Council, Harare, Zimbabwe, **5** Africaid, Harare, Zimbabwe, **6** Population Services International, Harare, Zimbabwe, **7** Ministry of Health and Child Welfare, Harare, Zimbabwe, **8** UNFPA, Harare, Zimbabwe

Abstract

Objective: Early HIV testing and diagnosis are paramount for increasing treatment initiation among children, necessary for their survival and improved health. However, uptake of pediatric HIV testing is low in high-prevalence areas. We present data on attitudes towards pediatric testing from a nationally representative survey in Zimbabwe.

Methods: All 18–24 year olds and a proportion of 25–49 year olds living in randomly selected enumeration areas from all ten Zimbabwe provinces were invited to self-complete an anonymous questionnaire on a personal digital assistant, and 16,719 people agreed to participate (75% of eligibles).

Results: Most people think children can benefit from HIV testing (91%), 81% of people who looked after children know how to access testing for their children and 92% would feel happier if their children were tested. Notably, 42% fear that, if tested, children may be discriminated against by some community members and 28% fear their children are HIV positive. People who fear discrimination against children who have tested for HIV are more likely than their counterparts to perceive their community as stigmatizing against HIV positive people (43% vs. 29%). They are also less likely to report positive attitudes to HIV themselves (49% vs. 74%). Only 28% think it is possible for children HIV-infected at birth to live into adolescence without treatment. Approximately 70% of people (irrespective of whether they are themselves parents) think HIV-infected children in their communities can access testing and treatment.

Conclusions: Pediatric HIV testing is the essential gateway to prevention and care services. Our data indicate positive attitudes to testing children, suggesting a conducive environment for increasing uptake of pediatric testing in Zimbabwe. However, there is a need to better understand the barriers to pediatric testing, such as stigma and discrimination, and address the gaps in knowledge regarding HIV/AIDS in children.

Editor: Sten H. Vermund, Vanderbilt University, United States of America

Funding: Funders: UNPFA Zimbabwe & Soul City. Soul City had no role in study design, data collection and analysis, decision to publish, or preparation of the manuscript. Clemens Benedikt from UNFPA provided substantive inputs into the study design and contributed to this manuscript.

Competing Interests: The authors have declared that no competing interests exist.

* E-mail: rbuzdugan@berkeley.edu

Introduction

An estimated 3.4 million children under the age of 15 were living with HIV globally in 2010 and 90% of them were living in Sub-Saharan Africa [1]. In Zimbabwe, 2.8% (138,642) of children are estimated to be living with HIV [2]. Given that most of these children acquired HIV from their mothers during pregnancy, labor or breastfeeding, and efficacious interventions for the prevention of mother-to-child HIV transmission have had limited coverage and impact, 330,000 children were newly infected with HIV in 2011, most of them living in sub-Saharan Africa [3].

In the absence of diagnosis and treatment, more than half of HIV infected children die by their second birthdate [4]. Initiating antiretroviral therapy (ART) of HIV positive children prior to their first year can reduce mortality by 76% and HIV progression by 75% [5], however only 456,000 children from low- and middle-income countries were receiving ART in 2010, an estimated 23% of the 2.02 million children in need of ART [1].

Early HIV testing and diagnosis are paramount for increasing ART initiation among children, necessary for their survival and improved health. However, uptake of HIV testing among children is low even in high HIV prevalence areas [6]. In Zimbabwe only 14% of infants born to HIV positive mothers were tested for HIV by two months of age [1] and data on uptake of HIV testing among older children is limited. Perception of pediatric HIV testing in terms of potential risks and benefits is an important factor in one's decision to have their child(ren) tested for HIV infection. For instance, fear of stigma and discrimination have been shown to negatively affect uptake of infant testing and care in Africa [7,8] and Zimbabwe in particular [9]. Previous studies have documented high acceptance of pediatric testing among Cote d'Ivoire health workers [10] and Zimbabwe adolescents [11] and low acceptance among Kenyan caregivers [12]. However, these have largely been small-scale studies focused on specific subpopulations. This paper presents data regarding knowledge and attitudes towards pediatric HIV testing, as reported during a nationally representative household survey of 18–49 years olds in Zimbabwe.

Methods

Survey Methodology

A cross-sectional survey of 18–49 year olds was conducted in all ten provinces in Zimbabwe in July 2011-January 2012, representing the final of three surveys conducted for the evaluation of Zimbabwe's National Behavioural Change Programme (NBCP). The evaluation of NBCP covered 16 districts from Mashonaland East, Masvingo, Matebeleland North and Midlands provinces (four districts selected per province) surveyed during the baseline survey (three randomly selected urban/peri-urban enumeration areas (EAs) and seven rural EAs per district). This survey was expanded beyond the geographic scope of the original evaluation to include all ten provinces in order to collect information on exposure to mass media messages nationally. (The expanded final survey also covered Manicaland, Mashonaland Central, Mashonaland West and Matebeleland South provinces (three urban/peri-urban EAs and seven rural EAs randomly selected per province), and Harare and Bulawayo cities (30 and 10 randomly selected EAs per city respectively)).

After enumerating all 18–49 year olds living in the selected EAs, all 18–24 year olds ("youth") and a proportion of 25–49 year olds ("adults") (approximately 40 per age group per EA) were invited to visit a centrally located survey site to self-complete an anonymous questionnaire on a personal digital assistant using audio-computer assisted self-interviewing software, following written informed consent. Complete questionnaires were collected among 16,719 people (75% of eligibles). The study procedures were approved by the institutional boards of University College London, United Kingdom and the Medical Research Council of Zimbabwe.

Data Analysis

The data were analyzed using Stata 12 (Stata Corp, College Station, TX, USA) after weighting through post-stratification to the 2002 Census. Specifically, the weights were developed by first calculating the percentage of the sample in each cross-classification of gender, age (youth vs. adults), urban/rural status and province. The corresponding percentages of the total population were derived from the census, and for each cross-classification a weight was calculated as the ratio of the census to sample percentages. However, for the four provinces where districts were initially selected and then EAs within these (see above), the post-stratification was performed at the district (rather than province) level and then participants were additionally weighted so that the proportion of the sample in these four provinces matched the population proportion derived from the census. The paper presents results of frequency distributions, cross-tabulations and tests of significance based on the survey functions in Stata.

We briefly explain how we derived some of the variables employed in the analysis. An index measuring HIV knowledge ranging from 0 to 6 was created by adding the answers (1 = yes, 0 = no/don't know) to six questions: 1) If you look carefully, you can know if someone has HIV (reverse coded); 2) Using condoms can prevent you from being infected by HIV; 3) A person who looks strong and healthy can have HIV; 4) A mother can transmit HIV through breastfeeding; 5) You can get HIV if you share utensils with someone who is infected (reverse coded); and 6) If a mosquito bites you it can infect you with HIV (reverse coded). The index was categorized into low (0–2), medium (3–4), and high knowledge (5–6).

Attitudes for HIV (specifically, expressed HIV-related stigma) were measured using an index computed by adding answers (1 = strongly agree/agree, 0 = strongly disagree/disagree) to 12 questions: 1) I would buy food from an HIV-positive shopkeeper; 2) HIV-positive teachers who are not ill should not be allowed to teach in school (reverse coded); 3) HIV-positive health workers should not be allowed to treat patients (reverse coded); 4) If a family member would become HIV-positive I would want it a secret (reverse coded); 5) HIV/AIDS is the result of sinning (reverse coded); 6) It is a waste of money to train/educate someone with HIV (reverse coded); 7) One would be foolish to marry someone with HIV (reverse coded); 8) People with HIV/AIDS should not be ashamed; 9) Health workers should treat people with AIDS as people with other illnesses; 10) People with HIV should be allowed to participated in social events; 11) It is reasonable for an employer to fire someone with AIDS (reverse coded); and 12) People with HIV/AIDS do not deserve any support (reverse coded). The index was categorized into mostly negative (0–4), medium (5–8), and mostly positive attitudes (9–12).

Perceived HIV-related stigma (1 = yes, 0 = no) in the community was coded 'yes' if the participant agreed with at least one of the following two statements: 1) Most people in this community would not buy vegetables from a shopkeeper or food seller if they knew that person had HIV; and 2) Most people in this community would want to remove the teacher in the school if they knew that this person had HIV though they were not sick.

Perceived community norms regarding HIV testing was assessed by adding the answers (1 = strongly agree/agree, 0 = strongly disagree/disagree) to 5 questions: 1) Most people in this community who want to get tested for HIV do not want other people to find out if they get tested (reverse coded); 2) Most people in this community who want to get tested for HIV will tell their spouses/partners that they want to get tested; 3) Most people in this community want to get tested for HIV; 4) Most people in this community get tested for HIV only if they are sick (reverse coded); and 5) In this community people think that young couples should go for an HIV test before getting married. The index was categorized into mostly negative (0–1), medium (2–3), and mostly positive perception scores (4–5).

Results

Awareness of Pediatric HIV/AIDS

Approximately 45% of people reported that they know children infected with HIV and 40% know children on ART (Table 1). One third of people know children who have been tested for HIV. With respect to perceived access to pediatric HIV testing and care, 68% of people think that HIV infected children in their communities can access testing and 70% that they can access ART.

Knowledge about Survival of HIV Infected Children

While the majority of people surveyed report being aware of HIV/AIDS among children and think that they can access testing and treatment, only 28% think it is possible for children HIV infected at birth to live into adolescence without treatment. Of these, 58% personally know such children.

Table 1. Pediatric HIV/AIDS indicators, Zimbabwe.

	Total (n = 17038)
Awareness of pediatric HIV/AIDS	
Know HIV positive children	44.3
Know HIV positive children on ART	39.5
Know children who have tested for HIV	33.0
Perceived access to HIV testing & care	
Think HIV positive children in their community can access HIV testing	
Yes	68.4
No	11.8
Don't know	19.8
Think HIV+ children in their community can access ART	
Yes	70.0
No	12.0
Don't know	18.1
Knowledge about survival of HIV infected children	
Think it is possible for some children infected with HIV at birth to live into adolescence without treatment	27.6
If yes, personally know such children	(n = 4691)
	57.9
Attitudes towards pediatric HIV testing	
Think that children can benefit from HIV testing	91.2
Afraid that if children are tested for HIV they may be discriminated against by some members of their community	41.9
Ever talked to their children about HIV testing	
Yes	39.6
No	40.6
Don't look after any children	19.8
Only those who look after children	(n = 13631)
Know how to access HIV testing for their children	80.8
Would feel happier if their children were tested for HIV	92.2
Fear that if their children were tested for HIV, they would be found positive	28.3

ART = antiretroviral treatment.

Attitudes Towards Pediatric HIV Testing

Most people think that children can benefit from being tested for HIV (91%). Moreover, 81% of parents/guardians know how to access HIV testing for their children and 92% would feel happier if their children were tested. However, only half of people who looked after children talked to them about HIV testing, although in many cases their children may have been too young for such discussions. Notably, 42% fear that, if tested, children may be discriminated against by some community members and 28% of parents/guardians fear that their children are HIV positive.

HIV Knowledge by Awareness of Pediatric HIV/AIDS

There appears to be an association between awareness of pediatric HIV/AIDS and knowledge about HIV and mother-to-child HIV transmission (Table 2). For example, 45% of people who personally know children on ART reported high knowledge about HIV compared to 35% of those who do not know children on ART. Similarly, 90% of people who know children on ART are aware that mothers can transmit HIV though breastfeeding compared to 79% of people who do not know children on ART. There is strong association between awareness of pediatric HIV and awareness of HIV in their community (where "HIV in the community" is generally synonymous with "adult HIV in the community", according to anecdotal evidence). Specifically, 90% of people who know HIV positive children also reported that they know someone with HIV, compared to 51% of people who do not know HIV positive children (Table 2). Table 3 indicates that people with better general knowledge about HIV/AIDS and mother-to-child HIV transmission are slightly more likely to know that some children infected with HIV at birth can live into adolescence without treatment, compared to those without such knowledge.

Figure 1 indicates substantial variation in the perceived access to pediatric HIV testing and care by province, but not by rural vs. urban status. For instance, 75% of people in Manicaland think parents can access HIV testing for their children compared to 56% in Matebeleland South. However, virtually the same percentage of people share this belief in urban (68%) and rural areas (69%). Similarly, 79% of people in Masvingo vs. 60% in Matebeleland South think parents can access ART for their children.

Table 2. HIV knowledge by awareness of pediatric HIV/AIDS.

	Know HIV positive children		Know HIV positive children on ART		Know children who tested for HIV	
	No	Yes	No	Yes	No	Yes
	(n = 9449)	(n = 7515)	(n = 10272)	(n = 6718)	(n = 11388)	(n = 5605)
HIV knowledge	p<0.001		p<0.001		p = 0.002	
Low (0–2)	13.8	5.1	13.6	4.3	10.8	8.2
Medium (3–4)	51.1	51.0	51.0	51.1	50.9	51.2
High (5–6)	35.1	44.0	35.4	44.7	38.3	40.5
A mother can transmit HIV through breastfeeding						
	p<0.001		p<0.001		p<0.001	
Yes	79.1	89.2	79.3	90.1	82.4	86.1
No	9.9	6.4	9.9	6.0	8.5	8.2
Don't know	10.9	4.3	10.7	3.9	9.1	5.7
An HIV positive mother can do something to prevent HIV infection of baby						
	p<0.001		p<0.001		p<0.001	
Yes	76.1	89.9	76.8	90.5	80.2	86.3
No	9.0	4.3	8.9	4.0	7.4	6.0
Don't know	14.8	5.8	14.3	5.5	12.4	7.6
Know someone who is HIV positive						
	p<0.001					
Yes	50.7	90.4				
No	49.3	9.6				
Know someone on ART			p<0.001			
Yes			48.2	90.2		
No			51.8	9.8		

ART = antiretroviral treatment.

HIV-related Stigma by Attitudes about Pediatric HIV Testing

People who think pediatric HIV testing is beneficial are more likely to have tested for HIV themselves (64% vs. 41%). Similarly, 68% of those who know how to access HIV testing for their children had tested for HIV compared to 54% of those who do not know (Table 4). Notably, people who fear discrimination against children who have been tested for HIV are more likely than their

Table 3. Knowledge about survival of HIV infected children by knowledge about HIV/AIDS.

		Think it is possible for children HIV infected at birth to live into adolescence without treatment	
		Yes	p value
HIV knowledge			0.010
Low (0–2)	(n = 1685)	24.3	
Medium (3–4)	(n = 8648)	27.2	
High (5–6)	(n = 6614)	29.0	
A mother can transmit HIV through breastfeeding			0.024
Yes	(n = 14206)	27.9	
No	(n = 1422)	28.5	
Don't know	(n = 1363)	23.3	
An HIV positive mother can do something to prevent HIV infection of baby			<0.001
Yes	(n = 13969)	28.7	
No	(n = 1184)	22.7	
Don't know	(n = 1842)	22.2	

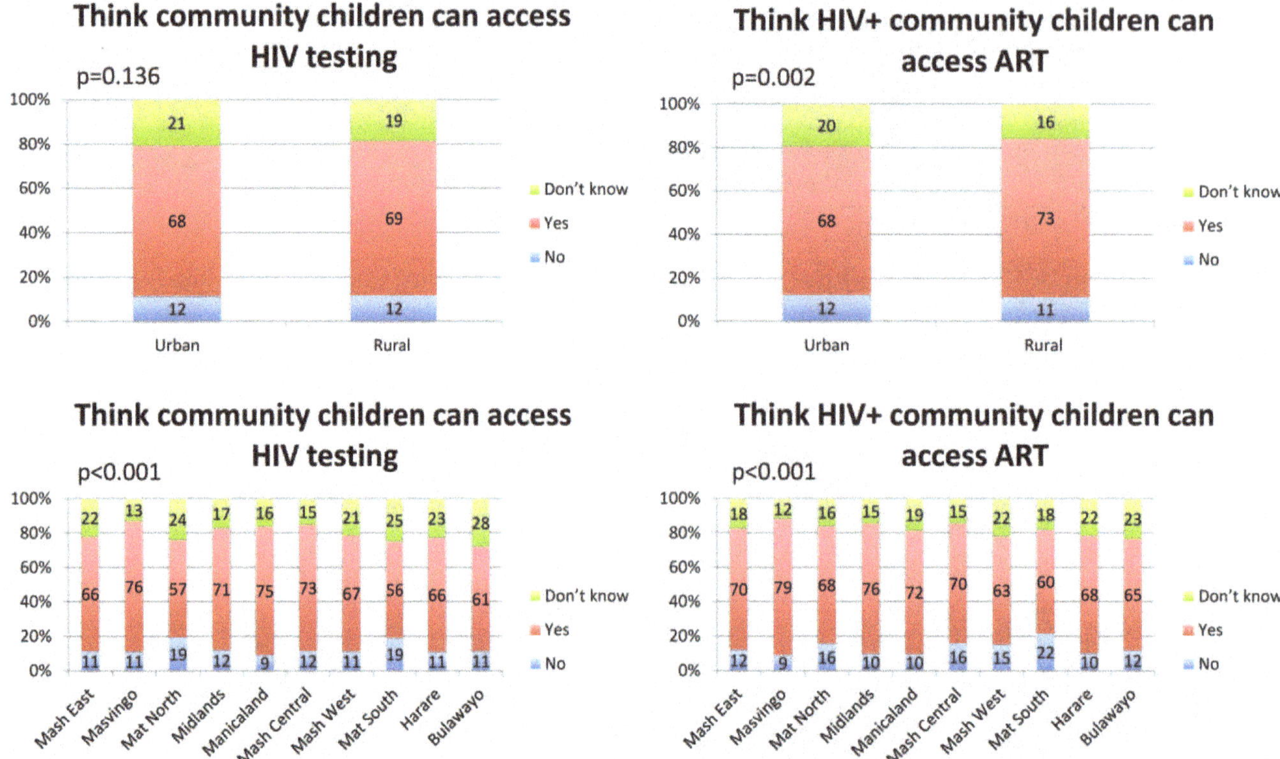

Figure 1. Perceived access to pediatric HIV testing and care by province and rural/ urban status.

counterparts to report HIV-related stigma in their communities (43% vs. 29%) and less likely to report positive HIV testing-related norms (11% vs. 19%). They are also less likely to report positive attitudes to HIV themselves (49% vs. 74%).

Fear about Pediatric HIV Testing by Own HIV Testing Behaviour

Table 5 examines associations between participants' reported fear that, if tested, their children would be found HIV positive and their self-perceived HIV risk and reported HIV status. There is only a weak association between fear that their children are HIV-infected and self-perceived HIV risk. People who have tested for HIV themselves are less likely to express fear that their children are HIV-infected (25% vs. 35% of those who have never tested for HIV themselves). Among those who tested for HIV, people who reported to be HIV positive are more likely to fear that they children are HIV-infected (33%) than those who reported being HIV negative (22%); 38% of those who tested for HIV but did not report their status fear that their children are HIV positive.

The associations discussed in this section were also observed for young men, young women, adult men and adult women separately (data not shown).

Discussion

We present data from a nationally representative survey from Zimbabwe that indicate positive attitudes towards HIV testing of children; most people think children can benefit from testing and would feel happier if their children (or the children in their care) had been tested. These findings, coupled with the fact that four fifths of people who look after children know where to access testing for their children, suggest a conducive environment for increasing uptake of pediatric testing. To the best of our knowledge, this is the first paper to present national-level data on attitudes to pediatric HIV testing from a high prevalence country.

High acceptance of pediatric testing was documented among health care workers from Cote d'Ivoire [10]. A study that examined actual uptake of pediatric testing, albeit in a much smaller sample, found that the majority of adolescents attending acute primary care services and offered provider initiated testing and counseling (PITC) in Harare, Zimbabwe accepted to be tested for HIV [11]. In contrast, almost half of caregivers from Western Kenya refused to have their high-risk children tested for HIV [12].

These data do suggest some potential barriers to pediatric testing, such as parents/guardians' fear of discrimination as a result of testing (42%) and fear that their children (or the children in their care) are HIV positive (28%). Notably, people who expressed fear that children tested for HIV would be discriminated against were less likely to have positive attitudes to HIV themselves, suggesting that for some people perceived stigma against children may be a "projection" of their own attitudes. Fear of discrimination has been shown to negatively affect uptake to HIV infant testing and care in the region [7,8], among other factors [13]. The decision to test one's child is clearly linked to parents' status and perceived risk, which complicates the decision-making process; people may not only fear discrimination against their tested children (or the children in their care), but also against themselves [9,14,15]. A study conducted in primary schools in Harare, Zimbabwe showed that biological parents feared their children's HIV test could disclose their own HIV status, while guardians did not share these concerns [9].

More than a quarter of people expressed fear that their children (or the children in their care) may be HIV seropositive, which is

Table 4. Reported HIV testing and HIV-related stigma in the community by attitudes about pediatric HIV testing.

	Think that children can benefit from HIV testing		Afraid that if tested for HIV children may be discriminated against		Know how to access HIV testing for their children	
	No	**Yes**	**No**	**Yes**	**No**	**Yes**
	(n = 1491)	**(n = 15472)**	**(n = 9866)**	**(n = 7122)**	**(n = 2611)**	**(n = 11014)**
Perceived HIV-related stigma in the community						
			$p<0.001$			
Yes			29.3	42.7		
No			70.7	57.4		
Perceived community norms regarding HIV testing						
			$p<0.001$			
0–1 (Mostly negative)			25.7	28.3		
2–3			55.4	60.7		
4–5 (Mostly positive)			18.9	11.1		
Attitudes to HIV						
			$p<0.001$			
0–4 (Mostly negative)			3.7	13.8		
5–8			22.6	37.0		
9–12 (Mostly positive)			73.7	49.3		
Ever been tested for HIV						
	$p<0.001$				$p<0.001$	
Yes	41.0	63.5			54.1	68.2
No	59.0	36.5			45.9	31.8

Table 5. Fear about pediatric HIV testing by self-perceived HIV risk and HIV testing.

		Fear that if tested for HIV their children would be found positive	
		Yes	p value
Self-perceived HIV risk			0.004
No risk	(n = 3040)	26.8	
Small or moderate	(n = 5545)	27.8	
Great	(n = 2749)	32.6	
Already know status	(n = 2291)	26.3	
Ever been tested for HIV			<0.001
No	(n = 4694)	34.6	
Yes	(n = 8930)	25.0	
Reported HIV status			<0.001
Negative	(n = 7018)	22.1	
Positive1	(n = 1227)	33.4	
Not reported	(n = 314)	38.2	

unlikely given that only 2.8% of Zimbabwean children are estimated to be HIV infected [2]. Therefore, most of these parents/guardians likely have an unfounded anxiety about the status of their children (or the children in their care). This fear is not associated with their perception of their own risk for HIV. People who have tested for HIV themselves and those who report being HIV-negative are less likely to fear that their children (or the children in their care) may be HIV-infected. These findings prompt additional questions beyond the available data, such as: Do parents think their children may be positive because they know the mother did not test for HIV or access care during her pregnancy? To what extent is perception of children's risk a reflection of their partners' perceived risk? A qualitative exploration of these fears and their underpinnings is needed to better understand why so many parents fear their children may be HIV-infected. At the same time, these figures may simply be a measure of people's fear of HIV rather than an indicator of their assessment of the status of their children (or the children in their care).

We document high perceived access to pediatric HIV testing and care. According to our data, perceived access to these services varies by province but not by urban/rural status, which may suggest regional variation in the availability of services. However, data from the Ministry of Health and Child Welfare (MOHCW) suggest that HIV testing and care services are widely available in Zimbabwe in both rural and urban settings and are free of charge. Specifically, the more efficacious regimen for the prevention of mother-to-child HIV transmission (PMTCT) recommended by the World Health Organization (which emphasizes the need for early infant diagnosis and children's enrollment into care) has been rolled out throughout the country since mid-2011. In addition, HIV testing for children over 18 months as well as adults is available at all health facilities in Zimbabwe, although for children under 16 years testing requires parental or guardian consent.

Over a quarter of people are aware that children infected with HIV at birth can live into adolescence without treatment, and almost 60% of them personally know such children, indicating the need for interventions to incorporate information about the chances of survival of HIV infected children in their materials and messaging. Although long-term survival following mother-to-child HIV transmission was underestimated during the early HIV epidemic, about a quarter of infected infants has been shown to live 10 years or more without ART [16]. Given high HIV prevalence in the absence of PMTCT interventions during the 1990s in many African countries, a substantial minority of children and adolescents are likely HIV positive [17]. Most long-term survivors of mother-to-child HIV transmission remain undiagnosed [16], partly because people are not aware that children can survive untreated mother-to-child HIV transmission [11]. Routine provider-initiated testing among hospitalized children is being advocated given that HIV is the most common cause of adolescent hospitalization in high prevalence countries [18–22].

Data indicates associations between awareness and knowledge about pediatric testing, and knowledge about HIV/AIDS in general. Moreover, positive attitudes about pediatric testing seem to be associated with parents/guardians' testing status. These data suggest that interventions aiming to increase HIV/AIDS knowledge and uptake of testing among adults may have a trickle-down effect on pediatric testing in the form of positive attitudes.

Reported findings are based on nationally representative data collected in all ten Zimbabwe provinces. However, weighting the data using 2002 Census indicators presents some limitations, given the high migration within Zimbabwe since 2002. While the examination of the above-mentioned associations disaggregated by gender and age groups indicated similar patterns, other underlying factors may explain some of the associations observed. All questions about pediatric testing asked about "children" generally, allowing a variation in participants' interpretation of the children's age range (e.g. including or excluding infants and/or older adolescents). We are unable to distinguish between the perceptions of biological parents and guardians or to take into account the age or HIV status of participants' children (or the children in their care), as these data were not collected as part of the survey.

Pediatric HIV testing is the essential gateway to prevention and care services for children. Our data indicate positive attitudes to testing children in Zimbabwe. However, positive attitudes to medical procedures do not always concretize as high uptake (as is the case for male circumcision as an HIV preventive method). Hence, there is a need to better understand the barriers to pediatric testing, such as stigma and discrimination, and address the gaps in knowledge regarding HIV/AIDS in children.

Author Contributions

Analyzed the data: RB. Wrote the paper: RB. Provided substantial feedback to the manuscript: CW JD OM LL NW KH GN OM CB AC FMC.

References

1. WHO UNICEF, UNAIDS (2011) Global HIV/AIDS Response. Epidemic update and health sector progress towards Universal Access. Progress report 2011. Geneva, Switzerland.
2. Zimbabwe Country Report (2012) Global AIDS Response Progress Report 2012.
3. Joint United Nations Programme on HIV/AIDS (2012) Together we will end AIDS.
4. Newell M-L, Brahmbhatt H, Ghys PD (2004) Child mortality and HIV infection in Africa: a review. AIDS 18: S27–34. doi:10.1097/01.aids.0000125981.71657.0d.
5. Violari A, Cotton MF, Gibb DM, Babiker AG, Steyn J, et al. (2008) Early antiretroviral therapy and mortality among HIV-infected infants. The New England Journal of Medicine 359: 2233–2244. Available: http://www.pubmedcentral.nih.gov/articlerender.fcgi?artid=2950021&tool=pmcentrez&rendertype=abstract.
6. Chhagan MK, Kauchali S, Arpadi SM, Craib MH, Bah F, et al. (2011) Failure to test children of HIV-infected mothers in South Africa: implications for HIV testing strategies for preschool children. Tropical Medicine & International Health 16: 1490–1494. Available: http://www.pubmedcentral.nih.gov/articlerender.fcgi?artid=3234311&tool=pmcentrez&rendertype=abstract. Accessed 8 March 2012.
7. Braitstein P, Songok J, Vreeman RC, Wools-Kaloustian KK, Koskei P, et al. (2011) "Wamepotea" (they have become lost): outcomes of HIV-positive and HIV-exposed children lost to follow-up from a large HIV treatment program in Western Kenya. Journal of Acquired Immune Deficiency Syndromes 57: e40–6. Available: http://www.ncbi.nlm.nih.gov/pubmed/21407085.
8. Donahue MC, Dube Q, Dow A, Umar E, Van Rie A (2012) "They Have Already Thrown Away Their Chicken": barriers affecting participation by HIV-infected women in care and treatment programs for their infants in Blantyre, Malawi. AIDS care. Available: http://www.ncbi.nlm.nih.gov/pubmed/22348314. Accessed 8 June 2012.
9. Bandason T, Langhaug L, Makamba M, Laver S, Hatzgold K, et al. (2011) Burden of HIV Infection and Acceptability of School-linked HIV Testing among Primary School Children in Harare, Zimbabwe. 18th Conference on Retroviruses and Opportunistic Infection (CROI). Boston, USA. p. Abstract no. 127.
10. Oga MA, Ndondoki C, Brou H, Salmon A, Bosse-Amani C, et al. (2011) Attitudes and Practices of Health Care Workers Toward Routine HIV Testing of Infants in Cote d'Ivoire: The PEDI-TEST ANRS 12165 Project. Journal of Acquired Immune Deficency Syndromes 57: S16–21.
11. Ferrand RA, Trigg C, Bandason T, Ndhlovu CE, Mungofa S, et al. (2011) Perception of risk of vertically acquired HIV infection and acceptability of provider-initiated testing and counseling among adolescents in Zimbabwe. American Journal of Public Health 101: 2325–2332. Available: http://www.ncbi.nlm.nih.gov/pubmed/22021300. Accessed 8 June 2012.
12. Vreeman RC, Nyandiko WM, Braitstein P, Were MC, Ayaya SO, et al. (2010) Acceptance of HIV testing for children ages 18 months to 13 years identified through voluntary, home-based HIV counseling and testing in western Kenya. Journal of Acquired Immune Deficiency Syndromes 55: e3–10. Available: http://www.ncbi.nlm.nih.gov/pubmed/20714272.
13. Yeap A, Hamilton R, Charalambous S, Dwadwa T, Churchyard G, et al. (2010) Factors influencing uptake of HIV care and treatment among children in South Africa - a qualitative study of caregivers and clinic staff. AIDS Care 22: 1101–1107. Available: http://www.ncbi.nlm.nih.gov/pubmed/20824563. Accessed 26 May 2012.
14. Berendes S, Rimal RN (2011) Addressing the slow uptake of HIV testing in Malawi: the role of stigma, self-efficacy, and knowledge in the Malawi BRIDGE Project. The Journal of the Association of Nurses in AIDS Care 22: 215–228. Available: http://www.ncbi.nlm.nih.gov/pubmed/21185751. Accessed 29 May 2012.
15. Ostermann J, Reddy E a, Shorter MM, Muiruri C, Mtalo A, et al. (2011) Who tests, who doesn't, and why? Uptake of mobile HIV counseling and testing in the Kilimanjaro Region of Tanzania. Plos One 6: e16488. Available: http://www.pubmedcentral.nih.gov/articlerender.fcgi?artid=3031571&tool=pmcentrez&rendertype=abstract. Accessed 20 March 2012.
16. Ferrand RA, Corbett EL, Wood R, Hargrove J, Ndhlovu CE, et al. (2009) AIDS among older children and adolescents in Southern Africa: projecting the time course and magnitude of the epidemic. AIDS 23: 2039–2046. Available: http://www.ncbi.nlm.nih.gov/pubmed/19684508. Accessed 8 June 2012.
17. Ferrand RA, Munaiwa L, Matsekete J, Bandason T, Nathoo K, et al. (2010) Undiagnosed HIV infection among adolescents seeking primary health care in Zimbabwe. Clinical Infectious Diseases 51: 844–851. Available: http://www.ncbi.nlm.nih.gov/pubmed/20804412. Accessed 12 April 2012.
18. Ferrand RA, Bandason T, Musvaire P, Larke N, Nathoo K, et al. (2010) Causes of acute hospitalization in adolescence: burden and spectrum of HIV-related morbidity in a country with an early-onset and severe HIV epidemic: a prospective survey. PLoS Medicine 7: e1000178. Available: http://www.pubmedcentral.nih.gov/articlerender.fcgi?artid=2814826&tool=pmcentrez&rendertype=abstract. Accessed 2 March 2012.
19. Kankasa C, Carter RJ, Briggs N, Bulterys M, Chama E, et al. (2009) Routine offering of HIV testing to hospitalized pediatric patients at university teaching hospital, Lusaka, Zambia: acceptability and feasibility. Journal of Acquired Immune Deficiency Syndrome 51: 202–208. Available: http://www.ncbi.nlm.nih.gov/pubmed/19504732.
20. McCollum ED, Preidis GA, Golitko CL, Siwande LD, Mwansambo C, et al. (2011) Routine inpatient human immunodeficiency virus testing system increases access to pediatric human immunodeficiency virus care in sub-Saharan Africa. The Pediatric Infectious Disease Journal 30: e75–81. Available: http://www.ncbi.nlm.nih.gov/pubmed/21297520. Accessed 8 June 2012.
21. Mutanga JN, Raymond J, Towle MS, Mutembo S, Fubisha RC, et al. (2012) Institutionalizing Provider-Initiated HIV Testing and Counselling for Children: An Observational Case Study from Zambia. PloS one 7: e29656. Available: http://www.pubmedcentral.nih.gov/articlerender.fcgi?artid=3335043&tool=pmcentrez&rendertype=abstract. Accessed 21 May 2012.
22. Wanyenze RK, Nawavvu C, Ouma J, Namale A, Colebunders R, et al. (2010) Provider-initiated HIV testing for paediatric inpatients and their caretakers is feasible and acceptable. Tropical medicine & international healt 15: 113–119. Available: http://www.ncbi.nlm.nih.gov/pubmed/19891756. Accessed 18 March 2012.

4

Cost-Effectiveness Analysis of Option B+ for HIV Prevention and Treatment of Mothers and Children in Malawi

Olufunke Fasawe[1], Carlos Avila[2*], Nathan Shaffer[3], Erik Schouten[4], Frank Chimbwandira[5], David Hoos[6], Olive Nakakeeto[7], Paul De Lay[8]

1 Master of International Health Management, Economics and Policy Program, SDA Bocconi School of Management, Milan, Italy, **2** Senior Health Economist, Principal Associate, Abt Associates, Bethesda, Maryland, United States of America, **3** PMTCT Technical Lead, HIV Department, World Health Organization, Geneva, Switzerland, **4** HIV Advisor, Management Sciences for Health, Lilongwe, Malawi, **5** Director of the HIV and AIDS Department, Ministry of Health, Lilongwe, Malawi, **6** Assistant Professor of Clinical Epidemiology, Senior Implementation Director, ICAP, Columbia University, Mailman School of Public Health, New York, New York, United States of America, **7** Health Economist, Independent Consultant, Saint-Genis-Poully, France, **8** Deputy Executive Director, Joint United Nations Programme on HIV/AIDS (UNAIDS), Geneva, Switzerland

Abstract

Background: The Ministry of Health in Malawi is implementing a pragmatic and innovative approach for the management of all HIV-infected pregnant women, termed Option B+, which consists of providing life-long antiretroviral treatment, regardless of their CD4 count or clinical stage. Our objective was to determine if Option B+ represents a cost-effective option.

Methods: A decision model simulates the disease progression of a cohort of HIV-infected pregnant women receiving prophylaxis and antiretroviral therapy, and estimates the number of paediatric infections averted and maternal life years gained over a ten-year time horizon. We assess the cost-effectiveness from the Ministry of Health perspective while taking into account the practical realities of implementing ART services in Malawi.

Results: If implemented as recommended by the World Health Organization, options A, B and B+ are equivalent in preventing new infant infections, yielding cost effectiveness ratios between US$ 37 and US$ 69 per disability adjusted life year averted in children. However, when the three options are compared to the current practice, the provision of antiretroviral therapy to all mothers (Option B+) not only prevents infant infections, but also improves the ten-year survival in mothers more than four-fold. This translates into saving more than 250,000 maternal life years, as compared to mothers receiving only Option A or B, with savings of 153,000 and 172,000 life years respectively. Option B+ also yields favourable incremental cost effectiveness ratios (ICER) of US$ 455 per life year gained over the current practice.

Conclusion: In Malawi, Option B+ represents a favorable policy option from a cost-effectiveness perspective to prevent future infant infections, save mothers' lives and reduce orphanhood. Although Option B+ would require more financial resources initially, it would save societal resources in the long-term and represents a strategic option to simplify and integrate HIV services into maternal, newborn and child health programmes.

Editor: Paula Braitstein, Indiana University and Moi University, United States of America

Funding: The authors have no support or funding to report.

Competing Interests: The authors have declared that no competing interests exist.

* E-mail: Carlos_Avila@abtassoc.com

Introduction

HIV continues to pose a serious health risk for pregnant women and their children in high prevalence settings. Vertical transmission, occurring during pregnancy, labour, delivery or breastfeeding [1], remains the main mode of HIV infection in children. An estimated 390 000 children globally acquired HIV from their mothers in 2010 with over 90% of these new infections occurring in sub-Saharan Africa [2]. While the majority of infants of HIV-infected mothers do not themselves become HIV-infected, they are nonetheless at risk of increased mortality and morbidity and vulnerable to orphanhood [3]. However, the use of antiretroviral drugs during and after pregnancy is a proven intervention to virtually eliminate the risk of HIV transmission to infants, as evidenced in high-income countries where new childhood HIV infections are now almost non-existent [4,5].

Malawi, a low-income country of 15 million people is one of the countries with the highest number of HIV-infected pregnant women; between 57,000 and 76,000 pregnant women (mid-point estimate 66,500) were HIV-infected and required antiretroviral prophylaxis for prevention of mother-to-child transmission (PMTCT) in 2010 [2]. There are approximately 663,000 annual births and a high mortality ratio (510/100,000 births); approximately 32% of maternal deaths are attributable to HIV [6].

Malawi has experienced successful national efforts in reducing disparities in safe motherhood with reductions in maternal mortality of approximately 50% in the last decade. More than 90% of pregnant women attend antenatal clinics at least once during their pregnancy [7], although the majority first attend during the second or third trimester. The Government of Malawi has implemented a decentralized approach to HIV prevention, care and treatment in order to reach the 85% of Malawi's population that live in rural areas [8]. Malawi has also had notable success in rapidly expanding ART (antiretroviral treatment) coverage in the general population; the number of ART sites across the country grew from 9 to 491 between 2003 and 2009, almost half of which are community-based health centres, and an estimated 49–57% of HIV-infected adults eligible by clinical or immunologic criteria were receiving ART by the end of 2010. By contrast, the coverage of antiretroviral prophylaxis for HIV-infected pregnant women was still very low in 2010, within the range of 23–31% [2]. Malawi's healthcare system remains overstretched, with one doctor for every 49 000 people and one nurse for every 1 800 people [7] which is ten times lower than the World Health Organization (WHO) recommended minimum standard.

The revised 2010 WHO guidelines for prevention of mother-to-child transmission of HIV recommend lifelong ART for women with CD4 counts at or lower than 350 cells/ μL. The guidelines recommend two prophylaxis regimens for women who are not clinically or immunologically eligible for ART [9]. Option A consists of antepartum zidovudine (AZT) from 14 weeks of pregnancy, single-dose nevirapine (sd-NVP) at the onset of labour and a dual-drug regimen of zidovudine (AZT) and lamivudine (3TC) until one week after delivery. The infant receives daily oral nevirapine from birth until all breastfeeding has ceased. In Option B, mothers receive triple-drug antiretroviral prophylaxis starting from 14 weeks of pregnancy until all exposure to breast milk has ended. Daily oral nevirapine to the infant is provided from birth until six weeks of age. Determination of which women are eligible for lifelong ART and which women receive prophylaxis is primarily through CD4 screening.

The Ministry of Health in Malawi proposed and has recently begun implementing a new approach termed Option B+ in which all pregnant women who test HIV positive are placed on ART for life, from 14 weeks gestation or first antenatal visit, and regardless of their CD4 count or clinical stage [10]. This simplified approach would facilitate the achievement of not only the Global Plan target of elimination of new paediatric HIV infections by 2015 [11], but also the target of universal access to HIV treatment for mothers in a setting where it is difficult to effectively distinguish between those mothers eligible for treatment and those needing prophylaxis. While CD4 testing should be available to guide the initiation of ART [12], Malawi, like many other low-income countries, suffers major constraints in the expansion of laboratory capacity, and specifically regarding access to CD4 testing [13]. The simplification of drug regimen options may also help to improve adherence to therapy and reduce the many bottlenecks within the cascade of PMTCT interventions as countries adopt the Treatment 2.0 framework of simplified HIV treatment [14]. Implementing Option B+ may be a more effective PMTCT strategy, as it can help overcome some of the individual, organizational and societal barriers associated with achieving high coverage levels of prophylaxis and treatment, and will ensure that most HIV-infected pregnant women are placed on treatment immediately following diagnosis leading to further reduction of MTCT [10].

The objective of this analysis was to determine if Option B+ represents a cost-effective policy option for the treatment of HIV-infected pregnant women and for PMTCT, as compared with WHO Options A and B. We assess the cost-effectiveness from the Ministry of Health perspective while taking into account the practical realities and costs of implementing ART services in Malawi.

Methods

Model Structure

A decision analytic model was developed to compare the costs, health outcomes and cost-effectiveness of WHO PMTCT Options A and B as well as Option B+ in Malawi for all HIV-infected pregnant women. The analysis was structured as a probability tree starting with an HIV-infected pregnant woman entering into contact with the health system for antenatal care, then receiving a cascade of interventions towards reducing the risk of transmission to her infant as well as care and treatment for her own health (Figure 1). The risk of transmission depends on the background HIV transmission rates during pregnancy, labour, delivery and breastfeeding, the efficacy of the antiretroviral drugs in preventing transmission, prophylaxis and treatment coverage and the level of adherence. The estimated number of HIV-infected pregnant women in Malawi was taken as the midpoint of the range reported for the end of 2010 [2] and this number, 66,500, was then used as an input to analyse as an annual cohort of HIV-infected pregnant women that, after surviving childbirth, was followed over a 10-year time horizon. This time horizon was thought to be sufficiently long enough to capture the effects of immediate or later access to treatment and to assess maternal survival outcomes.

The patterns of disease progression in HIV-infected pregnant women with and without ART were assumed to be similar to that documented in the general adult population. A Markov model was developed to simulate the natural history of HIV infection and project the 10-year maternal outcomes associated with the different options implemented. The model assumes that women are treatment naïve and in one of four transition states: (a) CD4 counts >350 cells/ μL; (b) CD4 counts 350–200 cells/ μL; (c) CD4 between 199–0 cells/ μL and (d) death, as the absorbing state. Women starting with high CD4 counts and subsequently becoming eligible for ART when their CD4 cell counts fall to 350 or below, would access ART services when they move into the eligible transition state, while women eligible for treatment receive life-long therapy and are accounted for in the PMTCT programme. As more women access ART services in the future, the background survival rates of HIV-infected mothers under Options A and B improve when compared to the no-treatment scenario.

Outcomes assessed include the number of infant infections averted, cost per infection averted, cost per disability adjusted life year (DALY) averted for infants, life years gained in HIV-infected mothers, cost per life year gained for the HIV-infected mothers and the incremental cost-effectiveness ratios for each outcome. DALYs were estimated using standard published methods [15].

Strategies being compared

We analyzed four strategies including; (1) Current practice in 2010, (2) Option A, (3) Option B, and (4) Option B+. For the current practice, we modelled the mix of interventions in Malawi including HIV testing and counselling and ARV prophylaxis for HIV-infected pregnant women at the reported coverage levels as of the end of 2010 [2].We modelled an ante-natal care (ANC) coverage of 91% according to the World Health Statistics report

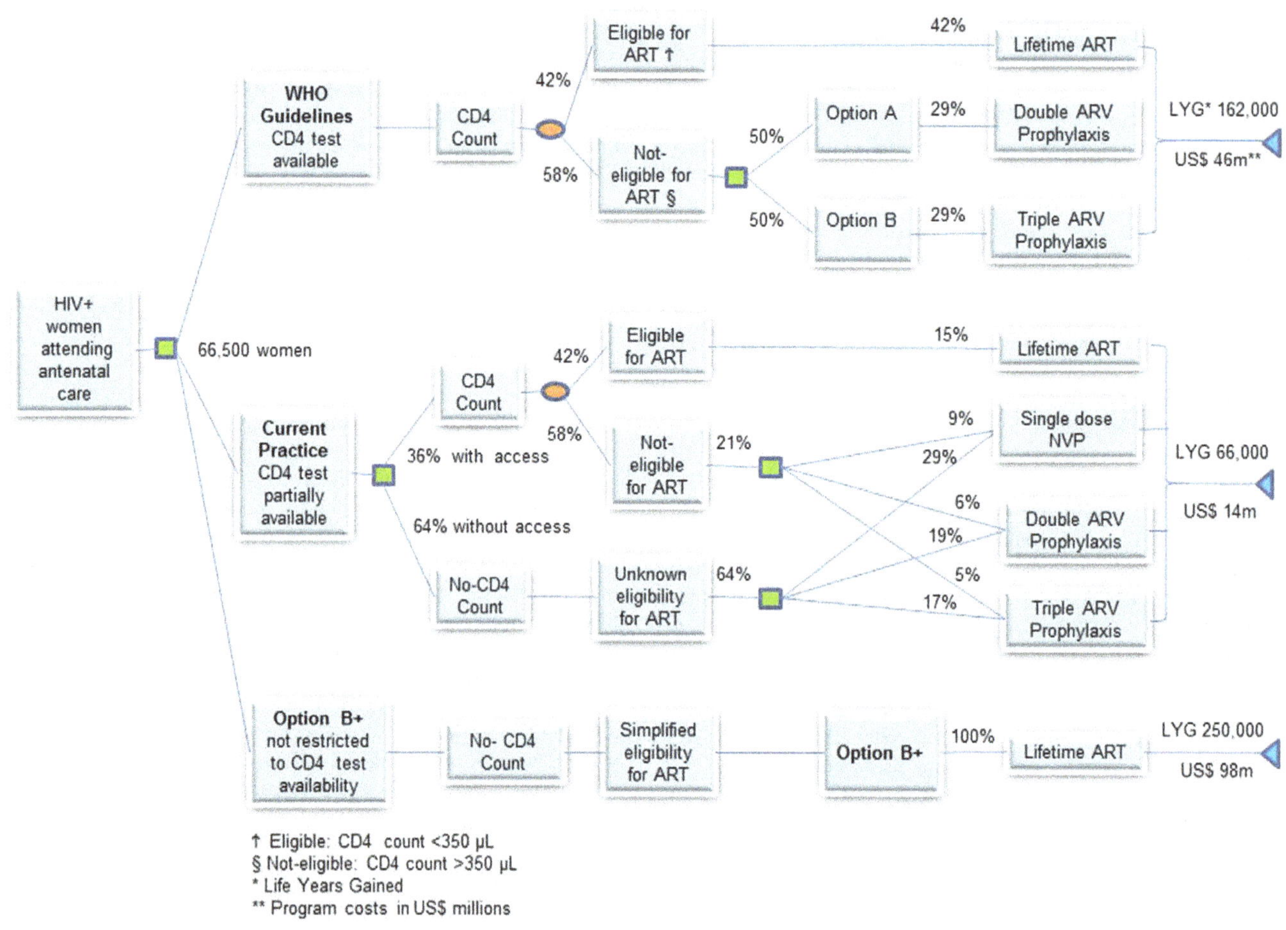

Figure 1. Abbreviated decision tree summarizing the analytical approach, policy options and results.

[7] with an HIV testing and counselling coverage of 66% in pregnant women [8]. Using data derived from a direct report from the Ministry of Health (MOH) in Malawi, of the 45% of HIV-infected pregnant women who received antiretrovirals for PMTCT in 2010, 38% received single-dose nevirapine (NVP), 25% received a dual-drug regimen containing zidovudine (AZT), 22% received triple-drug ARV prophylaxis and 15% received full ART [16]. These coverage rates were modelled as the current practice in 2010, prior to the start of the B+ programme. The options analysed and their components are shown in Table 1. In Option A, pregnant women not eligible for ART based on the disease stage were modelled to receive zidovudine from 14 weeks, a single dose of nevirapine at the onset of labour and a dual-drug regimen of zidovudine and lamivudine (AZT+3TC) for one week after delivery. In Option B, pregnant women not eligible for ART were modelled to receive triple-antiretroviral prophylaxis of tenofovir, lamivudine and efavirenz (TDF+3TC+EFV: this is the regimen adopted by Malawi) from 14 weeks until one week after all breastfeeding has stopped. In Option B+, treatment decisions are not based on CD4 count and therefore all HIV-infected pregnant women who receive HIV testing and are positive based on the prevalence rate assumptions, were modelled to initiate and continue lifelong ART. Infants receive prophylaxis with nevirapine until one week after all breastfeeding has stopped in Option A, while they receive nevirapine for six weeks after birth with current practice, Options B and B+.

For all strategies, it was assumed that 42% of HIV-infected pregnant women have CD4 counts at or less than 350 cells/ µL and are eligible for ART, based on findings of a population-based study in Malawi [13]. Therefore women eligible for ART under WHO Options A and B receive ART initially in the model and women who later become eligible after delivery and breastfeeding will start to receive ART according to their disease progression and at the coverage of ART in the general population [9]. For this analysis, full ANC coverage was assumed, and all pregnant women were assumed to receive HIV testing and counselling while ARV coverage rates for prophylaxis and treatment were assumed to be 90% for the three options while the 2010 coverage levels reported by the MOH were modelled for the current practice.

Input parameters

All the input parameters are presented in Table 2. For perinatal transmission rates, we used the recently revised mother-to-child transmission rates by the UNAIDS epidemiology reference group for use in Spectrum [17] along with published findings from the multicentre Kesho Bora study with rates of 2.7% for Option A and 1.7% for Options B and B+ for the postnatal transmission in all options [18]. Breastfeeding can contribute as much as 42% to the overall mother-to-child transmission [19]. The 2010 Demographic Health Survey for Malawi reports a mean breastfeeding duration of 23 months among all mothers [20] and study findings from Malawi report a median breastfeeding duration of 11.5 months among HIV-infected women. [21]. In this analysis, we assumed

Table 1. ARV regimens for HIV prevention and treatment of mothers and children compared in the analysis - Current Practice 2010, WHO Option A, WHO Option B and Malawi's Option B+.

ARV regimens for mothers who do not need treatment for their own health			**All HIV-infected mothers**
Current Practice 2010	**Option A**	**Option B**	**Option B+**
Mother	**Mother**	**Mother**	**Mother**
Depending on availability and setting, single-dose nevirapine (NVP), or dual-drug regimen containing zidovudine (AZT), or triple-drug ARV prophylaxis until cessation of breastfeeding	Antepartum twice-daily AZT starting from as early as 14 weeks of gestation and continued during pregnancy. At onset of labour, sd-NVP and initiation of twice daily AZT+3TC for 7 days postpartum (Note: If maternal AZT was provided for more than 4 weeks antenatally, omission of the sd-NVP and AZT+3TC tail can be considered; in this case, continue maternal AZT during labour and stop at delivery).	Triple ARV prophylaxis starting from as early as 14 weeks of gestation and continued until delivery, or, if breastfeeding, continued until 1 week after all infant exposure to breast milk has ended. Regimen: TDF+3TC+EFV	Antiretroviral therapy starting from as early as 14 weeks of gestation and continued for life. Preferred regimen: TDF+3TC+EFV
Infant	**Infant**	**Infant**	**Infant**
Irrespective of mode of infant feeding: Daily NVP or twice daily AZT from birth until 4 to 6 weeks of age.	For breastfeeding infants: Daily NVP from birth for a minimum of 4 to 6 weeks, and until 1 week after all exposure to breast milk has ended. **Infants receiving replacement feeding only:** Daily NVP or sd-NVP+twice−daily AZT from birth until 4 to 6 weeks of age.	**Irrespective of mode of infant feeding:** Daily NVP or twice daily AZT from birth until 4 to 6 weeks of age.	**Irrespective of mode of infant feeding:** Daily NVP or twice daily AZT from birth until 4 to 6 weeks of age.

that HIV-infected mothers would breastfeed for an average of 12 months. The monthly risk of postnatal HIV transmission through breastfeeding, in the absence of any intervention was assumed to be 1.04% which is the average of the rates reported for transmission in eligible and non-eligible women by the UNAIDS epidemiology reference group [18].

Survival estimates from the model were calibrated with results from the ART-LINC, which reported data from 36,615 patients on ART from 17 cohorts in Africa, Asia and South America [22]. Transition probabilities between adjacent states for untreated women were assumed to be similar to reported findings in other populations and were estimated from the published natural history studies [23–28] and calculated as the reciprocals of the mean waiting times in each CD4 cell state [29]. For women receiving ART, the transition probabilities from one state to the next lower one were calculated by applying the reported relative risk of disease progression with treatment compared to no treatment of 0.27 [30]. Weighted averages from studies reporting ART survival in low-income settings were used to determine the mortality rate in each state [31]. Women receiving ART could also progress from lower to higher states based on study findings on CD4 cell recovery for people on treatment [32], but these women are assumed to remain on treatment. The model incorporates possible treatment failures, which can result from poor adherence and loss to follow up (LTFU) during treatment. For the purpose of this analysis, an adherence rate of 90% was used, as reported adherence rates in resource-limited settings are comparable to those in developed countries [33–34].

Cost Estimates

The cost per patient-year in each Markov state was calculated by multiplying health care utilization by the cost per person per year, based on recent cost estimates in Malawi. All costs are shown in US dollars. The cost of rapid HIV testing was $3.50 per test and all pregnant women are assumed to undergo at least one HIV test during the first antenatal visit for Options A, B and B+ while the coverage rates for ANC and HIV testing and counselling were applied for the current practice. HIV-infected pregnant women undergo CD4 cell count testing with the Current Practice, Options A and B to determine eligibility for ART at a cost of US$ 20 per test. Costs of ARVs for Options A and B included 6 months during pregnancy and 12 months during breastfeeding. The cost of drugs per woman receiving Option A for 6 months of prophylaxis is US$ 76.20, consisting of $60 for AZT and AZT+3TC, $0.20 for NVP and $16 for infant Nevirapine for 12 months of breastfeeding. The annual cost of drugs per woman receiving Option B or Option B+ is US$ 193.60 per woman. Based on the percentage distribution of regimens under the current practice as previously described, the same costs of the various regimens were applied to the current practice. Total costs of ARV prophylaxis and ART for all options are calculated for the entire period of 10 years.

Other itemized costs for all the options and the current practice include early infant diagnosis testing, and cotrimoxazole prophylaxis for HIV-exposed infants. Ninety percent of all infants born to an HIV-infected mother are assumed to be tested with DNA PCR at a cost of US$ 32.50 [35]. Cotrimoxazole prophylaxis was assumed to be given to all HIV-exposed infants for a period of 12 months at a cost of US$5 per person per year to account for the time it takes to receive early-infant diagnosis (EID) results and place HIV-infected infants on treatment [36–37].

Costs are shown in Table 3. Cost estimates and prices were obtained directly from the Ministry of Health of Malawi, and supplemented with additional cost data from the World Health Organization Global Price Reporting Mechanism [38]. All costs are expressed in US dollars at a 2010 price base. Costs and benefits were discounted at 3% annually. The three options were compared to the current practice using incremental cost-effectiveness ratios, of US dollars per life-year gained and per disability-adjusted life-year averted.

Sensitivity analysis was performed to assess the robustness of the results to changes in the assumptions made. The efficacies of ARV prophylaxis and ART on reducing peripartum and postnatal

Table 2. Input parameters and plausible ranges used for sensitivity analysis and relevant references for the Malawi analysis (US $ 2010).

Parameters	Base-case	References
HIV Epidemiology		
1. Number of HIV-infected pregnant women	66,500 (57,000–76,000)	[2]
2. Percentage of pregnant women with CD4 count >350 cells/ μL (%)	58	[13]
3. Percentage of pregnant women with CD4 count 349–200 cells/ μL (%)	22	Same as above
4. Percentage of pregnant women with CD4 count <200 cells/ μL (%)	20	Same as above
MTCT transmission rates		
5. Background transmission rate without intervention (peripartum)%	22	[17]
6. Monthly post-natal transmission, no prophylaxis, breastfeeding (12 months)%	1.04	[17]
7. Peripartum transmission, Option A %	2.7	[17]
8. Monthly post-natal transmission with infant prophylaxis, breastfeeding (as per Option A)%	0.2	[17]
9. Peripartum transmission, Option B, Option B+ and eligible women on ART %	1.7	[17]
10. Monthly postnatal transmission with ART, breastfeeding (Options B and B+ and women on ART)%	0.2	[17]
Costs		
11. HIV Testing and counselling	$3.50	MOH Malawi
12. CD4 Screening	$20.00	MOH Malawi
13. Follow-up visit/clinical monitoring (per visit)	$2.00	MOH Malawi
14. Single-dose NVP	$0.20	MOH Malawi
15. AZT (6 months) and AZT+3TC (7 days)	$60	MOH Malawi
16. TDF+3TC+EFV (per year)	$193.6	MOH Malawi
17. Infant NVP including syringes (per year)	$16.00	MOH Malawi
18. Early infant diagnosis	$32.50	[35]
19. Cotrimoxazole prophylaxis (per year)	$5.00	[36,37]
21. Discounted lifetime cost for an HIV infected child on ART	$ 3195	[39,40]

transmission rates were varied using ranges reported in the literature to take into account clinical practice situations where adherence may be lower than reported in clinical trials.

Results

Using the current PMTCT practice and coverage in Malawi in 2010 as our base case, a cohort of HIV-infected pregnant women would result in an estimated 16,217 infant infections (24.4% transmission rate) after one year and an estimated 28% survival among HIV-infected mothers after ten years. Our counterfactual analysis showed that without any PMTCT interventions, an estimated 20,681 infections (31.1% transmission rate) would occur after 12 months of breastfeeding. In addition, if no antiretroviral treatment is provided to HIV-infected mothers, the natural HIV progression results in a 3% survival rate after 10 years or an estimated 1,920 women surviving from the initial cohort of HIV-infected women.

Cost-effectiveness analyses: preventing new paediatric infections

Table 3 shows the costs, outcomes and cost-effectiveness of different strategies modelled to prevent new child infections in the HIV-infected pregnant women. Our base case represents the current PMTCT practice and coverage in Malawi in 2010; at reported coverage levels, this resulted in 4,503 infections averted among infants, with a generalized cost effectiveness ratio of US$ 816 per infection averted.

If fully implemented, Option A averts 391 infections fewer than Options B and B+ and has a generalised cost-effectiveness ratio of $ 844 per infection averted; Option B, a generalised cost-effectiveness ratio of $1,331 per infection averted and Option B+ a generalised cost-effectiveness ratio of US$ 1,265 (from savings attributable to not carrying out CD4 testing). Generalized cost-effectiveness analysis for the three approaches resulted in costs per DALY of US$ 37 for Option A, US$ 60 for Option B and US$ 57 for Option B+.

The incremental cost effectiveness per DALY when compared to the current practice as the base case resulted in ratios of US$ 38 for Option A, US$ 68 for Option B and US$ 64 for Option B+. With comparable coverage and implementation, Option A emerges as the most cost-effective option to prevent new child infections among HIV-infected pregnant women following delivery and 12 months of breastfeeding.

Cost-effectiveness analysis: maternal health outcomes (10-year analysis of cohort of HIV-pregnant women)

Table 4 presents the assessment of the different options in terms of costs and maternal outcomes for the original annual cohort of HIV-infected pregnant women followed over a ten-year horizon. The total discounted cost of the current practice (limited coverage) amounts to US$ $14.3 million, which is a fraction of the most costly Option B+, at US$ 97.7 million. The current practice in 2010 results in a survival rate of 27.5%, with 18,267 of 66,500 HIV-infected mothers remaining alive after ten years and 66,289 life-years saved. Options A and B result in 152,966 and 171,543

Table 3. Costs and paediatric outcomes from preventing mother to child transmission programmatic interventions for 18 months of prophylaxis and treatment* (US $ 2010).

	Current Practice	Option A	Option B	Option B+
Programmatic Activity				
HIV testing and counseling	$ 139,789.7	$ 232,750	$ 232,750	$ 232,750
CD4 Testing	$ 455,314.9	$ 1,197,000	$ 1,197,000	$ 0**
Cost of ARVs for prophylaxis and treatment (including monitoring)	$ 2,984,,445.2	$ 8,860,309.6	$ 17,725,341.8	$ 17,725,341.8
Infant prophylaxis	$ 39,523.4	$ 844,603.2	$ 97,454.2	$ 97,454.2
Early infant diagnosis	$ 0.0	$ 1,906,222.5	$ 1,906,222.5	$ 1,906,222.5
Cotrimoxazole prophylaxis	$ 53,521.2	$ 131,969.3	$ 131,969.3	$ 131,969.3
Total PMTCT programme cost (18 months)	$ 3,672,594.3	$ 13,172,854.6	$ 21,290,737.8	$ 20,093,737.5
Pediatric outcomes				
Number of infants infected***	16,179	5,075	4,684	4,684
Number of infections averted	4,503	15,606	15,997	15,997
Lifetime costs of averted ART and hospital care among children	$ 14,385,762	$ 49,861,725	$ 51,110,042	$ 51,110,042
DALYS averted	101,308	351,139	359,930	359,930
Cost-effectiveness ratios				
Cost per infection averted	$ 816	$ 844	$ 1,331	$ 1,265
Cost per DALY averted	$ 37	$ 37	$ 60	$ 57
ICER per DALY (compared to the current practice)		$ 38	$ 68	$ 64

*Assumes 663,000 pregnant women, 66,500 HIV-infected pregnant women annually, and 90% (59,850) of those women reached by Option A, B and B+.
**Assumes no needed CD4 to start ART under the Malawi Option B+ approach; however, in practice some HIV-infected pregnant women will have access to CD4 testing as part of staging and response to treatment
***Background infections if no ARV interventions = 20,681

life-years saved respectively. However, Option B+ improves the survival and results in 249,576 life-years saved. The ICER per life-year gained, when each option is compared to the current practice, is US$ 314 for Option A, US$ 338 for Option B and US$ 455 for Option B+.

We evaluated a range of possible scenarios with increasing levels of service coverage for ARV prophylaxis and ART with the different Options and estimated the incremental cost-effectiveness among next best alternative strategies for Malawi. Figure 2 presents the relationship between level of investment and the effectiveness of the intervention expressed in Life Years Gained (LFG). The upward-sloped line represents the boundary and it is called the 'efficient frontier'. The efficient frontier offers the highest expected return for a given level of investment. The ICERs shown represent the incremental ratios from one alternative to the next best alternative outlined at the frontier line. Current practice represents our base case scenario or the status quo in 2010 and results in the lowest health gains. In terms of outcomes; Option A reaches the efficiency frontier by requiring fewer resources than option B and producing almost comparable outcomes. Full

Table 4. Costs, maternal health outcomes and cost-effectiveness ratios of options A and B and Malawi's Option B+ for the ten-year horizon (US $ 2010).

	Current Practice	Option A	Option B	Option B+
Costs				
PMTCT costs (first 18 months)	$ 3,672,594	$ 13,172,855	$ 21,290,738	$ 20,093,738
Cost of ART for eligible women (subsequent years)	$ 10,162,136	$ 26,639,260	$ 26,837,855	$ 73,852,060
Cost of follow up and monitoring	$ 448,525	$ 1,692,548	$ 1,692,548	$ 3,784,190
Total programme costs (10 years)	$ 14,283,255	$ 41,504,663	$ 49,821,141	$ 97,729,988
Outcomes				
Number of HIV infected women on ART and alive after ten years	18,267	28,567	30,057	42,137
Life years gained in HIV infected mothers after ten years	66,289	152,966	171,543	249,576
Cost-Effectiveness Ratios				
ICER per life year gained (compared to the current practice)	-	$ 314	$ 338	$ 455

Table 5. Results from sensitivity analyses on input parameters affecting outcomes in HIV-infected mothers; US$ per life year gained (compared to the current practice) and paediatric outcomes; US$ per DALY averted.

Model parameters	Option A	Option B	Option B+
Base case (US$/LYG in HIV-infected mothers)	314.1	337.6	455.3
ARV coverage among HIV-infected pregnant women			
Best case 100%	312.8	333.6	446.7
Worst case 30%	341.2	443.7	751.5
Coverage of CD4 testing			
Best case 90%	314.1	337.6	455.3
Break-even point–73%	320.1	320.4	455.3
Worst case 30%	328.1	305.0	455.3
Cost of Triple-drug regimen (ART)			
Best case $96.8	194.8	188.1	241.1
Break-even point - $ 105.6	217.8	217.0	282.5
Worst case $290	433.3	487.2	669.4
ART coverage in the general population			
Best case 90%	310.9	357.9	519.4
Worst case 49%	314.4	335.6	449.3
Base case (US$/DALY averted- infants)	37.2	69.0	64.3
Background transmission rate used (22%)			
Best case–15%	47.1	83.7	78.0
Worst case-40%	25.4	46.1	43.0
Peripartum transmission rate with Option A (2.7%)			
Best case–1.3%	36.2	68.1	63.5
Worst case–5.2%	41.7	68.1	63.5
Perinatal transmission rate with ART (1.7%)			
Best case–0.7%	37.7	65.3	60.9
Worst case–4.0%	38.9	75.7	70.5
Cost of ART (US$ 193.60)			
Best case-$96.8	30.6	40.5	69.0
Worst case-$ 290.4	45.5	95.8	57.9
Break-even point-$387	52.9	123.4	52.4

implementation of Option A coupled with the provision of ART to all eligible women results in rapid health gains, with 250 thousand life years over an investment of US$ 50 million. Doubling the investments to US$ 100 million, by providing full Option B+, results in an increase of 120 thousand life years gained.

Sensitivity analysis

Sensitivity analysis was performed to assess the robustness of the results. For infant outcomes, Option A remained the most cost-effective option with changes in the efficacy of antiretroviral drugs, changes in transmission rates and costs of antiretroviral drugs. The cost of ARVs was varied by 50% below and above the reported price. One-way sensitivity analyses were performed on key model parameters with the model being robust to most of the changes.

A break-even point between Option B+ and Option A occurs when the annual cost of antiretroviral treatment and care is reduced and reaches $387, with Option B+ becoming the more cost-effective option to prevent new infant infections and producing an ICER of $52.4 per DALY averted in infants. However, when considering outcomes for HIV- infected mothers, the model is sensitive to changes in the coverage of CD4 testing, ARV coverage among HIV-infected pregnant women, ART coverage in the general population and the cost of ART. Results are shown in Table 5. As the coverage of ART in the general population increases, the cost-effectiveness ratio of Option B+ increases while Options A and B become more cost-effective. Option B becomes the most cost-effective strategy when the coverage of CD4 testing is lower than 73% and if the cost of ART is reduced by 40%; with resultant ICERs of $320, and $217 per life year gained respectively. Figure 3 highlights results for the variables found to have the most effect on the ICER of Option B+ considering life years gained in HIV-infected mothers.

Discussion

We assessed the cost-effectiveness of the 2010 WHO mother-to-child transmission prevention strategies: Options A and B, and Malawi's Option B+. Analyzing both infant infection outcomes and long-term maternal health outcomes allows us to make a distinction between strategies to prevent mother-to-child transmission whose impact improves only child outcomes and those to treat mothers whose impacts improve both survival in HIV-

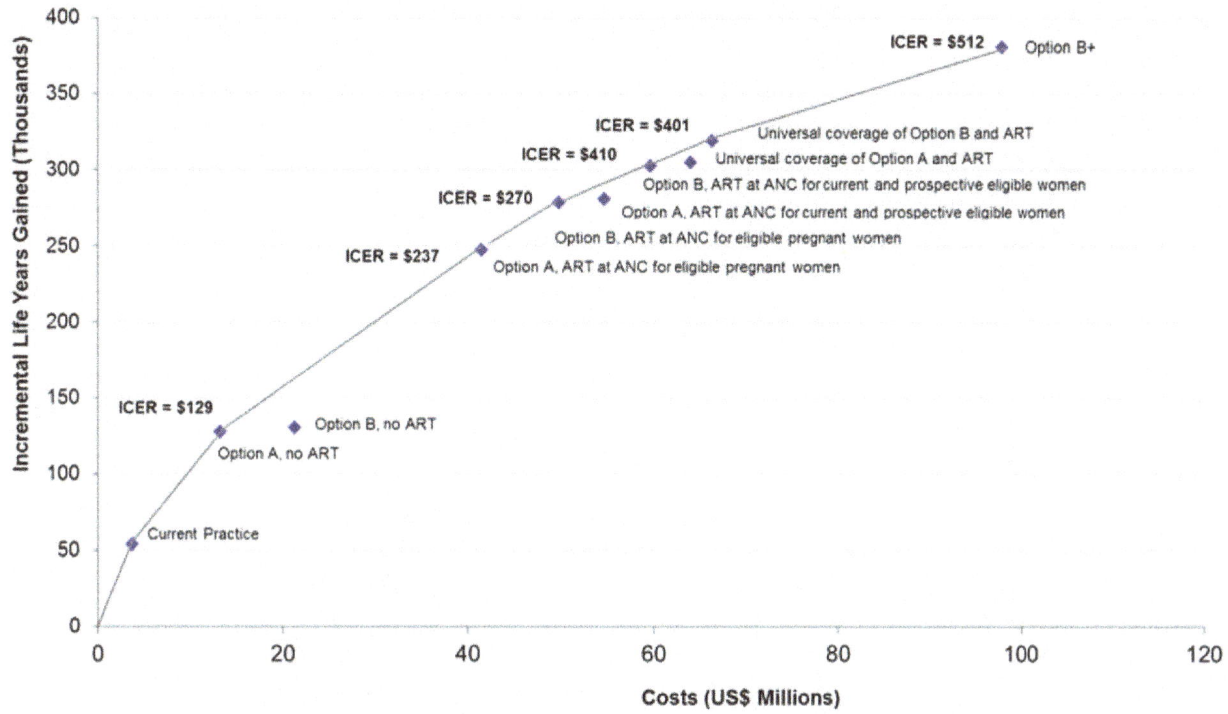

Figure 2. Cost effectiveness of various strategies for the prevention of new pediatric infections and the treatment of HIV-infected mothers in Malawi. Current practice represents our base case scenario or the status quo in 2010. The next set of scenarios highlight the cost effectiveness of incrementally expanding program implementation and service delivery coverage, and ranges from PMTCT only to the addition of integrated ART-ANC services for eligible pregnant women, both identified immediately and at a later time. Universal coverage implies the availability of HIV services for mother and children at any point of needing treatment. Option B+ offers ART to pregnant women regardless of CD4 count.

infected mothers and children. Option A is the most cost-effective alternative in our modelling where we have assumed an ideal scenario with universal CD4 screening available and very high rates of ARV coverage for prophylaxis and provision of ART to eligible women. However, in real-world situations such as Malawi, with low access to CD4 testing, and low levels of ART in treatment-eligible women with Option A, the cost-effectiveness favours Option B and B+. Using the WHO commission on Macroeconomics and health criterion for determining the cost-effectiveness of an intervention [41], we found that Option B+ represents a cost-effective strategy not only for preventing new HIV infections among infants, but also for improving the survival of HIV-infected mothers. In a recent programmatic update, WHO has encouraged countries to consider Option B+ [42].

The lower cost-effectiveness ratios (US $38–68 per DALY averted) derived in our analysis when compared to previous studies can be attributed to the current availability of less expensive and more effective regimens for PMTCT as well as improved coverage of services for HIV-infected mothers modelled here. Sweat and colleagues reported higher cost-effectiveness ratios with SD NVP up to US$ 310 per DALY averted, across eight countries in Sub-Saharan Africa [43]. Another study from Tanzania reported an incremental cost-effectiveness ratio of US$162 per DALY averted [44] for HAART compared to single-dose Nevirapine. A more

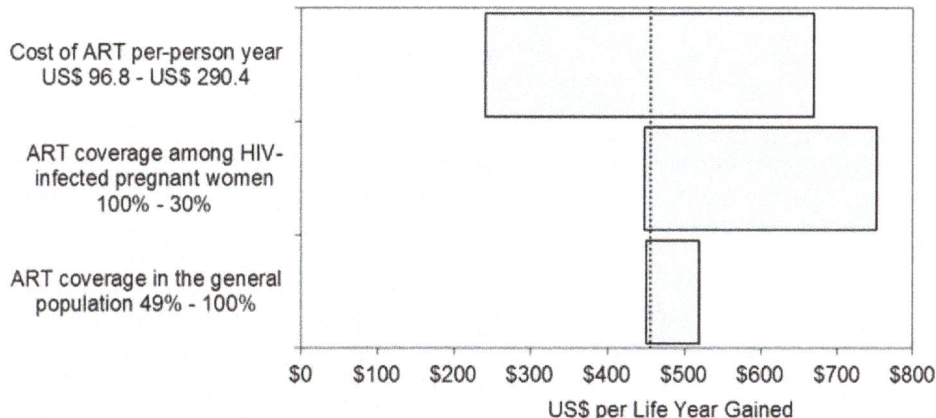

Figure 3. Tornado diagram for the ICER of Option B+, base case is $455 per life year gained shown with the dotted line.

recent study compares WHO option B with short course prophylaxis in Nigeria and reported an ICER of $111 per DALY averted if there was full PMTCT coverage among pregnant women [45].

From an economic perspective, each of the three options analyzed here results in enormous cost savings by averting new paediatric infections; thereby yielding significant returns on investment. For every dollar invested in the PMTCT programmes, between 2.5 and 4 dollars would be obtained in return from averted lifetime pediatric care, equivalent to saving nearly US$ 51 million from each annual birth cohort.

We believe that our study is the first economic evaluation to also assess maternal health outcomes when using ART regimens as part of prevention strategies for mother to child transmission. Integrating HIV services in the context of 'eliminating new infections among children and keeping their mothers alive' in Malawi, as the new Global Plan on MTCT elimination recommends [11], results in favourable outcomes for both mothers and infants while still yielding cost effective results. Under ideal settings where most women in need of ART for their own health and HIV-infected pregnant women who need ARV prophylaxis for PMTCT receive adequate drugs and clinical monitoring, the three options, A, B and B+ included in our analysis, when compared directly with the base case will result in incremental cost-effectiveness ratios that are less than three times the 2010 GDP per capita in Malawi of US$ 310 [41] and can be considered feasible policy options. After ten years of treatment, although Option B+ has significantly higher costs, the wider and earlier use of ART results in greater direct benefits, keeping the most women alive for the longest time, and yielding an incremental cost-effectiveness ratio of US $ 455 per life year gained over the current practice. In the Malawi context, where access to CD4 count and therefore targeted initiation of HIV-infected pregnant women on ART based upon CD4 results is unlikely to be successful given current limitations in CD4 test access, this approach represents a cost-effective policy option to prevent a child from being infected, improve HIV-free survival of infants, save mother's lives and reduce orphanhood.

Increasing access to treatment among pregnant women has several advantages. From a therapeutic point of view, it would reduce morbidity and mortality among HIV infected women. Treatment guidelines in North America and Europe recommend treatment initiation with higher CD4 counts [46] than those recommended for resource-limited settings. Recent results from the HPTN 052 study show that ART is 96% effective in preventing transmission to an uninfected sexual partner in discordant couples where the index case has CD4 counts between 350 and 550 cells/ µL [47] and ART during pregnancy and after may serve as a preventive strategy among discordant couples and to prevent sexual transmission more generally. Future modelling studies are needed to address the potential benefit of Option B+ as a strategy of early start of ART for prevention of new infections in the general population. Early ART is also known to reduce the risk of developing tuberculosis, the leading cause of mortality in HIV infected individuals, which increases with declining CD4 counts below 500cells/ µL [48]. Finally, evidence shows that women on ART before pregnancy can have lower mother-to-child transmission rates compared to those initiating ARV prophylaxis during pregnancy, as low as 0.5% during pregnancy [49] as some transmission can occur before the timing of prophylaxis protocols, and as women may often enter into antenatal care, and hence PMTCT late in pregnancy. Therefore, for countries like Malawi, which has a high fertility rate of 5.5 children per woman, the long-term effect of continuous ART would result in many more infections averted during subsequent pregnancies and improve the cost-effectiveness of Option B+.

As in any other modelling exercise, there are a number of limitations in relation to our assumptions. The successful implementation of these programmes rests on the capacity of overcoming many obstacles to increase access, especially in rural Malawi and at primary care level. The assumption about scaling programmes from their current levels to high aspiration targets should be taken with reservation. The costs and challenge of achieving such high coverage may be underestimated as the success of these programmes will require intensified community participation, human resources and the infrastructure necessary for service delivery. We made every effort to make explicit all the assumptions in our model, which we hope will be timely and critical to inform policy options. One simplifying assumption we made was that women would continue to receive the first-line ART regimen; this does not account for the realities that women face in terms of stigma, adherence and treatment failures requiring the switching of women to more expensive second- or third-line regimens. Finally, in the analysis, we have focused on the cost and cost-effectiveness of preventing new paediatric infections and on the health of the mother - we have not modelled the additional benefit and cost-benefit likely to result from the prevention of new adult infections in serodiscordant couples and partners. While we believe that our findings are robust and generalizable for many high burden countries, our results may not be applicable in some settings, particularly those with low prevalence, replacement feeding rather than breastfeeding for HIV-exposed infants and low fertility.

In conclusion, we present an economic analysis for the Malawi approach that places PMTCT within a continuum of care that integrates a comprehensive range of interventions, to make an impact on maternal, newborn and child health outcomes [10,50]. Our analysis suggests that Option B+ is a cost-effective strategy to integrate HIV prevention and treatment efforts towards achieving Millennium Development Goals 4, 5 & 6 [51] and ensuring universal access to ART. Careful monitoring of the Malawi approach is needed to assess the programmatic implications and will be critical for contributing to the evidence base for future global guidelines revisions. However, from an economic point of view, while this strategy will certainly require additional short-term financial resources, it has the potential to save significant societal resources in the long term.

Author Contributions

Conceived and designed the experiments: CA OF PDL. Performed the experiments: OF CA. Analyzed the data: OF CA NS. Contributed reagents/materials/analysis tools: OF CA ON. Wrote the paper: OF CA NS ES FC DH ON PDL.

References

1. UNAIDS (2011) Outlook Report: 30 years into the AIDS epidemic. Available: http://www.unaids.org/en/media/unaids/contentassets/documents/unaidspublication/2011/20110607_jc2069_30outlook_en.pdf.Accessed 2013 Feb 2.
2. WHO UNAIDS, UNICEF (2011) Global HIV/AIDS Response. Epidemic update and health sector progress towards Universal Access. Available: www.who.int/hiv/pub/progress_report2011/en/index.html.Accessed 2011 Nov 30.
3. Kuhn L, Kasonde P, Sinkala M, Kankasa C, Semrau K, et al. (2005) Does Severity of HIV Disease in HIV-Infected Mothers Affect Mortality and Morbidity among Their Uninfected Infants? Clin Infect Dis 41:1654–1661.

4. Townsend CL, Cortina-Borja M, Peckham CS, de Ruiter A, Lyall H, at al. (2008) Low rates of mother-to-child transmission of HIV following effective pregnancy interventions in the United Kingdom and Ireland, 2000–2006. AIDS 22:973–981.
5. McKenna MT, Hu XH (2007) Recent trends in the incidence and morbidity that are associated with perinatal human immunodeficiency virus infection in the United States. Am J Obstet Gynecol 197:S10–S16.
6. WHO UNICEF, UNFPA and World Bank (2010) Trends in Maternal Mortality:1990–2008; Estimates developed by the WHO, UNICEF,UNFPA and World Bank. Available: http://whqlibdoc.who.int/publications/2010/9789241500265_eng.pdf.Accessed 2011 Jun 21.
7. WHO (2011). World health Statictics 2011. Available: http://www.who.int/whosis/whostat/EN_WHS2011_Full.pdf.Accessed 2011 Aug 25.
8. Ministry of Health Malawi (2010) Making it Happen: Revising national policies to reflect changes in WHO recommendations for preventing vertical transmission of HIV. XVIII International AIDS Conference. Vienna.
9. WHO (2010) Antiretroviral drugs for treating pregnant women and preventing HIV infection in infants: recommendations for a public health approach 2010. Available: www.who.int/hiv/pub/mtct/antiretroviral/en/index.html.Accessed 2013 Feb 2.
10. Schouten EJ, Jahn A, Midiani D, Makombe SD, Mnthambala A, et al. (2011) Prevention of mother-to-child transmission of HIV and the health-related Millennium Development Goals: time for a public health approach. Lancet 378:282–284.
11. UNAIDS (2011) Global plan towards the elimination of new HIV infections among children by 2015 and keeping their mothers alive. Available: http://www.unaids.org/en/media/unaids/contentassets/documents/unaidspublication/2011/20110609_JC2137_Global-Plan-Elimination-HIV-Children_en.pdf.Accessed 2011 Jul 12.
12. Athan E, O'Brien DP, Legood R (2010) Cost-effectiveness of routine and low-cost CD4 T-cell count compared with WHO clinical staging of HIV to guide initiation of antiretroviral therapy in resource-limited settings. AIDS 24:1887–1895.
13. McGrath N, Kranzer K, Saul J, Crampin A, Malema S, et al (2007) Estimating the need for antiretroviral treatment and an assessment of a simplified HIV/AIDS case definition in rural Malawi. AIDS 21:S105–113.
14. Hirnschall G, Schwartlander B (2011) Treatment 2.0: catalysing the next phase of scale-up. Lancet 378:209–211.
15. Fox Rushby JA, Hanson K (2011) Calculating and presenting disability adjusted life years (DALYs) in cost-effectiveness analysis. Health Policy Plan 16: 326–331.
16. Ministry of Health of Malawi (2010). Quarterly HIV Programme Report. April–June 2010.
17. UNAIDS (2011) Expert group on vertical transmission rates: MTCT transmission rates for use in Spectrum. Working Paper on Mother-to-Child HIV Transmission Rates for use in Spectrum Available: http://www.epidem.org/Publications/MTCTratesworkingpaper.pdf.Accessed 2011 Jul 25.
18. The Kesho Bora Study Group (2011) Triple antiretroviral compared with zidovudine and single-dose nevirapine prophylaxis during pregnancy and breastfeeding for prevention of mother-to-child transmission of HIV-1: a randomised controlled trial. Lancet Infect Dis 11:171–180.
19. The Breastfeeding and HIV International Transmission Study Group (2004) Late Postnatal Transmission of HIV-1 in Breast-Fed Children: An Individual Patient Data Meta-Analysis. J Infect Dis 189:2154–2166.
20. National Statistical Office, Zomba, Malawi and ICF Macro, Calverton, Maryland, USA (2011) Malawi Demographic and Health Survey 2010. Available: http://www.measuredhs.com/pubs/pdf/FR247/FR247.pdf.Accessed 2013 Feb 9.
21. Miotti PG, Taha TET, Kumwenda NI, Broadhead R, Mtimavalye LAR, et al. (1999) HIV Transmission Through Breastfeeding. JAMA 282:744–749.
22. The eART-linc collaboration (2008) Duration from seroconversion to eligibility for antiretroviral therapy and from ART eligibility to death in adult HIV-infected patients from low and middle-income countries: collaborative analysis of prospective studies. Sex Transm Infect 84:i31–i36.
23. Currier JS, Spino C, Grimes J, Wofsy CB, Katzenstein DA, et al. (2000) Differences between women and men in adverse events and CD4+ responses to nucleoside analogue therapy for HIV infection. The AIDS Clinical Trials Group 175 Team. J Acquir Immune Defic Syndr 24:316–324.
24. Ekouevi D, Abrams EJ, Schlesinger M, Myer L, Phanuphak N, et al. (2012) Maternal CD4+ Cell Count Decline after Interruption of Antiretroviral Prophylaxis for the Prevention of Mother-to-Child Transmission of HIV. PLoS ONE 7:e43750. doi:10.1371/journal.pone.0043750
25. Longini IM Jr, Clark WS, Gardner LI, Brundage JF (1991) The dynamics of CD4+T-lymphocyte decline in HIV-infected individuals: a Markov modeling approach. J Acquir Immune Defic Syndr 4:1141–1147.
26. Mauskopf J (2000) Meeting the NICE requirements: a Markov model approach. Value Health 3:287–293.
27. Mauskopf J, Kitahata M, Kauf T, Richter A, Tolson J (2005) HIV antiretroviral treatment: early versus later. J Acquir Immune Defic Syndr 39:562–569.
28. Mauskopf J, Lacey L, Kempel A, Simpson K (1998) The cost-effectiveness of treatment with lamivudine and zidovudine compared with zidovudine alone: a comparison of Markov model and trial data estimates. Am J Manag Care 4:1004–1012.
29. Johansson K, Robberstad B, Norheim O (2010) Further benefits by early start of HIV treatment in low income countries: Survival estimates of early versus deferred antiretroviral therapy. AIDS Res Ther 7:3.
30. Mussini C, Cossarizza A, Sabin C, Babiker A, De Luca A, et al. (2011) Decline of CD4+T-cell count before start of therapy and immunological response to treatment in antiretroviral-naive individuals. AIDS 25:1041–1049
31. Lawn S, Little F, Bekker L, Kaplan R, Campbel E, et al. (2009) Changing mortality risk associated with CD4 cell response to antiretroviral therapy in South Africa. AIDS 23:335–342.
32. Hunt PW, Deeks SG, Rodriguez B, Valdez H, Shade SB, et al. (2003) Continued CD4 cell count increases in HIV-infected adults experiencing 4 years of viral suppression on antiretroviral therapy. AIDS 17:1907–1915.
33. Orrell C, Bangsberg DR, Badri M, Wood R (2003) Adherence is not a barrier to successful antiretroviral therapy in South Africa. AIDS 17:1369–1375.
34. Lanièce I, Ciss M, Desclaux A, Diop K, Mbodj F, et al. (2003) Adherence to HAART and its principal determinants in a cohort of Senegalese adults. AIDS 17:S103–S108.
35. Stevens W, Sherman G, Downing R, Parsons LM, Ou CY, et al. (2008) Role of the laboratory in ensuring global access to ARV treatment for HIV-infected children: consensus statement on the performance of laboratory assays for early infant diagnosis. Open AIDS J 2:17–25.
36. UNICEF (2010) Cotrimoxazole prophylaxis for HIV-exposed and HIV-infected infants and children; Practical approaches to implementation and scale up. 2010. Available: www.unicef.org/aids/files/CotrimoxazoleGuide_2009.pdf.Accessed 2013 Feb 2.
37. Ryan M, Griffin S, Chitah B, Walker AS, Mulenga V, et al. (2008) The cost-effectiveness of cotrimoxazole prophylaxis in HIV-infected children in Zambia. AIDS 22:749–757.
38. WHO (2010) Transaction prices for Antiretroviral Medicines and HIV Diagnostics from 2008 to March 2010. A summary report from the Global Price Reporting Mechanism. Available: www.who.int/hiv/amds/gprm/en.Accessed 2013 Feb 2.
39. Sansom SL, Anderson JE, Farnham PG, Dominguez K, Soorapanth S, et al. (2006) Updated Estimates of Healthcare Utilization and Costs Among Perinatally HIV-Infected Children. J Acquir Immune Defic Syndr 41:521–526
40. Orlando S, Marazzi MC, Mancinelli S, Liotta G, Ceffa S, et al. (2010) Cost-Effectiveness of Using HAART in Prevention of Mother-To-Child Transmission in the DREAM-Project Malawi. J Acquir Immune Defic Syndr 55:631–634
41. WHO (2001) Commission on Macroeconomics and Health. Investing in Health for Economic Development. Available: http://whqlibdoc.who.int/publications/2001/924154550x.pdf.Accessed 2013 Feb 2.
42. WHO (2012). Use of antiretroviral drugs for treating pregnant women and preventing HIV infection in infants. Programmatic update 2012. Available: http://whqlibdoc.who.int/hq/2012/WHO_HIV_2012.6_eng.pdf.Accessed 2013 Feb 2.
43. Sweat MD, O'Reilly KR, Schmid GP, Denison J, de Zoysa I (2004) Cost-effectiveness of nevirapine to prevent mother-to-child HIV transmission in eight African countries. AIDS 18:1661–1671.
44. Robberstad B, Evjen-Olsen B (2010) Preventing Mother to Child Transmission of HIV With Highly Active Antiretroviral Treatment in Tanzania-a Prospective Cost-Effectiveness Study. J Acquir Immune Defic Syndr 55:397–403.
45. Shah M, Johns B, Abimiku Al, Walker DG (2011) Cost-effectiveness of new WHO recommendations for prevention of mother-to-child transmission of HIV in a resource-limited setting. AIDS 25:1093–1102
46. Department of Health and Human Services (2011). Guidelines for the use of antiretroviral agents in HIV-1-infected adults and adolescents, 2011. Available: http://aidsinfo.nih.gov/contentfiles/lvguidelines/adultandadolescentgl.pdf.Accessed 2013 Feb 2.
47. Cohen MS, Chen YQ, McCauley M, Gamble T, Hosseinipour MC, et al., (2011) Prevention of HIV-1 Infection with Early Antiretroviral Therapy. N Engl J Med 365:493–505.
48. Harries AD, Zachariah R, Corbett EL, Lawn SD, Santos-Filho ET, et al., (2010) The HIV-associated tuberculosis epidemic: when will we act? Lancet 375:1906–1919.
49. Hoffman RM, Black V, Technau K, van der Merwe KJ, Currier J, et al. (2010) Effects of highly active antiretroviral therapy duration and regimen on risk for mother-to-child transmission of HIV in Johannesburg, South Africa. J Acquir Immune Defic Syndr 54:35–41.
50. Horton R (2009) What will it take to stop maternal deaths? Lancet 374:1400–1402.
51. UNDP. Millennium development goals: 4–5 and 6. Available: http://www.undp.org/content/undp/en/home/mdgoverview.html.Accessed 2013 Feb 2.

5

Phylogenetic and Phylodynamic Analyses of Human Metapneumovirus in Buenos Aires (Argentina) for a Three-Year Period (2009–2011)

Ana Julia Velez Rueda[1,2], Alicia Susana Mistchenko[1,2], Mariana Viegas[1,3]*

1 Laboratorio de Virología, Hospital de Niños "Dr. Ricardo Gutiérrez", Ciudad Autónoma de Buenos Aires, Argentina, 2 Comisión de Investigaciones Científicas (CIC), La Plata, Provincia de Buenos Aires, Argentina, 3 Consejo Nacional de Investigaciones Científicas y Técnicas (CONICET), Ciudad Autónoma de Buenos Aires, Argentina

Abstract

Human metapneumovirus, which belongs to the *Paramyxoviridae* family and has been classified as a member of the *Pneumovirus* genus, is genetically and clinically similar to other family members such as human respiratory syncytial virus. A total of 1146 nasopharyngeal aspirates from pediatric patients with moderate and severe acute lower respiratory tract infections, hospitalized at the Ricardo Gutierrez Childrens Hospital (Buenos Aires, Argentina), were tested by real time RT-PCR for human metapneumovirus. Results showed that 168 (14.65%) were positive. Thirty-six of these 168 samples were randomly selected to characterize positive cases molecularly. The phylogenetic analysis of the sequences of the G and F genes showed that genotypes A2 and B2 cocirculated during 2009 and 2010 and that only genotype A2 circulated in 2011 in Argentina. Genotype A2 prevailed during the study period, a fact supported by a higher effective population size (Neτ) and higher diversity as compared to that of genotype B2 (10.9% (SE 1.3%) vs. 1.7% (SE 0.4%), respectively). The phylogeographic analysis of the G protein gene sequences showed that this virus has no geographical restrictions and can travel globally harbored in hosts. The selection pressure analysis of the F protein showed that although this protein has regions with polymorphisms, it has vast structural and functional constraints. In addition, the predicted B-linear epitopes and the sites recognized by previously described monoclonal antibodies were conserved in all Argentine sequences. This points out this protein as a potential candidate to be the target of future humanized antibodies or vaccines.

Editor: Patricia V. Aguilar, University of Texas Medical Branch, United States of America

Funding: This work was supported by ANPCYT, Ministerio de Ciencia, Tecnología e Innovación Productiva de la Nación, Argentina (grant PICT1624/07). The funders had no role in study design, data collection and analysis, decision to publish, or preparation of the manuscript. No additional external funding was received for this study.

Competing Interests: The authors have declared that no competing interests exist.

* E-mail: viegasmariana@hotmail.com

Introduction

Human metapneumovirus (HMPV), which belongs to the *Paramyxoviridae* family and has been classified as a member of the *Pneumovirus* genus [1], is genetically and clinically similar to other family members such as human respiratory syncytial virus (HRSV) and human parainfluenza type 3 virus.

The HMPV genome is approximately 13.3 Kb in length and contains eight genes that are ordered 3′-N-P-M-F-M2-SH-G-L-5′ and encode nine different proteins. Three transmembrane glycoproteins protrude from its envelope: the attachment glycoprotein (G), the fusion protein (F) and the small hydrophobic protein (SH) [2]. The G and F proteins present great immunogenicity and can stimulate the production of neutralizing antibodies [3,4].

HMPV can be classified into two genetic groups (A and B) and each group can be further divided into two genotypes (A1 and A2, and B1 and B2, respectively) [5,6]. Although this grouping of genotypes is concordant regardless of which gene is studied (G or F), the G gene appears to allow the best discrimination (as observed for HRSV) [6]. The G protein is of particular interest because its variability at nucleotide and amino acid level is greater than of other proteins, both between and within groups and genotypes [1]. Recent publications have shown the possible cocirculation of groups and genotypes and the predominance of one of them within a geographic region [7].

HMPV infections are observed in all age groups, with a high incidence in pediatric patients, being children under 6 months of age the most affected ones. Serological studies have suggested that ~70% of children are infected with HMPV by the age of 5 years [1]. The nosocomial impact of HMPV is estimated to be as high as that for HRSV [8]. Children infected with HMPV typically present respiratory symptoms clinically indistinguishable from those elicited by HRSV, such as rhinorrhea, fever and cough as upper respiratory symptoms, and asthma exacerbations, bronchiolitis and pneumonia as the severe presentations of acute lower respiratory tract infections (ALRI) [9]. As with HRSV, infants at risk for severe respiratory infections with HMPV are those with congenital heart disease, chronic lung disease, immunocompromised infants and premature children [10,11].

Taking into account that there is yet no vaccine or prophylactic therapy to prevent HMPV infections, as there is for HRSV (Palivizumab), it is important to recognize the relevance of HMPV as an ALRI etiologic agent in children under one year of age and in high-risk patients.

In this study, we aimed to characterize the HMPV strains which produced moderate and severe ALRI in hospitalized children in Buenos Aires (Argentina) during a three-year period (2009–2011) by an exhaustive analysis of the G and F genes. In addition, based on the molecular analysis, we aimed to describe the global transmission chains of HMPV in order to deepen the general knowledge of the virus genetic background for the future development of potential treatments and/or vaccines.

Materials and Methods

Ethics Statement

Written informed consent was obtained from next of skin, caretakers, parents or guardians on the behalf of the minors/ children. The study was approved by the Medical Ethic and Research Committees of Dr. Ricardo Gutiérrez Children's Hospital (IRB N° 07-030). All samples were coded prior to analysis to ensure anonymity, according to the Declaration of Helsinki and the *Habeas Data* law on protection of personal data (Law N° 25326, Argentina).

Sample Collection

A total of 1146 nasopharyngeal aspirates (NPA) from pediatric patients with moderate and severe ALRI, hospitalized at the Ricardo Gutierrez Childrens Hospital of Buenos Aires (Argentina) during 2009–2011 were analyzed by real time RT-PCR for HMPV, as previously described [12].

According to the severity of the ALRI, patients were classified into two groups: moderate cases: patients with a diagnosis of bronchiolitis, pneumonitis or pneumonia, no requiring mechanical respiratory assistance; and severe cases: patients with diagnosis of bronchiolitis, pneumonitis and pneumonia or chronic lung disease (high risk patients), requiring intensive care and respiratory support.

The clinical samples with positive diagnosis for HMPV were kept frozen at $-70°C$ until molecular analysis.

RNA Extraction and Nucleotide Amplification of Partial G and F Genes of HMPV

Nucleic acids were extracted directly from clinical samples with a PureLink viral RNA/DNA minikit (Invitrogen Life Technologies, Carlsbad, CA, USA). RNA was reverse-transcribed and amplified using the Qiagen OneStep RT-PCR kit (Qiagen, GmbH, Hilden, Germany) following the manufacturer's instructions with the primers for both partial G and F genes, previously described [13].

The retrotranscription and amplification conditions for the G gene were: 50°C for 30 min; 95°C for 15 min; 94°C for 1 min, 59°C for 1 min, 72°C for 2 min for 34 cycles and 72°C for 7 min. For the F gene, the amplification protocol was the same but using an annealing temperature of 50°C and 39 cycles.

HMPV G and F Gene Sequences

PCR products were electrophoresed in a 1% agarose gel stained with ethidium bromide and purified with the Zymoclean^{TM} Gel DNA Recovery Kit (Applied Biosystems, Foster City, CA, USA). The purified PCR products were sequenced in forward and reverse directions by using the BigDye Terminator v3.1 cycle sequencing kit (Applied Biosystems, Foster City, CA, USA) on the ABI3500 genetic analyzer (Applied Biosystems).

The nucleotide sequences of the G protein gene and the F protein gene were manually edited with BioEdit v7.1.3 [14] and aligned with CLUSTAL W [15]. All these sequences were submitted to GenBank (accession numbers KC210054 to KC210091).

Phylogenetic Analyses

For the phylogenetic and evolutionary analyses, the G and F gene sequences of HMPV that largely represent the globally circulating strains were downloaded from GenBank (Table S1). Strains CAN83-97$_{A2}$ and CAN75-98$_{B2}$ from Canada (accession numbers AY485253 and AY297748/AY145289, respectively) and strains NL/1/99$_{B1}$, NL/17/00$_{A2}$ and NL/1/94$_{B2}$ from the Netherlands (accession numbers AY304361/AY2960347, AY296021, and AY304362/AY296040, respectively) were used as prototypes of each group and genotype. The most suitable nucleotide substitution model for the Bayesian Markov Chain Monte Carlo (MCMC), Maximum Likelihood (ML) and Neighbor joining (NJ) analyses was selected with MEGA v5.05 [16]. The Bayesian MCMC inference was performed with BEAST v1.7.4 (http: //beast.bio.ed.ac.uk) [17], whereas ML and NJ were performed with MEGA v5.05.

Evolutionary Rates, Population Dynamics and Phylogeographic Analyses

Nucleotide substitution rates, divergence times, demographic histories and a discrete phylogeographic analysis were estimated from the sequences stamped with date and location using the Bayesian approach with the BEAST v1.7.4 package. The results from BEAST were analyzed using Tracer v1.5 (http: //beast.-bio.ed.ac.uk/) to determine the time of the most recent common ancestor (tMRCA) and the nucleotide substitution rates and to plot the demographic histories (Bayesian Skyline Plots (BSP)). The BSP were used to estimate the changes in the population size. These results were also analyzed using Tree-Annotator v1.7.4 to infer a maximum clade credibility (MCC) tree. The trees were visualized and edited with FigTree v1.3.1 (http: //tree.bio.ed.ac.uk/ software/figtree). The SREAD (Spatial Phylogenetic Reconstruction of Evolutionary Dynamics) program [18] was used to summarize the discrete phylogeographic analysis in the diffusion dynamic plots and the interactive virtual global animations (KML files), played by Google Earth (http: earth.google.com).

Molecular Characterization: Adaptive Evolutionary Analysis

Estimates of genetic distances (number of nucleotide or amino acid substitutions per site obtained by averaging all sequence pairs) were used to calculate the divergence between sequences within each group, within genotypes and between years, using MEGA v5.05. Standard error estimates (SE) were obtained by the bootstrap method (1000 replicates). The DNAsp v5 (DNA Sequence Polymorphism) software as used to calculate the nucleotide sequence polymorphisms for both groups and both genes [19].

Natural selection on the HMPV G and F genes was estimated from the ratio of non-synonymous (dN) to synonymous (dS) substitutions per site (dN/dS) at every codon in the alignment and the overall $\omega = dN/dS$. The analysis was performed by using the following codon-based ML methods: SLAC [single likelihood ancestor counting], FEL [fixed effects likelihood], IFEL [internal fixed effects likelihood], and REL [random effects likelihood], at the specified significance levels ($P = 0.1$ and Bayes factor = 50), and using the procedures available in the HyPhy package and accessed through the Datamonkey web server [20,21].

The potential N-glycosylation sites were predicted with N-Glycosite, using the free public server available on line (http: //

www.hiv.lanl.gov/content/sequence/GLYCOSITE/glycosite.html) [22], whereas the O-glycosylation sites were predicted with NetOglyc, using the free public server available on line (http: //www.cbs.dtu.dk/services/NetOGlyc/) [23].

To predict potential B-linear epitopes, the AAP (Amino acid pair antigenicity predictor) and FBCPred (flexible length linear B-cell epitopes predictor) methods [24] (from BCPREDS B-cell epitope prediction server: http: //ailab.cs.iastate.edu/bcpreds/) were used. To perform comparable predictions, 14 epitope lengths were selected with a specificity of 75% and only non-overlapping predicted epitopes were informed.

The amino acid sequences required for the analyses were inferred using the universal genetic code.

Results

A total of 168 (14.65%) out of the 1146 NPA tested by real time RT-PCR were positive for HMPV. The annual frequencies were: 21.27% for 2009, 15.38% for 2010 and 10.52% for 2011. Most affected patients were children under 1 year of age (51.78%) and the circulation of HMPV during the study period was highest between epidemiology weeks 32 and 47 (late winter and spring) (Figure 1). The most frequent clinical ALRI presentations were bronchiolitis (53%) and pneumonia (36%).

To characterize positive cases molecularly, 36 out of the 168 positive cases were randomly selected each year of the study. Most selected patients corresponded to pneumonia and high risk patients (63%).

Phylogenetic Analysis

To typify the Argentine strains, a Bayesian phylogenetic reconstruction was performed with 30 Argentine G sequences and prototype A and B sequences downloaded from GenBank. Similar tree topologies and statistical support were obtained by ML and NJ inferences (data not shown). The analysis showed that 23 sequences clustered with group A and 7 with group B (trees upon request).

To define genetic clades and circulation patterns within each group, an exhaustive phylogenetic analysis was performed for each group separately. All the Argentine strains from group A clustered with genotype A2, whereas those from group B clustered with genotype B2 with high posterior probabilities (Figures 2a and 2b). Genotypes A2 and B2 cocirculated during 2009 and 2010, whereas only genotype A2 circulated in 2011. Genotype A2 prevailed during the study period. The same phylogenetic analyses were performed with eight Argentine F sequences and sequences downloaded from GenBank and similar genotype associations were obtained (trees upon request).

The phylogenetic analysis for group A also showed that there were some Argentine strains which remained circulating in our country during the study period supported by their association in the same genetic clade with high posterior probabilities (ARG7 and 10 from 2009, ARG4 from 2010, and ARG5, 6 and 8 from 2011; Figure 2a), and with a maximum mean distance between them of 3.4% (SE 1.1%), denoting microcirculation without evidence of annual alternation of genetic clades. Besides, the association of the Colombian strain COL3859 from 2009 in this genetic clade suggests that there was regional circulation of HMPV, supported by a maximum mean distance between the latter and the previously mentioned Argentine genetic clade of 2.7% (SE 0.9%). On the other hand, there was also an alternation of viral variants during the study period, evidenced by strains from 2009 and 2011 associated in a highly supported single genetic clade (ARG5 from 2009 and ARG1, ARG3, ARG9-12 and ARG14 from 2011) with a maximum mean distance between them of 2.5% (SE 0.9%), and a distance value of 6.7% (SE 1.7%) with Argentine strains from 2010 from a different genetic clade (ARG10 and ARG12) (Figure 2a). However, there was a close

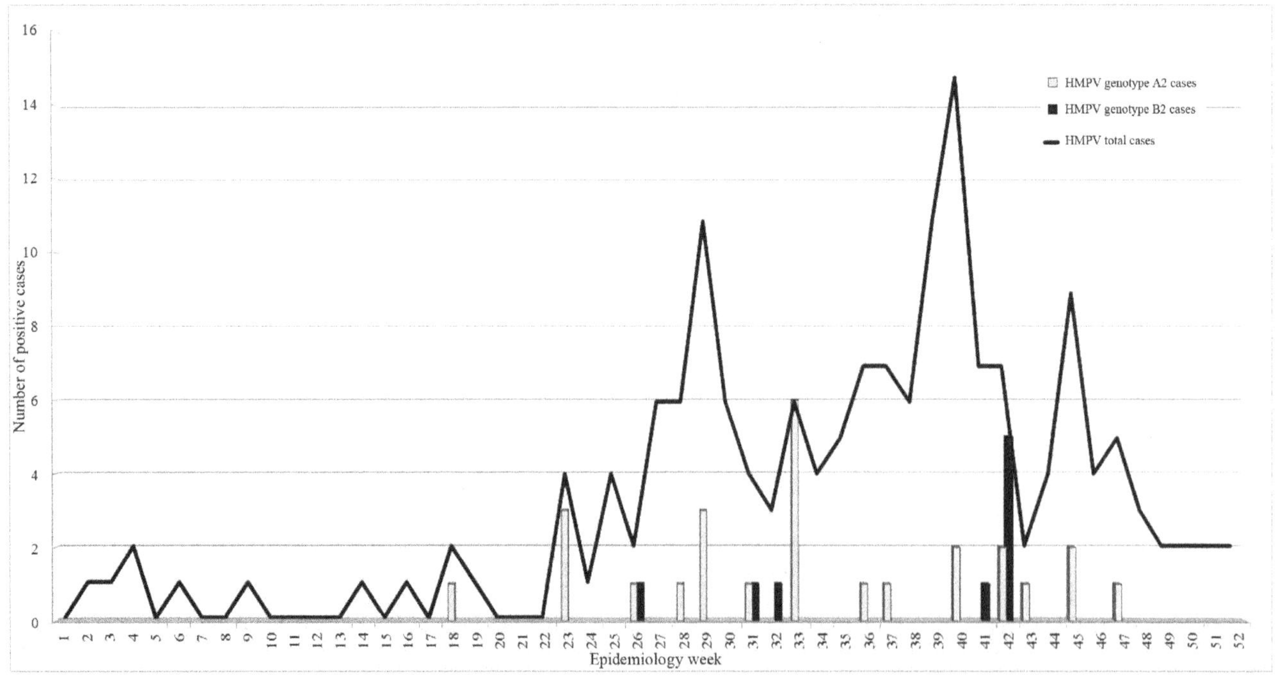

Figure 1. human metapneumovirus annual distribution. The total number of HMPV cases distributed in epidemiology weeks during the study period (2009–2011), are represented by a continuous line. Number of cases of genotype A2 and B2 are represented by gray bars and black bars, respectively.

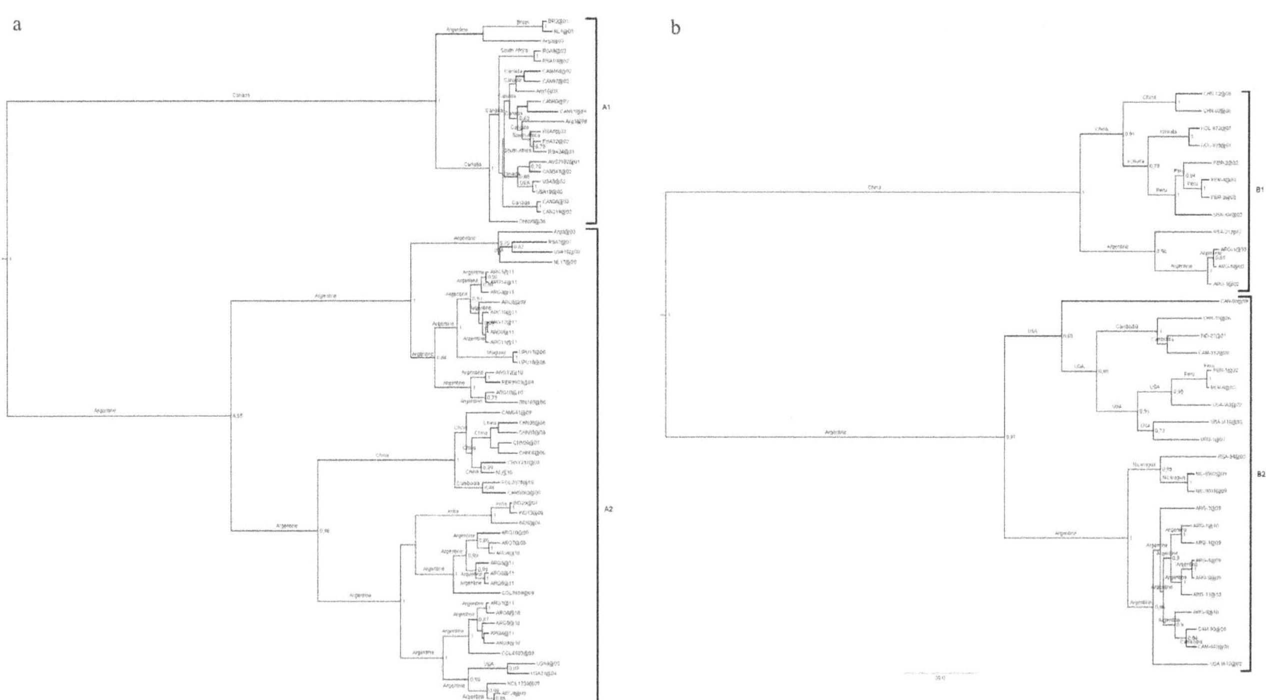

Figure 2. Maximum Clade Credibility trees. Phylogenetic analysis and discrete phylogeographic analysis. The Tamura-Nei 93 model with a discretized gamma distributed among-site rate variation (TN93+G) with four categories was used for all the analyses. Phylogeny was inferred with representative sequences retrieved from GenBank (Tree Coded Names, GenBank accession numbers, genotypes and countries of origin are listed in Table S1). The data set was analyzed assuming a relaxed (uncorrelated lognormal) molecular clock. Bayesian Markov Chain Monte Carlo (MCMC) chains were run for 10 million ngen, 1000 samplefreq and 1000 burnin to reach convergence (expected sample size>200). Only posterior probabilities above 0.7 are shown. The discrete phylogeographic analysis was estimated from the sequences stamped with date and location. Locations of ancestor strains for individual clades are indicated in each clade. **a)** HMPV group A and **b)** HMPV group B.

association of the Argentine strain ARG12 from 2010 with the Peruvian strain PER9903 from 2009, with a mean distance between them of 1.6% (SE 0.6%), supporting the idea of a regional circulation of the virus in successive outbreaks. Furthermore, a cosmopolitan circulation was denoted with a highly supported association between Argentine strains and other strains from more distant countries such as the USA, India, Cambodia, the Netherlands, and South Africa.

For group B, the phylogenetic analysis revealed that strains closely related to each other and also related to strains previously reported in Cambodia in 2008 circulated in Argentina during 2009–2010 (Figure 2b), with a maximum mean distance between them of 1.5% (SE 0.5%). At the regional level, the maximum mean distance between genotype B2 Uruguayan strains from 2007 and Argentine strains from 2009 and 2010 was 12% (SE 1.8%). However, Nicaraguan strains from 2009 (NIC8902 and NIC9019) were associated with Argentine strains of the same year (ARG2-4) in a well supported genetic clade and with a maximum mean distance between them of 3.4% (SE 1%), supporting the idea of regional movement of viral variants. Strikingly, strains of group B did not circulate in Argentina and, to our knowledge, no sequences of group B were reported in other parts of the world in 2011.

Evolutionary Rates, Population Dynamics and Phylogeographic Analyses

The discrete phylogeographic analyses depicted by the MCC trees and summarized in the diffusion dynamic plots show how the different viral variants were globally disseminated (Figures 2 and 3). The interactive animation for group A (Video S1) also suggests that Argentine viral variants spread locally to Peru and Colombia and globally to China, where new viral variants were originated and subsequently disseminated locally (to Cambodia) and globally (to Netherlands). The diffusion dynamic analysis for group B showed spreading patterns of viral variants similar to those observed for group A. Argentine viral variants spread to China and the USA, where new viral variants were originated and disseminated locally (to India and Canada) and globally (to Peru and Cambodia). The animation also shows that Argentina could act as a source and as a spreading node of new viral variants, such as those variants disseminated to Nicaragua (Figure 3b and Video S2).

The estimated tMRCA was 55 years (highest probability density (HPD) 95% 34 to 79) for group A and 36 years (HPD 95% 15 to 64) for group B. The Bayesian skyline plot analysis (Figures 4a and 4b) showed that the effective population size of group A remained above that of group B during the study period, although the population size of group A partially decreased after 2009.

Molecular Characterization: Adaptive Evolutionary Analysis

The global overall divergence analysis showed that the A sequences from the G gene were more diverse than the B sequences (22.0% (SE 2.7%) and 18.4% (SE 2.5%), respectively). In addition, at the local level, the B Argentine sequences showed less divergence than the A sequences (1.7% (SE 0.4%) and 10.9% (SE 1.3%), respectively). However, the mean substitution rate observed for both groups was similar (group A: 5.16×10^{-3} nucleotide substitutions/site/year (HPD 95%: 3.77×10^{-3} to

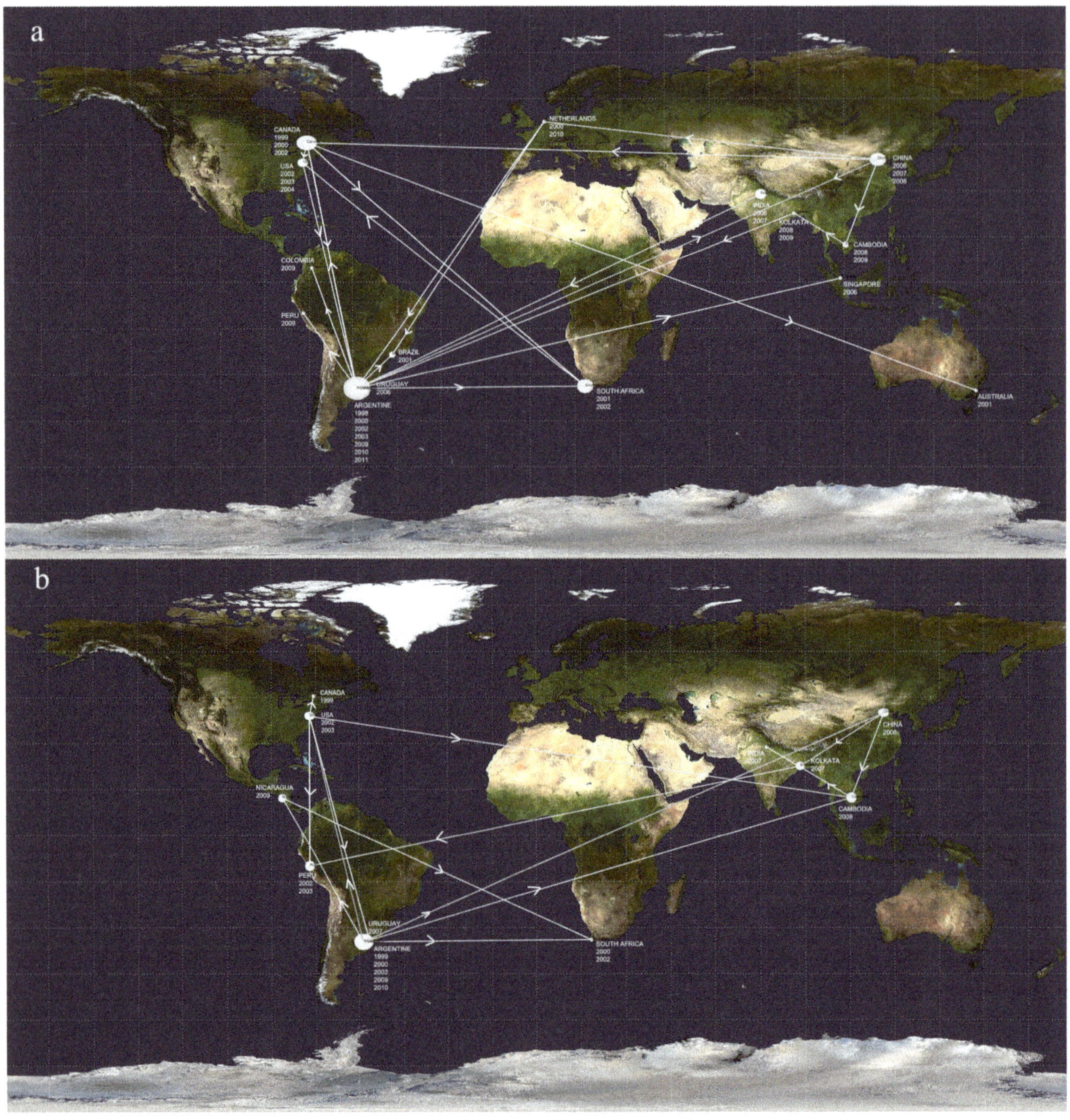

Figure 3. Discrete phylogeographic analysis. The date and location-annotated MCC trees based on the maximum clade credibility trees of HMPV A and B were summarized in the diffusion dynamic plots with SPREAD [18]. Lines between locations represent branches in the MCC tree along which the relevant location transition occurred. **a)** HMPV group A and **b)** HMPV group B.

6.59×10^{-3} nucleotide substitutions/site/year) and group B: 4.76×10^{-3} nucleotide substitutions/site/year (HPD 95%: 2.45×10^{-3} to 7.20×10^{-3}nucleotide substitutions/site/year)). The mean distance calculated for the A Argentine sequences from 2009 (9.4%, SE 1.2%) was lower than that calculated for sequences from 2010 (12.4%, SE 1.6%) and 2011 (10.2%, SE 1.3%). The analysis for group B also showed less diversity during 2009 (1.4%, SE 0.4%) than during 2010 (2.3%, SE 0.5%). In addition, the nucleotide overall mean distance for both groups was lower than the amino acid overall mean distance (group A: 10.9% (SE 1.3%) vs. 15.4% (SE 2.3%), and group B: 1.7% (SE 0.4%) vs. 3.1% (SE 0.8%)).

The polymorphisms of the nucleotide Argentine G sequences calculated separately for each group are shown in Figure 5. No conserved regions were found and the region between codons 131 and 178 showed the highest polymorphism. The selection pressure analysis revealed limited positive selection and abundant negative selection for group A. Indeed, only two positive sites (codons 161 and 176) were confirmed by FEL and IFEL and fifteen negative sites (codons 41, 46, 79, 110, 116, 120, 126, 143, 162, 183, 195,

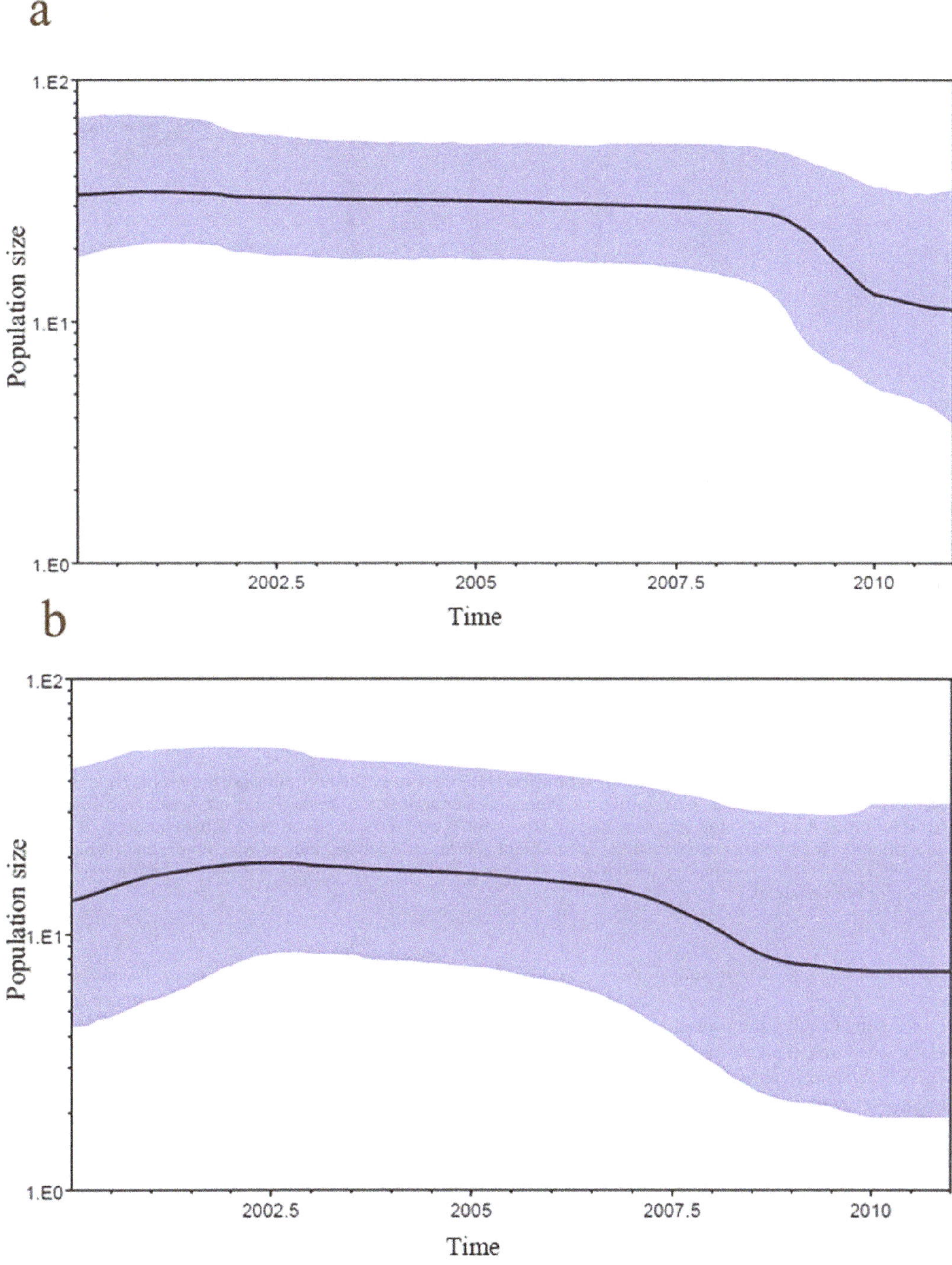

Figure 4. Population dynamics of genetic diversity in human metapneumovirus. Bayesian skyline plots. The horizontal axes represent time in years, the vertical axes represent the population sizes (Neτ), which are equal to the product of the effective population size (Ne) and the generation length in years (τ). The violet area gives the 95% highest probability density interval of these estimates. **a)** HMPV group A and **b)** HMPV group B.

197, 210, 211 and 218) were confirmed by three methods. Forty-six synonymous (*S*) and 53 non-synonymous (*N*) substitutions were found for group A and the overall ω ratio was 0.46 ($p<0.1$). No positive selection was found for group B but three negative sites (codons 27, 66, 158 and 230) were found and confirmed by at least two methods. Seven synonymous and 18 non-synonymous substitutions were found for group B and the overall ω ratio was 0.75 ($p<0.1$).

The prediction of potential B-linear epitopes for the G protein is represented in Figure 5. Most of the potential epitopes were in regions under selection pressure (mainly negative selection), and corresponded to sequence regions with low polymorphism. Codons 138, 160, 162, 195, 197 and 198 were predicted as potential O-glycosylation sites and are included in the predicted paratope binding regions. Only one epitope was predicted around codon 66 for group B, and no glycosylation was predicted at this

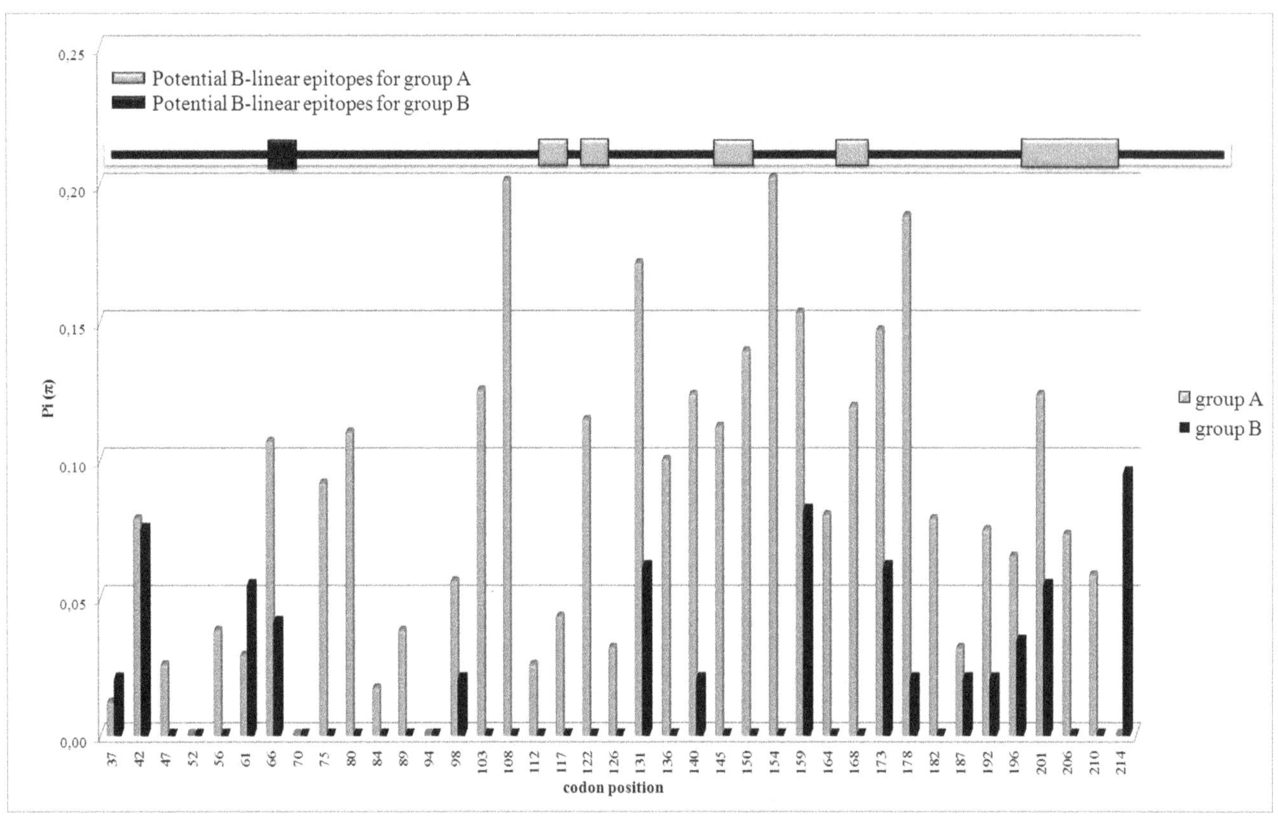

Figure 5. Sequence polymorphisms along the partial G protein of Argentine HMPV strains. The horizontal axe represents codons position in the G protein and the vertical axe represents sequence polymorphisms expressed as nucleotide diversity Pi (π) estimated with DNAsp [19]. Argentine sequence polymorphisms for group A are indicated with gray bars and for group B with black bars. The black square for group B, and gray squares and rectangles for group A placed in the black bar situated at the top of graph indicate the codons, around which there are the potential B-linear epitopes predicted with BCPREDS [24]. Non overlapping windows of 14 amino acids in lengths were selected to perform comparable predictions with a specificity of 75% for both analyses.

site. The frequency of O-glycosylation was higher than that of N-glycosylation for both groups.

In contrast with that observed for the G gene, the overall mean distance of the F gene nucleotide was lower than the amino acid overall mean distance (22.9% (SE 3.7%) for nucleotides and 2.7% (SE 0.6%) for amino acids). Only negative selected sites (codons 11, 35, 83, 102, 132, 157, 164, 191, 218 and 236) were found; the overall ω ratio was 0.05 ($p<0.1$). The region between codons 134 and 162 showed the highest polymorphism, whereas the fusion peptide and the protease cleavage site remained conserved in all Argentine strains. Eleven potential O-glycosylation sites and only two potential N-glycosylation sites were predicted for the F gene (Figure 6).

Seven potential B-linear epitopes around codons 14, 51, 69, 85, 203, 226 and 244 were predicted for the F gene (Figure 6). None of the predicted epitopes corresponded to sites under selection pressure. Two non-synonymous substitutions were found in regions that were previously described in monoclonal antibodies (MAb)-resistant mutants (MARMs) generated against MAb 1025 (K179R for ARG2@11) and MAb 757 (S132G for ARG6 and ARG10 from 2010). The region recognized by MAbs 234 and 338 (between codons 238 and 245) remained conserved in all Argentine strains [25].

Discussion

Since its discovery in 2001 [1], HMPV has become relevant as a respiratory pathogen in children under one year of age, having been reported as the second etiologic agent after HRSV in this age group [26]. Incidence values in China from January 2006 to December 2009 were of 9.1% [27], and those in Greece from June 2010 to June 2011 were of 3.7% [28]. A frequency of 14.7% was reported in Brazil from March 2008 to February 2009, regardless of the severity of ALRI [29]. In this study, we report frequencies as high as 21.57% in 2009. Since we analyzed only moderate and severe cases, these high frequency values demonstrate that HMPV is a significant etiologic agent in these cases. It is noteworthy the high frequency of HMPV found during the 2009 Influenza H1N1 pandemic. The reason of the high frequency might be the result of both the increase in surveillance of acute lower respiratory infections during the 2009 pandemic which continued in 2010 and the type of patients analyzed (hospitalized and mostly under one year of age), as was previously described in Brazil [29].

The phylogenetic analyses showed cocirculation of genotypes A2 and B2, as was reported in other Latin American countries such as Peru, and Brazil [29,30]. However, in contrast with previous reports [31], we found no changes in dominance of one group over the other (A and B), but the preponderance of genotype A2 during the study period. Although we observed no alternation of phylogenetic lineages at the level of genotypes or groups (defined by genetic distances ≥15%) between years, we observed alternation at the level of phylogenetic sublineages (defined by genetic distances ≤3.4%) [1].

Galiano *et al.* have reported cocirculation of genotypes A1 and B1/A2 and B1 in Argentina in previous years [32]. No A1 and B1 strains were detected in our study and A1 has not been detected

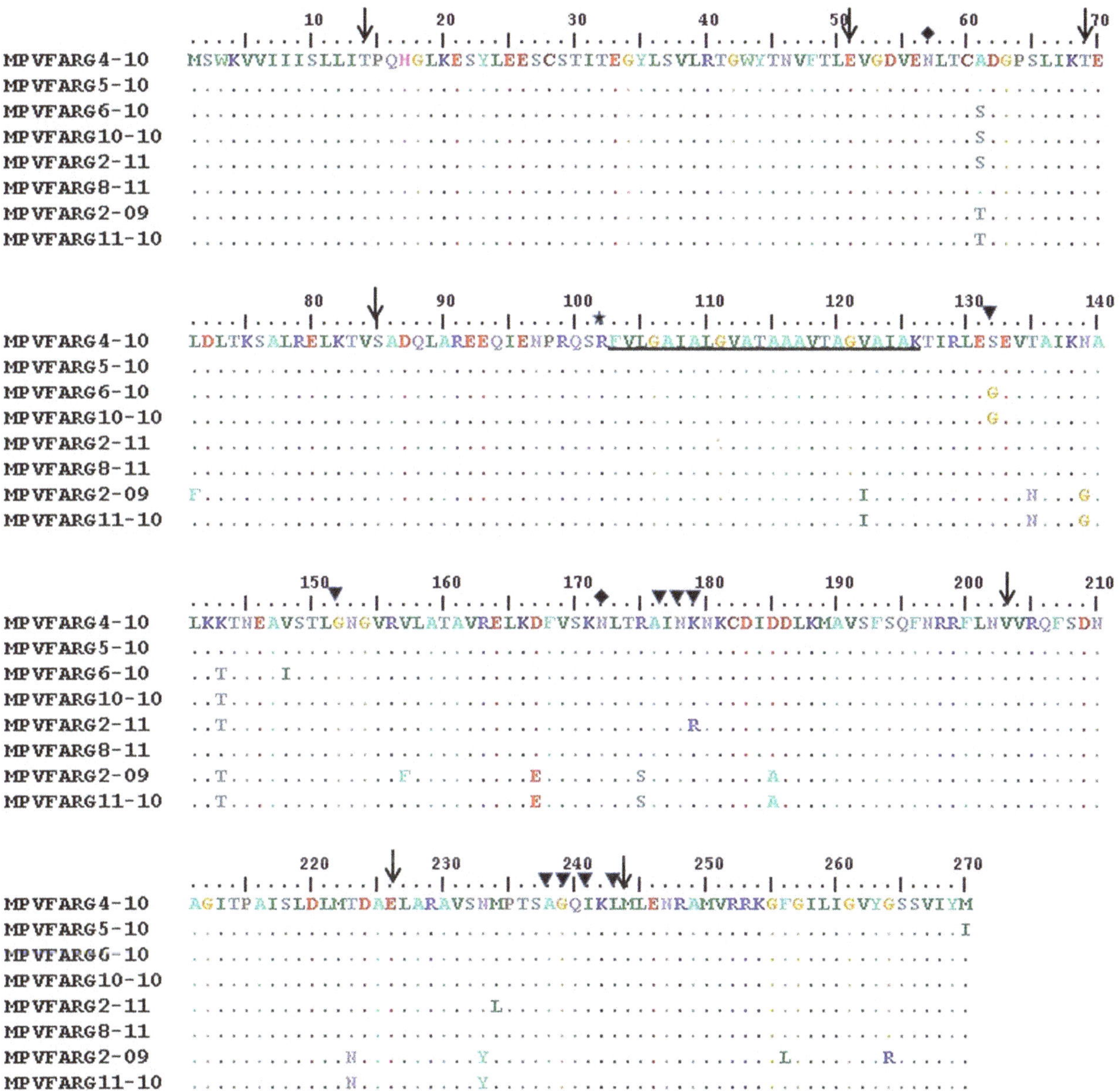

Figure 6. Amino acid alignment of partial F protein of Argentine HMPV strains. The sequences were aligned with CLUSTAL W [15]. Dots indicate identical residues. The first six sequences belong to group A, whereas the last two ones belong to group B. Black arrows indicate codons, around which there are the potential B-linear epitopes predicted with BCPREDS [24]. Black triangles indicate amino acids recognized by previously reported MAbs [38]. Black diamonds indicate potential N-glycosylation sites predicted with N-Glycosite [22]. The fusion peptide is underlined, and the protease cleavage site is indicated with a black star. Numbers indicate the amino acid position in the primary F open reading frame.

worldwide since 2004, supporting the idea that old lineages have been replaced by emerging genetic lineages [33–35].

Some researchers have reported no clinical differences between HMPV groups (A and B) [31], while others have found that greater severity of the illness is associated with group A [36]. Although we performed no analysis of association between genotypes and severity, genotype A2 was the genotype most frequently found in pneumonia cases or high-risk patients. However, the circulation of other genotypes cannot be rule out, and further studies are needed to analyze the strains that could be circulating in an outbreak from mild moderate and severe ALRI cases. The preponderance of genotype A2 over genotype B2 in 2009 and 2010 and the circulation of genotype A2 in 2011 only, in agreement with previous studies such as those reported by Li *et al* in China and García *et al* in Peru [7,30], suggest that genotype A2 has higher fitness than genotype B2. This hypothesis could be supported by higher values of effective population size and genetic distance of A2 over B2. Taking into account that the effective population size could be understood as a genetic diversity measure, the results previously exposed suggest the potential ability of local and global adaptation of genotype A2. The immune response could be less effective or may develop with insufficient speed to respond against virus with high diversity [37], such as those from genotype A2.

According to Holmes, the central tenet of the phylodynamics approach is that specific epidemiological processes, particularly rates of population growth and decline, the extent of population subdivision, and the strength and form of natural selection, are written into gene sequences and can be recovered using phylogenetic techniques [37]. Consequently, the branching structure of virus phylogenies provides a unique insight and temporal of the dynamics of viral populations that allow describing the transmission chains through phylogeographic analysis [38]. The phylogeographic analyses described in the present study allow inferring that some ancestor strains of several countries could act as a source of new viral variants that subsequently spread to other countries.

The transmission chains of viral variants described for HMPV through phylogeographic analysis have shown that its migratory events occur both globally and locally, in contrast to that found for other RNA viruses, such as dengue, in which migratory events occur mainly between neighboring countries [39]. These different migration features can be explained considering the mechanisms of transmission of both viruses. The spread of dengue, which is an arbovirus, is constrained by the presence of its vector in a given geographical region, while HMPV, which is transmitted by the respiratory route, has no geographical restrictions and can travel globally harbored in hosts.

The selection pressure analysis of the F protein showed that although it has regions with polymorphisms and mutations at sites recognized by monoclonal antibodies previously described [25], it has vast structural and functional constraints, denoted by both the fusion peptide and protease cleavage site conserved regions and numerous negative selection pressure sites, together with a very low overall ω ratio. Here we predict potential B-linear epitopes, which were conserved in all the sequences analyzed. Although an *in vitro* and *in vivo* analysis is necessary to confirm the functionality of these epitopes, they may contribute to the general knowledge of the F protein as candidate for future prophylactic therapies or vaccine development. In this regard, Ulbrandt *et al.* reported the production of two monoclonal antibodies, MAbs 234 and 338, against the HMPV F protein that neutralize all HMPV genotypes *in vitro* and *in vivo*, with neutralizing capacities comparable with those of palivizumab for HRSV [40]. Here, we report the conservation of the binding sites against these MAbs (234 and 338) in all the Argentine strains. Most of the strains reported here were the etiologic agents of severe ALRI in infants and high-risk patients, supporting the idea that the humanization of both antibodies may result in viable clinical candidates able to prevent HMPV infections in high-risk patients around the world.

The understanding of the evolutionary mechanisms and chains of viral transmission in the population and a comprehensive molecular characterization of the circulating viral variants are the first steps towards deciding which candidate proteins will be part of a vaccine or preventive therapy targets in the future.

Acknowledgments

We acknowledge Dra Paola Barrero for critical reading of the manuscript. We appreciate the excellent technical support of Patricia Riveiro for the receipt and administration of clinical samples, Viviana Viazzi for performing real time RT-PCR for HMPV diagnosis and Silvina Lusso for sequencing technical support.

Author Contributions

Contributed to the scientific discussions: AJVR ASM MV. Conceived and designed the experiments: AJVR MV. Performed the experiments: AJVR MV. Analyzed the data: AJVR ASM MV. Contributed reagents/ materials/analysis tools: AJVR ASM MV. Wrote the paper: AJVR MV.

References

1. van den Hoogen BG, de Jong JC, Groen J, Kuiken T, de Groot R, et al. (2001) A newly discovered human pneumovirus isolated from young children with respiratory tract disease. Nat Med 7: 719–724.
2. van den Hoogen BG, Bestebroer TM, Osterhaus AD, Fouchier RA (2002) Analysis of the genomic sequence of a human metapneumovirus.Virology 295: 119–132.
3. Orvell C, Norrby E, Mufson MA (1987) Preparation and characterization of monoclonal antibodies directed against five structural components of human respiratory syncytial virus subgroup B. J Gen Virol 68: 3125–3135.
4. Pavlin JA, Hickey AC, Ulbrandt N, Chan Y-P, Endy TP, et al. (2008) Human metapneumovirus reinfection among children in Thailand determined by ELISA using purified soluble fusion protein. J Infect Dis 198: 836–842.
5. Herfst S, de Graaf M, Schickli JH, Tang RS, Kaur J, et al. (2004) Recovery of human metapneumovirus genetic lineages A and B from cloned cDNA. J Virol 78: 8264–8270.
6. van den Hoogen BG, Herfst S, Sprong L, Cane PA, Forleo-Neto E, et al. (2004) Antigenic and Genetic Variability of Human Metapneumoviruses. Emerging Infect Dis 10: 658–666.
7. Li J, Ren L, Guo L, Xiang Z, Paranhos-Baccalà G, et al. (2012) Evolutionary dynamics analysis of human metapneumovirus subtype A2: genetic evidence for its dominant epidemic. PLoS ONE 7: e34544.
8. Schildgen V, van den Hoogen B, Fouchier R, Tripp RA, Alvarez R, et al. (2011)Human Metapneumovirus: lessons learned over the first decade. Clin Microbiol Rev 24: 734–754.
9. van den Hoogen BG, Osterhaus DM, Fouchier RA (2004) Clinical impact and diagnosis of human metapneumovirus infection.Pediatr Infect Dis J 23: S25–S32.
10. Boivin G, De Serres G, Côté S, Gilca R, Abed Y, et al. (2003)Human metapneumovirus infections in hospitalized children. Emerging Infect Dis 9: 634–640.
11. van den Hoogen BG, van Doornum GJJ, Fockens JC, Cornelissen JJ, Beyer WE, et al. (2003) Prevalence and clinical symptoms of human metapneumovirus infection in hospitalized patients. J Infect Dis 188: 1571–1577.
12. Kodani M, Yang G, Conklin LM, Travis TC, Whitney CG, et al. (2011) Application of TaqMan low-density arrays for simultaneous detection of multiple respiratory pathogens. J Clin Microbiol 49: 2175–2182.
13. Ludewick HP, Abed Y, van Niekerk N, Boivin G, Klugman KP, et al. (2005) Human metapneumovirus genetic variability, South Africa. Emerging Infect Dis 11: 1074–1078.
14. Hall TA (1999) BioEdit: A user-friendly biological sequence alignment editor and analysis program for Windows 95/98/NT. Nucleic Acids Symp Ser 41: 95–98.
15. Thompson JD, Higgins DG, Gibson TJ (1994) CLUSTAL W: improving the sensitivity of progressive multiple sequence alignment through sequence weighting, position-specific gap penalties and weight matrix choice. Nucleic Acids Res 22: 4673–4680.
16. Tamura K, Peterson D, Peterson N, Stecher G, Nei M, et al. (2011) MEGA5: molecular evolutionary genetics analysis using maximum likelihood, evolutionary distance, and maximum parsimony methods. Mol Biol Evol 28: 2731–2739.
17. Drummond AJ, Rambaut A (2007) BEAST: Bayesian evolutionary analysis by sampling trees. BMC Evol Biol 7: 214.
18. Bielejec F, Rambaut A, Suchard MA, Lemey P (2011) SPREAD: spatial phylogenetic reconstruction of evolutionary dynamics. Bioinformatics 27: 2910–2912.
19. Librado P, Rozas J (2009) DnaSP v5: a software for comprehensive analysis of DNA polymorphism data. Bioinformatics 25: 1451–1452.

20. Delport W, Poon AF, Frost SD, Kosakovsky Pond SL (2010) Datamonkey 2010: a suite of phylogenetic analysis tools for evolutionary biology. Bioinformatics 26: 2455–2457.
21. Kosakovsky Pond SL, Frost SD (2005) Not so different after all: a comparison of methods for detecting amino acid sites under selection. Mol Biol Evol 22: 1208–1222.
22. Zhang M, Gaschen B, Blay W, Foley B, Haigwood N, et al. (2004) Tracking global patterns of N-linked glycosylation site variation in highly variable viral glycoproteins: HIV, SIV, and HCV envelopes and influenza hemagglutinin. Glycobiology 14: 1229–1246.
23. Julenius K, Mølgaard A, Gupta R, Brunak S (2005) Prediction, conservation analysis, and structural characterization of mammalian mucin-type O-glycosylation sites. Glycobiology15: 153–164.
24. El-Manzalawy Y, Dobbs D, Honavar V (2008) On evaluating MHC-II binding peptide prediction methods. PLoS ONE 3: e3268.
25. Ulbrandt ND, Ji H, Patel NK, Barnes AS, Wilson S, et al. (2008) Identification of antibody neutralization epitopes on the fusion protein of human metapneumovirus. J Gen Virol 89: 3113–3118.
26. Klein MI, Coviello S, Bauer G, Benitez A, Serra ME, et al. (2006)The impact of infection with human metapneumovirus and other respiratory viruses in young infants and children at high risk for severe pulmonary disease. J Infect Dis193: 1544–1551.
27. Wang Y, Chen Z, Yan YD, Guo H, Chu C, et al. (2013) Seasonal distribution and epidemiological characteristics of human metapneumovirus infections in pediatric inpatients in Southeast China. Arch Virol 158: 417–424.
28. Kouni S, Karakitsos P, Chranioti A, Theodoridou M, Chrousos G, et al. (2012) Evaluation of viral co-infections in hospitalized and non-hospitalized children with respiratory infections using microarrays. Clin Microbiol Infect. doi: 10.1111/1469-0691.12015. [Epub ahead of print].
29. Souza JS, Watanabe A, Carraro E, Granato C, Bellei N (2013) Severe metapneumovirus infections among immunocompetent and immunocompromised patients admitted to hospital with respiratory infection. J Med Virol 85: 530–536.
30. Garcia J, Sovero M, Kochel T, Laguna-Torres VA, Gamero ME, et al. (2012) Human metapneumovirus strains circulating in Latin America. Arch Virol 157: 563–568.
31. Agapov E, Sumino KC, Gaudreault-Keener M, Storch GA, Holtzman MJ (2006) Genetic variability of human metapneumovirus infection: evidence of a shift in viral genotype without a change in illness. J Infect Dis 193: 396–403.
32. Galiano M, Trento A, Ver L, Carballal G, Videla C (2006) Genetic heterogeneity of G and F protein genes from Argentinean human metapneumovirus strains. J Med Virol 78: 631–637.
33. Huck B, Scharf G, Neumann-Haefelin D, Puppe W, Weigl J, et al. (2006) Novel human metapneumovirus sublineage. Emerging Infect Dis12: 147–150.
34. Aberle JH, Aberle SW, Redlberger-Fritz M, Sandhofer MJ, Popow-Kraupp T (2010) Human metapneumovirus subgroup changes and seasonality during epidemics. Pediatr Infect Dis J 29: 1016–1018.
35. Arnott A, Vong S, Sek M, Naughtin M, Beauté J, et al. (2011) Genetic variability of human metapneumovirus amongst an all ages population in Cambodia between 2007 and 2009. Infect Genet Evol Feb 1. [Epub ahead of print].
36. Vicente D, Montes M, Cilla G, Perez-Yarza EG, Perez-Trallero E (2006) Differences in clinical severity between genotype A and genotype B human metapneumovirus infection in children. Clin Infect Dis 42: e111–113.
37. Holmes EC (2009) RNA virus genomics: a world of possibilities. J Clin Invest 119: 2488–2495.
38. Holmes EC (2008) Evolutionary history and phylogeography of human viruses. Annu Rev Microbiol 62: 307–328.
39. Allicock OM, Lemey P, Tatem AJ, Pybus OG, Bennett SN, et al. (2012) Phylogeography and population dynamics of dengue viruses in the Americas. Mol Biol Evol 29: 1533–1543.
40. Ulbrandt ND, Ji H, Patel NK, Riggs JM, Brewah YA, et al. (2006) Isolation and characterization of monoclonal antibodies which neutralize human metapneumovirus in vitro and in vivo. J Virol 80: 7799–7806.

6

Linkage of HIV-Infected Infants from Diagnosis to Antiretroviral Therapy Services across the Western Cape, South Africa

Nei-Yuan Hsiao[1]*, Kathryn Stinson[2], Landon Myer[2]

1 Division of Virology, University of Cape Town and National Health Laboratory Service, Cape Town, South Africa, 2 Centre for Infectious Diseases Epidemiology and Research, School of Public Health and Family Medicine, University of Cape Town, Cape Town, South Africa

Abstract

Introduction: Early infant diagnosis (EID) of HIV infection is an important service to reduce paediatric morbidity and mortality related to HIV/AIDS. Although South Africa has a national EID programme based on PCR testing, there are no population-wide data on the linkage of infants testing HIV PCR-positive to HIV care and treatment services.

Methods: We conducted a retrospective analysis of all public sector laboratory data from across the Western Cape province between 2005 and 2011. We linked positive HIV PCR results to subsequent HIV viral load testing to determine the proportion of infants who were successfully linked to HIV care.

Results: A total of 83 698 unique infant HIV PCR tests were documented, of which 6322 (8%) were PCR positive. The proportion of PCR-positive children declined from 12% in 2005 to 3% in 2011. Of the children testing PCR-positive, 4105 (65%) had subsequent viral load testing indicating successful linkage to care. The proportion of successfully linked infants increased from 54% in 2005 to 71% in 2010, while the median delay in days to successful linkage decreased from 146 days in 2005 to 33 days in 2010.

Discussion: From 2005 to 2011 there has been a reduction in the proportion of children testing HIV PCR-positive, and an increase in the proportion of infected infants successfully linked to HIV care and treatment, in this setting. However a large proportion of infected infants remain unlinked to antiretroviral therapy services and there is a clear need for interventions to further strengthen EID programmes.

Editor: Grace C. John-Stewart, University of Washington, United States of America

Funding: Landon Myer is funded by the Elizabeth Glaser Pediatric AIDS Foundation. The funders had no role in study design, data collection and analysis, decision to publish, or preparation of the manuscript.

Competing Interests: The authors have declared that no competing interest exist.

* E-mail: marvin.hsiao@nhls.ac.za

Introduction

Across sub-Saharan Africa, mother-to-child-transmission (MTCT) of HIV infection remains an ongoing threat to child health. Despite the widespread implementation of PMTCT programmes, an estimated 390,000 infants were newly infected with HIV during 2010 alone [1]. Infant HIV infection often results in rapid HIV disease progression as approximately 50% of vertically-infected infants die in the first year of life [2]. In South Africa, where there were an estimated 40 000 new infant HIV infections during 2010, HIV contributes significantly towards preventable infant mortality [3,4].

Early identification of perinatally-infected infants and rapid referral for initiation of antiretroviral therapy (ART) is an important intervention to promote child health [5,6]. Early infant diagnosis (EID) of HIV by polymerase chain reaction (PCR) is routinely used to detect HIV infection in infants. Although EID is an important component of effective PMTCT programmes, HIV PCR testing is relatively expensive, requires specialised laboratory equipment, and is time consuming. This means the testing components of EID is firmly in the domain of centralised specialist laboratories. This in turn makes health systems issues and logistical considerations, such as conducting HIV testing in primary care facilities, transporting specimens to central reference laboratories, and return of results to primary care, a major concern [7,8].

Across Africa, non-retention of patients and delays in testing and referral are major operational concerns facing EID programmes [9]. Loss to follow-up of infants between HIV testing, the return of results, and referral of infected infants to paediatric ART services has been documented in several settings [10–13]. Even when infants are retained throughout these steps, the delays involved in testing and referring infants for ART may be unacceptable given the high mortality observed in infected infants who are not yet on ART [12–15]. But while EID services across Africa face important challenges, systems for monitoring EID programmes are not well developed; as a result, there are few population-level data on the performance of EID services in identifying HIV-infected infants and referring them to ART services [16].

In South Africa, there are few data on the performance of EID services in referring infected infants to long-term care. We used routinely collected HIV laboratory data to investigate the overall levels of MTCT in the Western Cape Province, and the performance of the EID service in referring infected infants for ART, between 2005 and 2011.

Materials and Methods

PMTCT and EID services operate at public sector primary care clinics and hospitals throughout the Western Cape province. HIV PCR testing is used for HIV screening in HIV-exposed infants attending routine postnatal immunization clinics as well as for HIV diagnosis in children who present to hospitals. Prior to 2008, newly diagnosed infants were referred to specialist paediatric infectious disease clinics operated in secondary and tertiary hospitals for ART initiation and follow-up; the provision of ART was based on the 2004 WHO recommendations [17]. Following the results of the Children with HIV Early Antiretroviral Therapy (CHER) study released in 2008, ART initiation for all infected infants became policy across the province, with ART delivered through hospitals as well as a growing number of primary care clinics. Throughout, HIV viral load testing was routinely performed by ART services prior to treatment initiation. This 'baseline' viral load serves as a confirmation of the positive HIV PCR result and is a tool for which subsequent treatment efficacy can be measured.

Study Objective

This study sought to describe the linkage of HIV-infected children to ART care using public sector laboratory testing data.

Sources of Data

Data for this analysis are all HIV PCR and HIV viral load testing results from public sector health services in the Western Cape Province between January 2005 and July 2011. Data came from the central data warehouse of the National Health Laboratory Service, the sole provider of pathology services for the public health sector in South Africa. The following data were available: patient name and provincial folder number; health facility; type and date of test and test result; and patient date of birth and gender. We identified the first positive HIV PCR result for each child under the age of 2 years, and the first HIV viral load for each child under the age of 5 years, for inclusion in the analysis. Test results related to quality assurance/quality control, and tests of patients enrolled into clinical trials, were excluded.

Data Analysis

Data were analysed used Stata Version 11.0 (Stata Corporation, College Station, Texas, USA). We used the date of a child's positive HIV PCR test result as the date of diagnosis, and used the date of the first HIV viral load as the date of first attendance at ART services. HIV PCR and viral load results for individual children were linked using combinations of folder number, name and date of birth. We defined 'definite' links as matching identical full surname or folder number in combination with an identical date of birth and 'probable' links as matching any combination of partial surname, date of birth and folder number. However, study findings did not differ appreciably between definitions, and the results presented here are based on all 'probable' linkages.

The delay in days between the first positive HIV PCR and the first HIV viral load test was used to estimate the delay between a PCR positive test result and a child's first attendance at an ART clinic. Children who were HIV PCR-positive but did not have a HIV viral load test were considered to have not attended ART services. A specialist hospital was defined as a hospital where a paediatrician with infectious diseases training was present, while the remaining facilities are primary and secondary care facilities administered by doctors and/or nurses without specific paediatric infectious disease training. An urban facility was defined as the site of testing within the greater Cape Town area; the remaining facilities in the province are considered rural facilities.

In analysis, continuous variables were described using medians and interquartile ranges (IQR) while proportions with exact binomial 95% confidence intervals (CI) were calculated for categorical variables. Logistic regression models were used to examine the independent predictors of (i) positive HIV PCR test results, and (ii) the successful referral of infected children to ART services; the results are presented as odds ratios (OR) with 95% CI. Variables in the model were selected based on a priori evidence and findings of descriptive statistics.

Ethics Statement

The study was approved by the National Health Laboratory Services and the Research Ethics Committee of the Faculty of Heath Sciences at the University of Cape Town.

Results

A total of 83 698 children less than 2 years of age underwent HIV PCR testing at public sector health care services in the Western Cape between 2005 and 2011. Of these, 6322 (7.6%) tested positive, 76 956 (91.9%) tested negative and 418 (0.5%) of PCR results were equivocal (Table 1). The number of HIV PCR tests almost doubled over time, while the proportion of PCR-positive children declined from 12% in 2005 to 3% in 2011. The median age of first HIV PCR testing was approximately 4 months (IQR 3.1–5 months) during 2005 and decreased to 1.5 months (IQR 1.4–2.1 months) during 2011.

In 2005, 303 health facilities conducted HIV PCR testing, increasing annually to 341 facilities in 2010. Thirteen percent of PCR testing came from hospitals with specialist paediatric services and 69% of PCR tests were from urban facilities around Cape Town. No significant changes in the proportions of specialist hospital and urban PCR testing were observed over the study period; however infants tested at specialist hospitals were much more likely to be PCR positive ($p<0.001$). Just over half of infants (51%) were tested under 3 months of age, the age targeted for the current EID programme.

During the same period, 11 653 first HIV viral load tests were carried out in children <5 years of age at public sector health care facilities. The median viral load of the samples with detectible HIV was 150 390 copies (IQR 12 975–990 000 copies/ml). The number of facilities that conducted HIV viral load testing rose from 91 in 2005 to 220 in 2010 (Table 2). Sixty-nine percent of the first time paediatric HIV viral load tests was performed in an urban facility; this proportion declined from 73% in 2005 to 60% in 2010.

Linkage of PCR-positive Children to ART Services

Using the 'definite' matching criteria, we found 3414 of 6322 (54%) children with first positive HIV PCR who also had a HIV viral load conducted prior to ART initiation and were thus considered successfully linked to care. Under the 'probable' matching criteria we were able to match a further 691 PCR-positive children to HIV viral load results, resulting in a total of 4105 children (65%) who were HIV PCR-positive and had laboratory evidence of attending ART services.

Table 1. Early infant diagnosis data, Western Cape, South Africa, 2005–2011.

		HIV PCR positive	HIV PCR negative	Total	Percent positive	OR (crude)	95%CI
Year	2005	1057	7594	8651	12%	1.0	(reference)
	2006	861	6193	7054	12%	1.00	0.91–1.10
	2007	1170	11416	12586	9%	0.74	0.67–0.80
	2008	1097	13279	14376	8%	0.59	0.54–0.65
	2009	1035	14640	15675	7%	0.51	0.46–0.56
	2010	793	14931	15724	5%	0.38	0.35–0.42
	2011*	311	8903	9214	3%	0.25	0.22–0.29
Sex	Female	3215	36648	39863	8%	1.0	(reference)
	Male	2848	36289	39137	7%	0.89	0.85–0.94
Facility	Primary care facility	3757	68605	72362	5%	1.0	(reference)
	Specialist Hospitals	2567	8351	10918	24%	5.61	5.31–5.93
Urban facilities	Rural	1953	22480	24433	8%	1.0	(reference)
	Urban	4372	54494	58866	7%	0.92	0.87–0.98
Age at time of PCR	≤2 months	1999	41151	43150	5%	1.0	(reference)
	>2 months	4326	35823	40149	11%	2.49	2.35–2.62

Factors associated with HIV PCR results amongst HIV-exposed children less than two years of age tested for the first time at public sector health facilities in the Western Cape Province of South Africa, January 2005 and July 2011.
*For 2011, results are from January to June.

The distribution of PCR-positive children who were and were not linked to ART services is shown in Table 3. Over the period, the proportion of linked children increased from 54% in 2005 to 71% in 2010. The linkage rate of children diagnosed HIV PCR-positive at specialist hospitals (69%) was substantially higher than at primary care centres (58%); despite contributing 13% of all PCR tests requested, the specialist hospitals accounted for 45% of all children successfully linked to ART services. In particular, Cape Town's largest paediatric hospital contributed 25% of all children linked to ART services in the province. Related to this, successful linkage of PCR-positive children to ART services was significantly more likely at urban health facilities (68%) compared to rural facilities (50%). This difference appeared independent of urban-rural variation (OR 1.89, 95%CI 1.68–2.14). In addition, children older than 2 months of age appeared to be less likely to be linked (OR 0.73, 95% CI 0.64–0.81) compared to younger infants; this association persisted after adjusting for potential confounding variables such as the year of testing and facility of testing (OR 0.82, 95% CI 0.72–0.92).

Table 2. Changes in early infant diagnosis, HIV viral load testing, and linkages to care over time.

		Year 2005	2006	2007	2008	2009	2010
Number of facilities testing	HIV PCR	271	276	312	330	322	343
	HIV Viral load	91	133	149	203	216	220
PCR tests done		8653	7065	12603	14416	15743	15922
Facility	Specialist Hospitals	1242	1430	1793	1941	1839	1761
	Primary care facility	7411	5634	10812	12477	13904	14161
	% from specialist care	*14*	*20*	*14*	*14*	*12*	*11*
Facilities	Urban	5752	4206	8997	10265	11159	11120
	Rural	2901	2858	3605	4153	4584	4802
	% Urban samples	*67*	*60*	*71*	*71*	*71*	*70*
Referral to care	Referred	576	483	662	758	703	566
	Not referred	481	378	508	337	332	227
	% referred	*54*	*56*	*57*	*69*	*68*	*71*

Changes in HIV PCR/VL testing facilities and linkage to care for HIV PCR positive children less than two years of age attending public sector health facilities in the Western Cape Province of South Africa, January 2005 to July 2010.

Table 3. Proportion of HIV PCR-positive infants linked to HIV treatment services.

		HIV PCR-positive children with linked VL					
		Linked	**Not linked**	**Total**	**Percent**	**OR (crude)**	**95%CI**
Year	2005	576	481	1057	54%	1.0	(reference)
	2006	483	378	861	56%	1.07	0.89–1.28
	2007	662	508	1170	57%	1.09	0.92–1.29
	2008	758	337	1095	69%	1.88	1.57–2.24
	2009	703	332	1035	68%	1.77	1.48–2.11
	2010	566	227	793	71%	2.08	1.71–2.53
Sex	Female	1924	1134	3058	63%	1.0	(reference)
	Male	1715	994	2709	63%	1.02	0.91–1.13
Facility	Primary care facility	2061	1488	3549	58%	1.0	(reference)
	Specialist Hospitals	1687	775	2462	69%	1.57	1.41–1.75
Urban facilities	Rural	954	936	1890	50%	1.0	(reference)
	Urban	2794	1327	4121	68%	2.07	1.85–2.31
Age at time of PCR	≤2 months	1257	599	1856	68%	1.0	(reference)
	>2 months	2491	1664	4155	60%	0.71	0.63–0.80

Factors associated with linkage of HIV PCR positive infants to antiretroviral therapy services among infants attending public sector health facilities in the Western Cape Province of South Africa, January 2005 to December 2010.

Delays from PCR-positive Diagnosis to ART Services

The median delay between the first positive HIV PCR test and the first viral load conducted as part of ART work-up was 146 days in 2005 (IQR 42–500 days) and decreased to 33 days (IQR 8–83 days) during 2010 (Figure 1). The largest decrease was observed during the period 2007–2008, as the delay halved from 81 days in 2007 to 39 days in 2008. Overall, 66% and 85% of these delays were less than 150 days and 365 days, respectively. In 2010, 83% of delays were less than 150 days compared to the 50% during 2005.

The shortest delays in linkage of PCR-positive children to ART services were observed at specialist paediatric hospitals. The median delay of children at these hospitals was 13 days (IQR 5–68 days) compared to all other children who experienced a median delay of 87 days (IQR 28–287 days, $p<0.001$). The overall trend of reductions in delays over calendar years was similar for the two main specialist hospitals and all other facilities. The major reduction in delays during the 2007/2008 period was observed at both specialist hospitals and primary care centres.

The median age of PCR-positive children undergoing their first attendance at ART clinics, as indicated by pre-ART HIV viral load testing, was 96 days over the entire study period (IQR 50–169 days). This age decreased from 119 days in 2005 to 60 days in 2010, with 2007/2008 being the year of the most significant decrease (from 103 days in 2007 to 73 days in 2008) (Figure 2a). However, the reduction in median age of HIV viral load was mainly observed outside the two specialist hospitals (Figure 2b); the age of first HIV viral load in two hospitals remained constant over the study period.

Discussion

These data demonstrate that only a fraction of children in this setting who test HIV PCR-positive within the PMTCT EID programme are successfully linked ART services. This proportion increased substantially during the period 2005–2010:71% of the HIV infected infants in 2010 had a subsequent HIV viral load indicating their attendance at ART services. In parallel, among HIV-infected children who were successfully linked to ART services, the time delay between HIV PCR-positive test results and first attendance at ART services decreased in each successive year, though the median delay remained greater than 1 month during 2010.

Our data demonstrate that the number of infants tested doubled over the six year period, while the proportion of infants testing PCR positive declined from 12% to 3%. The reduction in infant HIV prevalence is seen in both asymptomatic children in the primary care setting and infants tested in hospitals. This steady decline points to the successes of the PMTCT programme in the Western Cape province, mirroring gains nationally [18,19].

Linkage of HIV-infected Infants to ART Services

There are several factors that may contribute to the failure of children testing HIV PCR positive in the EID programme to be linked to ART services. First, an infant could demise before the caregiver received the test result and/or attended the ART clinic. For example one Tanzanian study showed that 14% of caregivers received the EID result after their child had already died [12]. Second, even if a child is alive, HIV PCR test results may not be returned to caregivers. A previous study done in South Africa had shown that of 584 infants undergoing HIV PCR testing for EID at a routine immunization clinic, only 332 mothers (57%) returned to receive the results [13]. This type of loss to follow-up (LTF) is a major challenge, as it increases the risk of morbidity and mortality in infants due to untreated HIV infection [20].

Some of the phenomenon of LTF of mother-infant pairs is likely due to migration patterns of women during pregnancy and postpartum, as there is widespread anecdotal evidence of women from rural areas migrating to urban centres for antenatal care and delivery, and then returning to rural homes early postpartum. This form of 'health migrancy' has been documented in many parts of Africa [21], and presents a major challenge to continuity of care in maternal and child health. In the setting of our study this migration between health services may negatively bias our linkage

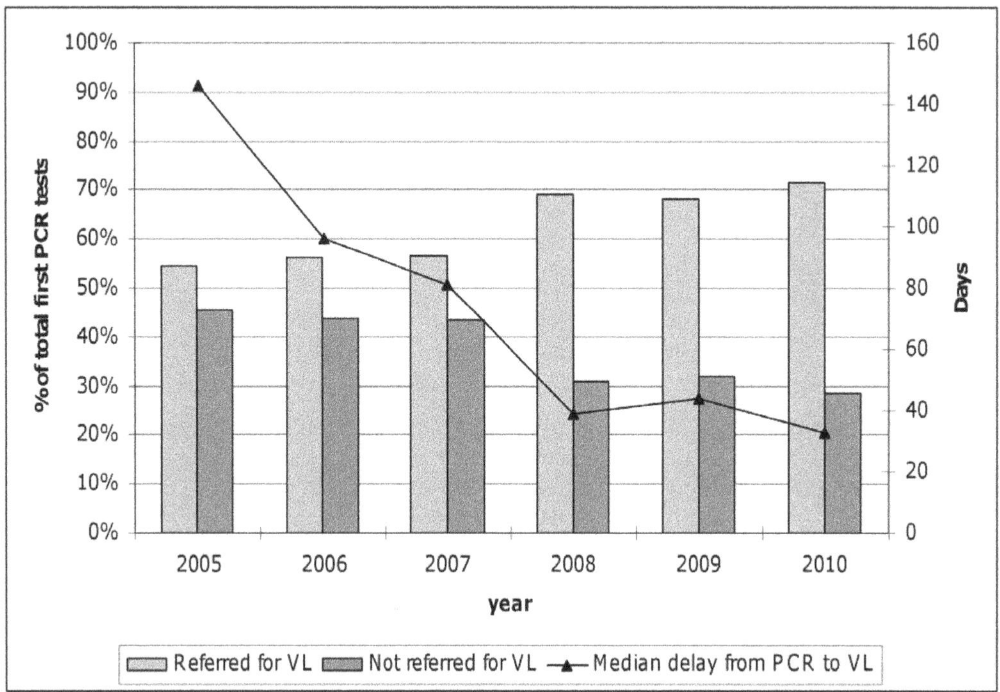

Figure 1. Linkage to antiretorivral therapy services. Proportion of infants testing positive on HIV PCR who are successfully linked to antiretroviral therapy services (as indicated by HIV viral load testing), with median delay between PCR and linked viral load (VL) testing.

to care estimate; the magnitude of this bias is difficult to estimate. An additional cause of phenomenon of LTF of mother-infant pairs operates at the level of health systems. In South Africa and elsewhere, EID testing is timed to coincide with the first infant immunization visit at 6 weeks of age, with results commonly returned to caregivers at the second immunization visit 10 weeks postpartum. Although this integration of EID into immunization services may reduce the burden of clinic visits for the caregiver, the 4-week interval between testing and receiving results may increase LTF and alternative systems for returning HIV PCR results need urgent consideration. For example, cellphone technology has been used to deliver EID results with some success in Zambia and warrants further investigation [22].

A third concern is LTF of caregiver/infant pairs who are diagnosed as HIV-positive but LTF before attending ART services. Prior to 2008 in this setting all HIV-infected infants were referred to specialist hospitals for ART care, and the time and cost of attending these hospital visits may present a barrier to many caregivers, particularly in rural areas [23]. Since 2008 there has been a shift towards paediatric ART services delivered through community-based primary care services, although since not all clinics offering EID also provide paediatric ART the separation of diagnostic and treatment services remains a barrier to rapid ART initiation in infants. In order to overcome these challenges in paediatric HIV care, a re-engineering of the current health systems to integrate the PMTCT, EID and infant HIV treatment is required. For instance, delivery of HIV specific services at immunization clinics instead of general paediatric clinics had been found to achieve superior uptake in Malawi [24].

Delays in Attending ART Services

The time delay between positive HIV PCR test results and presentation to ART services decreased between 2005 and 2010 but remained more than 5 weeks in the most recent period. Several factors contribute to these delays. First, the number of primary care facilities that provide paediatric ART has increased during the past few years, reducing delays related to geographically distant referrals. Second, HIV testing for EID is based on PCR technology in central laboratories, creating delays around the transport of specimens, testing and return of results; thereafter, infants with positive test results may require referral to separate facilities for ART screening (including baseline HIV viral load testing) and initiation. In light of the steps required, a 4–5 week delay may approach the minimum possible delay under the current system.

The development of point-of-care EID assays based on HIV PCR [25] or HIV p24 antigen detection [26] may play a valuable role in further reducing these delays. Having access to the EID result on the same day using point-of-care testing could mean that appropriate counseling and clinical management can be initiated during the same clinic visit. This could have a positive impact on the proportion of children starting ART as well as the delay between diagnosis and treatment, and this possibility warrants further research.

Strengths and Limitations

The interpretation of these data is subject to a number of limitations. While we included all HIV PCR tests conducted in public sector health facilities across the province, the coverage of the EID programme may not be complete, and the number of HIV-exposed infants who are not tested in the province is unknown. The EID coverage in low- and middle-income countries had been estimated to be around 15% [27]. However this is likely an underestimate for South Africa as more recent local data suggest the coverage in South Africa to be around 68% [1]. Second, we have used 'baseline' HIV viral load testing as a marker of attendance at ART services, which presumes that paediatric ART services adhere to policy guidelines and conduct viral load

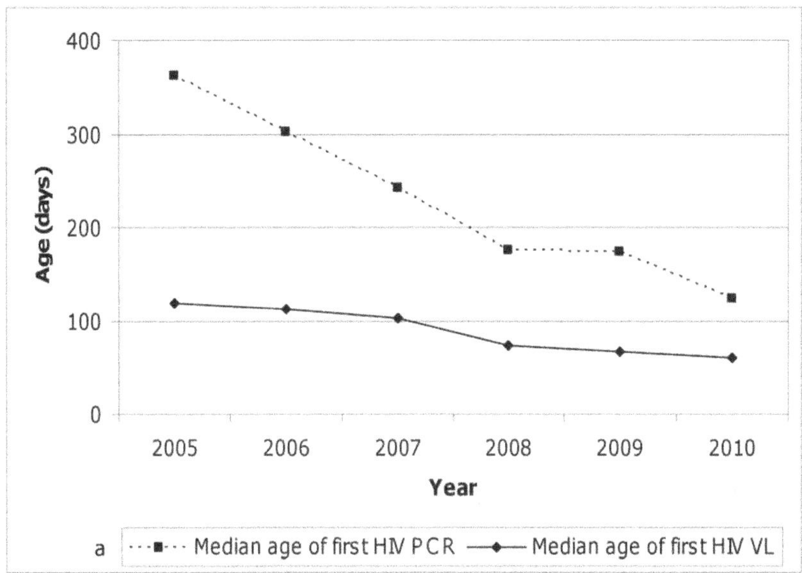

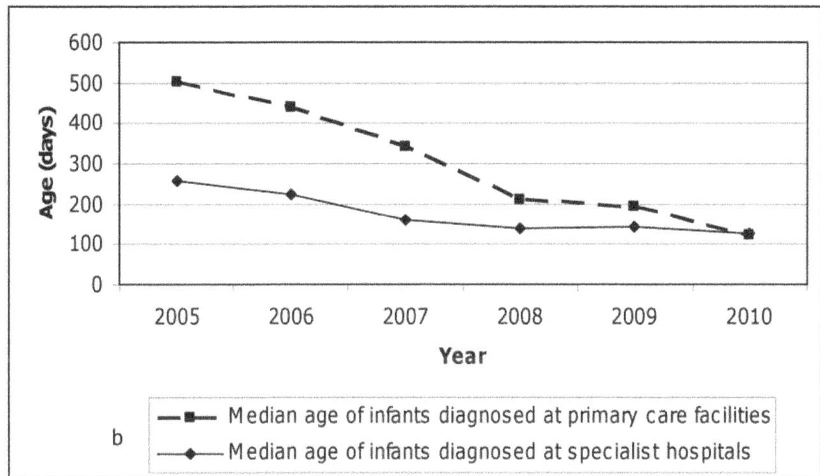

Figure 2. Age of children accessing early infant diagnosis and antiretroviral therapy services. 2a. The age children (in days) at the time of HIV PCR testing and attendance at antiretroviral therapy clinics (as indicated by HIV viral load testing), by year, among children attending public sector services in the Western Cape province, 2005–2010. The median age of first HIV viral load represent a small subset infants starting ART. This median age is mostly in the first 6 months due to the nature history of HIV disease progression in children. The median age of PCR reflects the age at which PCR testing are being used in all HIV exposed children, including much older children. 2b. The age children (in days) at the time of HIV viral load testing and attendance at antiretroviral therapy clinics, by year, among children attending public sector services in the Western Cape province, 2005–2010. The dotted line represents children diagnosed at primary care facility and the solid like represent children diagnosed at specialist facilities. The time to HIV diagnosis in primary care facilities had shown a great improvement over time, likely due to improved access to EID program. The diagnosis at specialist facilities represents children presenting with disease progression. In order to avoid HIV related paediatric mortality, the age of diagnosis at primary cares sites should be below the age of diagnosis at specialist hospitals.

testing at an infant's first ART clinic visit. While deviations from national guidelines for paediatric ART have not been documented, it is possible that some children were seen at ART clinics but do not have a viral load test; if this is the case, we may underestimate slightly the proportion of infected children who go on to start ART. It is also possible that children may access ART in the private sector and thus are not captured by our method, however private paediatric services account for a very small minority HIV related care in this setting, and thus this phenomenon is unlikely to impact our study findings. Third, as described above, there are multiple steps required for a child to be diagnosed as HIV PCR-positive and linked to ART services. Using laboratory data, we are unable to tell which specific barriers between EID and ART services are most important, and additional research is required to explore these in detail. Finally, these data should be generalized with caution, as the coverage of EID and ART services, and the strength of health systems more generally, varies widely between settings.

In summary, these data demonstrate that the proportion HIV-exposed infants testing PCR positive in the Western Cape province of South Africa has decreased dramatically since 2005. During the same period the proportion of HIV PCR-positive infants who subsequently attended ART services has increased substantially but remains suboptimal. While additional research is required to understand the barriers to successful ART referral, there is a clear need for interventions that facilitate linkage of infants diagnosed as HIV-infected to paediatric ART programmes. As the number of infant HIV infections decline, the absence of a direct system to trace HIV-infected infants and 'fast track' them onto ART is emerging as an important need in this setting as elsewhere in South Africa.

Acknowledgments

We would like to acknowledge the South African National Health Laboratory Service for providing the data for the study.

Author Contributions

Conceived and designed the experiments: LM KS NH. Performed the experiments: NH. Analyzed the data: NH. Wrote the paper: LM KS NH.

References

1. World Health Organisation, The Joint United Nations Programme on HIV/AIDS, and The United Nations Children's Fund (2012) Global HIV AIDS response - Epidemic update and health sector progress towards Universal Access - Progress report 2011. Geneva, Switzerland: WHO.
2. Chilongozi D, Wang L, Brown L, Taha T, Valentine M, et al. (2008) Morbidity and mortality among a cohort of human immunodeficiency virus type 1-infected and uninfected pregnant women and their infants from Malawi, Zambia, and Tanzania. Pediatr Infect Dis J 27: 808–814.
3. Bourne DE, Thompson M, Brody LL, Cotton M, Draper B, et al. (2009) Emergence of a peak in early infant mortality due to HIV/AIDS in South Africa. AIDS 23: 101–106.
4. Dramowski A, Coovadia A, Meyers T, Goga A (2012) Identifying missed opportunities for early intervention among HIV-infected paediatric admissions at Chris Hani Baragwanath hospital, Soweto, South Africa. Southern African Journal of HIV Medicine 12: 16–23.
5. Violari A, Cotton MF, Gibb DM, Babiker AG, Steyn J, et al. (2008) Early antiretroviral therapy and mortality among HIV-infected infants. N Engl J Med 359: 2233–2244.
6. World Health Organisation (2010) WHO recommendations on the diagnosis of HIV infection in infants and children. Geneva, Switzerland: WHO.
7. Creek TL, Sherman GG, Nkengasong J, Lu L, Finkbeiner T, et al. (2007) Infant human immunodeficiency virus diagnosis in resource-limited settings: issues, technologies, and country experiences. Am J Obstet Gynecol 197: S64–S71.
8. Tejiokem MC, Faye A, Penda IC, Guemkam G, Ateba NF, et al. (2011) Feasibility of early infant diagnosis of HIV in resource-limited settings: the ANRS 12140-PEDIACAM study in Cameroon. PLoS One 6: e21840.
9. Ciaranello AL, Park JE, Ramirez-Avila L, Freedberg KA, Walensky RP, et al. (2011) Early infant HIV-1 diagnosis programs in resource-limited settings: opportunities for improved outcomes and more cost-effective interventions. BMC Med 9: 59.
10. Hassan AS, Sakwa EM, Nabwera HM, Taegtmeyer MM, Kimutai RM, et al. (2012) Dynamics and Constraints of Early Infant Diagnosis of HIV Infection in Rural Kenya. AIDS Behav 16: 5–12.
11. Lofgren SM, Morrissey AB, Chevallier CC, Malabeja AI, Edmonds S, et al. (2009) Evaluation of a dried blood spot HIV-1 RNA program for early infant diagnosis and viral load monitoring at rural and remote healthcare facilities. AIDS 23: 2459–2466.
12. Nuwagaba-Biribonwoha H, Werq-Semo B, Abdallah A, Cunningham A, Gamaliel JG, et al. (2010) Introducing a multi-site program for early diagnosis of HIV infection among HIV-exposed infants in Tanzania. BMC Pediatr 10: 44.
13. Rollins N, Mzolo S, Moodley T, Esterhuizen T, van Rooyen H (2009) Universal HIV testing of infants at immunization clinics: an acceptable and feasible approach for early infant diagnosis in high HIV prevalence settings. AIDS 23: 1851–1857.
14. Creek T, Tanuri A, Smith M, Seipone K, Smit M, et al. (2008) Early diagnosis of human immunodeficiency virus in infants using polymerase chain reaction on dried blood spots in Botswana's national program for prevention of mother-to-child transmission. Pediatr Infect Dis J 27: 22–26.
15. Braun M, Kabue MM, McCollum ED, Ahmed S, Kim M, et al. (2011) Inadequate coordination of maternal and infant HIV services detrimentally affects early infant diagnosis outcomes in Lilongwe, Malawi. J Acquir Immune Defic Syndr 56: e122–e128.
16. Chatterjee A, Tripathi S, Gass R, Hamunime N, Panha S, et al. (2011) Implementing services for Early Infant Diagnosis (EID) of HIV: a comparative descriptive analysis of national programs in four countries. BMC Public Health 11: 553.
17. Gilks CF, Crowley S, Ekpini R, Gove S, Perriens J, et al. (2006) The WHO public-health approach to antiretroviral treatment against HIV in resource-limited settings. Lancet 368: 505–510.
18. Goga AE, Dinh TH, Jackson DJ for the SAPMTCTE study group (2012) Evaluation of the Effectiveness of the National Prevention of Mother-to-Child Transmission (PMTCT) Programme Measured at Six Weeks Postpartum in South Africa, 2010. South African Medical Research Council, National Department of Health of South Africa and PEPFAR/US Centers for Disease Control and Prevention. 2012.
19. Grimwood A, Fatti G, Mothibi E, Eley B, Jackson D (2012) Progress of preventing mother-to-child transmission of HIV at primary healthcare facilities and district hospitals in three South African provinces. S Afr Med J 102: 81–83.
20. Becquet R, Marston M, Dabis F, Moulton LH, Gray G, et al. (2012) Children who acquire HIV infection perinatally are at higher risk of early death than those acquiring infection through breastmilk: a meta-analysis. PLoS One 7: e28510.
21. Vearey J (2012) Learning from HIV: exploring migration and health in South Africa. Glob Public Health 7: 58–70.
22. Seidenberg P, Nicholson S, Schaefer M, Semrau K, Bweupe M, et al. (2012) Early infant diagnosis of HIV infection in Zambia through mobile phone texting of blood test results. Bull World Health Organ 90: 348–356.
23. Silal SP, Penn-Kekana L, Harris B, Birch S, McIntyre D (2012) Exploring inequalities in access to and use of maternal health services in South Africa. BMC Health Serv Res 12: 120.
24. McCollum ED, Johnson DC, Chasela CS, Siwande LD, Kazembe PN, et al. (2012) Superior Uptake and Outcomes of Early Infant Diagnosis of HIV Services at an Immunization Clinic Versus an "Under-Five" General Pediatric Clinic in Malawi. J Acquir Immune Defic Syndr 60(4): e107–e110.
25. Jangam SR, Yamada DH, McFall SM, Kelso DM (2009) Rapid, point-of-care extraction of human immunodeficiency virus type 1 proviral DNA from whole blood for detection by real-time PCR. J Clin Microbiol 47: 2363–2368.
26. Parpia ZA, Elghanian R, Nabatiyan A, Hardie DR, Kelso DM (2010) p24 antigen rapid test for diagnosis of acute pediatric HIV infection. J Acquir Immune Defic Syndr 55: 413–419.
27. World Health Organisation, The Joint United Nations Programme on HIV/AIDS, and The United Nations Children's Fund (2010) Towards universal access: Scaling up priority HIV/AIDS interventions in the health sector - Progress report 2010. Geneva, Switzerland: WHO.

7

Conserved B-Cell Epitopes among Human Bocavirus Species Indicate Potential Diagnostic Targets

Zhuo Zhou[1§], Xin Gao[1§], Yaying Wang[1], Hongli Zhou[1], Chao Wu[1], Gláucia Paranhos-Baccalà[2], Guy Vernet[2], Li Guo[1]*, Jianwei Wang[1]*

1 MOH Key Laboratory of Systems Biology of Pathogens and Christophe Mérieux Laboratory, IPB, CAMS-Fondation Mérieux, Institute of Pathogen Biology (IPB), Chinese Academy of Medical Sciences (CAMS) & Peking Union Medical College (PUMC), Beijing, People's Republic of China, **2** Fondation Mérieux, Lyon, France

Abstract

Background: Human bocavirus species 1–4 (HBoV1–4) have been associated with respiratory and enteric infections in children. However, the immunological mechanisms in response to HBoV infections are not fully understood. Though previous studies have shown cross-reactivities between HBoV species, the epitopes responsible for this phenomenon remain unknown. In this study, we used genomic and immunologic approaches to identify the reactive epitopes conserved across multiple HBoV species and explored their potential as the basis of a novel diagnostic test for HBoVs.

Methodology/Principal Findings: We generated HBoV1–3 VP2 gene fragment phage display libraries (GFPDLs) and used these libraries to analyze mouse antisera against VP2 protein of HBoV1, 2, and 3, and human sera positive for HBoVs. Using this approach, we mapped four epitope clusters of HBoVs and identified two immunodominant peptides–P1 (^{1}MSDTDIQDQQPDTVDAPQNT^{20}), and P2 (^{162}EHAYPNASHPWDEDVMPDL^{180})–that are conserved among HBoV1–4. To confirm epitope immunogenicity, we immunized mice with the immunodominant P1 and P2 peptides identified in our screen and found that they elicited high titer antibodies in mice. These two antibodies could only recognize the VP2 of HBoV 1–4 in Western blot assays, rather than those of the two other parvoviruses human parvovirus B19 and human parvovirus 4 (PARV4). Based on our findings, we evaluated epitope-based peptide-IgM ELISAs as potential diagnostic tools for HBoVs IgM antibodies. We found that the P1+P2-IgM ELISA showed a higher sensitivity and specificity in HBoVs IgM detection than the assays using a single peptide.

Conclusions/Significance: The identification of the conserved B-cell epitopes among human bocavirus species contributes to our understanding of immunological cross-reactivities of HBoVs, and provides important insights for the development of HBoV diagnostic tools.

Editor: Fausto Baldanti, Fondazione IRCCS Policlinico San Matteo, Italy

Funding: This study was supported in part by the International Science and Technology Cooperation Program of China (2010DFB33270) (http://www.cistc.gov.cn) and by the National Major Science & Technology Project for Control and Prevention of Major Infectious Diseases of China (2012ZX10004-206) (http://www.nmp.gov.cn). The funders had no role in the study design, data collection and analysis, decision to publish, or preparation of the manuscript. No additional external funding was received for this study.

Competing Interests: The authors have declared that no competing interests exist.

* E-mail: wangjw28@163.com (JW); gnyny0803@163.com (LG)

§ These authors contributed equally to this work.

Introduction

Human bocavirus (HBoV) was first identified in nasopharyngeal samples of children with acute respiratory-tract infections (ARTIs) in 2005. This first virus was later designated as HBoV species 1 (HBoV1) [1]. HBoV1 is frequently detected in respiratory tract samples of children with upper or lower respiratory tract infections (URTIs/LRTIs) [2–5]. Three additional human bocavirus species, HBoV2, 3, and 4 were recently identified in fecal samples, but appear to be rare in respiratory tract samples and less prevalent in the population [6–10].

HBoV is frequently co-detected with other viruses and persists in the nasopharynx [11,12]. Thus, the extent of correlation between HBoV infection and human diseases remains elusive. However, severe HBoV infections have been recently reported in pediatric patients [13–15]. Mitui et al. reported that HBoV1 and HBoV2 DNA was the only pathogen nucleic acid detected in the cerebrospinal fluid specimens from children with severe encephalitis in Bangladesh [13], and Körner et al. confirmed HBoV infection in an 8-month-old girl with hypoxia, respiratory distress, wheezing, cough, and fever in Germany [14]. In addition, a case of life-threatening HBoV infection has been described in a pediatric patient with pneumothorax and acute respiratory failure in Slovenia [15]. These cases indicate that HBoVs may be etiological agents that can lead to severe and life-threatening diseases. In addition, a more recent longitudinal study of healthy children from infancy to early adolescence indicated that HBoV1 primary infection is significantly associated with ARTIs and otitis [16]. In light of these studies, convenient diagnostic tools for HBoV infections will be helpful for assessing the role HBoVs play in respiratory infections.

The most efficient and effective diagnostic tests should be capable of detecting multiple HBoV species in a single sample. One way to develop such a test is through the identification of an immunogenic epitope that is conserved across many HBoV species. The HBoV genome encodes four proteins–two nonstructural proteins (NS1 and NP1) and two overlapping capsid proteins (VP1 and VP2) [1]. In fact, recent evidence suggests that common immunoreactive epitopes among HBoVs may exist within the VP2 protein. For example, the VP2 protein contains the major antigen of HBoV and can form empty virus-like particles (VLPs). HBoV VLPs, which are similar in morphology and antigenicity to virions, have been successfully used as antigens for detecting antibodies against HBoVs [10,17,18]. Additionally, the homologies of the amino acid (aa) sequences of the HBoV1–4 VP2 are high – aa sequence identities of VP2 are about 77–78% between HBoV1 and HBoV2–4, 88–90% between HBoV2 and HBoV3–4,and 90.7% between HBoV3 and HBoV4. Further, recent studies have shown strong serological cross-reactivities among HBoV1–4 VP2 VLPs [9,10]. These data suggest that common immunoreactive epitopes among HBoVs may exist and highlight the potential for its use as a diagnostic tool for HBoV infection. However, the epitopes in the HBoV VP2 proteins have not been finely mapped.

Gene fragment phage display libraries (GFPDLs) have become a powerful tool to identify and map antigen epitopes following natural exposure to or vaccination against pathogens, and has contributed largely to infectious disease diagnostics, vaccine designs, and antibody repertoires evaluation [19–21]. In this study, we constructed HBoV1–3 GFPDLs to identify the VP2 epitopes recognized by mouse and human antisera. By comparing the epitope recognition maps, we identified conserved VP2 epitopes that demonstrated the potential of HBoV peptides for undifferentiating, single-well detection of antibodies against any of the four known HBoV species.

Results

HBoV VP2 epitopes identified by GFPDL panning

To identify antigenic clusters, we performed panning of GFPDLs with mouse antisera against VP2 protein of HBoV1, 2 and 3, as well as human sera positive for HBoVs. In the GFPDL screening, the phage clones that harbor inserts encoding epitopes, which can be recognized by mouse and human sera, were obtained in the affinity selections and were amplified by PCR for sequencing. Only the clones with a frequency of ≥ 2 in the panning were regarded as the positive clone [20]. Using these methods, we identified four antigenic clusters (I–IV), distributed across the VP2 protein (Figure 1). Of note, the sequences we identified share similar positions in HBoV1, 2, and 3. In addition, we found that the epitopes located at aa 1–20 (designated P1) in cluster I, and aa 162–180 (designated P2) in cluster II were present in HBoV1, 2, and 3. However, the epitopes in cluster III (P3) were only present in HBoV1 and HBoV3, and the epitopes in cluster IV (P4) were only present in HBoV1 and HBoV2. These results suggest that P1 and P2 may be conserved immunoreactive epitopes among HBoV species.

Immunogenicity of the immunodominant HBoV peptides

To test the immunogenicity of the VP2 segments identified by GFPDL panning, we synthesized two immunodominant peptides–P1 and P2, and used the keyhole limpet hemocyanin (KLH) conjugates of these peptides to immunize mice (Table 1). After three rounds of immunization, we effectively generated specific IgG antibodies against P1 and P2, and achieved titers as high as 1:160,000 (Figure 2A), indicating that the P1 and P2 peptides are strongly immunogenic peptides.

Conservation of P1 and P2 among HBoV species

To verify whether the peptides of P1 and P2 are conserved epitopes among the known HBoV species (HBoV1–4), we subjected the purified VP2 VLPs of HBoV1–4, human parvovirus B19 (B19), and human parvovirus 4 (PARV4) to Western blot analysis using mouse sera against P1 and P2. We found that the polyclonal antibodies against the two peptides reacted with HBoV1–4 VLPs rather than with the VLPs of B19 and PARV4 (Figure 2B). These results suggest that the peptides of P1 and P2 are HBoV specific and conserved among HBoV1–4.

To confirm the conservation of P1 and P2 among different HBoV species further, we aligned the amino acid sequences of P1 and P2 with the corresponding amino acid sequences of HBoV1–4. We found that ^{1}MS^{2} and ^{6}IQDQQP^{11} in the P1 epitope have 100% amino acid sequence identities among HBoV1, 2, 3, and 4; while ^{162}EHAYPNA^{168}, ^{170}HPWDEDVMP^{178}, and L^{180} in the P2 epitope showed 100% amino acid sequence identities among HBoV1, 2, 3, and 4 (Figure.3). These findings further indicate that the aa sequence of P1 and P2 are conserved among HBoV1–4.

Precise mapping of the HBoV epitopes

To precisely map the epitopes contained in P1 and P2, we performed a peptide-inhibition ELISA assay to examine the abilities of a panel of short peptides derived from P1 and P2 to inhibit the binding of mouse antisera to the parent peptides.

We found that the binding of P1 to anti-P1 was inhibited by the shorter peptides ^{1}MSDTDIQDQQPDTVD^{15} and ^{6}IQDQQPDTVDAPQNT^{20} (Figure 4A). However, the peptides ^{1}MSDTDIQDQQ^{10} and ^{11}PDTVDAPQNT^{20} lost the ability to block the binding of anti-P1 antibody to P1, which suggests that the peptide ^{6}IQDQQPDTVD^{15} is likely the critical peptide fragment for P1 antigenecity. Subsequently, we synthesized peptide ^{6}IQDQQPDTVD^{15} to confirm its ability to block the binding of anti-P1 antibody to P1 by peptide-inhibition ELISA. We found that the ^{6}IQDQQPDTVD^{15} peptide could inhibit the binding of anti-P1 to P1, though inhibition was less than that achieved with P1. To clarify whether the deleted N and C terminal amino acids could provide part of role in the binding to P1 antibody, we used peptide ^{5}DIQDQQPDTVDA^{16} to perform a peptide-inhibition ELISA. We found that the peptide ^{5}DIQDQQPDTVDA^{16} achieves inhibition that is comparable to P1 (Figure 4A), indicating that the deleted N and C terminal amino acids participate in the binding of P1 to anti-P1.

Furthermore, we observed that the binding of anti-P2 to P2 was blocked by the shorter peptide ^{167}NASHPWDEDVMPD^{180} (Figure 4C). However, the peptides ^{172}WDEDVMPDL^{180} and ^{162}EHAYPNASHPWDED^{175} lost the ability to inhibit the binding of anti-P2 to P2, which suggests that the peptides ^{167}NASHP^{171} and ^{176}VMPDL^{180} are also likely a critical part of the binding site for P2 antibody. To confirm their ability to block antibody binding, the peptides ^{167}NASHP^{171} and ^{176}VMPDL^{180} were used in a peptide-inhibition ELISA assay. We found that the peptides of ^{167}NASHP^{171} or ^{176}VMPDL^{180} alone was not able to block the binding of anti-P2 antibody to P2 (Figure 4C), suggesting additional amino acids among the peptides are also involved in the binding of P2 antibody.

To verify these findings in human humoral responses, we performed P1 and P2 peptide-inhibition ELISA assays using human sera positive for HBoVs. Interestingly, we achieved similar results with human and mouse sera (Figure 4B, 4D), except that the inhibition of antibody binding was less than that achieved with

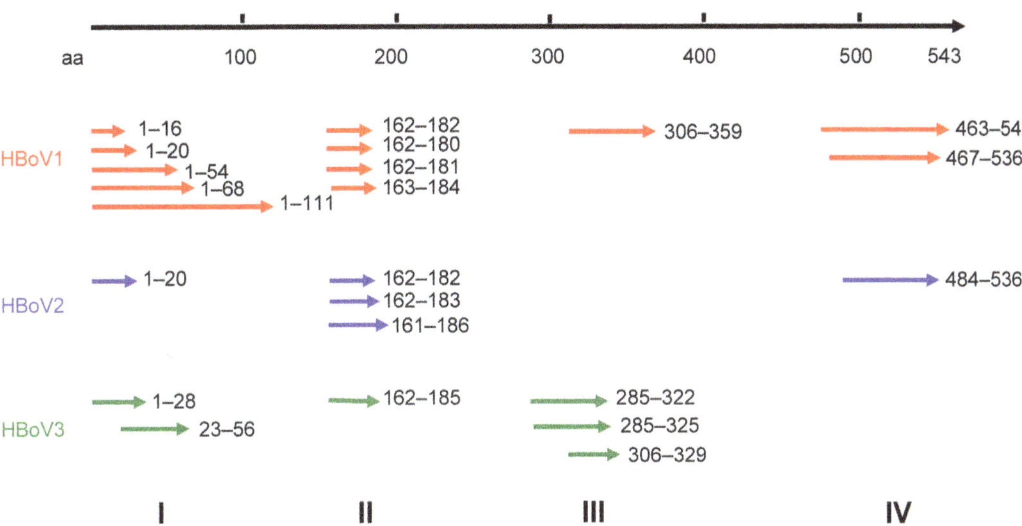

Figure 1. Epitopes identified in HBoV VP2 proteins by GFPDL screening. HBoV epitopes were identified by GFPDL panning using mouse sera obtained after immunization with HBoV1, 2, and 3 VP2, and human sera positive for HBoVs. Amino acid numbers correspond to HBoV strain 111-BJ07 (GenBank accession number JQ240469).

mouse sera. These results suggest that the P1 and P2 peptides can also stimulate humoral responses in humans. However, epitopes recognized and presented in the process of antigen presentation may be different in humans and mice, leading to differences in antigen structures essential for antibody binding.

Performance of peptide-IgM ELISA for HBoV antibody detection

As the P1 and P2 epitopes are antigenic and conserved among HBoV species, we developed an ELISA to detect IgM against HBoV and assessed its performance as a diagnostic tool by using clinical serum samples. Based on the findings from our epitope mapping experiments, P1 and P2 were used as coating antigens to keep the binding capacity of the epitopes. We compared the performance of P1, P2, or P1+P2 in detecting IgM (P1-IgM ELISA, P2-IgM ELISA, P1+P2-IgM ELISA), respectively. Acute-phase serum samples were obtained from 89 children with acute LRTIs from day 1 to 3 after onset of fever. The HBoV VLP IgM ELISA test was used as a positive control. Overall, results from the P1 and P2 IgM ELISAs were comparable to those achieved with the VLP IgM ELISA. Specifically, results matched 94.4% for P1-IgM ELISA, 95.5% for P2-IgM ELISA, and 95.5% for P1+P2-IgM ELISA (Table 2), indicating that the two methods have good correlation. However, the sensitivity and specificity of P1-, P2-, and P1+P2-IgM ELISA versus HBoV VLPs IgM ELISA was 72.7% and 97.4%, 72.2% and 98.7%, and 90% and 97.4%,

Table 1. Sequences of the peptides conjugated with KLH carrier for mice immunization.

Designation	Position	Sequence
P1-KLH	1–20[a]	KLH-CMSDTDIQDQQPDTVDAPQNT
P2-KLH	162–180[a]	KLH-CEHAYPNASHPWDEDVMPDL

[a]Indicated as the position corresponding to the VP2 protein of HBoV1 strain 111-BJ07
(GenBank accession number JQ240469).

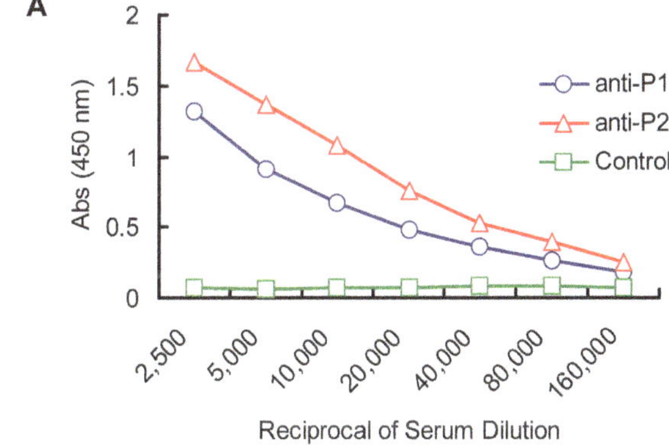

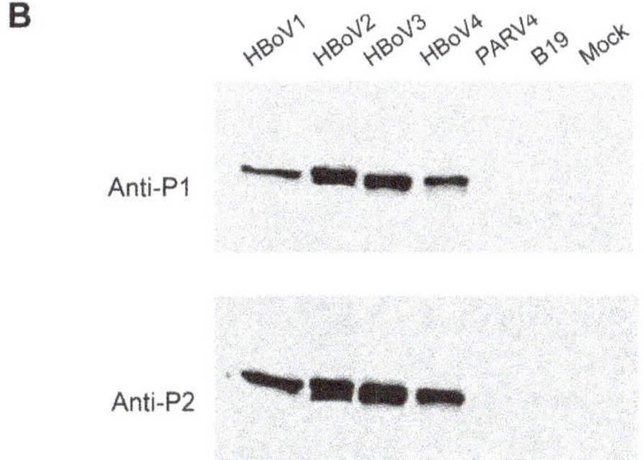

Figure 2. Antigenic characterization of potential HBoV epitopes P1 and P2. (A) Titers of IgG antibody against P1 and P2 in mouse sera. The titers of mice sera were determined as a series of two-fold dilutions by ELISA. (B) The immunological cross-reactivity was analyzed between mice antisera against P1 or P2 with virus-like particles (VLPs) of HBoV1, 2, 3, and 4 by Western blot. The VLPs of human parvovirus B19 and PARV4 were used as controls.

A

Strain name	GenBank number	aa1 … aa20
HBoV1 111-BJ07	JQ240469	M S D T D I Q D Q Q P - D T V D A P Q N T
HBoV1 ST1	DQ000495	. . . . - . . . . A
HBoV1 ST2	DQ000496	. . . . - . . . .
HBoV2 211-BJ07	JQ240470	. . E N E . . . . . . S . S M E E R G G G
HBoV2 277-BJ07	JQ240471	. . E N E . . . . . . S . S M E E R G G G
HBoV2 PK-2255	FJ170279	. . E N E . . . . . . S G S M E E R G G G
HBoV2 W153	EU82213	. . E N E . . . . . . S . S M E E R G G G
HBoV3 46-BJ07	HM132056	. . E N E . . . . . . S E P N . G Q R G G
HBoV3 W471	EU918736	. . E N E . . . . . . S E P N . G Q R G G
HBoV3 W855	EU948861	. . E N E . . . . . . S E P N . G Q R G G
HBoV4 NI385	FJ973561	. . E N E . . . . . . S . S M . G Q R G G

B

Strain name	GenBank number	aa162 … aa180
HBoV1 111-BJ07	JQ240469	E H A Y P N A S H P W D E D V M P D L
HBoV1 ST1	DQ000495	. . . .
HBoV1 ST2	DQ000496	. . . .
HBoV2 211-BJ07	JQ240470	. . . . T . . . . E .
HBoV2 277-BJ07	JQ240471	. . . . T . . . . E .
HBoV2 PK-2255	FJ170279	. . . . T . . . . E .
HBoV2 W153	EU82213	. . . . T . . . . E .
HBoV3 46-BJ07	HM132056	. . . . T . . . . E .
HBoV3 W471	EU918736	. . . . T . . . . E .
HBoV3 W855	EU948861	. . . . T . . . . E .
HBoV4 NI385	FJ973561	. . . . T . . . . E .

Figure 3. Alignment between the amino acid sequences of the peptides P1 and P2 with the corresponding representative VP2 sequences of HBoV species 1–4. Sequences of aa1 to 20, 162 to 180, according to the VP2 protein of HBoV strain 111-BJ07 (GenBank accession number JQ240469), are aligned with the corresponding region of multiple VP2 proteins of HBoV1–4 species using MEGA 4.0 software [28].

respectively. These data suggest that the P1+P2-IgM ELISA methods have stronger potential to detect IgM antibody against HBoVs than the assays using a single peptide.

Discussion

In this study, we identified immunodominant epitopes of HBoV VP2 proteins using the GFPDL assay. Our findings show that peptides P1 (aa 1–20) and P2 (aa 162–180) contain conserved epitopes among HBoV1–4, and elicit high titer antibodies in mice. They were also recognized by human polyclonal antibody. We also showed that though either P1 or P2 can be used in an ELISA to detect the IgM antibodies against HBoVs in acute phase sera from ARTI patients, the P1+P2-IgM ELISA showed higher sensitivity and specificity than the assays using single peptide alone. Thus, in addition to mapping the linear cross-reactive B cell epitopes areas among the four known HBoV species, our studies provide the basis for a potential diagnostic tool for HBoV infections.

Many patients show HBoVs persistence in the nasopharynx, which makes PCR-based diagnosis problematic [22]. Hence, immunological assays can be a useful method for diagnosing HBoV infections. Whereas peptide-based detection of antibodies involves relatively straightforward techniques, conventional VLP-based IgM and IgG ELISAs require laborious antigen preparation. As such, virus epitope-based peptide antigens have proven to be useful for laboratory diagnosis of some viral infections, including Influenza A virus [23], Dengue virus [24], and West Nile virus [25], etc. The results of the peptide ELISA tests in our study support the use of epitope-based peptides as serological reagents in the diagnosis of HBoV infection and suggest that the combination of two epitope-based peptides may increase the sensitivity of this method. In addition, we performed peptide P3- and P4- IgM ELISAs using acute-phase serum samples from children with acute LRTIs. However, we found that the sensitivity of these ELISA assays was low (45.4% for P3 and 54.5% for P4, respectively). As such, peptides P3 and P4 were not pursued as an approach for antibody detection.

In this study, we only screened the IgM antibody against HBoV from acute LRTI patients, as we would like to develop an alternative diagnostic tool for acute HBoV infections. Thus, the performance of this assay for IgG tests should be verified in future studies. Furthermore, we found that the absorption values at 450 nm of the peptide-based ELISA assay used to detect HBoV-infected serum samples were lower than that of HBoV VLP-based ELISA, as is the case of a serologic test based on Dengue virus B-cell epitopes [24]. Hence, it will be necessary to improve the detection sensitivity of the peptide ELISA method in future studies. For instance, conjugating the HBoV peptides to a carrier protein, such as bovine serum albumin (BSA), may be helpful to increase the absorbance in the ELISA assay [26].

In summary, we have identified two immunodominant epitopes that are conserved among all known HBoV species. These findings provide insight into the cross-reactivities of HBoV1–4. The study also provides a basis for developing new diagnostic tools for HBoV.

Materials and Methods

HBoV polyclonal antibodies and serum samples

Mouse antisera against the VP2 proteins of HBoV1, 2 and 3 were produced as previously described [10]. The human sera were

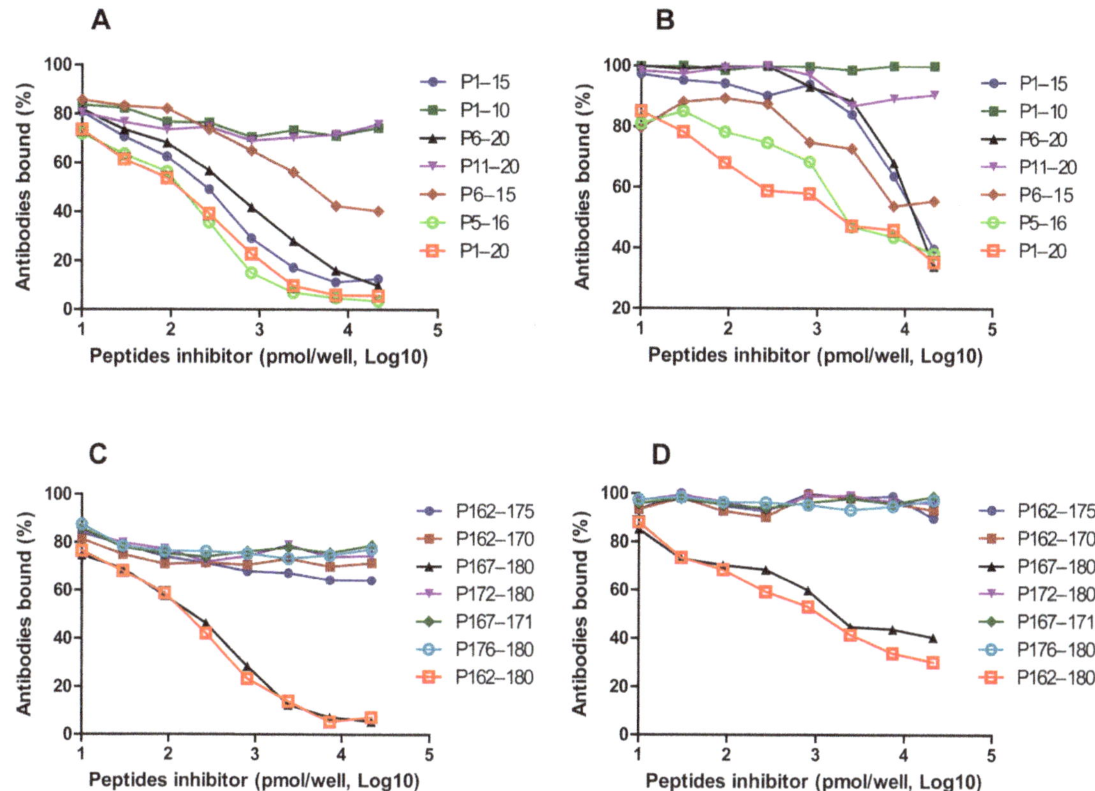

Figure 4. Inhibition of the binding of serum against P1 and P2 to parental peptide P1 and P2 by peptide homologs. Mouse antiserum samples induced by the P1-KLH/P2-KLH conjugate were tested by ELISA for their ability to bind to the P1/P2 peptide in the presence of dilutions of short peptide homologs to the P1 (A) and P2 (C) peptides. Human serum samples positive for HBoVs were tested by ELISA for their ability to bind to the P1/P2 peptide in the presence of dilutions of short peptide homologs to the P1 (B) and P2 (D) peptides.

identified as positive for HBoVs using VLP ELISA [10]. Acute-phase serum samples (taken within 3 days after the onset of fever) were collected from 89 children (median age 14 months; range of 1 month to 13 years) with acute lower respiratory tract infections (LRTIs) when they were hospitalized at the Beijing Children's Hospital.

Table 2. Comparison of peptide ELISA and VLP ELISA in detection of HBoV IgM antibodies.

	VLP		
P1	**Positive**	**Negative**	**Total**
Positive	8	2	10
Negative	3	76	79
Total	11	78	89
P2			
Positive	8	1	9
Negative	3	77	80
Total	11	78	89
P1+P2			
Positive	10	3	13
Negative	1	75	76
Total	11	78	89

Written informed consent was obtained from all guardians on behalf of children. This study was approved by the ethical review committee of the Institute of Pathogen Biology, the Chinese Academy of Medical Sciences, and by Beijing Children's Hospital.

Panning of GFPDLs

As the HBoV1, 2 and 3 are the major HBoV species detected in humans, we screened the epitopes in VP2 by GFPDLs using the full-length VP2 genes of HBoV1, 2 and 3 (GenBank accession numbers: JQ240469, JQ240470 and HM132056, respectively) [10]. The gIIIp display-based phage vector pCom3XV (a gift from Dr. Yuxian He at MOH Key Laboratory of Systems Biology of Pathogens, IPB, CAMS) was used to express the desired polypeptide as a gIIIp fusion protein. The library affinity selection was performed as previously described using mouse antisera against VP2 proteins of HBoV1, 2 and 3, and human polyclonal sera [19]. For GFPDL panning using mouse and human antisera, equal volumes of sera collected from five mice or five humans were pooled.

Peptides and conjugates

The immunodominant peptides –P1 (^{1}MSDTDIQDQQPDTVDAPQNT^{20}), and P2 (^{162}EHAYP-NASHPWDEDVMPDL^{180}), corresponding to the VP2 protein of HBoV1 strain 111-BJ07 (GenBank accession number JQ240469), were selected for immunization experiments (Table 1). To improve their immunogenicity, these peptides were synthesized and conjugated to KLH (Sigma, St. Louis, MO). To fine tune the epitope map of antibody binding sites on P1 and P2 peptides, a series of short peptides (unconjugated) homologous to the P1 and P2 peptides were synthesized by Sangon Biotech (Shanghai, China). Each peptide was purified to achieve a purity of ≥95% by high performance liquid chromatography. Each peptide was then verified by mass spectrometry.

Animal immunizations

Female BALB/c mice, six to eight weeks old, were subcutaneously immunized with 100 μg peptide-KLH conjugates in Freund's complete adjuvant (Sigma). The mice were boosted twice at 2-week intervals with 50 μg peptide-KLH conjugates in Freund's incomplete adjuvant (Sigma). Serum samples were collected two weeks after the last immunization. This study was carried out in strict accordance with Chinese government's animal experiment regulations. All animal experiments were performed in the facilities of the Institute of Laboratory Animal Sciences, Chinese Academy of Medical Sciences (ILAS, CAMS), and all experimental procedures were approved and supervised by the Animal Protection and Usage Committee of ILAS, CAMS.

ELISA

Indirect ELISA was used to detect mouse antibodies against P1 and P2, as described elsewhere [23]. Briefly, ninety six-well microtiter plates (Corning Costar, Acton, MA) were coated with peptides P1 and P2 at 1 μg/well in 0.1 M carbonate buffer (pH 9.6) at 4°C overnight.

Peptide-inhibition ELISA assays were performed to evaluate the reactivity of the P1- and P2-derived short peptides with the corresponding antibody against P1 and P2, as described elsewhere [23].

The reactivities of the synthetic P1 and P2 peptides (1 μg/well) with acute-phase serum samples from acute LRTI patients were also determined by ELISA. ELISA performed using coating antigens of HBoV1–4 VLPs (VLP ELISA) were used as positive controls, where 50 ng/well of each HBoV species VLPs were used to coat 96-well microtiter plates (Corning Costar) in 0.1 M carbonate buffer (pH 9.6) at 4°C overnight. The plates coated with peptides or VLPs were then blocked with 300 μL 1% (w/v) bovine serum albumin (BSA, Sigma) in PBS at 37°C for 2 h. Acute-phase serum samples (100 μL) were tested at 1:100 dilutions with HBoV peptides or HBoV1–4 VLPs, simultaneously. After washing five times with PBST (300 μL; PBS containing 0.5% Tween-20), HRP-conjugated goat anti-human IgM (100 μL; Sigma) was added to the plates at a dilution of 1:40,000 and the plates were incubated at 37°C for 1 h. Plates were washed five times with PBST (300 μL) and developed with substrate solutions A and B (100 μL; Wantai Biotech, Beijing, China). The absorbance of each serum sample was read at 450 nm using a multifunctional microplate reader, SpectraMax M5 (Molecular Devices, Sunnyvale, CA). As the VLP ELISA is designed to test for all four HBoV species in one well, a positive result indicates that the sample is infected with at least one of the four HBoVs (HBoV1, HBoV2, HBoV3 or HBoV4) and a negative result indicates that the serum sample is negative for all four HBoVs.

To determine the cut-off value, all the absorbance values below a provisional cut-off of 0.20 were taken and their mean and standard deviations (SD) were calculated as previously reported by Kahn and Hustedt [18,27]. All samples with values above 0.18 and 0.15 (mean + 3 SD) were considered positive for HBoV VLPs IgM ELISA and peptide IgM ELISA.

Western blot analysis

HBoV1–4 VLPs, B19 VLPs, and PARV4) VLPs were expressed and purified, as described previously [10]. The VLPs of HBoV1–4, B19, and PARV4 were loaded on a 12% SDS-PAGE gel. The gels were transferred to a nitrocellulose membrane (Pall, Port Washington, NY) and blocked with 5% nonfat dry milk. The P1 and P2 peptide antibodies produced in mice were applied followed by incubation with the corresponding goat anti-mouse IRDye Fluor 800-labeled IgG secondary antibody (1:10,000) (Li-Cor, Lincoln, NE). The membranes were scanned by the Odyssey Infrared Imaging System (Li-Cor) and analyzed with Odyssey software.

Acknowledgments

We thank Beijing Children's Hospital for providing the blood samples, and Dr. Yuxian He of MOH Key Laboratory of Systems Biology of Pathogens, IPB, CAMS for providing plasmid pCom3XV.

Author Contributions

Conceived and designed the experiments: ZZ XG YW GPB GV LG JW. Performed the experiments: ZZ XG YW LG HZ CW. Analyzed the data: ZZ XG LG JW. Contributed reagents/materials/analysis tools: ZZ XG LG JW. Wrote the paper: LG ZZ XG JW. Contributed to the scientific discussions: LG JW.

References

1. Allander T, Tammi MT, Eriksson M, Bjerkner A, Tiveljung-Lindell A, et al. (2005) Cloning of a human parvovirus by molecular screening of respiratory tract samples. Proc Natl Acad Sci U S A 102: 12891–12896.
2. Allander T, Jartti T, Gupta S, Niesters HG, Lehtinen P, et al. (2007) Human bocavirus and acute wheezing in children. Clin Infect Dis 44: 904–910.
3. Kesebir D, Vazquez M, Weibel C, Shapiro ED, Ferguson D, et al. (2006) Human bocavirus infection in young children in the United States: molecular epidemiological profile and clinical characteristics of a newly emerging respiratory virus. J Infect Dis 194: 1276–1282.
4. Lau SK, Yip CC, Que TL, Lee RA, Au-Yeung RK, et al. (2007) Clinical and molecular epidemiology of human bocavirus in respiratory and fecal samples from children in Hong Kong. J Infect Dis 196: 986–993.
5. Guo L, Gonzalez R, Xie Z, Zhou H, Liu C, et al. (2011) Bocavirus in children with respiratory tract infections. Emerg Infect Dis 17: 1775–1777.
6. Kapoor A, Slikas E, Simmonds P, Chieochansin T, Naeem A, et al. (2009) A newly identified bocavirus species in human stool. J Infect Dis 199: 196–200.
7. Arthur JL, Higgins GD, Davidson GP, Givney RC, Ratcliff RM. (2009) A novel bocavirus associated with acute gastroenteritis in Australian children. PLoS Pathog 5: e1000391.
8. Kapoor A, Simmonds P, Slikas E, Li L, Bodhidatta L, et al. (2010) Human bocaviruses are highly diverse, dispersed, recombination prone, and prevalent in enteric infections. J Infect Dis 201: 1633–1643.
9. Kantola K, Hedman L, Arthur J, Alibeto A, Delwart E, et al. (2011) Seroepidemiology of human bocaviruses 1-4. J Infect Dis 204: 1403–1412.
10. Guo L, Wang Y, Zhou H, Wu C, Song J, et al. (2012) Differential seroprevalence of human bocavirus species 1-4 in Beijing, China. PLoS One 7: e39644.
11. Blessing K, Neske F, Herre U, Kreth HW, Weissbrich B (2009) Prolonged detection of human bocavirus DNA in nasopharyngeal aspirates of children with respiratory tract disease. Pediatr Infect Dis J 28: 1018–1019.
12. Martin ET, Fairchok MP, Kuypers J, Magaret A, Zerr DM, et al. (2010) Frequent and prolonged shedding of bocavirus in young children attending daycare. J Infect Dis 201: 1625–1632.
13. Mitui MT, Tabib SM, Matsumoto T, Khanam W, Ahmed S, et al. (2012) Detection of human bocavirus in the cerebrospinal fluid of children with encephalitis. Clin Infect Dis 54: 964–967.
14. Körner RW, Söderlund-Venermo M, van Koningsbruggen-Rietschel S, Kaiser R, Malecki M, et al. (2011) Severe human bocavirus infection, Germany. Emerg Infect Dis 17: 2303–2305.
15. Ursic T, Steyer A, Kopriva S, Kalan G, Krivec U, et al. (2011) Human bocavirus as the cause of a life-threatening infection. J Clin Microbiol 49: 1179–1181.

16. Meriluoto M, Hedman L, Tanner L, Simell V, Mäkinen M, et al. (2012) Association of human bocavirus 1 infection with respiratory disease in childhood follow-up study, Finland. Emerg Infect Dis 18: 264–271.
17. Lin F, Guan W, Cheng F, Yang N, Pintel D, et al. (2008) ELISAs using human bocavirus VP2 virus-like particles for detection of antibodies against HBoV. J Virol Methods 149: 110–117.
18. Kahn JS, Kesebir D, Cotmore SF, D'Abramo A Jr, Cosby C, et al. (2008) Seroepidemiology of human bocavirus defined using recombinant virus-like particles. J Infect Dis 198: 41–50.
19. Khurana S, Suguitan AL Jr, Rivera Y, Simmons CP, Lanzavecchia A, et al. (2009) Antigenic fingerprinting of H5N1 avian influenza using convalescent sera and monoclonal antibodies reveals potential vaccine and diagnostic targets. PLoS Med 6: e1000049.
20. Verma N, Dimitrova M, Carter DM, Crevar CJ, Ross TM, et al. (2012) Influenza virus H1N1pdm09 infections in the young and old: evidence of greater antibody diversity and affinity for the hemagglutinin globular head domain (HA1 Domain) in the elderly than in young adults and children. J Virol 86: 5515–5522.
21. Khurana S, Wu J, Verma N, Verma S, Raghunandan R, et al. (2011) H5N1 virus-like particle vaccine elicits cross-reactive neutralizing antibodies that preferentially bind to the oligomeric form of influenza virus hemagglutinin in humans. J Virol 85: 10945–10954.
22. Kantola K, Hedman L, Allander T, Jartti T, Lehtinen P, et al. (2008) Serodiagnosis of human bocavirus infection. Clin Infect Dis 46: 540–546.
23. Zhao R, Cui S, Guo L, Wu C, Gonzalez R, et al. (2011) Identification of a highly conserved H1 subtype-specific epitope with diagnostic potential in the hemagglutinin protein of influenza A virus. PLoS One 6: e23374.
24. Wu HC, Huang YL, Chao TT, Jan JT, Huang JL, et al. (2001) Identification of B-cell epitope of dengue virus type 1 and its application in diagnosis of patients. J Clin Microbiol 39: 977–982.
25. Sun EC, Ma JN, Liu NH, Yang T, Zhao J, et al. (2011) Identification of two linear B-cell epitopes from West Nile virus NS1 by screening a phage-displayed random peptide library. BMC Microbiol 11: 160.
26. Dubois ME, Hammarlund E, Slifka MK (2012) Optimization of peptide-based ELISA for serological diagnostics: a retrospective study of human monkeypox infection. Vector Borne Zoonotic Dis 12: 400–409.
27. Hustedt JW, Christie C, Hustedt MM, Esposito D, Vazquez M (2012) Seroepidemiology of human bocavirus infection in Jamaica. PLoS One 7: e38206.
28. Tamura K, Dudley J, Nei M, Kumar S (2007) MEGA4: Molecular Evolutionary Genetics Analysis (MEGA) software version 4.0. Mol Biol Evol 24: 1596–1599.

8

High Drug Resistance Prevalence among Vertically HIV-Infected Patients Transferred from Pediatric Care to Adult Units in Spain

Miguel de Mulder[1], Gonzalo Yebra[1], Adriana Navas[2], María Isabel de José[3], María Dolores Gurbindo[4], María Isabel González-Tomé[5], María José Mellado[6], Jesús Saavedra-Lozano[4], María Ángeles Muñoz-Fernández[7], Santiago Jiménez de Ory[7], José Tomás Ramos[8], África Holguín[1]*, on behalf of the Madrid Cohort of HIV-Infected Children¶

1 HIV-1 Molecular Epidemiology Laboratory, Microbiology and Parasitology Department, Hospital Universitario Ramón y Cajal, IRYCIS and CIBER-ESP, Madrid, Spain, **2** Pediatrics Department, Hospital Universitario Infanta Leonor, Madrid, Spain, **3** Pediatrics Department, Hospital Universitario La Paz, Madrid, Spain, **4** Pediatrics Department, Hospital General Universitario Gregorio Marañón, Madrid, Spain, **5** Pediatrics Department, Hospital Universitario Doce de Octubre, Madrid, Spain, **6** Pediatrics Department, Hospital Carlos III, Madrid, Spain, **7** Molecular Immunobiology Laboratory, Hospital General Universitario Gregorio Marañón, Madrid, Spain, **8** Pediatrics Department, Hospital Universitario de Getafe, Madrid, Spain

Abstract

Background: Antiretroviral treatment (ART) has contributed to increased life expectancy of HIV-1 infected children. In developed countries, an increasing number of children reaching adulthood are transferred to adult units. The objectives were to describe the demographic and clinical features, ART history, antiviral drug resistance and drug susceptibility in HIV-1 perinatally infected adolescents transferred to adult care units in Spain from the Madrid Cohort of HIV-1 infected children.

Methods: Clinical, virological and immunological features of HIV-1 vertically infected patients in the Madrid Cohort of HIV-infected children were analyzed at the time of transfer. *Pol* sequences from each patient were recovered before transfer. Resistance mutations according to the International AIDS Society 2011 list were identified and interpreted using the Stanford algorithm. Results were compared to the non-transferred HIV-1 infected pediatric cohort from Madrid.

Results: One hundred twelve infected patients were transferred to adult units between 1997 and 2011. They were mainly perinatally infected (93.7%), with a mean nadir CD4+-T-cells count of 10% and presented moderate or severe clinical symptoms (75%). By the time of transfer, the mean age was 18.9 years, the mean CD4+T-cells count was 627.5 cells/ml, 64.2% presented more than 350 CD4+T-cells/ml and 47.3% had ≤200 RNA-copies/ml. Most (97.3%) were ART experienced receiving Highly Active ART (HAART) (84.8%). Resistance prevalence among pretreated was 50.9%, 76.9% and 36.5% for Protease Inhibitors (PI), Nucleoside Reverse Transcriptase Inhibitors (NRTI) and Non-NRTI (NNRTI), respectively. Resistance mutations were significantly higher among transferred patients compared to non-transferred for the PI+NRTI combination (19% *vs.* 8.4%). Triple resistance was similar to non-transferred pediatric patients (17.3% *vs.* 17.6%).

Conclusion: Despite a good immunological and virological control before transfer, we found high levels of resistance to PI, NRTI and triple drug resistance in HIV-1 infected adolescents transferred to adult units.

Editor: Douglas F. Nixon, University of California San Francisco, United States of America

Funding: This work was supported in part by grants from Fondo de Investigaciones Sanitarias (FIS) from Ministerio de Ciencia e Innovación (grants PI09/00284 and PI07/0236) and from Fundación para la Investigación y Prevención del SIDA en España (FIPSE, grant 360829/09). MDM is supported by PI09/00284 and PI07/0236. GY is supported by Consejería de Educación de la Comunidad de Madrid and Fondo Social Europeo (FSE). AH is supported by Agencia Laín Entralgo. The funders had no role in study design, data collection and analysis, decision to publish, or preparation of the manuscript.

Competing Interests: The authors have declared that no competing interests exist.

* E-mail: aholguin.hciii@salud.madrid.org

¶ Membership of the Madrid Cohort of HIV-Infected Children is provided in the Acknowledgments

Introduction

By the end of 2010, of the 34 million people living with human immunodeficiency virus (HIV), there were 3.4 million children below the age of 15 years [1]. During 2010, 390.000 children were infected with HIV and 250.000 died from AIDS related causes [1]. In Western Europe and North America the HIV epidemic has remained stable since 2004. In 2010, one million infected individuals lived in Western and Central Europe, including 6,000 infected children [1]. In the WHO European Region of the 646 children who acquired the HIV infection through mother-to-child transmission (MTCT) [2], 19% of them originated from countries with generalized epidemics (in sub-Saharan Africa, the Caribbean and Asia).

Due to the expanded access to highly active antiretroviral treatment (HAART) and prevention efforts in HIV testing, prenatal care, formula feeding, elective Caesarean and pregnancy monitoring [3–5], few children were newly infected with HIV (<500) or died from AIDS-related illnesses (<500) in Western Europe in 2010. This reflects the extensive provision of services that can prevent MTCT of HIV [6,7]. Despite the success of preventive measures, MTCT still occurs in high-income countries [8–10] mainly due to infected immigrants from countries with a high HIV prevalence and within social compartments that refuse pregnancy monitoring and HIV testing. A total of 80.827 cases of AIDS had been declared in Spain [11] by the end of 2010; these 958 were children infected through MTCT. During 2010, a total of 2907 new HIV infections cases were notified in Spain, twelve of them caused by MTCT (0.4%) mainly (8/12 cases) among foreign patients. In the region of Madrid, a total of 805 HIV infection cases were reported in 2010, 2 of them caused by MTCT [11].

In developed settings with access to HAART, perinatally acquired HIV-1 infection has become a chronic disease of childhood with increasing numbers of adolescents surviving to adulthood and transitioning from pediatric to adult services. Perinatally infected adolescents have been heavily pretreated, have a long history of treatment with many switches and variable levels of adherence to the treatment have been reported. Sub-optimal treatments and non-complete compliance can increase the prevalence of drug resistance mutations in HIV thus, compromising the success of present and future treatment options.

Successful transition to adult services has become a necessity in these heavily pretreated patients. Teenagers growing up with HIV/AIDS have common problems related to social difficulties and to side-effects of HIV and HAART which play an impact on their growth and development. The objectives of this study were to describe the demographic and clinical features, antiretroviral therapy (ART) history, antiviral drug resistance and susceptibility to drugs in HIV-1 perinatally infected adolescents transferred to adult units in Spain from the Madrid Cohort of HIV-1 infected children.

Patients and Methods

Study Population

Since the beginning of the HIV epidemic in Spain, a total of 534 patients have been registered in the Madrid cohort of HIV-infected children established in 2003. By the end of December 2011, 175 of them still remained under clinical follow-up in pediatric units, 112 had been transferred to adult units, 62 had been lost to follow-up and 185 had died. In this study we selected the 112 patients from the cohort that had reached adolescence and been transferred to adult units in 8 public hospitals from 1997 to December 2011. Clinical and epidemiological features of all transferred patients were recorded from the database of the cohort.

An additional cohort of HIV-1 infected patients was used to compare results on drug resistance and drug sensitivity. The selected cohort consisted of the HIV Madrid cohort of non-transferred perinatally infected patients previously described [12,13].

This study was part of a project approved by the review board of the Hospital Universitario Ramón y Cajal Clinical Research Ethical Committee. It was designed to protect the right of all subjects involved under the appropriate local regulations. To maintain subject confidentiality, a unique number was assigned to each specimen, and written consent obtained for each patient by clinicians.

Drug Resistance Analysis

For the drug resistance study, we selected those transferred patients according to *pol* sequence, genotypic resistance profile or sample availability by December 2011. Most genetic sequences and genotypic resistance profiles were previously reported [12,13] or recovered from clinical routine drug-resistance tests performed in hospitals where patients were or had been under follow-up. When more than one sample was available per patient, we selected the closest and previous to the time of transference to adult units among transferred subjects and the most recent for non-transferred patients.

Previously reported genotypes were performed from infected samples (immortalized DNA, plasma or peripheral blood mononuclear cells, PBMCs) kindly provided by the HIV BioBank integrated in the Spanish AIDS Research Network (RIS) [14,15]. Samples from patients were processed following current procedures and frozen immediately after their reception. Sample collection, processing and storing were performed under international guidelines for biological storing and under supervision of a Scientific and Ethical Committee. HIV-1 subtyping of new sequences was performed by phylogenetic analysis (phy) as previously described [13].

The prevalence of transmitted drug resistance among naïve patients was defined according to the list of mutations for Transmitted Drug Resistances (TDR) surveillance, as recommended by the WHO [16] using the Calibrated Population Resistance tool [17]. Drug-resistance mutations (DRM) in pretreated patients were defined by the International AIDS Society-USA list (IAS) [18]. Drug susceptibility was estimated for each available antiretroviral according to the HIVdb Interpretation Algorithm version 6.0.11 (Stanford University, Palo Alto, CA, USA) [19].

Statistical Analysis

Prevalence was expressed in percentage with a 95% confidence interval (CI). CI tests were performed with Epidat 3.1 (Pan American Health Organization). Statistical significance was set at $p<0.05$.

Results

Baseline Features of the Transferred Population

A total of 112 patients of the Madrid cohort of HIV-infected children transferred from pediatric services to adult units in different hospitals in Madrid between 1997 and December 2011 were selected for this study. Baseline characteristics of the non-transferred (n = 131), total transferred (n = 112), and transferred patients with available genotypic profile (n = 63) are summarized in **Table 1**. All transferred patients were HIV-1 diagnosed at childhood (mean 2 years of age), the majority were born in Spain (91.9%) and mainly infected through MTCT (93.7%). Only a few (12.5%) were adopted. Most (81.3%) were diagnosed along the 1985–1994 period. The median duration of follow-up was 13.2 (Standard Deviation, SD 5.2), 15.6 (SD 4.5), and 16.7 (SD 3.6) years for non-transferred, transferred (n = 112) and transferred with available resistance genotypic profile, respectively.

Advanced stages of immunosuppression were observed as a result of the long term infection and scarce effective antiretroviral availability before 1996. Over two thirds of transferred patients reached less than 15% CD4+ cell counts and half (57.1%) reached <200 cells/mm^3. The mean nadir CD4+ T-cells count was 10%. Monotherapy was the first ARV treatment in 59.8%, mainly with AZT (79.1%), 23.2% started with combined therapy (including AZT backbone in 88.4% of them) and only 14.3% with HAART.

Table 1. Baseline characteristics of the non-transferred, transferred and transferred with available genotypic profile patients.

Features	Non-transferred n = 131	Transferred n = 112	Transferred with genotype* n = 63
	[n (%)]	[n (%)]	[n (%)]
Adopted	31 (23.7)	14 (12.5)	8 (12.7)
Female gender	76 (58)	60 (53.6)	34 (54)
Median age until diagnosis (years)	0.5	2	1.4
Non-B variants prevalence (%)	11.6	–	1.9
Demographics			
Caucasian	100 (76.3)	98 (87.5)	59 (93.6)
Hispanic	6 (4.6)	4 (3.5)	2 (3.2)
Romani	4 (3.1)	3 (2.7)	1 (1.6)
African**	18 (13.7)	2 (1.8)	–
Other	2 (1.5)	2 (1.8)	1 (1.6)
Unknown	1 (0.8)	3 (2.7)	–
Origin[a]			
Europe	112 (85.5)	105 (93.7)	61 (96.8)
North America	1 (0.8)	–	–
South and Central America	8 (6.1)	5 (4.5)	2 (3.2)
North Africa	2 (1.5)	–	–
Sub-Saharan Africa	7 (5.3)	2 (1.8)	–
Asia	1 (0.8)	–	–
Year of HIV diagnosis			
1985–1989**	1 (0.8)	31 (27.7)	16 (25.4)
1990–1994**	37 (28.2)	60 (53.6)	39 (61.9)
1995–1999**	54 (41.2)	18 (16)	7 (11.1)
2000–2004**	28 (21.4)	3 (2.7)	1 (1.6)
2005–2009	10 (7.6)	–	–
Unknown	1 (0.8)	–	–
Route of infection			
Perinatally	127 (96.9)	105 (93.7)	61 (96.8)
Transfusion	3 (2.3)	5 (4.5)	2 (3.2)
Unknown	1 (0.8)	2 (1.8)	–
Year of transfer			
1997–1999	–	3 (2.7)	–
2000–2002	–	9 (8)	1 (1.6)
2003–2005	–	27 (24.1)	13 (20.7)
2006–2008	–	33 (29.5)	21 (33.3)
2009–2011	–	40 (35.7)	28 (44.4)
Nadir CD4 count achieved		Mean 10%	Mean 11%
<15%	67 (51.1)	75 (67)	43 (68.3)
15–24%	42 (32.1)	24 (21.4)	13 (20.6)
≥25%	19 (14.5)	13 (11.6)	7 (11.1)
Unknown	3 (2.3)	–	–
Nadir CD4 count achieved (cells/mm^3)			
<200**	35 (26.7)	64 (57.1)	31 (52.4)
200–499	63 (48.1)	37 (33)	26 (38.1)
≥500**	30 (22.9)	11 (9.9)	6 (9.5)
Unknown	3 (2.3)	–	–

[a]Origin of patients by country: Spain (n = 103), Portugal (n = 1), Romania (n = 1), Honduras (n = 2), Argentina (n = 1), Mexico (n = 1), Peru (n = 1), Cape Verde (n = 1), Equatorial Guinea (n = 1).

*Transferred to adult units with available resistance genotyping profile.

**Statistical differences ($p<0.05$) have been found between transferred and non-transferred patients for these features. HIV-1 non-B variants include HIV-1 non-B subtypes and recombinants.

In the transferred cohort compared to the non-transferred, a statistical significant lower number of African patients were found (1.8% *vs.* 13.7%, p<0.05), a significant higher number of children reached nadir CD4-Tcell values below 200 (57.1 *vs.* 26.7, p<0.05) and a lower number of patients achieved CD4 T-cells over 500 (9.9% *vs.* 22.9%, p<0.05). No statistical differences were found in the baseline studied characteristics between transferred patients with and without available genotype (**Table 1**).

Features of the Population at the Time of Transfer

Characteristics of the study population at the time of transfer to adult units are shown in **Table 2**. By the time of transfer, the mean age was 18.9 years and the mean CD4+T-cells count 627.5 cells/ml. 5.4% presented less than 15% CD4+T-cells, 66% more than 25% and 55.3% more than 500 CD4+ cells/ml counts. Nearly all (98.2%) had presented signs and symptoms of AIDS according to CDC classification [20], which were severe in 34.8% of cases. Immunological status at the time of the transfer revealed an immunologically severe suppression in 66.9% (CDC stage 3). Among the 102 patients with available viral load data, 56.2% had ≤500 RNA-copies/ml and 38.4% undetectable viraemia (≤50 RNA-copies/ml).

Comparison among transferred and non-transferred patients by December 2011 revealed that transferred patients had a worst immunological-virological profile comparing to the non-transferred group. A lower number of transferred patients were categorized in clinical status A (23.2% *vs.* 37.4%, p<0.05) and achieved undetectable levels of viraemia (38.4% *vs.* 64.9%, p<0.05). T-cell CD4 counts (either ≥25% or >500 CD4+ T-cells) were also lower among transferred and a lower number of transferred were on HAART (84.8% *vs.* 94.6%, p<0.05). No statistical differences were found in studied clinical features by December 2011 between transferred patients with and without available genotype (**Table 2**).

ART Experience among Transferred Patients

The transferred cohort started any type of ART with a median age of 5.6 years (SD 3.5 years) and the median duration of ART was 11.5 years (SD 4.8 years). Only 3 (2.7%) of the 112 transferred individuals remained drug naïve at transfer and the rest (97.3%) were ART experienced. Most (84.8%) were receiving HAART, 9.8% had stopped treatment and 2.7% were receiving combined therapy at the transfer time according to clinical reports. The most commonly used HAART combinations in our cohort were 2NRTI+1NNRTI (32.6%) and 2NRTI+1PI (28.4%). The pretreated patients presented a long treatment history and had experienced several different ART combinations; the mean number of regimens was five, with at least 3 HAART regimens in 48% of them. The main ART families were NRTI, PI and NNRTI, 94.6%, 84.8%, and 72.3% respectively (**Table 2**). Triple class experience was found in almost two-thirds of patients. Use of other drug families was scarce and only three transferred patients had experience with the fusion inhibitor, enfuvirtide and one of them also had received raltegravir, an integrase inhibitor. Adherence history was assessed according to clinical charts data but was not available in all cases.

High Prevalence of HIV-1 Resistant Variants in Pretreated Transferred Patients

Among the 112 patients transferred before the end of December 2011, only in 63 (56.2%) subjects drug resistance genotypes could be analyzed. Among them, in 48 (76.2%) cases the *pol* sequence had been previously reported by our group [12,13]. In the remaining 15 patients, six patients had an available plasma specimen stored in the HIV-1 Spanish Biobank and new HIV-1 *pol* sequences were newly generated as previously reported [13]. Other 9 patients presented a genotypic resistance profile derived from *pol* sequences obtained from plasma specimens recovered from clinical routine drug-resistance tests performed in hospitals where the patients were or had been under follow-up. However, no fasta format sequences of any profile were available. Clinical specimens in all 63 genotyped samples were obtained before the transfer time to adult units: during 1993–1999 (5 genotypes), 2000–2004 (27 genotypes) and 2005–2010 (31 genotypes). The median age of patients when genotypic data was generated was 14.7 years old (SD 4.4). The 63 patients with available genotypic data included five genotypes (accession numbers HQ426734, HQ426806, HQ426860, HQ426867, HQ426893) performed before treatment was initiated. Out of these five, only 2 patients remained drug naïve until they were transferred to adult units while the other 3 received any ART during their follow-up. None of these sequences harboured TDR mutations.

Among the 63 transferred patients of the Madrid cohort of HIV-infected children with available *pol* sequences or resistance profiles, the prevalence of HIV drug resistance mutations was analyzed according to the drug class family. Fifty-eight were pretreated and 5 remained drug-naïve at sampling time. No TDR mutations were found among the *pol* sequences from the 5 transferred naïve subjects. The most prevalent DRM found in the 58 transferred ART-experienced patients were: for PI, L90M (27.5%), V82A (15.7%), M46I (13.7%) and D30N (9.8%); for NRTI, M41L (48.1%), D67N (40.4%), T215Y (40.4%), L210W (34.6%), M184V (25%), T69D (23.1%), and K219Q (23.1%); and for NNRTI, K103N (19.2%), Y181C (7.7%) and G190A (7.7%).

Global resistance prevalence among the 58 transferred ARV-exposed pretreated patients with available *pol* sequences or resistance profiles was 50.9% for PI, 76.9% for NRTI and 36.5% for NNRTI (**Table 3**). No primary drug resistance mutations were found among naïve subjects. According to our data, no statistical differences were found between the resistance rate and the duration of treatment (data not shown).

Higher Prevalence of Drug Resistance Mutations Among Transferred Patients than in Non-transferred

Besides assessing the global prevalence of DRM in the 58 pretreated patients of the transferred cohort, prevalence of DRM was also compared to the non-transferred cohort. The first included the 58 transferred and pretreated patients with available genotypic data compared to the 131 non-transferred pretreated pediatric patients from the Madrid cohort of HIV-1 infected children (**Table 3**). All 131 non-transferred pediatric patients had available resistance genotype, previously reported [12,13] and with available GenBank accession numbers.

Transferred patients tended to present higher DRM prevalence when compared to non-transferred children (**Table 3**). Drug resistance mutations were found in a higher number of transferred patients than in the non-transferred pretreated population under follow up in Madrid for PI (50.9% *vs.* 36.8%, p = NS) and for NRTI, 76.9% *vs.* 62.1%, p = NS) and lower for NNRTI (36.5% vs. 40.5%, p = NS). However, resistance prevalence was significantly higher among transferred patients for the PI+NRTI combination (19% *vs.* 8.4%, p<0.05). Triple resistance was similar to non-transferred pediatric patients (17.3% *vs.* 17.6%, p = NS).

Table 2. Characteristics of the non-transferred, transferred and transferred with available genotypic profile patients by December 2011.

Features	Non-transferred n = 131	Transferred n = 112	Transferred with genotype* n = 63
Mean age (years)	14.7	18.9	18.5
LTNP [n (%)]	1 (0.8)	5 (4.5)	2 (3.2)
Median ART duration [years (SD)]	12 (4.5)	11.5 (4.8)	13.5 (4.1)
Median follow-up [years SD)]	13.2 (5.2)	15.6 (4.5)	16.7 (3.6)
Immunological status [n (%)]			
1	8 (6.1)	4 (3.6)	2 (3.2)
2	41 (31.3)	31 (27.7)	18 (28.5)
3	79 (60.3)	75 (66.9)	43 (68.3)
Unknown	3 (2.3)	2 (1.8)	-
Clinical status [n (%)]			
N	-	2 (1.8)	1 (1.6)
A**	49 (37.4)	26 (23.2)	14 (22.2)
B**	35 (26.7)	45 (40.2)	23 (36.5)
C	43 (32.8)	39 (34.8)	25 (39.7)
Unknown	4 (3.1)	-	-
CD4 count (%) [n (%)]			
<15%	3 (2.3)	6 (5.4)	3 (4.8)
15–24%	18 (13.7)	26 (23.2)	15 (23.8)
≥25%**	105 (80.2)	74 (66)	43 (68.2)
Unknown	5 (3.8)	6 (5.4)	2 (3.2)
CD4 count (cells/ml) [n (%)]			
	Mean 770.5 cells/ml	Mean 627.5 cells/ml	Mean 654 cells/ml
≤200	3 (2.3)	4 (3.6)	1 (1.6)
201–350	6 (4.6)	7 (6.3)	5 (7.9)
351–500	13 (9.9)	10 (8.9)	4 (6.4)
>500**	99 (75.6)	62 (55.3)	36 (57.1)
Unknown	10 (7.6)	29 (25.9)	17 (27)
Viral load (HIV-1 RNA-copies/ml) [n (%)]			
≤20**	41 (31.3)	12 (10.7)	9 (14.2)
21–50	44 (33.6)	31 (27.7)	23 (36.5)
51–200	10 (7.6)	10 (8.9)	4 (6.4)
201–500	7 (5.3)	10 (8.9)	2 (3.2)
501–1,000	-	4 (3.6)	3 (4.8)
1,001–10,000	12 (9.2)	19 (17)	9 (14.3)
>10,000	13 (9.9)	16 (14.3)	11 (17.4)
Unknown	4 (3.1)	10 (8.9)	2 (3.2)
ART experience [n (%)]			
Drug naive	1 (0.8)	3 (2.7)	2 (3.2)
PI-experienced	116 (88.6)	95 (84.8)	54 (85.7)
NRTI-experienced**	130 (99.2)	106 (94.6)	59 (93.6)
NNRTI-experienced	99 (75.6)	81 (72.3)	47 (74.6)
FI-experienced	-	3 (2.7)	1 (1.6)
InI-experienced	-	1 (0.9)	1 (1.6)
PI+NRTI+NNRTI-experienced	88 (67.2)	72 (64.3)	42 (66.7)
Treatment status [n (%)]			
HAART**	124 (94.6)	95 (84.8)	54 (85.7)
Stopped-treatment	3 (2.3)	11 (9.8)	6 (9.5)
Naive	1 (0.8)	3 (2.7)	2 (3.2)

Table 2. Cont.

Features	Non-transferred n = 131	Transferred n = 112	Transferred with genotype* n = 63
Monotherapy	1 (0.8)		
Combined	2 (1.5)	3 (2.7)	1 (1.6)

SD, standard deviation; ART, antiretroviral therapy; PI, protease inhibitors; NRTI, nucleoside reverse transcriptase inhibitors; NNRTI, non-NRTI; FI, fusion inhibitors, InI; integrase inhibitors.
*Transferred to adult units with available resistance genotyping profile.
**Statistical differences ($p<0.05$) have been found between transferred and non-transferred patients for these features.

Higher Predicted Level of Resistance to PI and NRTI among Transferred Patients

Figure 1 shows the comparison of the predicted level of resistance to each drug in all pretreated patients from the two study cohorts. Analysis of the genotypic resistance interpretation revealed that transferred adolescents presented a significantly higher predicted level of resistance to all drugs from the PI and NRTI families probably explained by the long-term therapy history of these patients. Half of the transferred patients carried infecting HIV-1 variants resistant to NFV, followed by AZT and d4T (nearly 40% of them). Similar predicted resistance was observed for 3TC and FTC in the non-transferred and transferred study groups (around 20%). Between nearly 20% and 30% of the adolescents in Madrid were infected with variants resistant to the remaining PI drugs, except for TPV/r and DRV/r, the new PI drug generation. EFV and NVP were the NNRTI with the most compromised susceptibility in both cohorts (around 20–30%), being higher in non-transferred patients. Data revealed a low (2–5%) predicted resistance level to etravirine and rilpivirine, the new NNRTI drugs; resistance levels to these drugs remained low in a gap between 2% and 5% for both studied cohorts.

Low Prevalence of HIV-1 Non-B Variants in Transferred Patients

Most (98.1%) of the transferred patients were infected by subtype B, the most prevalent HIV-1 variant in North America and Western Europe, including Spain [13,21]. Only one transferred perinatally infected female carried a "pure" sub-subtype A2. She was a white-Caucasian, vertically infected and born of Spanish parents in 1992. Prevalence of HIV-1 non-B variants among the 54 transferred patients with available *pol* sequence was low (1.9%, 1/54), compared to the 11.5% (15 patients) found among the 131 non-transferred children of the same pediatric cohort (**Table 1**) or the 12.2% reported n the Spanish cohort of antiretroviral treatment-naïve HIV-infected patients [21]. Of interest, recombinant viruses were absent in transferred patients although found in 60% (9/15) of infections caused by non-B variants in the non-transferred pediatric cohort, respectively.

Sequence Data

Pol (PR and/or RT) sequences from 48 (88.8%) of the 54 transferred patients included in this study had been previously submitted to GenBank [13]: HQ426715, HQ426719, HQ426725, HQ426728, HQ426734, HQ426766, HQ426768, HQ426779, HQ426780, HQ426788, HQ426799, HQ426806, HQ426807, HQ426818, HQ426826, HQ426840, HQ426842, HQ426847,

Table 3. Comparison of HIV drug resistance mutations prevalence according to drug class family in the non-transferred and the transferred pediatric cohorts.

	Transferred patients[a] (n = 58)	Non-transferred children[b] (n = 131)
Patients with available PR	51	125
Patients with available RT	52	116
Prevalence of drug resistance mutations (%) [95% CI][c]		
Global (to any class)	81.0 [70.1–92]	69.5 [61.2–77.7]
To PIs	50.9 [36.3–65.7]	36.8 [27.9–45.7]
To NRTIs	76.9 [64.5–89.3]	62.1 [52.8–71.3]
To NNRTIs	36.5 [22.5–50.6]	40.5 [31.2–49.9]
To NRTI+NNRTI	12.1 [2.8–21.3]	12.2 [6.2–18.2]
To PI+NRTI**	19 [8–29.9]	8.4 [3.3–13.5]
To PI+NNRTI	–	0.8 [0.02–4.2]
To PI+NRTI+NNRTI	17.3 [6.7–27.8]	17.6 [10.7–24.5]

[a]Selected patients from the Madrid cohort of HIV-1 infected children that have been transferred to adult units by December 2011.
[b]Pretreated patients selected from the Madrid cohort of HIV-1 infected children excluding those transferred to adult units.
[c]Prevalence of drug resistance mutations was determined following the IAS-USA 2011 list [18]. PR, protease; RT, reverse transcriptase; NRTI, nucleoside reverse transcriptase inhibitors; NNRTI, non-NRTI; PI, protease inhibitors.
**Statistical difference ($p<0.05$) has been found between transferred and non-transferred patients for this feature.

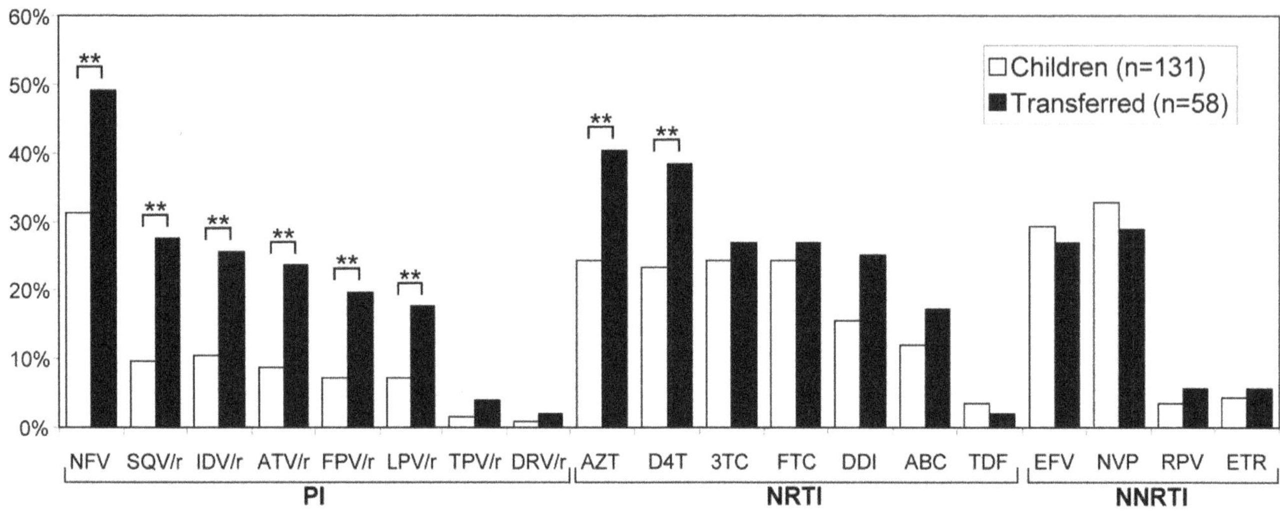

Figure 1. Predicted resistance level to antiretroviral drugs in pretreated patients from the two studied cohorts. Resistance level was estimated according to the HIVdb Interpretation Algorithm (Stanford University, Palo Alto, CA, USA) [19]. PI, protease inhibitors: nelfinavir (NFV), saquinavir/r (SQV/r), indinavir/r (IDV/r), atazanavir/r (ATV/r), fosamprenavir/r (FPV/r), lopinavir/r (LPV/r), tipranavir/r (TPV/r) and darunavir/r (DRV/r), where "/r" indicates co-administration with low-dose ritonavir (RTV) for pharmacological "boosting". NRTI, nucleoside reverse transcriptase inhibitors: zidovudine (AZT), stavudine (d4T), lamivudine (3TC), emtricitabine (FTC), didanosine (DDI), abacavir (ABC), tenofovir (TDF). NNRTI, non-nucleoside reverse transcriptase inhibitors: efavirenz (EFV), nevirapine (NVP), rilpivirine (RPV), etravirine (ETR). **Statistical differences ($p<0.05$) in resistance levels have been found between transferred and non-transferred patients for these drugs.

HQ426850, HQ426857, HQ426860, HQ426861, HQ426866, HQ426867, HQ426868, HQ426869, HQ426874, HQ426879, HQ426880, HQ426883, HQ426889, HQ426890, and HQ426893. In reference [12]: JQ351951, JQ351960, JQ351984, JQ351986, JQ351988, JQ351989, JQ351995, JQ351997, JQ352005, JQ352006, JQ352010-JQ352012, JQ352014, and JQ352021. The 6 newly generated *pol* sequences for this study were submitted to GenBank with the following accession numbers: JQ828989-JQ828994. GenBank accession numbers for the 131 sequences from non-transferred children were previously reported [12,13].

Discussion

Due to the low number of new cases of HIV infection caused by MTCT in developed countries [2], perinatally infected cohorts will tend to reduce. However, several studies have assessed the current state of adolescent survivors of perinatally or early acquired HIV infection [22–33]. As ART becomes more widely available in the developing world, increasing the effective viral suppression with immunologic reconstitution, we can expect a steady increase in the number of children being transferred into adult units, as reported in European [24–26] and North American pediatric [22,29,32] cohorts. This recent process described in high income regions could eventually occur in developing countries, if the access to optimal treatment is maintained.

High Rate of Perinatally HIV-1 Infected Patients Transferred to Adults Units in Madrid

Features of the transferred patients from the Madrid cohort of HIV-1 infected children have been scarcely studied [34]. Among the 534 patients from the Madrid cohort of HIV-1 infected children by the end of December 2011, a total of 112 (21%) had reached adolescence and were transferred to adult units from 1997 through 2011. The first patient was transferred in 1997. The high percentage of transferred patients, even higher than in the British pediatric HIV CHIPS cohort [23] (n = 103; 16% *vs.* n = 112; 21%), is directly related to the high number of HIV-1 infections occurring in Spain in the early nineties due to the so called "heroin epidemic". The abuse of heroin during the 1980s and 1990s in Spain had a special impact in women, reaching the highest AIDS incidence and prevalence in Western Europe, which led to a high incidence of MTCT in children born between 1980 and 1990 [11,35]. Future transitioning programs will include a smaller number of patients due to the low number of new diagnoses [2,9] of HIV-1 among children in high income countries.

Higher Prevalence of Drug Resistant Strains among Transferred and Non-transferred Patients

The emergence of drug resistance due to incomplete viral suppression and incomplete adherence are the major obstacle for an effective ART [36]. Adolescents with perinatally acquired HIV are heavily pretreated, have a long history of treatment with many regimen switches, and present variable levels of adherence to the treatment, mainly during adolescence. However, there are few data about disease progression, response to ART and drug resistance prevalence in vertically HIV-infected adolescents in the era of effective therapy, even though their number is increasing in developed countries where ARV therapy is guaranteed. The results presented showed that two thirds of transferred patients from the Madrid cohort of HIV-1 infected children to adult units were triple class-experienced, higher than in other cohorts as in the UK (64.3% *vs.* 47%, respectively) [23]. Results may be explained by longer exposure to older, less efficacious treatments. In fact, HIV infected patients during childhood in our cohort were mainly infected during the early 1990's, and had to face the monotherapy and dual therapy regimens available at the time, thus increasing the risk of virological failures due to resistance development. The first patient reached adulthood in 1997 and thus had received previous, less efficacious treatments during his childhood.

Interestingly, DRM prevalence to all 3 drug classes among transferred patients was higher than for non-transferred infected children. This fact could be caused by regimen switches due to therapeutic failure or because of the availability of new drugs during the infection period. As a consequence of their long treatment history and the treatment switches they have experimented, 81% of the patients transferred to adult units harboured resistant virus to at least one of the drug classes, higher than in non-transferred children (69.5%) mainly for NRTI, the first available drug class for clinical use, and for PI. This high rate of resistance could have compromised the susceptibility found in our data from both the PI and NRTI families.

In fact, the pediatric population (transferred and non-transferred) infected by viruses carrying triple resistance mutations was significantly higher than in pretreated adults from Madrid (17% *vs.* 8.6%), and moreover, was higher than in adolescents from the UK and Ireland (12%) [23] and the COHERE pediatric cohort of perinatally infected children in Western Europe aged less than 16 years (10%) [37]. On the other hand, DRM to NNRTI was slightly higher in the Madrid cohort of HIV-1 infected children than in the transferred group, so reflecting their preferential use in the pediatric population during the study period. These results on prevalence highlight the potential problem that clinicians have and will face in the near future with HIV-1 adolescents who are highly resistant to all drug classes.

Possible Candidates to Rescue Transferred Highly Pretreated Patients

Treatment failure in children during ART is frequent, develops fast and with more extensive drug resistance than in adults, leading to detectable viral loads and immunological damage [37–42]. Thus, keeping a close surveillance of adherence has to be a priority in these heavily pretreated adolescents requiring treatment for life [42,43]. Moreover resistance studies are also required to optimize ARV regimens. According to the predicted drug susceptibility, our data revealed than TDF (NRTI) and the new PI (TPV/r and DRV/r) and NNRTI (ETR and RPV) drugs could be good alternatives for inclusion in future ARV regimens to control the viraemia in highly pretreated transferred adolescents in Madrid. Adolescents could also benefit from the newly licensed drugs to treat HIV-1 infection for adults. Other drug families (cell-entry and integrase inhibitors), could be good candidates to control viraemia among pretreated transferred patients in Madrid due to their previous scarce exposure (<1%). However, the presence of X4-tropic variants in over 80% of the cohort of antiretroviral-experienced children and adolescents with vertical HIV-1 infection in Madrid has recently been reported [44]. The authors indicate a very limited role for CCR5 antagonists as part of salvage regimens for highly treatment-experienced vertically infected patients with extensive antiretroviral drug resistance [44]. Thus, integrase inhibitors could be the best rescue alternative in the cases of therapeutic failure with multiresistance, although additional genetic resistance studies should be performed to guarantee their usefulness.

Low Prevalence of HIV-1 Non-B Variants Infection among Transferred Patients

Epidemiological differences related to the nature of HIV-1 infecting variants were found between the non-transferred cohort of HIV infected children (11.4%) and with those transferred to adult units (1.9%). Pediatric patients that reached adulthood and were transferred to adult units were mainly infected by subtype B (98.2%). This fact is explained by the long term infection of our patients (mean age of 18.9 years), reflecting the local epidemiological situation in Spain at the time in which circulating variants other than B had not yet been detected in Spain.

Previous studies in the Madrid cohort of HIV-1 infected children and adolescents reported a non-B prevalence of 10% [12,13]. In fact, in Madrid an increase of HIV-1 non-B infections after year 2000 was reported among infected children [12] and among newly HIV infected adults [14]. Interestingly, the increasing complexity of the epidemic reported in HIV-infected adults [21,45] and in the pediatric population in Madrid [13] was not observed among the transferred population, in whom no recombinant strains were found. As a limitation, only half (n = 54) of the transferred cohort had an available *pol* sequence to perform HIV-1 variant characterization. Prevalence of HIV-1 non-B variants infecting children and adults from Madrid has been estimated as about 10% [12,13,21]. Similar results have been published for other pediatric cohorts, where non-B infections ranged from 5 to 15% [46,47].

Conclusions

Understanding the progress of HIV-1 infected children through pediatric care until they reach adolescence in developed countries could help to improve and plan adequate clinical and psychological transitioning services for the HIV-1 infected children that will reach adolescence [23,24,26,33] in the future. The increasing resistance prevalence among the HIV-infected-pediatric population in Spain highlights the importance of specific drug-resistance and drug-susceptibility surveillance in long-term pretreated children to optimize treatment regimens. Clinicians in Spain should consider that young adults infected during childhood do not present same clinical features as those young adults infected by other routes and that they require a specific clinical follow up.

Acknowledgments

We thank all the members of the Madrid cohort of HIV-infected children: Navarro ML, Delgado R, Martín-Fontelos P, Guillén S, Martínez J, Roa MA, Beceiro J, Blázquez D, Fernández-Silveira L, Medín G, Rojo P, Prieto L, García-Hortelano M, Jiménez B, Calvo C, Rubio B, Gonzalez-Granado I, Bellón-Cano JM, Penin-Antón JM, García I and Medin G.

Author Contributions

Conceived and designed the experiments: MDM GY AN JTR AH. Performed the experiments: MDM. Analyzed the data: MDM GY AN AH JTR. Wrote the paper: MDM AH GY AN. Provided clinical records of the study population: MIDJ MDG MIGT MJMJSL. Provided clinical samples from HIV-1 biobank: MAMF. Provided statistical analysis and cohort data: SJDO.

References

1. World Health Organization (WHO) Global HIV/AIDS response. Epidemic update and health sector progress towards universal access. Progress report 2011. Available: http://whqlibdoc.who.int/publications/2011/9789241502986_eng.pdf. Accessed 2012 Nov 16.
2. European Centre for Disease Prevention and Control/WHO Regional Office for Europe. HIV/AIDS surveillance in Europe 2010. Stockholm: European Centre for Disease Prevention and Control; 2011. Available: http://ecdc.europa.eu/en/publications/Publications/1111_SUR_Annual_Epidemiological_Report_on_Communicable_Diseases_in_Europe.pdf. Accessed 2012 Nov 16.
3. European Collaborative Study. Mother-to-child transmission of HIV infection in the era of highly active antiretroviral therapy. Clin Infect Dis 2005; 40: 458–465.
4. Welch S, Sharland M, Lyall EG, Tudor-Williams G, Niehues T, et al. (2009) PENTA 2009 guidelines for the use of antiretroviral therapy in paediatric HIV-1 infection. HIV Med 10: 591–613.

5. US Public Health Service Task Force. Recommendations for use of antiretroviral drugs in pregnant HIV-infected women for maternal health and interventions to reduce perinatal HIV transmission in the United States. Available: http://aidsinfo.nih.gov/contentfiles/PerinatalGL.pdf. Accessed 2012 Nov 16.
6. Townsend CL, Cortina-Borja M, Peckham CS, de Ruiter A, Lyall H, et al. (2008) Low rates of mother-to-child transmission of HIV following effective pregnancy interventions in the United Kingdom and Ireland, 2000–2006. AIDS 22: 973–981.
7. European Collaborative Study (2005) Mother-to-child transmission of HIV infection in the era of highly active antiretroviral therapy. Clin Infect Dis 40: 458–465.
8. Fernández-Ibieta M, Ramos Amador JT, Guillén Martín S, González-Tomé MI, Navarro Gómez M, et al. (2007) Why are HIV-infected infants still being born in Spain? An Pediatr (Barc) 67: 109–115.
9. Guillén S, Prieto L, Jiménez de Ory S, González-Granado I, González-Tomé MI, et al. (2012) New diagnosis of HIV infection in children. Enferm Infecc Microbiol Clin 30: 131–136.
10. Frange P, Burgard M, Lachassinne E, le Chenadec J, Chaix ML, et al. (2010) Late postnatal HIV infection in children born to HIV-1-infected mothers in a high-income country. AIDS 24: 1771–1776.
11. SINIVIH (2011) Área de Vigilancia de VIH y Conductas de Riesgo. Vigilancia Epidemiológica del VIH/sida en España: Sistema de Información sobre Nuevos Diagnósticos de VIH y Registro Nacional de Casos de Sida. Secretaría del Plan Nacional sobre el Sida/Centro Nacional de Epidemiología. Madrid. (Updated November 2011). Available: http://www.msps.es/novedades/docs/InformeVIH-sida_Junio2011.pdf Accessed 16 November 2012.
12. de Mulder M, Yebra G, Navas A, Martín L, de Jose MI, et al. (2012) Dynamics of drug resistance prevalence and susceptibility in the Madrid cohort of HIV-1 infected children: 1993–2010 analysis. Pediatr Infect Dis J 11: e213–e221.
13. de Mulder M, Yebra G, Martín L, Prieto L, Mellado MJ, et al. (2011) Drug resistance prevalence and HIV-1 variant characterization in the naive and pretreated HIV-1-infected paediatric population in Madrid, Spain. J Antimicrob Chemother 10: 2362–2371.
14. García-Merino I, de Las Cuevas N, Jiménez JL, García A, Gallego J, et al. (2010) Pediatric HIV BioBank: a new role of the Spanish HIV BioBank in pediatric HIV research. AIDS Res Hum Retroviruses 26: 241–244.
15. García-Merino I, de Las Cuevas N, Jiménez JL, Gallego J, Gómez C, et al. (2009) Spanish HIV BioBank. The Spanish HIV BioBank: a model of cooperative HIV research. Retrovirology 6: 27.
16. Bennett DE, Camacho RJ, Otelea D, Kuritzkes DR, Fleury H, et al. (2009) Drug resistance mutations for surveillance of transmitted HIV-1 drug-resistance: 2009 update. PLoS One 4: e4724.
17. Gifford RJ, Liu TF, Rhee SY, Kiuchi M, Hue S, et al. (2009) The calibrated population resistance tool: standardized genotypic estimation of transmitted HIV-1 drug resistance. Bioinformatics 25: 1197–1198.
18. Johnson VA, Calvez V, Gunthard HF, Paredes R, Pillay D, et al. (2011) 2011 update of the drug resistance mutations in HIV-1. Top Antivir Med 19: 156–164.
19. Liu TF, Shafer RW (2006) Web resources for HIV type 1 genotypic-resistance test interpretation. Clin Infect Dis 42: 1608–1618.
20. Center for Disease Control (1994) Revised classification system for human immunodeficiency virus infection in children less than 13 years of age; Official authorized addenda: human immunodeficiency virus infection codes and official guidelines for coding and reporting ICD-9-CM. MMWR 1994; 43 (RR-12): 1–10. Available: http://www.cdc.gov/mmwr/PDF/rr/rr4312.pdf. Accessed 2012 Nov 16.
21. Yebra G, de Mulder M, Martín L, Rodríguez C, Labarga P, et al. (2012) Most HIV type 1 non-B infections in the Spanish cohort of antiretroviral treatment-naïve HIV-infected patients (CoRIS) are due to recombinant viruses. J Clin Microbiol 50: 407–413.
22. Patel K, Hernán MA, Williams PL, Seeger JD, McIntosh K, et al. (2008) Long-term effectiveness of highly active antiretroviral therapy on the survival of children and adolescents with HIV infection: a 10-year follow-up study. Clin Infect Dis 46: 507–515.
23. Foster C, Judd A, Tookey P, Tudor-Williams G, Dunn D, et al. (2009) Young people in the United Kingdom and Ireland with perinatally acquired HIV: the pediatric legacy for adult services. AIDS Patient Care STDS 23: 159–166.
24. Judd A, Doerholt K, Tookey PA, Sharland M, Riordan A, et al. (2007) Morbidity, mortality, and response to treatment by children in the United Kingdom and Ireland with perinatally acquired HIV infection during 1996–2006: planning for teenage and adult care. Clin Infect Dis 45: 918–924.
25. Schmid J, Jensen-Fangel S, Valerius NH, Nielsen VR, Herlin T, et al. (2005) Demographics in HIV-infected children in Denmark: results from the Danish Paediatric HIV Cohort Study. Scand J Infect Dis 37: 344–349.
26. Dollfus C, Le Chenadec J, Faye A, Blanche S, Briand N, et al. (2010) Long-term outcomes in adolescents perinatally infected with HIV-1 and followed up since birth in the French perinatal cohort (EPF/ANRS CO10). Clin Infect Dis 51: 214–224.
27. Kenny J, Williams B, Prime K, Tookey P, Foster C (2012) Pregnancy outcomes in adolescents in the UK and Ireland growing up with HIV. HIV Med 13: 304–308.
28. Foster C, Fidler S (2010) Optimizing antiretroviral therapy in adolescents with perinatally acquired HIV-1 infection. Expert Rev Anti Infect Ther 8: 1403–1416.
29. Gordon DE, Ghazaryan LR, Maslak J, Anderson BJ, Brousseau KS, et al. (2012) Projections of diagnosed HIV infection in children and adolescents in New York State. Paediatr Perinat Epidemiol 26: 131–139.
30. Nglazi MD, Kranzer K, Holele P, Kaplan R, Mark D, et al. (2012) Treatment outcomes in HIV-infected adolescents attending a community-based antiretroviral therapy clinic in South Africa. BMC Infect Dis 12: 21.
31. Judd A, Ferrand RA, Jungmann E, Foster C, Masters J, et al. (2009) Vertically acquired HIV diagnosed in adolescence and early adulthood in the United Kingdom and Ireland: findings from national surveillance. HIV Med 10: 253–256.
32. Kapogiannis BG, Soe MM, Nesheim SR, Abrams EJ, Carter RJ, et al. (2011) Mortality trends in the US Perinatal AIDS Collaborative Transmission Study (1986–2004). Clin Infect Dis 53: 1024–1034.
33. Andiman WA (2011) Transition from pediatric to adult healthcare services for young adults with chronic illnesses: the special case of human immunodeficiency virus infection. J Pediatr 159: 714–719.
34. Saavedra-Lozano J, Navarro M, Rojo P, Gonzalez-Granado I, De Jose MI, et al. Status of vertically-acquired HIV-infected children at the time of their transfer to an adult clinic. 18th Conference on Retroviruses and Opportunistic Infections; February 27 - March 3 2011, Boston, MA USA. Abstract 693. Available: http://retroconference.org/2011/Abstracts/42269.htm. Accessed 2012 Nov 16.
35. Palladino C, Bellón JM, Perez-Hoyos S, Resino R, Guillén S, et al. (2008) Spatial pattern of HIV-1 mother-to-child-transmission in Madrid (Spain) from 1980 till now: demographic and socioeconomic factors. AIDS 22: 2199–2205.
36. Ammaranond P, Sanguansittianan S (2012) Mechanism of HIV antiretroviral drugs progress toward drug resistance. Fundam Clin Pharmacol 26: 146–161.
37. Castro H, Judd A, Gibb DM, Butler K, Lodwick RK, et al. (2011) Risk of triple-class virological failure in children with HIV: a retrospective cohort study. Lancet 377: 1580–1587.
38. Ding H, Wilson CM, Modjarrad K, McGwin G Jr, Tang J, et al. (2009) Predictors of suboptimal virologic response to highly active antiretroviral therapy among human immunodeficiency virus-infected adolescents. Arch Pediatr Adolesc Med 163: 1100–1105.
39. Rutstein RM, Gebo KA, Flynn PM, Fleishman JA, Sharp VL, et al. (2005) Immunologic function and virologic suppression among children with perinatally acquired HIV infection on highly active antiretroviral therapy. Med Care 2005; 43: 15–22.
40. Germanaud D, Derache A, Traore M, Madec Y, Toure S, et al. (2010) Level of viral load and antiretroviral resistance after 6 months of non-nucleoside reverse transcriptase inhibitor first-line treatment in HIV-1-infected children in Mali. J Antimicrob Chemother 65: 118–124.
41. Charpentier C, Gody JC, Mbitikon O, Moussa S, Matta M, et al. (2012) Virological response and resistance profiles after 18 to 30 months of first- or second-/third-line antiretroviral treatment: a cross-sectional evaluation in HIV type 1-infected children living in the Central African Republic. AIDS Res Hum Retroviruses 28: 87–94.
42. van Rossum AM, Fraaij PL, de Groot R (2002) Efficacy of highly active antiretroviral therapy in HIV-1 infected children. Lancet Infect Dis 2: 93–102.
43. Bain-Brickley D, Butler LM, Kennedy GE, Rutherford GW (2011) Interventions to improve adherence to antiretroviral therapy in children with HIV infection. Cochrane Database Syst Rev 12:CD009513.
44. Briz V, García D, Méndez-Lagares G, Ruiz-Mateos E, de Mulder M, et al. (2012) High prevalence of X4/DM-tropic variants in children and adolescents infected with HIV-1 by vertical transmission. Pediatr Infect Dis J 31: 1048–1052.
45. Holguín A, Lospitao E, López M, de Arellano ER, Pena MJ, et al. (2008) Genetic characterization of complex inter-recombinant HIV-1 strains circulating in Spain and reliability of distinct rapid subtyping tools. J Med Virol 80: 383–391.
46. Karchava M, Pulver W, Smith L, Philpott S, Sullivan TJ, et al. (2006) Prevalence of drug-resistance mutations and nonsubtype B strains among HIV-infected infants from New York State. J Acquir Immune Defic Syndr 42: 614–619.
47. Descamps D, Chaix ML, Montes B, Pakianather S, Charpentier C, et al. (2010) Increasing prevalence of transmitted drug resistance mutations and non-B subtype circulation in antiretroviral-naive chronically HIV-infected patients from 2001 to 2006/2007 in France. J Antimicrob Chemother 65: 2620–2627.

Clinical Features of Coxsackievirus A4, B3 and B4 Infections in Children

Chia-Jie Lee[1], Yhu-Chering Huang[1,2]*, Shuan Yang[2,3], Kuo-Chien Tsao[2,3], Chih-Jung Chen[1,2], Yu-Chia Hsieh[1,2], Cheng-Hsun Chiu[1,2], Tzou-Yien Lin[1,2]

1 Department of Pediatrics, Chang Gung Memorial Hospital at Linkou, Kweishan, Taoyuan, Taiwan, **2** Chang Gung University College of Medicine, Kweishan, Taoyuan, Taiwan, **3** Department of Laboratory Medicine, Chang Gung Memorial Hospital at Linkou, Kweishan, Taoyuan, Taiwan

Abstract

Background: Clinical features of coxsackievirus A4 (CA4), B3 (CB3) and B4 (CB4) infections in children have not been comprehensively described.

Methods/Principal Findings: From January 2004 to June 2012, a total of 386 children with culture-proven CA4, CB3 and CB4 infections treated at Chang Gung Memorial Hospital, including 296 inpatients (CA4, 103; CB3, 131; CB4, 62) and 90 outpatients (CA4, 55; CB3, 14; CB4, 21), were included. From outpatients, only demographics were extracted and from inpatients, detailed clinical and laboratory data were collected retrospectively. The mean age was 32.1±30.2 months; male to female ratio was 1.3:1. Children with CB3 infection were youngest (76.6% <3 years of age), and had a highest hospitalization rate (90.3%) and a longest duration of hospitalization (mean ± SD, 7.5±6.2 days). Herpangina (74.8%) was the most common presentation for children with CA4 infection, aseptic meningitis (26.7%) and young infant with fever (23.7%) for those with CB3 infection, and herpangina (32.3%) and tonsillitis/pharyngitis (27.4%) for children with CB4 infection. Almost all the inpatients had fever (97.6%). Twelve out of thirteen (92.3%) children with complications and ten of 11 children with long-term sequelae had CB3 infections. Two fatal cases were noted, one due to myocarditis with CA4 infection and CB3 were detected from the other case which had hepatic necrosis with coagulopathy. The remaining 285 children (96.3%) recovered uneventfully.

Conclusion: CA4, CB3 and CB4 infections in children had different clinical disease spectrums and involved different age groups. Though rare, severe diseases may occur, particularly caused by CB3.

Editor: Eng Eong Ooi, Duke-National University of Singapore Graduate Medical School, Singapore

Funding: This study was supported by a grant from Chang Gung Memorial Hospital (CMRPG 490112). The funders had no role in study design, data collection and analysis, decision to publish, or preparation of the manuscript.

Competing Interests: The authors have declared that no competing interests exist.

* E-mail: ychuang@adm.cgmh.org.tw

Introduction

Enterovirus are common pathogens in pediatric infectious disease and traditionally classified into poliovirus, coxsackievirus A (CA), coxsackievirus B (CB), echovirus, and the enteroviruses named with numbers such as enterovirus 68 to 71 [1]. International Committee on Taxonomy of Viruses adopted a new classification of human enteroviruses (HEVs) in 2000 and then HEVs are subgrouped into five species: poliovirus, HEV-A, HEV-B, HEV-C, and HEV-D; according to the similarities in their viral structure protein (VP) genes [2].

Non-polio enteroviruses can cause a wide range of clinical diseases, including herpangina, hand, foot and mouth disease (HFMD), respiratory infections, enteritis, and non-specific febrile illness. In severe cases, enterovirus can lead to aseptic meningitis, encephalitis, myocarditis, and even death.

Enterovirus activity was closely monitored by Centers for Diseases Control of Taiwan (CDC-Taiwan). The most commonly reported serotypes changed each year, as did the ranking of individual serotypes. However, according to the data from CDC-Taiwan during 2001–2008, coxsackievirus A4 (CA4), B3 (CB3) and B4 (CB4) were usually among the five most common enterovirus serotypes in Taiwan [3]. These three coxsackievirus are classified as HEV-A(CA4) and HEV-B(CB3 and CB4), respectively, based on their viral genomic structure. However, detailed clinical features of CA4, CB3 and CB4 infections in children have not been described. In order to better characterize the clinical features of coxsackievirus A4 (CA4), B3 (CB3) and B4 (CB4) infections in children, we conducted this retrospective study.

Materials and Methods

Ethical Approval

This study was approved by the Institutional Review Board of Chang Gung Memorial Hospital and the written inform consent was waived since the nature of this study was retrospective chart review.

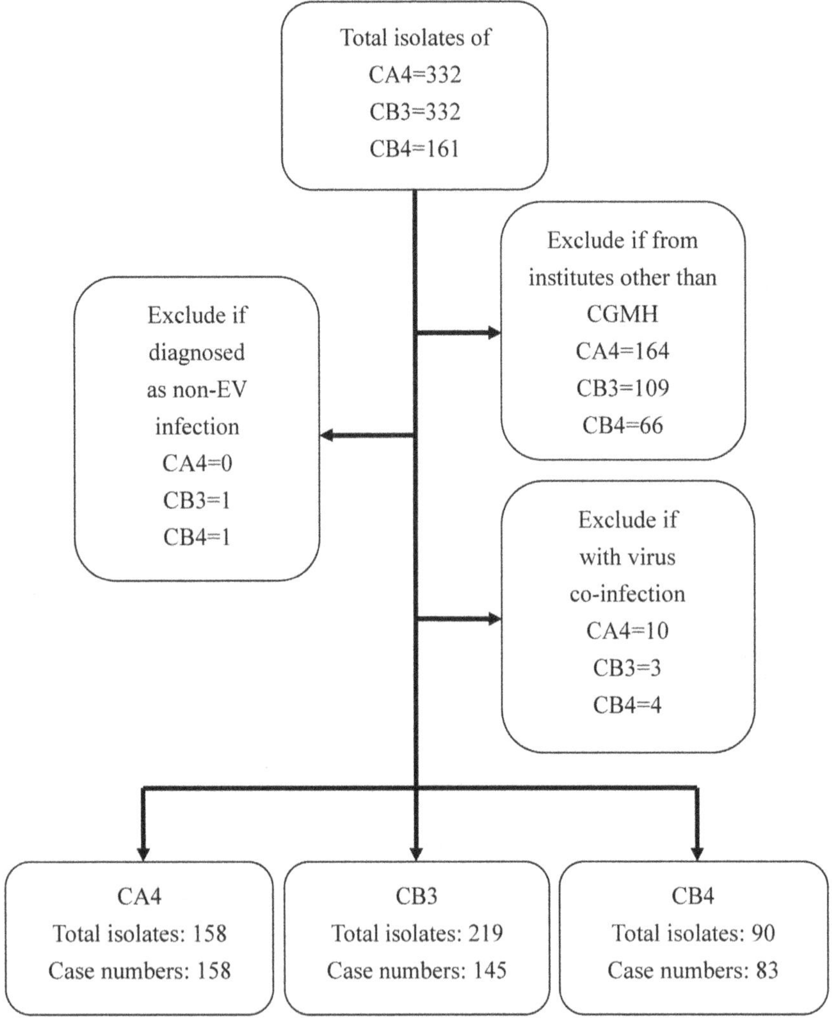

Figure 1. Flow chart of the patients enrolled in this study. CA4, coxsackievirus A4; CB3, coxsackievirus B3; CB4, coxsackievirus B4.

Isolation and Identification of Coxsackievirus A4 (CA4), B3 (CB3) and B4 (CB4)

Chang Gung Memorial Hospital (CGMH) is a 3500-bed university-affiliated medical center located in northern Taiwan. Virus isolation from clinical specimens was routinely carried out by the department of laboratory medicine [4]. Specimens were inoculated into human embryonic fibroblast (MRC-5), MDCK, HEp-2 and RD. All cultures were observed daily for cytopathic effects (CPEs). Indirect fluorescent staining with panenteroviral antibody (Chemicon International, Temecula, CA, USA) was performed to identify the enterovirus when CPE involved more than 50% of the cell monolayer. All positive specimens were further confirmed by neutralization with type-specific pools of immune sera. The monoclonal antibodies, including18 serotypes (Poliovirus 1–3; coxsackievirus A9, A16, A24; coxsackievirus B1–6; echovirus 4, 6, 9, 11, 30; EV71), were from a commercial kit (Chemicon International, Temecula, CA, USA), and monoclonal antibodies against coxsackievirus A2, A4, A5, A6 and A10 were provided by CDC–Taiwan since 2006 [5].

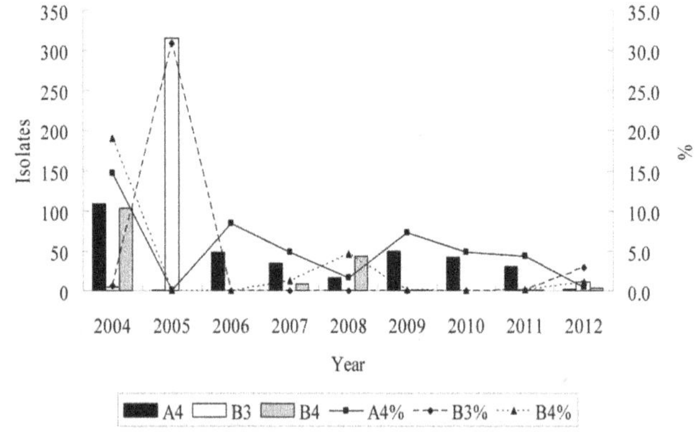

Figure 2. Isolates and percentage of Coxsackie A4, B3 and B4 isolates from January, 2004 to June, 2012 in Chang Gung Memorial Hospital, Taiwan.

Case Enrollment and Data Collection

From January 2004 to June 2012, a total of 825 isolates of CA4, CB3 and CB4 were identified via an electronic database of virologic laboratory. The virologic laboratory of CGMH was also a contracted laboratory of CDC-Taiwan, which provided the service for viral surveillance in northern part of Taiwan. Patients who didn't receive treatment at CGMH, or with concomitant viral infection or with a final diagnosis unrelated to enterovirus infection were excluded. Medical records of these cases were reviewed. For outpatients, only demographic data were collected. Inpatients were enrolled for further analysis of clinical manifestations, clinical diagnosis, laboratory data, treatment course and outcomes.

Definitions

Herpangina was defined as presence of oral ulcers over anterior tonsillar pillars, soft palate, buccal mucosa, or the uvula. Patients with hand, foot and mouth disease (HFMD) had oral ulcers and typical rash over palms, soles, knees, or the buttocks. Diagnosis of tonsillitis/pharyngitis was based on clinical features, such as injected tonsil/throat or presence of exudate. Lower respiratory tract infection (LRTI) included bronchiolitis, bronchopneumonia and pneumonia. Acute gastroenteritis was defined as patients having symptoms of diarrhea and vomiting without other identified viral or bacterial pathogens. Patients younger than three months of age who had fever greater than 38°C but without other symptoms were classified as young infant with fever.

A diagnosis of aseptic meningitis was made when enterovirus was isolated from cerebrospinal fluid (CSF) or pleocytosis in the CSF (leukocyte count in the CSF exceeded 30 cells/mm^3 in neonates or greater than 5 cells/mm^3 beyond the neonatal age), with a negative bacterial culture in CSF. Patients who had symptoms and signs of meningeal irritation, such as headache, vomiting, meningeal signs or fever, but no available CSF for analysis or negative results for CSF studies were categorized as meningismus. The diagnosis of encephalitis depended on altered consciousness or focal neurological signs with abnormal findings in neuro-imaging or electroencephalogram (EEG).

Complications included disseminated intravascular coagulopathy, myocarditis, respiratory distress, shock and hepatic necrosis with coagulopathy The diagnosis of disseminated intravascular coagulopathy was confirmed by the scoring system proposed by International Society on Thrombosis and Haemostasis [6]. Myocarditis was defined as an elevation in the cardiac fraction of creatine kinase and ejection fraction less than 50% on echocardiogary or arrhythmia on electrocardiography. Respiratory distress was defined as requiring mechanical ventilation, which included noninvasive modes (e.g., bilevel positive airway pressure, or continuous positive airway pressure) and invasive modes (e.g., pressure-control ventilation, high frequency oscillatory ventilation). Patients who needed inotropic agents due to profound hypotension and accompanied with at least two end-organ injuries were categorized as shock. Hepatic necrosis with coagulopathy was defined as aspartate aminotransferase more than three times the upper limit of normal value plus platelet count less than 10^5/mm^3.

Statistics

The descriptive statistics was performed with SPSS 18.0. The categorical variables were compared by ANOVA and chi-square test. Statistical significance was defined as $p<0.05$.

Results

From January 2004 to June 2012, a total of 802 patients less than 18 year of ages with 825 isolates of CA4, CB3 and CB4 which were collected from throat, rectal or CSF were enrolled. 339 patients who didn't receive treatment at CGMH were excluded. 17 patients were excluded because of other virus co-infection. One patient admitted due to chronic myopathy and the other admitted because of vasculitis were excluded due to no clinical symptoms of enterovirus infection (Fig. 1).

A total of 386 children treated at Chang Gung Memorial Hospital, including 296 inpatients (CA4, 103; CB3, 131; CB4, 62) and 90 outpatients (CA4, 55; CB3, 14; CB4, 21), were included in this study. Figure 2 showed the annual distribution and the percentage of CA4, CB3 and CB4 among the total enterovirus isolates which were identified from CGMH during the study period. CA4 and CB4 both had one peak in 2004 and accounted for 14.7% and 19% of the total enterovirus isolates in CGMH, respectively. CB3 constituted 30.9% of the total enterovirus isolates in 2005. On average, from January 2004 to June 2012, CA4 and CB3 each accounted for 5% and CB4 accounted for 2.4% of the overall enterovirus isolates. CA4, CB3 and CB4 were most commonly detected between May and July. The monthly distribution of these three virus during the study period is shown in Figure 3.

The median age of infected children was 25 [10, 49] months (median [IQR]); male to female ratio was 1.3:1. Children with CB3 infection were youngest (76.6% <3 years of age; 40.7% <3 months of age), and had a highest hospitalization rate (90.3%) and a longest duration of hospitalization (median [IQR], 6 [4,9] days) (Table 1).

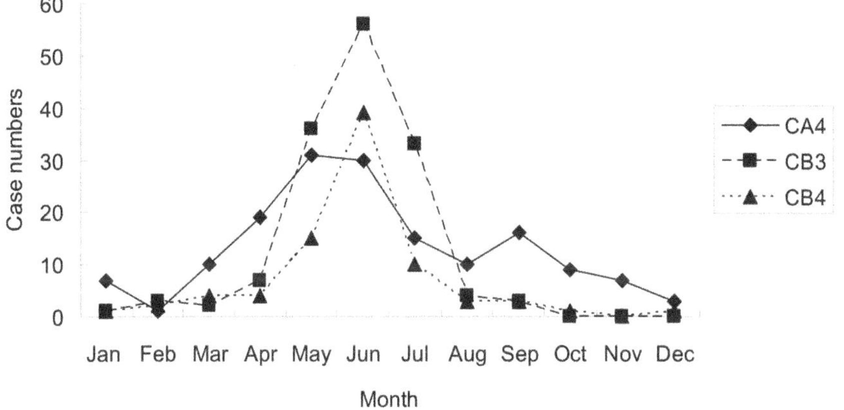

Figure 3. Monthly distribution of coxsackievirus A4 (CA4), B3 (CB3) and B4 (CB4) isolates from January, 2004 to June, 2012 in Chang Gung Memorial Hospital, Taiwan.

Table 1. Demographics of 386 children with Coxsackievirus A4, B3 and B4 infections in Chang Gung Memorial Hospital, January, 2004–June, 2012.

Characteristics	No. (%)				*p* value
	Coxsackie A4	Coxsackie B3	Coxsackie B4	Total	
Total	158	145	83	386	
Male gender	81 (51.3)	88 (60.7)	49 (59)	218 (56.5)	.222
Age, months (median [IQR])	30.5 [17.8, 48]	11 [1.2, 33.5]	35 [12, 56]	25 [10,49]	.000
≦3 years	92 (58.2)	111 (76.6)	42 (50.6)	245 (63.5)	.000
≦3 months	1 (0.63)	59 (40.7)	13 (15.7)	73(18.9)	.000
Admission rate (%)	65.2	90.3	74.7	76.7	.000
Specimens					
Throat	158	128	81	367	
Rectum	0	60	8	68	
Cerebrospinal fluid	0	30	0	30	
Others	0	1[a]	1[b]	2	
Multiple sites (≥2 sites)	0	52	7	59	
Inpatients	103	131	62	296	
Male gender	54(52.4)	78(59.5)	38(45.8)	170(57.4)	.434
Age, months (median [IQR])	27 [15, 45]	8 [0.9, 32]	24 [7, 53.3]	21 [5,46]	.001
≦3 years	69(67)	105(80.2)	39(62.9)	213(72)	.017
≦3 months	1(1)	59(45)	12(19.3)	72(24.7)	.000
Days of hospital stay (median [IQR])	4 [3,5]	6 [4,9]	5 [3,9]	5 [3,7]	.000
Underlying diseases	11(10.7)	22(16.8)	12(19.4)	45(15.2)	.257
Prematurity	3	13	6	22	
Allergy	2	4	1	7	
Neurological	3	5	1	9	
Congenital anomaly	1	2	2	5	
Others	0	1	2	3	

[a]Culture from urine.
[b]Culture from pleural effusion.

Clinical manifestations and laboratory data of the 296 inpatients are displayed in Table 2 and 3. Of these inpatients, the positive samples for enteroviruses were obtained within three days of hospitalization in all but five patients. The diagnoses of these five patients on admission included herpangina for one, acute tonsillitis for two and lower respiratory tract infection for two. The most common symptoms in the 296 inpatients were fever (97.6%). Children with CA4 infection usually presented with a high-grade fever (75.5%) and those infected with CB3 had a longer duration of fever (55.1% patients had fever greater than 3 days). Patients who were infected by CA4 usually had oral ulcers (80.6%), which is a typical symptom of herpangina, and decreased oral intake (86.4%). Respiratory symptoms were less common in CB3 group. No statistically difference was found for gastrointestinal and neurologic symptoms.

Leukocytosis (leukocyte count ≥15000/μL) and higher C-reactive protein (>40 mg/L) were both more frequently seen in children with CA4 infection (34% and 40.6%, respectively). CB3 infection was more likely to develop anemia and thrombocytopenia (22.3% and 12.3%, respectively). 35 patients diagnosed as aseptic meningitis were all infected by CB3. Of them, 31 patients had pleocytosis in CSF and the mean WBC count was 170±193/μL without lymphocyte or netrophil predominance(17.7±27.7% and 18.6±21.4%, respectively). Elevated protein level (mean ± SD, 93.9±51.8 mg/dL) and lower sugar level (mean ± SD, 48.5±10.5 mg/dL) were observed.

Herpangina (74.8%) was the most common diagnosis for children with CA4 infection, aseptic meningitis (26.7%) and young infant with fever (23.7%) for those with CB3 infection, and herpangina (32.3%) and tonsillitis/pharyngitis (27.4%) for children with CB4 infection (Table 4.). Of the 38 patients diagnosed as LRTI, 11 patients were infected by CA4, 17 patients by CB3 and 10 patients by CB4 (Table 5.). Among these patients, most plain chest radiography films were interpreted as having bronchopneumonia (CA4, 90.9%; CB3, 94.1%; CB4, 80%). Positive urine pneumococcus antigen was identified in one patient, 3 patients probably were coinfected with *Mycoplasma pneumoniae* which was supported by either serology or polymerase chain reaction (PCR), and 2 patients had MRSA isolated from sputum cultures.

Children with CB3 infection had the highest complication rate (9.2%), with disseminated intravascular coagulopathy being the most common syndrome, followed by respiratory distress, shock and hepatic necrosis with coagulopathy. CB3 infection had a highest rate of receiving antibiotics or IVIG treatment (58.8% and

Table 2. Clinical manifestations in 296 hospitalized children with coxsackievirus A4, B3 and B4 infections stratified by serotypes.

Symptoms and signs	No. (%)			*p* value
	Coxsackie A4 (n = 103)	Coxsackie B3 (n = 131)	Coxsackie B4 (n = 62)	
Constitutional				
Fever[a]	102 (99)	126 (96.2)	61 (98.4)	.330
High fever (>39°C)	74 (75.5)	65 (55.1)	32 (57.1)	.011
Days of fever (median [IQR])	3 [2,3]	4 [3,5]	4 [2,5]	.001
Fever>3 days	23 (23.5)	65 (55.1)	28 (50.9)	.000
Poor oral intake	89 (86.4)	65 (49.6)	34 (54.8)	.000
Poor activity	56 (54.3)	61 (46.6)	26 (41.9)	.261
Mucocutaneous[b]				
Oral ulcer	83 (80.6)	29 (22.1)	25 (40.3)	.000
Skin rash	11 (10.7)	4 (3.1)	3 (4.8)	.039
Respiratory				
Cough	51 (49.5)	43 (32.8)	28 (45.1)	.028
Rhinorrhea	38 (36.9)	25 (19.1)	20 (32.2)	.008
Gastrointestinal				
Diarrhea	17 (16.5)	12 (9.2)	11 (17.7)	.145
Vomiting	27 (26.2)	27 (20.6)	20 (32.2)	.205
Neurologic				
Myoclonic jerk	11 (10.7)	13 (9.9)	8 (12.9)	.823
Headache	2 (1.9)	10 (7.6)	5 (8.1)	.121
Limb weakness	0 (0)	0 (0)	1 (1.6)	.151
Febrile seizure	3 (2.9)	4 (3.1)	3 (4.8)	.773
Afebrile seizure	2 (1.9)	7 (5.3)	1 (1.6)	.247

[a]Fever was defined as body temperature greater than 38°C.
[b]Typical mucocutaneous manifestations of enteroviral infections.

10.7%, respectively). 10 of 11 children with long-term sequelae were also caused by CB3. Two fatal cases were noted, one due to myocarditis caused by CA4 and t CB3 was detected from the other case which had hepatic necrosis with coagulopathy. The remaining 285 children (96.3%) recovered uneventfully.

In CB4 group, enterovirus was isolated from pleural effusion and throat swab in a case of necrotizing pneumonia. This 4-year-old boy was admitted due to pneumonia complicated with pleural effusion and subsequent chest computed tomography found necrotizing lung tissue during hospitalization. Echo-guided thoracentesis was performed and the results were compatible with an exudate (lactate dehydrogenase 621 IU/mL) according to Light's criteria. Etiology survey found positive urine pneumococcus antigen, but gram stain, pneumococcus antigen and bacterial culture from pleural effusion were all negative. However, virus culture from pleural effusion and throat specimen which was collected about one week later both yielded CB4. The patient recovered uneventfully without surgical intervention.

In present study, CB3 infection was found to have more severe clinical presentation. We classified patients into CB3 and non-CB3 infection groups for multiple logistic regression analysis. The results showed that patient's age (adjusted odds ratio, 0.982; 95% confidence interval [CI], 0.971 to 0.992; $P = .001$) and fever duration (adjusted odds ratio, 1.18; 95% confidence interval [CI], 1.06 to 1.314; $P = .003$) were significantly related to CB3 infection. Aseptic meningitis was more frequently diagnosed in CB3 group (adjusted odds ratio, 19.829; 95% confidence interval [CI], 4.876 to 80.649; $P = .000$) as well as complication or mortality (adjusted odds ratio, 13.558; 95% confidence interval [CI], 1.302 to 141.135; $P = .029$). However, length of hospital stay didn't reach statistic significance (adjusted odds ratio, 1.032; 95% confidence interval [CI], 0.954 to 1.116; $P = .433$).

Discussion

Results from the present study showed that from January 2004 to June 2012, CA4, CB3 and CB4 each accounted for 2.4–5% of the overall enterovirus isolates. CA4 and CB4 both had a peak in 2004 while CB3 was predominant in 2005. Since 2006, CA4, CB3 and CB4 played less important roles in the enterovirus epidemics. These results were consistent with those from CDC of Taiwan, which revealed that in 2004, the most prevalent serotype was CA4, accounting for 23.8% of total enterovirus isolates, and CB3 constituted 30.6% in 2005 [7]. Whereas, CA4, CB3 and CB4 each constituted 0 to 1.8% of total enterovirus isolates from 1998 to 2007 in Spain, 0.9–2.6% from 2005 to 2006, and 0–3.2% from 2008–2009 in Korea [8–10]. From 1970–2005, Khetsuriani N et al. conducted a study based on data from the National Enterovirus Surveillance System in United States, they found CA4, CB3 and CB4 each constituted 0.4%, 3.9% and 4.2% of total enterovirus isolates. CB3 and CB4 were both consistently appeared among the 15 most common enteroviruses [11].

Coxsackieviruses have various serotypes and can cause distinct disease spectrum. In a previous study, Yen FB et al. reported

Table 3. Laboratory findings in 296 hospitalized children with Coxsackievirus A4, B3 and B4 infections stratified by serotypes.

Laboratory data	No. (%)			p value
	Coxsackie A4 (n = 103)	Coxsackie B3 (n = 131)	Coxsackie B4 (n = 62)	
Blood				
WBC (×1000/μL) on admission	13.9±6.1	11.3±4.0	12.4±5.3	.000
Leukocytosis (peak)[a]	35 (34)	21 (16)	18 (29)	.000
Leukopenia (nadir)[b]	2 (2)	2 (1.5)	1 (1.61)	.745
Hb (g/dL) on admission	11.8±1.2	12.1±2.1	11.8±1.4	.273
Hb<10 g/dL (nadir)	5 (4.9)	29 (22.3)	6 (9.7)	.003
Platelet (1000/μL) on admission	262.1±70.4	299.2±140.5	312.0±127.0	.014
Platelet<150000/μL (nadir)	0 (0)	16 (12.3)	4 (6.5)	.007
CRP (mg/L) on admission	40.5±37.0	20.6±25.9	30.1±53.5	.000
CRP>40 mg/L(peak)	41 (40.6)	22 (16.9)	12 (20)	.000
Cerebrospinal fluid findings in aseptic meningitis				
Case numbers	0	35	0	
Pleocytosis[c]		31		
WBC (/μL)	-	170±193	-	
Neutrophil (%)	-	17.7±27.7	-	
Lymphocyte (%)	-	18.6±21.4	-	
Protein (mg/dL)	-	93.9±51.8	-	
Sugar (mg/dL)	-	48.5±10.5	-	
Lactate (mg/dL)	-	17.1±4.2	-	
Positive virus culture	-	29	-	

[a]Leukocytosis was defined as WBC count ≥15000/μL in patients older than 1-month-old and ≥30000/μL in patients young than 1-month-old.
[b]Leukopenia was defined as WBC count <4500/μL.
[c]Pleocytosis was defined as WBC count in CSF greater than 30 cells/mm^3 in neonates or greater than 5 cells/mm^3 beyond the neonatal age.

higher hospital admission rate in CB infection than patients with CA infection. CA was commonly related to herpangina while respiratory symptoms were more prominent in CB infection [12]. In another epidemic report in northern Taiwan, Hsu CH et al. not only observed this trend but also identified the association between Human enteroviruses B (including CB1, CB3, CB4, CB5, CA9, Echo3, Echo4, Echo6, Echo25, and Echo30) and aseptic meningitis [13], which was consistent with previous findings [14].

In this study, we found CA4 usually caused herpangina with high grade fever, leukocytosis and higher CRP but rarely caused complications. CB3 tended to infect young children. In the present study, 76.6% patients with CB3 infection were younger than 3 years and half of them were younger than 3 months, which resulted in more frequent usage of empiric antibiotic therapy for these young infants. Aseptic meningitis and young infant with fever were the most common diagnosis and more complications, mostly DIC (9 out of 12 patients with complications developed DIC) were found. In contrast, herpangina and pharyngitis/tonsillitis were the most common diagnosis for CB4 infection and rare complications were noted.

From the enterovirus outbreak in 2005, we learned that CB3 often occurred in infants younger than 3-month-old and caused various manifestations, including fever, meningitis, hepatitis, and sepsis [15]. In this study, we found 35 patients with aseptic meningitis proven by lumbar puncture and all of them were infected by CB3. Most of these patients (91.4%) were younger than 3-month-old (data not shown).

Hepatic necrosis with coagulopathy (HNC) is another important issue in neonatal enteroviral disease. We only collected patients with CA4, CB3 and CB4 infections in this study but already found 6 patients with HNC among 37 neonates and CB3 was detected from all of these cases. In a previous study, Lin et al reported 42 cases had HNC among 146 neonates in northern Taiwan with non-polio entrovirus infections [16]. Another single-center study showed much smaller proportion, from 1999–2006 only one patient with CB3 had developed HNC [12]. Further study is needed to clarify the prevalence of HNC in neonatal enteroviral disease.

Correlations between respiratory tract infections and enterovirus have been reported previously [17,18]. According to a previous surveillance data of respiratory viral infections among pediatric patients in northern Taiwan, enterovirus is one of the most common viruses identified from pediatric outpatients with acute, febrile URTIs [4]. Tsai et al showed 12.7% children with respiratory tract infections, including upper and lower RTIs, were caused by enterovirus and enterovirus was identified from 20% of viral pneumonia cases [19]. In a study discussing the role of enteroviruses for community acquired pneumonia in adults, Hohenthal et al indicated that enteroviruses could be identified in 5% of the patients [20]. In the present study, 38 patients were diagnosed as LRTIs based on clinical symptoms and chest radiographs. Most children had increased infiltrations on chest radiographs, but patchy opacity and pleural effusion were found in three and one patients, respectively. 25 out of the patients were younger than three years of age. CB4 isolate was identified from

Table 4. Diagnosis, treatment, complications and outcomes of 296 hospitalized children with coxsackievirus A4, B3 and B4 infections stratified by serotypes.

Clinical parameters	No. (%)			*p* value
	Coxsackie A4 (n = 103)	Coxsackie B3 (n = 131)	Coxsackie B4 (n = 62)	
Diagnosis				
Herpangina	77 (74.8)	22 (16.8)	20 (32.3)	.000
Hand-foot-mouth disease	5 (4.9)	2 (1.5)	2 (3.2)	.337
Tonsillitis/pharyngitis	14 (13.6)	18 (13.7)	17 (27.4)	.035
LRTI	11 (10.7)	17 (13)	10 (16.1)	.552
Acute gastroenteritis	2 (1.9)	5 (3.8)	11 (17.7)	.000
Young infant with fever	0 (0)	31 (23.7)	9 (14.5)	.000
Aseptic meningitis	0 (0)	35 (26.7)	0 (0)	.000
Meningismus	1 (1)	7 (5.3)	3 (4.8)	.585
Encephalitis	0 (0)	6 (4.6)	0 (0)	.021
Others	8 (7.8)	9 (6.9)	5 (8.1)	.945
More than one diagnosis	14 (13.6)	18 (13.7)	14 (22.6)	
Treatment				
Antibiotics	19 (18.4)	77 (58.8)	28 (45.2)	.000
IVIG	2 (1.9)	14 (10.7)	2 (3.2)	.012
Complications	1 (1)	12 (9.2)	0 (0)	
DIC	1 (1)	9 (6.9)	0 (0)	.012
Myocarditis	1 (1)	1 (0.8)	0 (0)	.752
Respiratory distress	1 (1)	7 (5.3)	0 (0)	.041
Shock	1 (1)	6 (4.6)	0 (0)	.076
HNC	0 (0)	6 (4.6)	0 (0)	.013
Other	0 (0)	3 (2.3)[a]	0 (0)	.148
Outcomes				
Total recovery	102 (99)	121 (92.4)	62 (100)	.006
Long-term sequelae	1 (1)	10 (7.6)	0 (0)	.006
Mortality	1 (1)	1 (0.8)	0 (0)	.752
Requiring ECMO	1 (1)	1 (0.8)	0 (0)	.752

URTI, upper respiratory tract infection; LRTI, lower respiratory tract infection; IVIG, intravenous immunoglobulin; DIC, disseminated intravascular coagulopathy; HNC, hepatic necrosis and coagulopathy; ECMO, extracorporeal membrane oxygenation.
[a]Two patients complicated with renal failure and one patient had rhabdomyolysis.

pleural effusion from a previously healthy child with necrotizing pneumonia, which was not reported previously, though enteroviruses isolated from lung tissue and bronchoalveolar lavage in immunocompromised patients have been reported [21,22]. Although concurrent infection couldn't be excluded, it could be a more direct evidence for enterovius in LRTIs. However, the role of enteroviruses in lower respiratory tract infection is still undetermined, since it is difficult to distinguish colonization from true pathogen without performing simultaneous serologic results. Further studies are needed to address this issue.

There are some limitations in this study. First, this is a retrospective study. Inevitably, there are some missing records or laboratory findings in the medical charts. Second, the presence of clinical features was based on medical records and thus inter-observer's variation may exist. Third, we generated these data from a single medical center situated in northern Taiwan and the virus cultures were clinical diagnostics requested by treating physicians. Therefore, the results may not be able to apply to other populations. Fourth, because CGMH is a tertiary care center, most severe cases were referred to our hospital and this could be misleading as to the extent of disease spectrums.

In conclusion, we analyzed the clinical features and laboratory findings in children with CA4, CB3 and CB4 infection and found each serotype had distinct clinical presentations. Enteroviruses are common pathogens in children and sometimes can cause morbidity and mortality. A better understanding of the clinical symptoms of enteroviruses infections will be helpful for patient management.

Author Contributions

Conceived and designed the experiments: YC Huang. Performed the experiments: CJL SY KCT. Analyzed the data: CJL YC Huang. Contributed reagents/materials/analysis tools: CJC YC Hsieh CHC YC Huang TYL. Wrote the paper: CJL YC Huang.

Table 5. Chest X ray findings and results of etiology survey in hospitalized lower respiratory tract infection (LRTI) patients.

	No. (%)			*p* value
	Coxsackie A4	**Coxsackie B3**	**Coxsackie B4**	
Case numbers of LRTI	11	17	10	.552
CXR				
Increased perihilar infiltrates	10 (90.9)	16 (94.1)	8 (80)	
Patch consolidation	1 (9.1)	1 (5.9)	1 (10)	
Pleural effusion	0 (0)	0 (0)	1 (10)	
Survey for bacterial co-infections				
Positive urine pneumococcus antigen	0 (0)	0 (0)	1 (33.3)	
Mycoplasma pneumoniae[a]	0 (0)	2 (33.3)	1 (20)	
MRSA[b]	0 (0)	2 (100)	0 (0)	
RSV antigen (NP)[c]	0 (0)	0 (0)	0 (0)	

[a]Including mycoplasma serology or mycoplasma DNA PCR.
[b]MRSA, methicillin-resistant Staphylococcus aureus; confirmed by sputum culture.
[c]RSV, respiratory syncytial virus; nasopharyngeal aspirate examined by immunofluorescent aassay.

References

1. Muir P, Kammerer U, Korn K, Mulders MN, Poyry T, et al. (1998) Molecular typing of enteroviruses: current status and future requirements. The European Union Concerted Action on Virus Meningitis and Encephalitis. Clin Microbiol Rev 11: 202–227.
2. Kiang D, Newbower EC, Yeh E, Wold L, Chen L, et al. (2009) An algorithm for the typing of enteroviruses and correlation to serotyping by viral neutralization. J Clin Virol 45: 334–340.
3. Lo SH, Huang YC, Huang CG, Tsao KC, Li WC, et al. (2011) Clinical and epidemiologic features of Coxsackievirus A6 infection in children in northern Taiwan between 2004 and 2009. Journal of Microbiology Immunology and Infection 44: 252–257.
4. Lin TY, Huang YC, Ning HC, Tsao KC (2004) Surveillance of respiratory viral infections among pediatric outpatients in northern Taiwan. J Clin Virol 30: 81–85.
5. Lin TL, Li YS, Huang CW, Hsu CC, Wu HS, et al. (2008) Rapid and highly sensitive coxsackievirus a indirect immunofluorescence assay typing kit for enterovirus serotyping. J Clin Microbiol 46: 785–788.
6. Taylor FB, Jr., Toh CH, Hoots WK, Wada H, Levi M (2001) Towards definition, clinical and laboratory criteria, and a scoring system for disseminated intravascular coagulation. Thromb Haemost 86: 1327–1330.
7. Tseng FC, Huang HC, Chi CY, Lin TL, Liu CC, et al. (2007) Epidemiological survey of enterovirus infections occurring in Taiwan between 2000 and 2005: analysis of sentinel physician surveillance data. J Med Virol 79: 1850–1860.
8. Trallero G, Avellon A, Otero A, De Miguel T, Perez C, et al. (2010) Enteroviruses in Spain over the decade 1998–2007: virological and epidemiological studies. J Clin Virol 47: 170–176.
9. Baek K, Park K, Jung E, Chung E, Park J, et al. (2009) Molecular and epidemiological characterization of enteroviruses isolated in Chungnam, Korea from 2005 to 2006. J Microbiol Biotechnol 19: 1055–1064.
10. Baek K, Yeo S, Lee B, Park K, Song J, et al. (2011) Epidemics of enterovirus infection in Chungnam Korea, 2008 and 2009. Virol J 8: 297.
11. Khetsuriani N, Lamonte-Fowlkes A, Oberst S, Pallansch MA (2006) Enterovirus surveillance–United States, 1970–2005. MMWR Surveill Summ 55: 1–20.
12. Yen FB, Chang LY, Kao CL, Lee PI, Chen CM, et al. (2009) Coxsackieviruses infection in northern Taiwan–epidemiology and clinical characteristics. J Microbiol Immunol Infect 42: 38–46.
13. Hsu CH, Lu CY, Shao PL, Lee PI, Kao CL, et al. (2011) Epidemiologic and clinical features of non-polio enteroviral infections in northern Taiwan in 2008. J Microbiol Immunol Infect 44: 265–273.
14. Cherry JD, Krogstad P. Enteroviruses and parechoviruses. In: Feigin & Cherry, eds. Textbook of Pediatric Infectious Diseases. 6th edi. Philadelphia, PA: WB Saunders; 2009: 2110–2170.
15. Ju-Hsin Chen T-LL, En-Tzu Wang, Nan-Chang Chiu, Kun-Bin Wu (2007) An analysis of Coxsackie B3 enterovirus outbreaks in Taiwan in 2005. The Fourth TEPHINET Southeast Asia and Western Pacific Bi-Regional Scientific Confernce.
16. Lin TY, Kao HT, Hsieh SH, Huang YC, Chiu CH, et al. (2003) Neonatal enterovirus infections: emphasis on risk factors of severe and fatal infections. Pediatr Infect Dis J 22: 889–894.
17. Jennings LC, Anderson TP, Werno AM, Beynon KA, Murdoch DR (2004) Viral etiology of acute respiratory tract infections in children presenting to hospital: role of polymerase chain reaction and demonstration of multiple infections. Pediatr Infect Dis J 23: 1003–1007.
18. Jacques J, Moret H, Minette D, Leveque N, Jovenin N, et al. (2008) Epidemiological, molecular, and clinical features of enterovirus respiratory infections in French children between 1999 and 2005. J Clin Microbiol 46: 206–213.
19. Tsai HP, Kuo PH, Liu CC, Wang JR (2001) Respiratory viral infections among pediatric inpatients and outpatients in Taiwan from 1997 to 1999. J Clin Microbiol 39: 111–118.
20. Hohenthal U, Vainionpaa R, Nikoskelainen J, Kotilainen P (2008) The role of rhinoviruses and enteroviruses in community acquired pneumonia in adults. Thorax 63: 658–659.
21. Oberste MS, Maher K, Schnurr D, Flemister MR, Lovchik JC, et al. (2004) Enterovirus 68 is associated with respiratory illness and shares biological features with both the enteroviruses and the rhinoviruses. J Gen Virol 85: 2577–2584.
22. Gonzalez Y, Martino R, Badell I, Pardo N, Sureda A, et al. (1999) Pulmonary enterovirus infections in stem cell transplant recipients. Bone Marrow Transplant 23: 511–513.

Age-Related Expansion of Tim-3 Expressing T Cells in Vertically HIV-1 Infected Children

Ravi Tandon[1]*, Maria T. M. Giret[3], Devi SenGupta[2], Vanessa A. York[2], Andrew A. Wiznia[4], Michael G. Rosenberg[4], Esper G. Kallas[3], Lishomwa C. Ndhlovu[1]❡, Douglas F. Nixon[2]❡

1 Hawaii Center for AIDS, Department of Tropical Medicine, John A. Burns School of Medicine, University of Hawaii, Honolulu, Hawaii, United States of America, **2** Division of Experimental Medicine, University of California San Francisco, San Francisco, California, United States of America, **3** Division of Clinical Immunology and Allergy, University of São Paulo, São Paulo, Brazil, **4** Albert Einstein College of Medicine, Bronx, New York, United States of America

Abstract

As perinatally HIV-1-infected children grow into adolescents and young adults, they are increasingly burdened with the long-term consequences of chronic HIV-1 infection, with long-term morbidity due to inadequate immunity. In progressive HIV-1 infection in horizontally infected adults, inflammation, T cell activation, and perturbed T cell differentiation lead to an "immune exhaustion", with decline in T cell effector functions. T effector cells develop an increased expression of CD57 and loss of CD28, with an increase in co-inhibitory receptors such as PD-1 and Tim-3. Very little is known about HIV-1 induced T cell dysfunction in vertical infection. In two perinatally antiretroviral drug treated HIV-1-infected groups with median ages of 11.2 yr and 18.5 yr, matched for viral load, we found no difference in the proportion of senescent $CD28^-CD57^+CD8^+$ T cells between the groups. However, the frequency of Tim-3^+CD8^+ and Tim-3^+CD4^+ exhausted T cells, but not PD-1^+ T cells, was significantly increased in the adolescents with longer duration of infection compared to the children with shorter duration of HIV-1 infection. PD-1^+CD8^+ T cells were directly associated with T cell immune activation in children. The frequency of Tim-3^+CD8^+ T cells positively correlated with HIV-1 plasma viral load in the adolescents but not in the children. These data suggest that Tim-3 upregulation was driven by both HIV-1 viral replication and increased age, whereas PD-1 expression is associated with immune activation. These findings also suggest that the Tim-3 immune exhaustion phenotype rather than PD-1 or senescent cells plays an important role in age-related T cell dysfunction in perinatal HIV-1 infection. Targeting Tim-3 may serve as a novel therapeutic approach to improve immune control of virus replication and mitigate age related T cell exhaustion.

Editor: Xu Yu, Massachusetts General Hospital, United States of America

Funding: Award Number R56AI083112 from the National Institute of Allergy and Infectious Diseases supported this work (http://www.niaid.nih.gov/Pages/default.aspx). The project was also supported by National Institutes of Health grant (AI60397)(http://www.nih.gov/).The funders had no role in study design, data collection and analysis, decision to publish, or preparation of the manuscript.

Competing Interests: The authors have declared that no competing interests exist.

* E-mail: rtandon@hawaii.edu

❡ These authors contributed equally to this work.

Introduction

Since the advent of antiretroviral drugs, perinatally HIV-1-infected children have grown up into the adolescent age with lower rates of AIDS related mortality and morbidity [1,2,3,4,5]. Despite combination antiretroviral therapy (cART), perinatally HIV-1 infected subjects have striking differences in HIV-1 disease progression compared to adults and adolescents and have higher viral load (VL) and lower virological responses rates than adults [6,7,8,9]. This is primarily as a consequence of poor adherence to drugs over a lifetime, underdosing, treatment fatigue, altered pharmacokinetics, novel toxicities, caregiver-related problems and high rates of psychiatric illness including the complications of long-standing infection and the deleterious effects of cART [6,10,11,12]. In horizontally infected adults with chronic treated HIV-1 infection, it is evident that mortality due to non-AIDS events is more common than mortality due to AIDS-related events [13] and this could potentially occur in perinatally infected children earlier. As perinatally HIV-1-infected children age with HIV-1, deleterious consequences to protective T cell immunity may persist or develop despite cART [6,14]. The exact nature of these immunological events and the association with disease progression in vertically infected patients remain unclear.

On encountering antigen, $CD8^+$ T cells differentiate from the least differentiated (naive or early memory) stage to the most mature (memory/effector) stage. In this process, cell surface receptors are progressively downregulated (CD45RA, CCR7, CD28, CD27, CD127) or upregulated (CD57 and CD45RA) as $CD8^+$ T cells differentiate [15,16,17,18]. In adults with HIV-1 infection, T cells fail to fully mature into effector T cells [19,20,21]. We have previously shown that the differentiation status of HIV-1 specific T cells in adults were not readily altered by cART despite declines in T cell activation suggesting that cART does not reverse T cell effector defects [14]. We further showed that in perinatally infected children, T cell effector maturation induced by HIV-1 infection was markedly weaker compared to adults, even in those on cART [22]. As HIV-1 specific T cells develop increased CD57 expression, they have replicative senescence [23], and remain senescent despite suppressive cART.

During many chronic viral infections a distinct terminal state of T cell differentiation, or T cell exhaustion arises [24,25]. Such functionally impaired T cells are characterized by abnormally low cytokine production, poor proliferative capacity with the upregulation of several inhibitory receptors including Programmed Death-1 (PD-1) and T-cell immunoglobulin and mucin domain-containing molecule-3 (Tim-3) among others [26,27,28,29]. These receptors not only mark but also induce inhibitory signals to dampen T cell immune responses. In HIV-1 infection, PD-1, a CD28 family member, is increased on $CD8^{+}$ T cells in progressive HIV-1 disease [30,31]. Tim-3, an immunoglobulin (Ig) superfamily member, initially identified as a negative regulator of Th1 response through the Tim-3/Galectin-9 pathway in several inflammatory disease states [32,33], is also elevated in HIV-1 disease [30] and associated with disease progression. cART can reduce PD-1 levels in T cells in HIV-1 infected adults, and in some subjects Tim-3 expression is also reduced [30,34]. Several combinations of markers are therefore used to discriminate differentiated and senescent T cells. However, whether there are common mechanisms regulating them remain unclear [35].

In the setting of treated HIV-1 disease in adults, T cell function remains perturbed with $CD8^{+}$ T cell activation, defined by $CD38^{+}$ or $CD38^{+}HLA\text{-}DR^{+}$ coexpression, at higher levels than in uninfected subjects [14,36,37]. Immune activation occurs in perinatally infected children and the degree of immune activation present as early as 1–2 months of age can be used to predict which children will become long-term non-progressors [38,39]. In children, the relationship between HIV-1 viral load and immune activation appears to be less clear-cut than in adults, in whom a higher level of viremia is predictably associated with higher levels of activation [38,39,40]

As adults with HIV-1 infection age, it appears that alterations in immune profile or immunosenescence begin to resemble those of much older uninfected subjects, and is now referred to as "premature aging" [41,42,43]. Phenotypic and functional T cell alterations observed during advancing human age lead to poor responses to and efficacy of vaccines, and increased susceptibility to new infections and tumors in the elderly [44,45]. With an acceleration of aging and T cell decline induced by HIV-1 infection, a similar impact on T cell immunity could occur in perinatal HIV-1 infected children as they age into adolescenthood.

In this study we sought to assess the effects of HIV-1 infection on T cell differentiation, senescence and exhaustion in two age groups of perinatally HIV-1-infected subjects with shorter and longer durations of infection that present with persistently high HIV viremia despite access to cART, and determine the associations with markers for disease progression (viral load, immune activation) to improve our understanding of how these parameters may modulate the ability of protective T cell immunity to control HIV infection in children.

Materials and Methods

Ethics Statement

The research involving human participants reported in this study was approved by University of California, San Francisco (UCSF) and Albert Einstein College of Medicine (AECOM) institutional review boards (IRBs), with the approval numbers 10-04893 (UCSF) and 1999-255-000 (AECOM). The legal guardians (biological parent, adoptive parent etc.) provided written informed consent for these patients. For children above 12 years of age, signed consent on the regular informed consent document along with their legal guardians was obtained; for children between the ages of 7 through 12, child assent was also required and obtained; for children less than 7 years old, only the legal guardian provided written consent. The research was conducted according to the Declaration of Helsinki.

Study Population

The study population included 16 perinatally HIV-infected subjects from the Jacobi Medical Center, Bronx, New York. Whole blood samples were collected in EDTA tubes from the subjects during their scheduled monthly visit after obtaining informed consents. Peripheral blood mononuclear cells (PBMC) were purified using Ficoll-Paque™ PLUS density gradient centrifugation (Amersham Pharmacia Biotech, Uppsala, Sweden). Cells were frozen in media containing 90% fetal bovine serum (HyClone, Logan, UT) and 10% dimethyl sulfoxide (Sigma Aldrich, St. Louis, MO) and stored in liquid nitrogen. All subjects were under the care of pediatricians at the Jacobi Medical Center, Bronx, New York.

Measurement of Viral Load

Plasma HIV-1 viral load (VL) was measured with Amplicor HIV-1 Monitor with a lower limit of detection of 50 copies of RNA/ml (Roche Diagnostic Systems, Branchburg, NJ).

Flow Cytometry Assessment

Cryopreserved PBMC were thawed in 37°C water bath, washed in RPMI-1640 medium (HyClone, Logan, UT) supplemented with 10% fetal bovine serum. The PBMC were used in two different panels for surface staining. Briefly, 1×10^{6} PBMC were washed in FACS buffer (PBS+0.02% EDTA and 1% BSA) and transferred to a 96-well V-bottom plate, surface stained for different surface markers for 30 minutes on ice followed by washing in FACS buffer twice and then fixing in 1% paraformaldehyde (Polysciences, Niles, IL) on ice. Finally, cells were analyzed on a LSRII flow cytometer (Becton Dickinson, San Jose, CA). The data was analyzed with FlowJo software, version 9.0 (Tree Star, Ashland, OR). Panel 1 included PE-anti-CD38 (BD Biosciences, San Jose, CA), FITC-anti-HLA-DR (BD Biosciences), Alexa 700-anti-CD4 (BD Biosciences), Qdot 605-anti-CD8 (Invitrogen, Carlsbad, CA), ECD-anti-CD3 (Beckman Coulter, Brea, CA). Panel 2 had PE-anti-Tim-3 (R&D System, Minneapolis, MN) APC-anti-PD-1 (Biolegend, San Diego, CA), Alexa 700-anti-CD4 (BD Biosciences), ECD-anti-CD3 (Beckman Coulter), APC Cy7-anti-CD8 (BD Biosciences), PE-Cy7-anti-CD28 (eBiosciences, San Diego, CA), and FITC-anti-CD57 (BD Biosciences). An amine aqua dye (Invitrogen) was also included in both panels to discriminate between live and dead cells.

Statistical analysis

Statistical analysis was performed using GraphPad Prism statistical software (GraphPad Software, San Diego, CA). The nonparametric Mann-Whitney U was used for comparison tests, and the Spearman Rank test was used for correlation analyses.

Results

Human Subjects

Sixteen HIV-1-infected pediatric subjects of Hispanic and Black ethnicity were divided into two groups based on age. The median age of the two groups consisting children (n = 6) and adolescents (n = 10) was 11.2 and 18.5 years, respectively (Table 1). The two groups were matched for viral load and CD4 count (Table 1). All except three subjects in adolescents were on cART with variable

Table 1. Numbers, CD4 count, viral load, CD8+ T cell activation, and age of subjects in each group.

Measurement	Children	Adolescents	P-value
N	6	10	
Median $CD4^{+}$T cell count (cells/mm^3 [IQR])	547 (299–1,223)	380.5 (338.5–426.5)	0.41
Median HIV-1 viral load (log10 c/ml [IQR])	3.8 (2.8–4.7)	4.5 (4.0–4.8)	0.18
Median $CD8^{+}$ T cell activation (% CD38, HLA-DR [IQR])	33.05 (19.95–37.98)	16.15 (16.17–29.63)	0.103
Median age (yr [IQR])	11.2 (11.0–11.8)	18.5 (17.4–19.9)	0.0002*

adherence to antiretroviral treatment. The characteristics of both groups are displayed in table 2.

There are similar proportions of $CD28^{-}/CD57^{+}$ T cells in children and adolescents

T cell immunosenescence is characterized by the complete and permanent loss of $CD28^{+}$ T cells [16,17] and elevated expression of CD57 on $CD8^{+}$ T cells [18]. To analyze the effect of the duration of HIV-1 infection and aging process on the T cell immune response, we assessed T cell differentiation and senescence ($CD28^{+}$, $CD57^{+}$, and $CD57^{+}CD28^{-}$) of both $CD4^{+}$ and $CD8^{+}$ T cells in two perinatally HIV-1 infected age groups on cART. We observed that $CD8^{+}$ and $CD4^{+}$ T cells did not show any difference in their senescence level between children and adolescents with shorter and longer duration of HIV-1 infection respectively, as observed by $CD57^{+}$ (CD8: median 34.83%; IQR 22.84, 47.83 versus median 29.33%; IQR 21.29, 37.10; $p = 0.367$, figure 1A and B; CD4: median 1.18%; IQR 0.81, 5.87 versus median 1.84%; IQR 1.20, 4.88; $p = 0.493$, figure 2A and B), $CD28^{-}$ (CD8: median 55.27%; IQR 36.42, 66.60 versus median 65.22%; IQR 54.66, 72.59; $p = 0.263$ figure 1A and B; CD4: median 2.21%; IQR 1.31, 6.67 versus median 0.38%; IQR 0.18, 5.97; $p = 0.117$, figure 2A and B) and $CD57^{+}CD28^{-}$ (CD8: median 31.55%; IQR 18.64, 39.52 versus median 24.61%; IQR 19.81, 31.88; $p = 0.427$, figure 1A and B; CD4: median 0.36%; IQR 0.10, 3.14 versus median 0.23%; IQR 0.07, 2.48; $p = 0.792$, figure 2A and B) levels.

Expansion of $Tim\text{-}3^{+}CD4^{+}$ and $CD8^{+}$ T cells in perinatally HIV-1 infected adolescents

In contrast to HIV-1 infection in adults, we did not observe any age related alterations in CD57 or CD28 T cell expression [18,46]. We next assessed the expression of the inhibitory receptors, Tim-3 and PD-1. Compared to younger group, the frequency of Tim-3 in older group was increased in both $CD8^{+}$ (median 18.35%; IQR 13.14, 20.95 versus median 23.93%; IQR 18.19, 32.94; $^{*}p = 0.045$, figure 1C and D) and $CD4^{+}$ (median 11.94%; IQR 10.04, 13.51 versus median 21.34%; IQR 16.47, 23.51; $^{**}p = 0.003$, figure 2C and D) T cells. There was no significant difference in $PD\text{-}1^{+}CD8^{+}$ (median 40.05%; IQR 27.68, 55.80

Table 2. Subject characteristics.

Group	Patient ID	Age (in yrs)	R/E*	Sex	ART§	Notes
Children	S1	11.0	W/H	M	ABC, 3TC, ATV/r	-
	S2	11.0	B/NH	F	ddl, 3TC, LPV/r	Variable adherence.
	S3	11.1	W/H	M	d4T, EFV, LPV/r	Excellent adherence.
	S4	11.4	B/H	F	ABC, 3TC, ATV/r	-
	S5	11.8	W/H	F	ZDV, 3TC	Long term PTI patient.
	S6	12.0	B/NH	F	ZDV, 3TC	-
Adolescents	P1	19.3	W/H	M	On etravirine study	Complete non-adherence to ART.
	P2	19.6	W/H	F	ZDV, 3TC, LPV/r	2nd trimester pregnancy, improved adherence.
	P3	21.2	B/NH	M	EFV-based HAART	Variable adherence.
	P4	22.8	W/H	M	TDF, FTC, ddl, ATV	-
	P5	18.5	W/H	M	ZDV, 3TC	-
	P6	18.6	W/H	F	No ARVs	Off ARVs for >2 yrs.
	P7	18.0	B/NH	F	No ARVs	AIDS, HIV nephropathy, on hemodialysis, non-adherence.
	P8	17.7	W/H	F	ZDV, 3TC, ABC, TDF, ATV/r	Complete non-adherence to ART.
	P9	16.5	W/H	M	No ARVs	Off ARVs for >2 yrs.
	P10	16.3	W/H	F	ZDV, 3TC, ABC, RTV	Poor adherence.

R/E = Race/Ethnicity, W/H = White/Hispanic, B/NH = Black/Non-Hispanic,
§ART = Antiretroviral treatment, ZDV = Zidovudine, 3TC = Lamivudine (2′, 3′-dideoxy-3′-thiacytidine), ABC = Abcavir, TDF = Tenofovir disoproxil fumarate, ATV/r = Atazanavir/ritonavir, LPV/r = Lopinavir/ritonavir, ddl = Didanosine, EFV = Efavirenz.

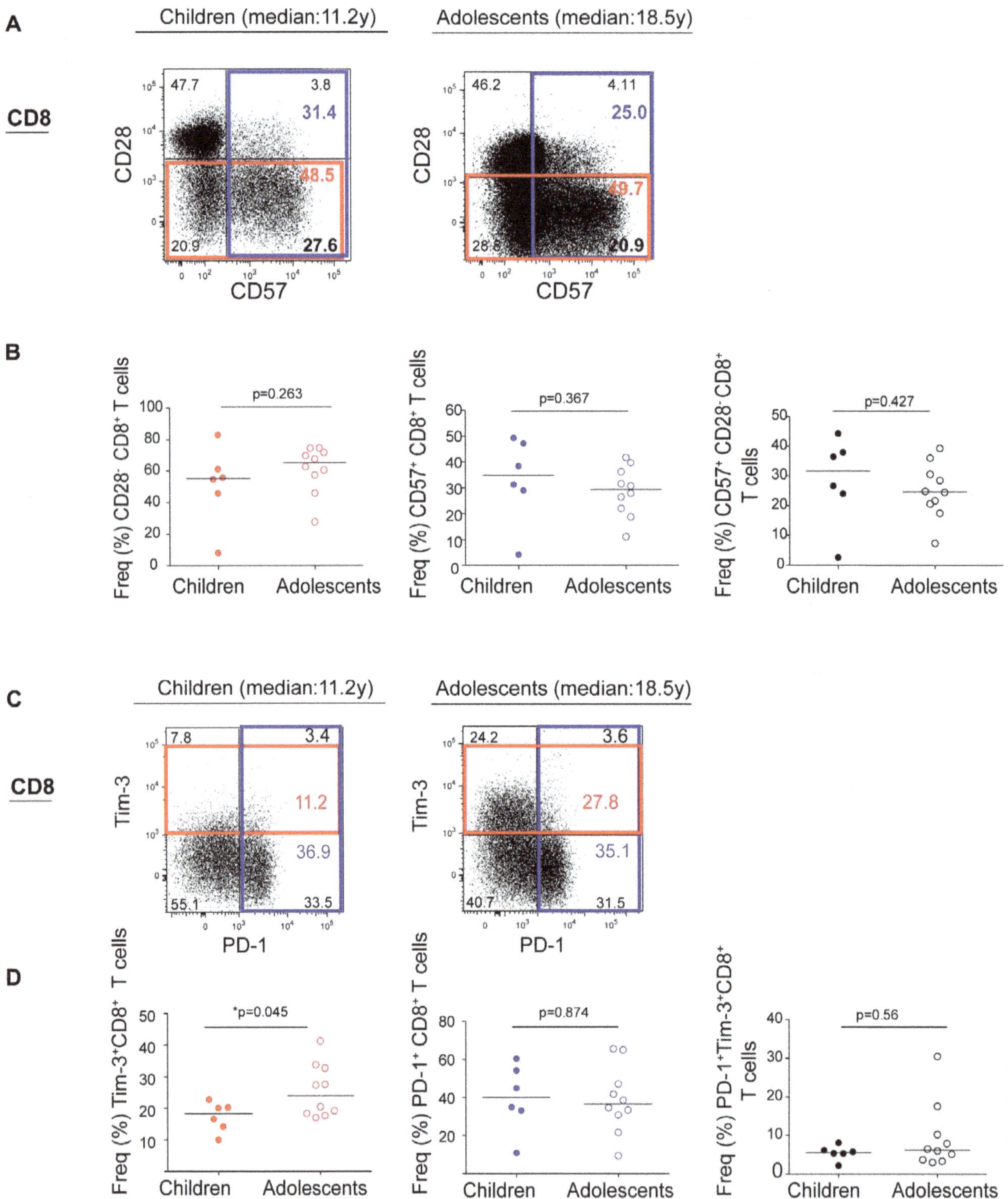

Figure 1. Expansion of Tim-3$^+$CD8$^+$ T cells in perinatally HIV-1-infected adolescents. (A) Flow dot plots show CD8$^+$ T cell surface expression of CD28 and CD57 in perinatally HIV-1-infected children with shorter duration of HIV-1 infection (median: 11.2 y) and adolescents with longer duration of HIV infection (median:18.5 y). (B) Frequencies of CD28$^-$, CD57$^+$, and CD57$^+$CD28$^-$ CD8$^+$ T cells in perinatally HIV-1-infected children and adolescents. (C) Flow dot plots show CD8$^+$ T cell surface expression of PD-1 and Tim-3 in perinatally HIV-1-infected children with shorter duration of HIV infection (median: 11.2 y) and adolescents with longer duration of HIV-1 infection (median: 18.5 y). (D) Frequencies of Tim-3$^+$, PD-1$^+$, and PD-1$^+$ Tim-3$^+$CD8$^+$ T cells in perinatally HIV-1-infected children and adolescents. A significant increase in Tim-3$^+$CD8$^+$ T cell (*p = 0.045) population was observed with age. P values were obtained using two-tailed Mann-Whitney *U* test. Flow dot plots are representative of all subjects in respective groups.

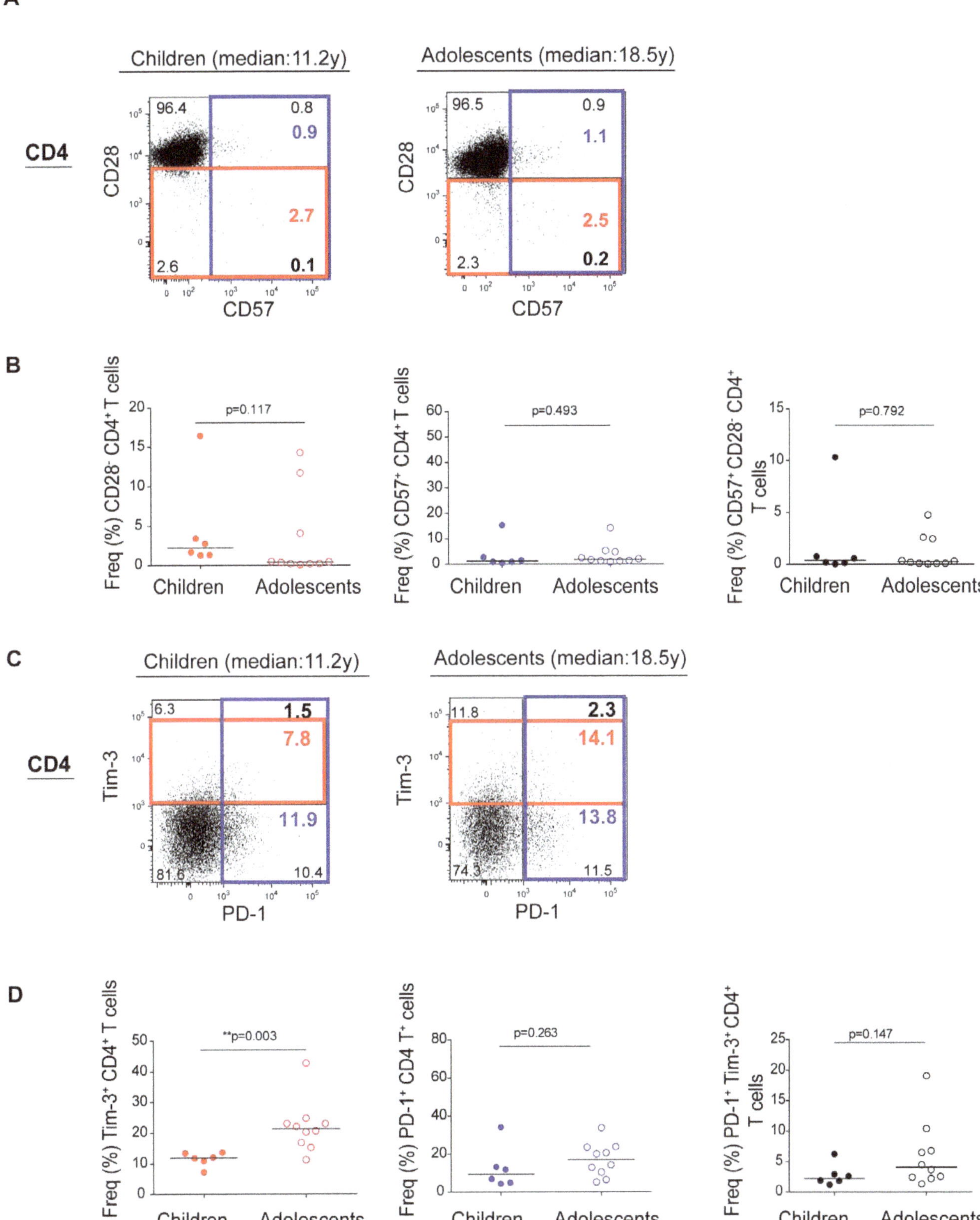

Figure 2. Expansion of Tim-3$^+$ CD4$^+$ T cells in perinatally HIV-1-infected adolescents. (A) Flow dot plots show CD4$^+$ T cell surface expression of CD28 and CD57 in perinatally HIV-1-infected children with shorter duration of HIV-1 infection (median: 11.2 y) and adolescents with longer duration of HIV infection (median:18.5 y). (B) Frequencies of CD28$^-$, CD57$^+$, and CD57$^+$CD28$^-$ CD4$^+$ T cells in perinatally HIV-1-infected children and adolescents. (C) Flow dot plots show CD4$^+$ T cell surface expression of PD-1 and Tim-3 in perinatally HIV-1-infected children with shorter duration of HIV infection (median: 11.2 y) and adolescents with longer duration of HIV-1 infection (median: 18.5 y). (D) Frequencies of Tim-3$^+$, PD-1$^+$, and PD-1$^+$ Tim-3$^+$CD4$^+$ T cells in perinatally HIV-1-infected children and adolescents. A significant increase in Tim-3$^+$CD4$^+$ T cell (**p = 0.003)

population was observed with age. P values were obtained using two-tailed Mann-Whitney *U* test. Flow dot plots are representative of all subjects in respective groups.

versus median 36.75%; IQR 28.58, 51.71; p = 0.874, figure 1C and D) or PD-1^+CD4^+ (median 9.43%; IQR 4.82, 18.46 versus median 17.14%; IQR 9.48, 23.58; p = 0.263, figure 2C and D) and Tim-3^+PD-1^+CD8^+ (median 5.55%; IQR 4.52, 6.67 versus median 6.23%; IQR 3.59, 12.07; p = 0.56, figure 1C and D) or Tim-3^+PD-1^+CD4^+ T cell (median 2.26%; IQR 1.69, 3.76 versus median 4.08%; IQR 2.39, 7.67; p = 0.147, figure 2C and D) T cell population between groups. This suggests that Tim-3^+ T cell expansion and not PD-1 is potentially driven by infection duration and possibly by age, and serves as a better marker for age related T cell dysfunction in the context of perinatal HIV-1 infection.

Tim-3^+CD8^+ T cell expression and not PD-1^+ is associated with HIV-1 viral load in adolescents with longer infection

We and others previously observed that Tim-3 and PD-1 on CD8^+ T cells are associated with HIV-1 viral load in adults [47]. We next determined whether the levels of Tim-3 or PD-1 on T cells were associated with HIV-1 plasma viral load. Interestingly, Tim-3^+CD8^+ T cells showed a significant direct association with HIV-1 plasma viral load in the adolescents (Figure 3B, *p = 0.017, *r* = 0.74), while no such association existed in the children (Figure 3A). PD-1^+CD8^+ T cells did not associate with HIV-1 plasma viral load in either of age groups (Figure 3C and D). Tim-3^+CD4^+ T cells did not show any association with HIV-1 plasma viral load in both children (Figure S1A) and adolescents (Figure S1B). However PD1^+CD4^+ T cells were directly associated with HIV-1 plasma viral load in children (Figure S1C, *p = 0.033, *r* = 0.88) but not in adolescents (Figure S1D).

Infection duration and age related decline in CD8^+ T cell activation in the adolescents with longer HIV infection

T cell activation, as defined by the expression of HLA-DR and CD38, is the marker of HIV-1 disease progression [37,48,49]. In perinatally HIV-1 infected children, CD38 expression in CD8^+ T cells predicts virological failure despite antiretroviral therapy [50]. We determined next whether the levels of CD38 and HLA-DR or CD38 alone were associated with T cell activation. Given that perinatally HIV-1 children have a high HIV-1 load and poor adherence to cART, we hypothesized that perinatally HIV-1-infected children would show higher immune activation with advancing age. However, when we looked at treatment-experienced subjects from the two groups, we observed a decrease in immune activation in the adolescent group only, despite no significant change in viral load and CD4^+ count in both groups.

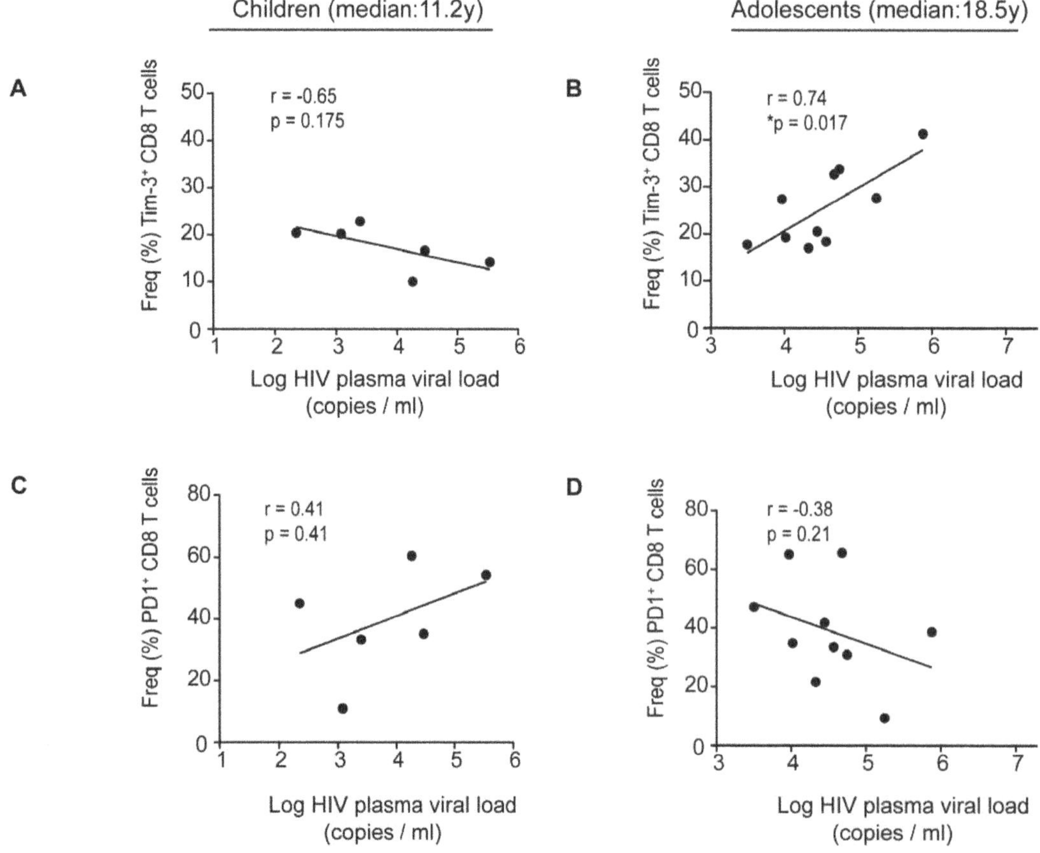

Figure 3. A positive correlation between Tim3^+CD8^+ T cells and HIV-1 plasma viral load (VL) in adolescents. Scatter plots showing correlation between HIV plasma viral load (VL) and Tim-3^+CD8^+ T cells (A and B), and PD-1^+CD8^+ T cells (C and D) in children (left) and adolescents (right) subjects. Tim-3^+CD8^+ T cells show a significant direct correlation with HIV-1 plasma viral load (VL) in adolescents (Spearman r = 0.74, *p = 0.017).

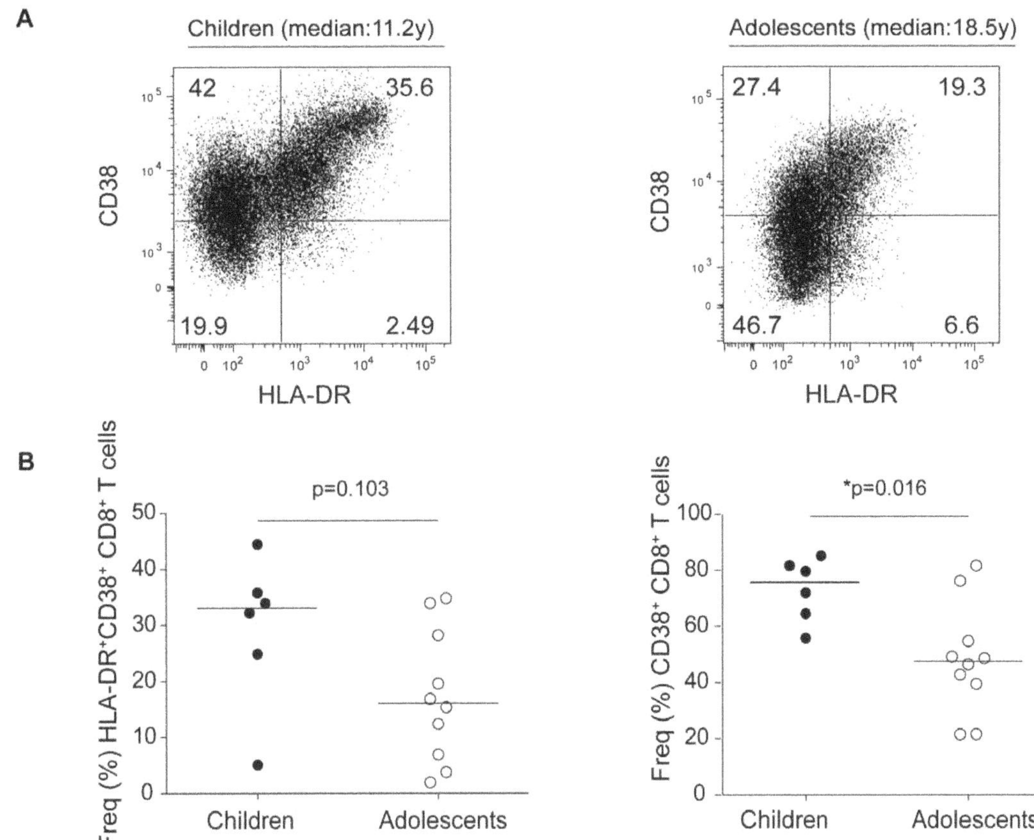

Figure 4. Infection duration and age related decrease in CD8$^+$ T cell activation in adolescents. (A) Flow dot plots show CD8 surface expression of CD38 and HLA-DR in perinatally HIV-1 infected children (median: 11.2 y) and adolescents (median: 18.5 y). Dot plots are representative of all subjects in respective groups. (B) Frequencies of HLA-DR$^+$CD38$^+$CD8$^+$ T cells and CD38$^+$CD8$^+$ T cells in perinatally HIV-1-infected children and adolescents. A significant decrease in CD38$^+$CD8$^+$ T cell (*p = 0.016) and a marginal decrease in HLA-DR$^+$CD38$^+$CD8$^+$ T cell (p = 0.103) populations were observed with the duration of HIV infection. P values were obtained using two-tailed Mann-Whitney *U* test.

There was a marginal decrease in HLA-DR$^+$CD38$^+$CD8$^+$ T cells in adolescents, while CD38$^+$CD8$^+$ T cells were significantly (*p = 0.016) decreased in adolescents (Figure 4A and B). The changes in immune activation were independent of HIV-1 plasma viral load (data not shown).

PD-1$^+$CD8$^+$ T cells are associated with T cell activation but not viral load

We next assessed the relationship between T cell exhaustion and immune activation. Intriguingly, PD-1$^+$CD8$^+$ T cells had a direct strong significant association with HLA-DR$^+$CD38$^+$CD8$^+$ T cells in children (r = 0.947, **p = 0.004) as well as in the adolescents (r = 0.70, *p = 0.026). This suggests that there is a possibility that PD-1 expression may be driven by immune activation (Figure 5A and B). Tim-3 did not show any association with immune activation in either group (Figure 5C and D).

Discussion

Despite access to cART, children aging with HIV-1 infection are unable to control HIV-1 infection adequately [51]. Therefore, it is imperative to determine better correlates of protective immunity. This study shows that markers of T cell senescence do not appear to change with the duration of infection. However, there was an expansion of immune exhausted Tim-3$^+$CD8$^+$ T cells, but not PD-1$^+$ T cells, in adolescents compared to younger children in the setting of high viremia. More importantly, these high levels of Tim-3$^+$CD8$^+$ T cells had a significant direct association with HIV-1 plasma viral load.

The expression of the inhibitory molecules Tim-3 and PD-1 on CD8 T cells has been associated with T cell exhaustion during chronic HIV-1 infection in adults. Their expression results in inhibition of T cell expansion and cytokine production [29,30,47], and associate with disease progression. A recent study has shown that PD-1 increased on T cells derived from older mice compared to younger mice [52], suggesting these exhaustion markers may contribute to age-related declines in immunity. Our data suggest that Tim-3 plays an important role in age-related T cell dysfunction in perinatal HIV-1 infection. By contrast, neither PD-1$^+$ nor PD1$^+$Tim-3$^+$ T cells showed any difference in the two age groups in our study. While we did not observe differential PD-1 expression, this may be due to the small differences in age between the two groups in our study, or may reflect differences in the dynamics of PD-1 and Tim-3 expression.

T cell activation is undoubtedly the best marker of HIV-1 disease in adults. We and others have shown that HIV-1 viral load directly associates with T cell activation (HLA-DR$^+$CD38$^+$ or CD38$^+$) in adults [53,54], but this does not appear to occur in pediatric vertical infection which has also been confirmed by others [55]. Tim-3$^+$ CD8$^+$ T cells are not associated with T cell activation [30]. Our results are consistent with a recent report that shows a positive association between CD8$^+$ T cell activation and

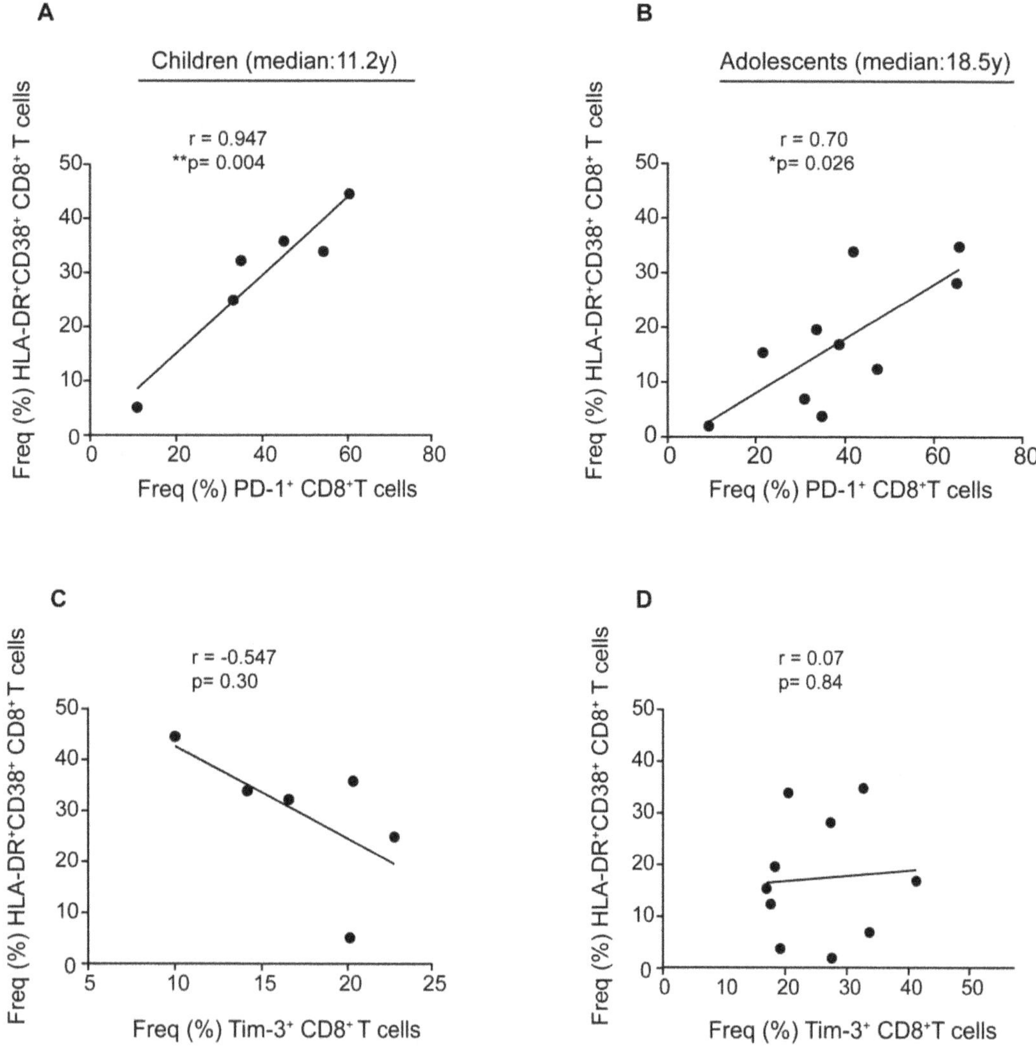

Figure 5. PD-1$^+$CD8$^+$ T cells have a strong significant correlation with immune activation in both age groups. Scatter plots showing a correlation between immune activation and PD-1$^+$ or Tim3$^+$CD8$^+$ T cells. (A) and (B) show a significant strong correlation between HLA-DR$^+$CD38$^+$CD8$^+$ T cell and PD-1$^+$CD8$^+$ T cells in children with shorter duration of HIV-1 infection (Spearman $r = 0.947$, $^{**}p = 0.004$) and adolescents with longer duration of HIV-1 infection (Spearman $r = 0.70$, $^{*}p = 0.026$) respectively. (C) and (D) show a correlation between HLA-DR$^+$CD38$^+$ CD8$^+$ T cells and Tim-3$^+$CD8$^+$ T cells in both age groups.

the frequency of PD-1$^+$CD8$^+$ T cells in HIV-1 infected untreated younger children [56]. PD-1 may thus serve as a marker of T cell activation and our results build on this observation. Our previous study revealed that CD38 is associated with HIV-1 viral load [53]. We found that CD38 alone was lower in the adolescents with longer duration of HIV-1 infection despite both age groups having similar matched HIV-1 viral load.

T cell immunosenescence is characterized by the complete and permanent loss of CD28$^+$ T cells and elevated expression of CD57 on CD8$^+$ T cells [41,43]. Compared to age-matched controls, HIV-1-infected adults have noticeable increase in CD28$^-$ and CD57$^+$ CD8$^+$ T cell population [57,58,59]. In addition, CD28$^-$CD8$^+$ T cells have been shown to be significantly associated with the CD4$^+$ T cell loss, and lymphocyte apoptosis in perinatally HIV-1-infected children [60]. In our present study, we expected an accumulation of CD57$^+$CD28$^-$ T cells in the adolescents with longer duration of infection. However, unlike adult HIV-1 infection, we did not observe any changes in these cell subsets in pediatric HIV-1 infection. These observations suggest that the previous published senescent markers (CD28, CD57) in adults may not reflect age related changes in perinatally HIV-1-infected children. Instead, Tim-3 may be a better marker of T cell immunosenescence in children and adolescents.

Due to the complexities in the management of perinatal HIV infection, and its accompanying specific treatment related issues, novel strategies are needed. Earlier initiation of cART follow by partial treatment interruption (PTI) is being reconsidered and envisioned to permit functional maturity of protective T-cell based immunity before introduction of a PTI regimen [61]. A recent study showed that adherence rates to antiretroviral therapy remained the same between PTI and continuous therapy (CT) [62]. Our previous work has shown that PTI was ineffective in controlling HIV-1 replication [63]. We propose that defining effective phenotypic profile of protective T cell immunity and reinvigorating T cell immunity by targeting age dependent pathways like Tim-3 may help induce effective anti-HIV-1 immune responses in children on either CT or PTI and be considered as an adjunctive therapy.

It is still debated whether T cell senescence and exhaustion are related or unrelated processes in compromised immunity. Detailed assessment of the signaling pathways that regulate T cell senescence and exhaustion suggest that they appear to be distinct processes [35]. Our study design did not permit the assessment of multiple age groups to determine the shifts in the profiles of the T cell differentiation and exhaustion markers over time in both HIV-1-infected and uninfected children. Therefore, further studies are needed to address these longitudinal changes in a large pediatric cohort. Our findings reveal the importance of the Tim-3 marker in pediatric HIV-1 infection and suggests that Tim-3 upregulation in the older age group was driven by HIV-1 viral replication, increased age, and longer duration of infection. The use of reagents targeting Tim-3 or its ligand could potentially reverse immunosenescence or exhaustion and other possible age-related complications. We have shown that blocking Tim-3-Tim-3L pathway either by addition of recombinant soluble Tim-3 (sTim-3) glycoprotein as a competitor for Tim-3 ligand(s) or using a blocking anti-Tim-3 mAB in vitro, increased expansion of antigen specific CD8^{+}T cells and T cell proliferation responses [30]. Furthermore, we are now beginning to unravel the Tim-3 signaling pathway mediating T cell inhibition [64,65], which could unveil potential targets that reverse Tim-3 mediated events. Applying these strategies to target Tim-3 in context of perinatal HIV-1 infection together with improved cART delivery strategies may therefore serve as a novel therapeutic to suppress viral replication and mitigate age-related complications offering further alternative treatment options in perinatal HIV-1 infection.

Acknowledgments

We thank Glen Chew and Tsuyoshi Fujita for help with specimens' preparations. Part of this work was presented at the HIV Vaccines Keystone Symposia, Keystone, CO, USA in March 2012 (R.T.).

Author Contributions

Conceived and designed the experiments: RT MTMG AAW MGR EGK LCN DFN. Performed the experiments: RT MTMG DS VAY. Analyzed the data: RT MTMG DS MGR EGK LCN DFN. Contributed reagents/materials/analysis tools: RT MTMG DS VAY AAW MGR EGK LCN DFN. Wrote the paper: RT MTMG DS VAY MGR LCN DFN.

References

1. Gibb DM, Duong T, Tookey PA, Sharland M, Tudor-Williams G, et al. (2003) Decline in mortality, AIDS, and hospital admissions in perinatally HIV-1 infected children in the United Kingdom and Ireland. Bmj 327: 1019.
2. Judd A, Doerholt K, Tookey PA, Sharland M, Riordan A, et al. (2007) Morbidity, mortality, and response to treatment by children in the United Kingdom and Ireland with perinatally acquired HIV infection during 1996–2006: planning for teenage and adult care. Clinical infectious diseases: an official publication of the Infectious Diseases Society of America 45: 918–924.
3. Violari A, Cotton MF, Gibb DM, Babiker AG, Steyn J, et al. (2008) Early antiretroviral therapy and mortality among HIV-infected infants. The New England journal of medicine 359: 2233–2244.
4. Reddi A, Leeper SC, Grobler AC, Geddes R, France KH, et al. (2007) Preliminary outcomes of a paediatric highly active antiretroviral therapy cohort from KwaZulu-Natal, South Africa. BMC pediatrics 7: 13.
5. Sutcliffe CG, van Dijk JH, Bolton C, Persaud D, Moss WJ (2008) Effectiveness of antiretroviral therapy among HIV-infected children in sub-Saharan Africa. The Lancet infectious diseases 8: 477–489.
6. Kahana SY, Rohan J, Allison S, Frazier TW, Drotar D (2012) A Meta-Analysis of Adherence to Antiretroviral Therapy and Virologic Responses in HIV-Infected Children, Adolescents, and Young Adults. AIDS and behavior.
7. Sabin CA, Smith CJ, d'Arminio Monforte A, Battegay M, Gabiano C, et al. (2008) Response to combination antiretroviral therapy: variation by age. AIDS 22: 1463–1473.
8. MJ O (1994) Vertically acquired HIV infection in the United States. In: Pizzo PA, Wilfert CM, eds. . 3–20 p.
9. Levy JA (1993) Pathogenesis of human immunodeficiency virus infection. Microbiological reviews 57: 183–289.
10. Amaya RA, Kozinetz CA, McMeans A, Schwarzwald H, Kline MW (2002) Lipodystrophy syndrome in human immunodeficiency virus-infected children. The Pediatric infectious disease journal 21: 405–410.
11. Menson EN, Walker AS, Sharland M, Wells C, Tudor-Williams G, et al. (2006) Underdosing of antiretrovirals in UK and Irish children with HIV as an example of problems in prescribing medicines to children, 1997–2005: cohort study. Bmj 332: 1183–1187.
12. Leonard EG, McComsey GA (2003) Metabolic complications of antiretroviral therapy in children. The Pediatric infectious disease journal 22: 77–84.
13. Mocroft A, Reiss P, Gasiorowski J, Ledergerber B, Kowalska J, et al. (2010) Serious fatal and nonfatal non-AIDS-defining illnesses in Europe. Journal of acquired immune deficiency syndromes 55: 262–270.
14. Barbour JD, Ndhlovu LC, Xuan Tan Q, Ho T, Epling L, et al. (2009) High CD8+ T cell activation marks a less differentiated HIV-1 specific CD8+ T cell response that is not altered by suppression of viral replication. PloS one 4: e4408.
15. Cao W, Jamieson BD, Hultin LE, Hultin PM, Effros RB, et al. (2009) Premature aging of T cells is associated with faster HIV-1 disease progression. Journal of acquired immune deficiency syndromes 50: 137–147.
16. Valenzuela HF, Effros RB (2002) Divergent telomerase and CD28 expression patterns in human CD4 and CD8 T cells following repeated encounters with the same antigenic stimulus. Clinical immunology 105: 117–125.
17. Nociari MM, Telford W, Russo C (1999) Postthymic development of CD28−CD8+ T cell subset: age-associated expansion and shift from memory to naive phenotype. Journal of immunology 162: 3327–3335.
18. Merino J, Martinez-Gonzalez MA, Rubio M, Inoges S, Sanchez-Ibarrola A, et al. (1998) Progressive decrease of CD8high+ CD28+ CD57− cells with ageing. Clinical and experimental immunology 112: 48–51.
19. van Baarle D, Kostense S, Hovenkamp E, Ogg G, Nanlohy N, et al. (2002) Lack of Epstein-Barr virus- and HIV-specific CD27− CD8+ T cells is associated with progression to viral disease in HIV-infection. AIDS 16: 2001–2011.
20. van Baarle D, Kostense S, van Oers MH, Hamann D, Miedema F (2002) Failing immune control as a result of impaired CD8+ T-cell maturation: CD27 might provide a clue. Trends Immunol 23: 586–591.
21. Addo MM, Draenert R, Rathod A, Verrill CL, Davis BT, et al. (2007) Fully differentiated HIV-1 specific CD8+ T effector cells are more frequently detectable in controlled than in progressive HIV-1 infection. PloS one 2: e321.
22. Sandberg JK, Fast NM, Jordan KA, Furlan SN, Barbour JD, et al. (2003) HIV-specific CD8+ T cell function in children with vertically acquired HIV-1 infection is critically influenced by age and the state of the CD4+ T cell compartment. Journal of immunology 170: 4403–4410.
23. Brenchley JM, Karandikar NJ, Betts MR, Ambrozak DR, Hill BJ, et al. (2003) Expression of CD57 defines replicative senescence and antigen-induced apoptotic death of CD8+ T cells. Blood 101: 2711–2720.
24. Zajac AJ, Blattman JN, Murali-Krishna K, Sourdive DJ, Suresh M, et al. (1998) Viral immune evasion due to persistence of activated T cells without effector function. The Journal of experimental medicine 188: 2205–2213.
25. Gallimore A, Glithero A, Godkin A, Tissot AC, Pluckthun A, et al. (1998) Induction and exhaustion of lymphocytic choriomeningitis virus-specific cytotoxic T lymphocytes visualized using soluble tetrameric major histocompatibility complex class I-peptide complexes. The Journal of experimental medicine 187: 1383–1393.
26. Banerjee P, Feuer G, Barker E (2007) Human T-cell leukemia virus type 1 (HTLV-1) p12I down-modulates ICAM-1 and -2 and reduces adherence of natural killer cells, thereby protecting HTLV-1-infected primary CD4+ T cells from autologous natural killer cell-mediated cytotoxicity despite the reduction of major histocompatibility complex class I molecules on infected cells. Journal of virology 81: 9707–9717.
27. Bengsch B, Seigel B, Ruhl M, Timm J, Kuntz M, et al. (2010) Coexpression of PD-1, 2B4, CD160 and KLRG1 on exhausted HCV-specific CD8+ T cells is linked to antigen recognition and T cell differentiation. PLoS pathogens 6: e1000947.
28. Baitsch L, Legat A, Barba L, Fuertes Marraco SA, Rivals JP, et al. (2012) Extended co-expression of inhibitory receptors by human CD8 T-cells

depending on differentiation, antigen-specificity and anatomical localization. PloS one 7: e30852.
29. Jin HT, Anderson AC, Tan WG, West EE, Ha SJ, et al. (2010) Cooperation of Tim-3 and PD-1 in CD8 T-cell exhaustion during chronic viral infection. Proceedings of the National Academy of Sciences of the United States of America 107: 14733–14738.
30. Jones RB, Ndhlovu LC, Barbour JD, Sheth PM, Jha AR, et al. (2008) Tim-3 expression defines a novel population of dysfunctional T cells with highly elevated frequencies in progressive HIV-1 infection. The Journal of experimental medicine 205: 2763–2779.
31. Golden-Mason L, Palmer BE, Kassam N, Townshend-Bulson L, Livingston S, et al. (2009) Negative immune regulator Tim-3 is overexpressed on T cells in hepatitis C virus infection and its blockade rescues dysfunctional CD4+ and CD8+ T cells. Journal of virology 83: 9122–9130.
32. Chou FC, Shieh SJ, Sytwu HK (2009) Attenuation of Th1 response through galectin-9 and T-cell Ig mucin 3 interaction inhibits autoimmune diabetes in NOD mice. Eur J Immunol 39: 2403–2411.
33. Zhu C, Anderson AC, Schubart A, Xiong H, Imitola J, et al. (2005) The Tim-3 ligand galectin-9 negatively regulates T helper type 1 immunity. Nature immunology 6: 1245–1252.
34. Kassu A, Marcus RA, D'Souza MB, Kelly-McKnight EA, Palmer BE (2011) Suppression of HIV replication by antiretroviral therapy reduces TIM-3 expression on HIV-specific CD8(+) T cells. AIDS research and human retroviruses 27: 1–3.
35. Akbar AN, Henson SM (2011) Are senescence and exhaustion intertwined or unrelated processes that compromise immunity? Nature reviews Immunology 11: 289–295.
36. Sinclair E, Ronquillo R, Lollo N, Deeks SG, Hunt P, et al. (2008) Antiretroviral treatment effect on immune activation reduces cerebrospinal fluid HIV-1 infection. Journal of acquired immune deficiency syndromes 47: 544–552.
37. Hunt PW, Brenchley J, Sinclair E, McCune JM, Roland M, et al. (2008) Relationship between T cell activation and CD4+ T cell count in HIV-seropositive individuals with undetectable plasma HIV RNA levels in the absence of therapy. The Journal of infectious diseases 197: 126–133.
38. Mekmullica J, Brouwers P, Charurat M, Paul M, Shearer W, et al. (2009) Early immunological predictors of neurodevelopmental outcomes in HIV-infected children. Clinical infectious diseases: an official publication of the Infectious Diseases Society of America 48: 338–346.
39. Paul ME, Mao C, Charurat M, Serchuck L, Foca M, et al. (2005) Predictors of immunologic long-term nonprogression in HIV-infected children: implications for initiating therapy. J Allergy Clin Immunol 115: 848–855.
40. Giorgi JV, Hultin LE, McKeating JA, Johnson TD, Owens B, et al. (1999) Shorter survival in advanced human immunodeficiency virus type 1 infection is more closely associated with T lymphocyte activation than with plasma virus burden or virus chemokine coreceptor usage. J Infect Dis 179: 859–870.
41. Effros RB, Dagarag M, Spaulding C, Man J (2005) The role of CD8+ T-cell replicative senescence in human aging. Immunological reviews 205: 147–157.
42. Appay V, Almeida JR, Sauce D, Autran B, Papagno L (2007) Accelerated immune senescence and HIV-1 infection. Experimental gerontology 42: 432–437.
43. Desai S, Landay A (2010) Early immune senescence in HIV disease. Current HIV/AIDS reports 7: 4–10.
44. McElhaney JE (2009) Prevention of infectious diseases in older adults through immunization: the challenge of the senescent immune response. Expert review of vaccines 8: 593–606.
45. Nikolich-Zugich J (2008) Ageing and life-long maintenance of T-cell subsets in the face of latent persistent infections. Nature reviews Immunology 8: 512–522.
46. Sadat-Sowti B, Debre P, Idziorek T, Guillon JM, Hadida F, et al. (1991) A lectin-binding soluble factor released by CD8+CD57+ lymphocytes from AIDS patients inhibits T cell cytotoxicity. European journal of immunology 21: 737–741.
47. Day CL, Kaufmann DE, Kiepiela P, Brown JA, Moodley ES, et al. (2006) PD-1 expression on HIV-specific T cells is associated with T-cell exhaustion and disease progression. Nature 443: 350–354.
48. Deeks SG, Kitchen CM, Liu L, Guo H, Gascon R, et al. (2004) Immune activation set point during early HIV infection predicts subsequent CD4+ T-cell changes independent of viral load. Blood 104: 942–947.
49. Liu Z, Cumberland WG, Hultin LE, Prince HE, Detels R, et al. (1997) Elevated CD38 antigen expression on CD8+ T cells is a stronger marker for the risk of chronic HIV disease progression to AIDS and death in the Multicenter AIDS Cohort Study than CD4+ cell count, soluble immune activation markers, or combinations of HLA-DR and CD38 expression. Journal of acquired immune deficiency syndromes and human retrovirology: official publication of the International Retrovirology Association 16: 83–92.
50. Resino S, Bellon JM, Gurbindo MD, Munoz-Fernandez MA (2004) CD38 expression in CD8+ T cells predicts virological failure in HIV type 1-infected children receiving antiretroviral therapy. Clinical infectious diseases: an official publication of the Infectious Diseases Society of America 38: 412–417.
51. Tandon R, SenGupta D, Ndhlovu LC, Vieira RG, Jones RB, et al. (2011) Identification of human endogenous retrovirus-specific T cell responses in vertically HIV-1-infected subjects. Journal of virology 85: 11526–11531.
52. Shimada Y, Hayashi M, Nagasaka Y, Ohno-Iwashita Y, Inomata M (2009) Age-associated up-regulation of a negative co-stimulatory receptor PD-1 in mouse CD4+ T cells. Experimental gerontology 44: 517–522.
53. Ndhlovu LC, Loo CP, Spotts G, Nixon DF, Hecht FM (2008) FOXP3 expressing CD127lo CD4+ T cells inversely correlate with CD38+ CD8+ T cell activation levels in primary HIV-1 infection. Journal of leukocyte biology 83: 254–262.
54. Agarwal A, Sankaran S, Vajpayee M, Sreenivas V, Seth P, et al. (2007) Correlation of immune activation with HIV-1 RNA levels assayed by real-time RT-PCR in HIV-1 subtype C infected patients in Northern India. Journal of clinical virology: the official publication of the Pan American Society for Clinical Virology 40: 301–306.
55. Romeiro JR, Pinto JA, Silva ML, Eloi-Santos SM (2012) Further Evidence That the Expression of CD38 and HLA-DR+ in CD8+ Lymphocytes Does Not Correlate to Disease Progression in HIV-1 Vertically Infected Children. Journal of the International Association of Physicians in AIDS Care 11: 164–168.
56. Prendergast A, O'Callaghan M, Menson E, Hamadache D, Walters S, et al. (2011) Factors Influencing T Cell Activation and Programmed Death 1 Expression in HIV-Infected Children. AIDS research and human retroviruses.
57. Kalayjian RC, Landay A, Pollard RB, Taub DD, Gross BH, et al. (2003) Age-related immune dysfunction in health and in human immunodeficiency virus (HIV) disease: association of age and HIV infection with naive CD8+ cell depletion, reduced expression of CD28 on CD8+ cells, and reduced thymic volumes. The Journal of infectious diseases 187: 1924–1933.
58. Le Priol Y, Puthier D, Lecureuil C, Combadiere C, Debre P, et al. (2006) High cytotoxic and specific migratory potencies of senescent CD8+ CD57+ cells in HIV-infected and uninfected individuals. Journal of immunology 177: 5145–5154.
59. Appay V, Dunbar PR, Callan M, Klenerman P, Gillespie GM, et al. (2002) Memory CD8+ T cells vary in differentiation phenotype in different persistent virus infections. Nat Med 8: 379–385.
60. Brugnoni D, Airo P, Timpano S, Malacarne F, Ugazio AG, et al. (1997) CD8+CD28− T cells in vertically HIV-infected children. Clinical and experimental immunology 109: 412–415.
61. Goulder PJ, Prendergast AJ (2011) Approaches towards avoiding lifelong antiretroviral therapy in paediatric HIV infection. Advances in experimental medicine and biology 719: 25–37.
62. Harrison L, Ananworanich J, Hamadache D, Compagnucci A, Penazzato M, et al. (2012) Adherence to Antiretroviral Therapy and Acceptability of Planned Treatment Interruptions in HIV-Infected Children. AIDS and behavior.
63. Legrand FA, Abadi J, Jordan KA, Davenport MP, Deeks SG, et al. (2005) Partial treatment interruption of protease inhibitors augments HIV-specific immune responses in vertically infected pediatric patients. AIDS 19: 1575–1585.
64. Lee J, Su EW, Zhu C, Hainline S, Phuah J, et al. (2011) Phosphotyrosine-dependent coupling of Tim-3 to T-cell receptor signaling pathways. Molecular and cellular biology 31: 3963–3974.
65. van de Weyer PS, Muehlfeit M, Klose C, Bonventre JV, Walz G, et al. (2006) A highly conserved tyrosine of Tim-3 is phosphorylated upon stimulation by its ligand galectin-9. Biochem Biophys Res Commun 351: 571–576.

11

Short-Term In-Vitro Expansion Improves Monitoring and Allows Affordable Generation of Virus-Specific T-Cells against Several Viruses for a Broad Clinical Application

René Geyeregger[1]*, Christine Freimüller[1], Stefan Stevanovic[4], Julia Stemberger[1], Gabor Mester[4], Jasmin Dmytrus[1], Thomas Lion[2,3], Hans-Georg Rammensee[4], Gottfried Fischer[5], Britta Eiz-Vesper[6], Anita Lawitschka[2,7], Susanne Matthes[2,7], Gerhard Fritsch[1,2]

1 Department of Clinical Cell Biology and FACS Core Unit, Children's Cancer Research Institute (CCRI), Vienna, Austria, **2** Department Pediatrics, Medical University of Vienna, Vienna, Austria, **3** Department of Molecular Microbiology, Children's Cancer Research Institute (CCRI), Vienna, Austria, **4** Department of Immunology, Institute for Cell Biology, Eberhard-Karls-Universität Tübingen, Tübingen, Germany, **5** Department of Blood Group Serology and Transfusion Medicine, Medical University of Vienna, Vienna, Austria, **6** Institute for Transfusion Medicine, Hannover Medical School, Hannover, Germany, **7** Department of Stem Cell Transplantation, St. Anna Children's Hospital, Vienna, Austria

Abstract

Adenoviral infections are a major cause of morbidity and mortality after allogeneic hematopoietic stem cell transplantation (HSCT) in pediatric patients. Adoptive transfer of donor-derived human adenovirus (HAdV)-specific T-cells represents a promising treatment option. However, the difficulty in identifying and selecting rare HAdV-specific T-cells, and the short time span between patients at high risk for invasive infection and viremia are major limitations. We therefore developed an IL-15-driven 6 to 12 day short-term protocol for *in vitro* detection of HAdV-specific T cells, as revealed by known MHC class I multimers and a newly identified adenoviral CD8 T-cell epitope derived from the E1A protein for the frequent HLA-type A*02:01 and IFN-γ. Using this novel and improved diagnostic approach we observed a correlation between adenoviral load and reconstitution of $CD8^+$ and $CD4^+$ HAdV-specific T-cells including central memory cells in HSCT-patients. Adaption of the 12-day protocol to good manufacturing practice conditions resulted in a 2.6-log (mean) expansion of HAdV-specific T-cells displaying high cytolytic activity (4-fold) compared to controls and low or absent alloreactivity. Similar protocols successfully identified and rapidly expanded CMV-, EBV-, and BKV-specific T-cells. Our approach provides a powerful clinical-grade convertible tool for rapid and cost-effective detection and enrichment of multiple virus-specific T-cells that may facilitate broad clinical application.

Editor: Natalia Lapteva, Baylor College of Medicine, United States of America

Funding: This work was supported in part by grants from Eurostars Grant E! 5744 (FFG 829495), Clinical Trial Investigator Driven (CTID)-RG-Matthes and the German Children's Cancer Foundation. The funders had no role in study design, data collection and analysis, decision to publish, or preparation of the manuscript. No additional external funding received for this study.

Competing Interests: The authors have declared that no competing interests exist.

* E-mail: rene.geyeregger@ccri.at

Introduction

Adenovirus (HAdV), cytomegalovirus (CMV), Epstein-Barr-Virus (EBV), and polyoma-Virus (BKV) are responsible for serious morbidity and mortality in patients after hematopoietic stem cell transplantation (HSCT) [1,2,3,4]. HAdV represents one of the most frequent and dangerous infections post transplant [5,6], especially after haploidentical HSCT [1,5,7] and, therefore, is a front-ranking target for early preemptive antiviral therapy [8]. Unfortunately, prophylactic treatment with anti-viral drugs is of limited effectiveness, expensive and associated with substantial toxicity, and may result in overtreatment of patients [1,6,9,10]. Recently, it has been shown that reconstitution of HAdV-specific T-cell response correlates with clearance of ADV infection [11,12,13,14]. In patients who showed no virus-specific immune reconstitution after HSCT, donor-derived virus-specific T-cells against different viruses including HAdV were administered with impressive clinical results [15,16,17,18,19,20,21,22]. As a prerequisite for the monitoring of virus-specific T-cells in donors and patients, immunodominant viral epitopes have to be identified. Altough we focused only on the monitoring of HAdV-specific T cells, new epitopes could also be used for adoptive therapy, i.e. for the magnetic isolation of HAdV-mulitmer+ T cells [22]. Certain sequences of the major capsid protein hexon are highly conserved among human HAdV which currently comprise more than 55 sybtypes divided into 7 different species (A–G)[23]. This provides the basis for "cross-reactivity" of HAdV-specific T-cells facilitating broad recognition and protection against several species [24]. It is known that most $CD4^+$ and $CD8^+$ ADV-specific T-cells recognize predominantly hexon protein structures or overlapping 15-mer peptide pools. The IFN-γ secretion induced by appropriate stimulation enables their detection by the IFN-γ -cytokine secretion assay (CSA) [25,26]. Alternatively, virus-specific T-cells can be identified and isolated using different types of MHC class I multimers including tetramers, pentamers or streptamers [24]. To date, only few HAdV-specific immunodominant $CD8^+$ T-cell epitopes have been identified that are presented in the context of the common HLA-types A*01, A*24, B*07 and B*35 [14,27] thus greatly limiting the number of available HAdV-multimers. Using these four multimers, the probability to detect ADV-specific T-cells within the Caucasian population is about 73%. According to an algorithm presented by Schipper et al [28], this percentage could be increased to 95%, if a functional A*02-based multimer were available. Our primary aim was therefore to identify new promising ADV-specific epitopes for the HLA-types A*01 and A*24, and particularly for the frequent HLA-type A*02, by analyzing the main structural proteins of the virus, including hexon and protein II, as well as the E1A protein expressed very early after infection.

The utility of HAdV-specific multimers for diagnostic applications is further supported by the recent observation that, in patients who cleared HAdV-infection after HSCT, apart from $CD4^+$-, also $CD8^+$ T-cells were present. [14]. However, in most healthy donors and HSCT-patients, HAdV-specific T-cells were reliably detectable only after *in vitro* culture with HAdV-antigen [14,29]. Due to the low frequency of circulating the HAdV-specific T-cells, their exact phenotype remains to be elucidated.

Current clinical immunotherapy protocols are based on either long-term *in vitro* expansion, excluding [15] or including transfected antigen-presenting cells (APCs) [16,17]. Alternatively, direct magnetic selection of virus-specific T-cells using the IFN-γ -CSA [18,20], tetramers [19] or pentamers [22] is employed. More recently good manufacturing practice (GMP)-compliant removable streptamers became available that represent the only therapy presently not considered as an "Advanced Therapy Medicinal Product (ATMP)" [21]. Although all studies referenced above reported prevention of overt viral disease and only mild or no graft versus host disease (GvHD), they have a number of important limitations: some are very time-consuming (10–14 weeks), technically demanding and cost intensive, others involve gene therapy, require large volumes of blood, or are limited to those patients that express HLA alleles for which multimers are available. These constraints represent a major impediment to broad clinical application of these adoptive immunotherapy approaches [30]. The first attempt to use only synthetic peptide mixes and cytokines to rapidly generate virus-specific T-cells within 9–16 days was recently published [31]. A major focus of this study was to evaluate optimal conditions for T-cell expansion by testing different viral peptide concentrations and cytokines (preferential IL-4 and IL-7). However, relevant cytolytic activity ($<10\%$) of e.g. expanded HAdV-specific T-cells was only shown after 16 days of expansion. In our study, fresh/frozen PBMCs were stimulated twice within only 12 days by using GMP-compliant adaptable peptide mixes and a consciously delayed supplementation of IL-15, which resulted in high numbers of functional and cytolytically active virus-specific T-cells against HAdV, CMV, EBV and BKV. In addition, for the first time, no or only low alloreactivity was evaluated very detailed by several different assays to further proof the safety of these cells.

Materials and Methods

Epitope prediction

Epitope candidates were predicted using the SYFPEITHI software (www.syfpeithi.de) [32,33]. Protein sequences were derived from the SwissProt database (www.uniprot.org release 2010_06): P03277 for hexon Ad2, P04133 for hexon Ad5, P03254 for E1A Ad2, P03255 for E1A Ad5, P03280 for pVIII Ad2, and P24930 for pVIII Ad5.

Peptide synthesis

Peptides were synthesized by standard Fmoc chemistry using an ABI 433A Synthesizer (Applied Biosystems, Darmstadt, Germany), or an Economy Peptides Synthesizer EPS 221 (ABIMED, Langen, Germany). Synthesis products were analyzed by HPLC (Varian Star, Zinsser Analytics, Munich, Germany) and MALDI-TOF (G2025A, Agilent Technologies, Santa Clara, CA) or electron spray ionization-time of flight (Q-TOF I, Micromass, Manchester, UK) mass spectrometry.

Cells from donors and patients

PBMCs were isolated by standard Ficoll (PAA, Pasching, Austria) gradient separation and used directly or cryopreserved in fetal calf serum (PAA) or 2% Octaplas (OP, Octapharma, Vienna, Austria) with 10% Dimethylsulfoxide (DMSO, CryoSure, Dessau-Tornau, Germany) until further analysis. Monocytes (purity 70 to 95%) were either positively selected by using CD14 MicroBeads (Miltenyi Biotec, Bergisch Gladbach, Germany) according to the manufacturers instructions or isolated after adherence to plastic flasks for 2 h at 37°C in AIM-V medium (Invitrogen, Carlsbad, CA) (1% OP) as described [34], depending on the assay used (see below). To obtain Phytohemagglutinine- (PHA-L; Sigma-Aldrich, St Louis, MO) blasts as targets for the cytotoxicity assay, PBMCs (2×10^6/ml) were cultured for 6 days in AIM-V supplemented with 2% OP, 2 mM L-Glutamine and 25 mM HEPES, designated as AIM−V+, in the presence of PHA (5 µg/ml). In addition, IL-2 (PeproTech, Rocky Hill, NY) (5 ng/ml) was added on day 3.

Magnetic selection of ADV-specific T-cells from patients

Five to 8×10^6 PBMCs were stained with HAdV-specific streptamers according to manufactures instructions (IBA Technologies, Göttingen, Germany), incubated with anti-phycoerythrin(PE) MicroBeads (Miltenyi), magnetically selected by MS-columns (Miltenyi) according to manufacturers instructions (Miltenyi) and analyzed by flow cytometry.

HLA typing of blood donors and patients

Low and high resolution HLA typing of healthy blood donors and patients was performed at the Institute of Transfusion Medicine (Tübingen, Germany) or the Department of Blood Group Serology (Vienna, Austria) with the donors and patients written consent.

Virus-specific and control antigens

Peptides used for multimer analyses are shown in the Table S2 in File S1. Peptide pools for EBV (EBNA-3A) and BKV (LT-Ag) were purchased from JPT (JPT Peptide Technologies, Berlin, Germany) and used at a final concentration of 10 µg/ml for stimulation or pulsing of cells. The final concentration of HAdV (subgroup C-derived Hexon AdV5), EBV (EBNA-1, BZLF-1 and LMP-2) and CMV (pp65) PepTivator (Miltenyi) in the cell suspension was 0.6 nmol for each pepide per ml.

Quantitative real-time-PCR analysis of viruses from patients

Routine HAdV virus screening of patientss stool and blood samples was performed by real-time quantitative (RQ) PCR. Viral DNA isolation followed by RQ-PCR were done as described [1].

In vitro expansion of virus-specific T-cells

For ELIspot analysis, IL-2-expanded peptide-specific T-cells were generated as follows: thawed PBMCs were washed and cultured in Iscove's modified Dulbecco's medium (IMDM) (Lonza,

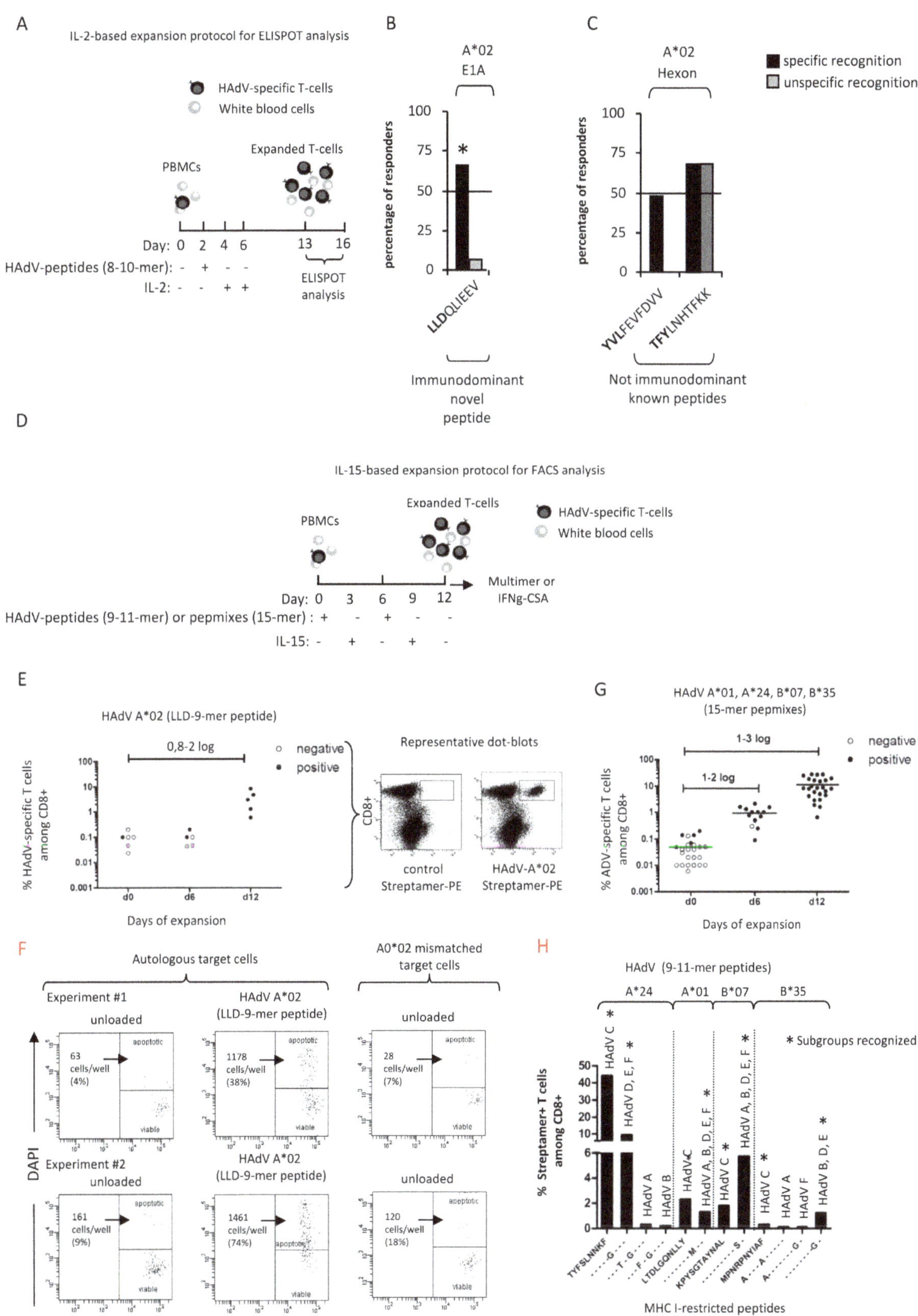

Figure 1. Frequency of responses to novel and known HAdV peptides by ELIspot. Frequency of HAdV-specific T-cells in donors before and after short-term *in vitro* expansion analyzed by multimers and IFNg-CSA. A) Schematic drawing of the IL-2-based *in vitro* expansion protocol for ELIspot analysis. Percentage of donors responding to novel B) and known C) A*02-based peptides by ELIspot assay. Black bars represent donors

positive, gray bars those negative for the respective allele. Significant differences are indicated (*, $p>0.05$, Fishers exact test). D) Schematic drawing of the IL-15-based *in vitro* expansion protocol for FACS analysis. E) Percentages of A*02 ADV-streptamer$^+$ T-cells including representative dot plots are given. F) Specific lysis is shown of autologous and allogeneic A*02 mismatched PHA-blasts (target cells), unloaded- or HAdV-A*02 (LLD) peptide-loaded, induced by A*02-multimer-sorted HAdV-T-cells. The total number of "dying" target cells/well and percentage values were evaluated from each sample. Two representative dot plots are shown. G) A*01, A*24, B*07, and B*35 HLA- dependent ADV-specific multimer$^+$ (streptamer or pentamer) T-cells among CD8$^+$ T-cells, before (day0) and after 6 and 12 days of expansion are shown. Notably, for some donors, multimer analyses were only performed at day 0, 6 and/or 12. H) Subgroup C-derived streptamer staining of PBMCs stimulated with specific peptides for 12 days, representing different adenoviral subgroups, as indicated. The percentage of streptamer$^+$ T cells among CD8$^+$ is shown. Asterisks represent subgroup recognition.

Basel, Switzerland) supplemented with 2% heat-inactivated human serum produced in the laboratory (Tübingen), 50 μM β-mercaptoethanol (Roth), 50 U/ml penicillin, 50 μg/ml streptomycin (both Lonza), and 20 μg/ml gentamicin (Cambrex, Baltimore, USA), and stimulated with peptides (1 μg/ml) on day 2. On days 4 and 6, IL-2 (Promokine) was added at 2 ng/ml. PBMCs were analyzed on day 13 by ELIspot.

For the generation of IL-15-based short-term expanded virus-specific T-cells (seVirus-T-cells), fresh or frozen PBMCs were cultured in AIM−V+ and stimulated with the appropriate peptide pools from HAdV (AdV5-PepTivator), EBV (BZLF-1- and EBNA-1-PepTivator), CMV (pp65-Peptivator), or BKV (LT-Ag-pepmix) antigens for 6 days. On day 6, cultured cells were added to 5×10^6 post-thaw and adherent monocytes and re-stimulated with a peptide pool. In addition, IL-15 (R&D Systems) was added at 5 ng/ml on days 3 and 9. On day 12, seVirus-T-cells were harvested and used for several analyses. To determine cross-reactivity with other strains of adenovirus, PBMCs were stimulated and expanded as described for the seVirus-T-cells, with the exception that different subgroup-specific peptides were used prior to streptamer analysis. For the monitoring of virus-specific T-cells in donors and patients, PBMCs were mostly stimulated for 6 days, without a second re-stimulation step and IL-15 treatment.

IFN-γ ELIspot assays

Five $\times10^5$ IL-2 (20 IU/ml)-expanded T-cells/well (see above and Fig. 1A) were seeded and stimulated for 24 h with pools of ADV-derived peptides (1 μg/ml each) or HIV peptide (1 μg/ml) as negative control. As positive control, 10 μg/ml PHA-L (Roche Applied Science, Indianapolis, IN) was used. IFN-γ was detected using the Human IFN-γ ELIspot kit (MabTech, Nacka Strand, Sweden) according to the manufacturer's instructions. Pools eliciting positive responses were split into reactions containing individual peptides and tested again against the respective donor. The cut-off value for a positive response was more than 5 spots per 10^5 cells exceeding background levels.

Flow cytometry

PBMCs or seVirus-T-cells were counted on a Sysmex KX21 hematology analyzer (Sysmex, Hyogo, Japan). At least 2.5×10^5 cells/sample were washed with PBS (PAA), resuspended in 50 μl washing buffer (WB; 0.1% sodium azide, 0.1% BSA in PBS) and incubated with either 7 μl PE-labeled Pentamers (Proimmune, Oxford, UK) or streptamers comprising 1 μl MHC class I and 1.25 μl Strep-Tactin-PE (IBA) for 45 min at 4°C. After two washing steps, cells were resuspended in 50 μl WB, stained with antibodies for 15 min at 4°C, washed again, transferred to Trucount™ tubes (BD Biosciences, San Diego, CA) (optional), and analyzed by flow cytometry. All multimers used are described in Table S2 in File S1. In general, between 95×10^3 and 500×10^3 events were acquired. For flow cytometry analyses, the following antibodies were purchases from BD: PE-TR (Texas Red)-labeled anti-CD3 (UCHT1), PerCP-labeled anti-CD3 (SK7), PE-Cy7-labeled anti-CD4 (SK3), Horizon™ V500-labeled anti-CD8 (RPA-T8), APC-Cy7- or PerCP-labeled anti-CD8 (SK1), APC-Cy7-labeled anti-CD19 (SJ25C1), APC-Cy7-labeled anti-CD20 (L27), PE-TR-labeled anti-CD45RA (HI100), Horizon™ V450-labeled anti-CD62L (DREG-56), FITC-labeled anti-CD107a (H4A3), PE-labeled anti-CD137 (1HA2) and FITC-labeled anti-CD56. The PE-labeled anti-CD3 (UCHT1) and PerCP-eFlour® 710-labeled anti-CD4 (SK3) were purchased from DAKO (Glostrup, Denmark) and eBiosciense (San Diego, CA, USA), respectively. For the IFN-γ-CSA, 5×10^5 cells were washed, resuspended in 100 μl AIM−V+, cultured over night (o/n), and stimulated with the appropriate peptide pools for 4 h. For functional assays, virus-specific T-cell lines (8×10^5) were mixed at a ratio of 5:1 with autologous monocytes obtained by CD14 positive selection, and stimulated with the ADV-PepTivator for either 4 h or o/n, depending on whether CD107a or CD137 were analyzed. The subsequent procedure was performed according to the manufacturers instructions (Miltenyi). For the intracellular staining of IFN-γ and TNF-α, cells were stimulated for 4 h with the HAdV-peptide pools and stained according to the manufacturers instructions (BD Biosciences). Samples without stimulation or stimulated with 1 μg/ml of SEB (Sigma-Aldrich) served as controls.

General gating strategy and cut-off values

First, beads (if used) were defined. Viable cells were addressed by their appropriate position in the SSC versus FSC plot. Notably, for multimer analysis, CD19$^+$ B cells were excluded to avoid false positive results. The analyses were performed either on a FACS LSRII or a LSRFortessa, and the FACSDiva (all BD, Biosciences, CA) was used for data evaluation. The limit of detection for the multimers and the IFN-γ-CSA was defined as >10 positive events and a 5-fold increase compared to the individual negative control.

CFSE labeling

PBMCs or PHA blasts (10^7/ml) were resuspended in PBS (0.1% BSA,, Sigma-Aldrich) and labeled with 3 μM CFSE (Sigma-Aldrich) for 10 min at 37°C. The reaction was quenched with 1 ml of Octaplas for 5 min at room temperature (RT). Cells were washed twice with PBS and adjusted to a density of 10^6 cells/ml in AIM-V+. After incubation o/n at 37°C/5% CO_2 they were used for proliferation or cytotoxicity assays.

Proliferation assay

CFSE-labeled PBMCs (2.5×10^6) were expanded for 12 days according to the IL-15-based *in vitro* expansion protocol described above (Fig. 1D), with the exception of using Cell Proliferation Dye (CPD) eFluor 670 (Ebioscience, San Diego, CA)-labeled monocytes instead of unlabeled monocytes, which enabled exclusion by gating. On day 12, cells were scraped, washed and analyzed by flow cytometry using Trucount™ tubes to determine the percentage and absolute cell number of viable proliferating cells.

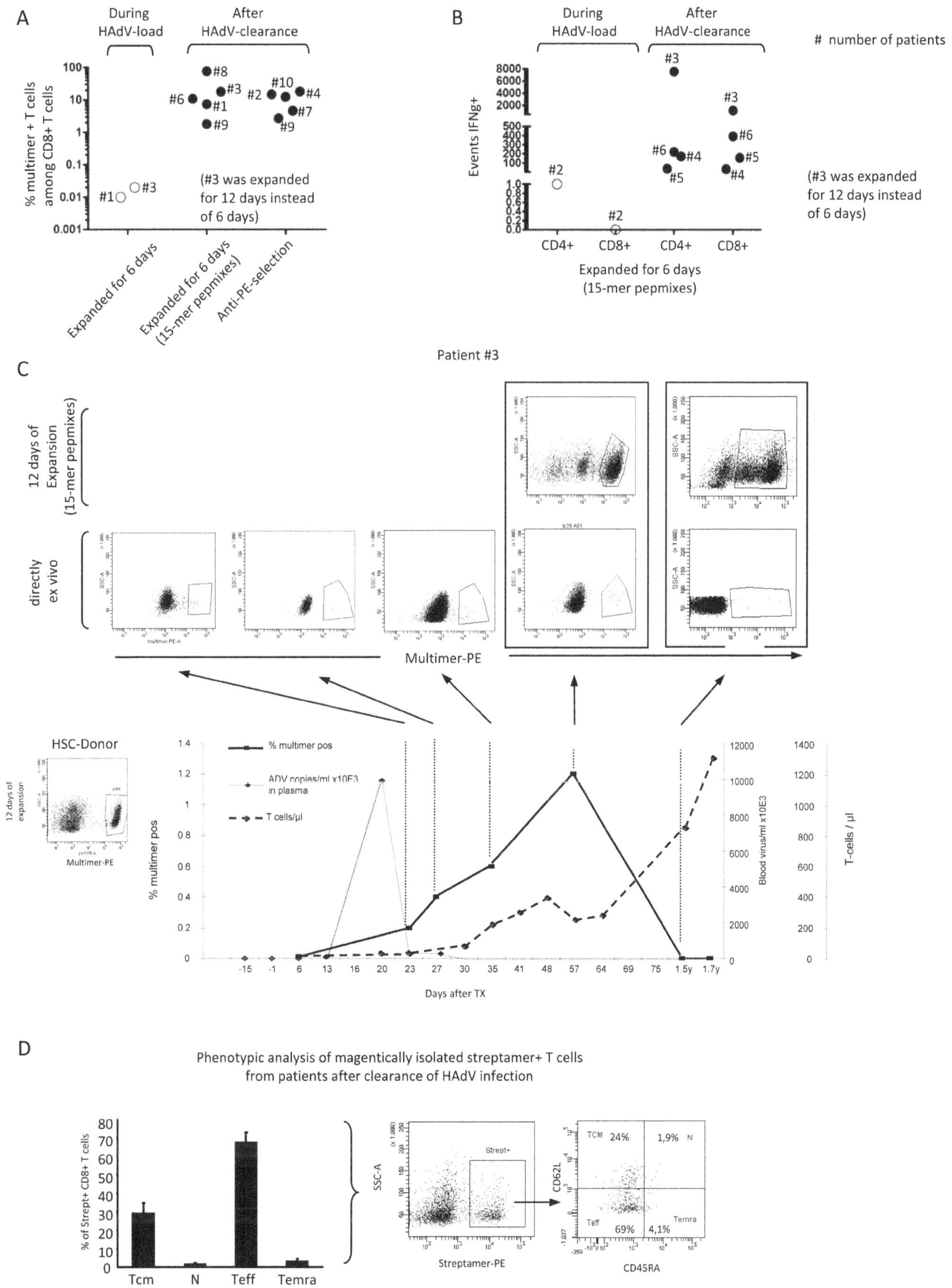

A

During HAdV-load

After HAdV-clearance

% multimer + T cells among CD8+ T cells

100, 10, 1, 0.1, 0.01, 0.001

#1 #3 #6 #8 #3 #1 #9 #2 #10 #4 #7 #9

(#3 was expanded for 12 days instead of 6 days)

Expanded for 6 days

Expanded for 6 days (15-mer pepmixes)

Anti-PE-selection

B

During HAdV-load

After HAdV-clearance

number of patients

Events IFNg+

#2 #2 #3 #6 #4 #5 #3 #6 #5 #4

CD4+ CD8+ CD4+ CD8+

Expanded for 6 days (15-mer pepmixes)

(#3 was expanded for 12 days instead of 6 days)

C

Patient #3

12 days of Expansion (15-mer pepmixes)

directly ex vivo

Multimer-PE

HSC-Donor

12 days of expansion

Multimer-PE

% multimer pos

ADV copies/ml x10E3 in plasma

T cells/µl

% multimer pos

Blood virus/ml x10E3

T-cells / µl

-15 -1 6 13 16 20 23 27 30 35 41 48 57 64 69 75 1.5y 1.7y

Days after TX

D

Phenotypic analysis of magentically isolated streptamer+ T cells from patients after clearance of HAdV infection

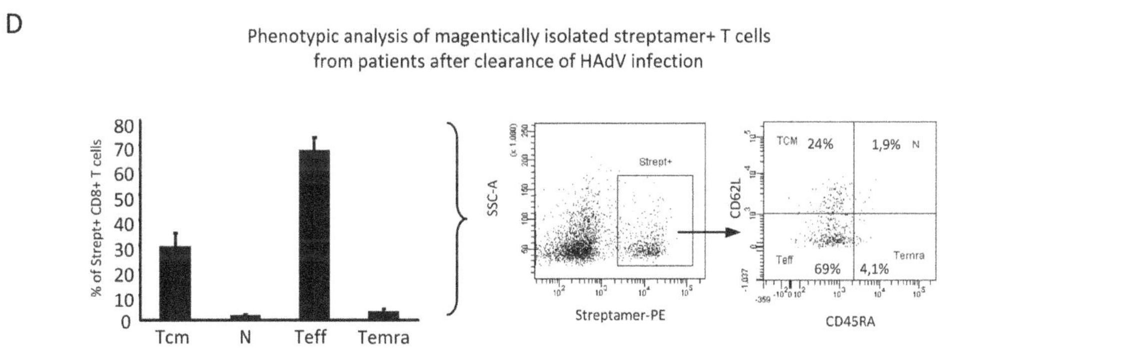

Figure 2. Analysis of HAdV-specific T-cells in patients during and after allogeneic SCT. The presence of 6 day expanded or magnetically isolated HAdV-specific T-cells was assessed by A) the percentage of multimer$^+$ T-cells among CD8$^+$ and by B) events of IFN-γ secreting CD4$^+$ and CD8$^+$ T-cells during HAdV load, or after ADV clearance in 10 patients. Of note, for most patients, either multimer or IFN-γ assays before or after viral load were performed. Each dot refers to the appropriate patient number, as indicated.C) Detailed analysis of ADV-multimer$^+$ T-cells of patient No. 3 and the representative HSC-donor are shown. Dot plots show the percentage of HAdV-multimer$^+$ T-cells among CD8$^+$ at several time points after clearance of HAdV plasma load. For the last two stainings, cells were measured directly *ex vivo* and after a 12 instead of 6 day expansion period. The graphs show percentage of HAdV-multimer$^+$ T-cells among CD8$^+$ (bold line, rectangle), HAdV copies per ml serum (dotted line, diamond) and number of CD3$^+$ T-cells/μl blood (bold line, diamond). D) A summarizing diagram + SEM (of patients No. 2, 4, 7, 9 and 10) including representative dot plots of magnetically isolated HAdV-streptamer$^+$ T-cells and percentages of their 4 subsets of naïve (N), central (TCM), effector memory (TEM) and effector memory CD45RA$^+$ (TEMRA) T-cells are shown.

MLR

10^5 CFSE-labeled PBMCs or seHAdV-T-cells were incubated with 10^5 autologous or allogeneic 30Gy-irradiated PBMCs in 100 μl AIM−V+ in a 96 well (round bottom) microtiter plate. On day 7, the cell suspension was transferred into Trucount^{TM} tubes and residual alloreactivity, represented by the total number of viable proliferating (CFSE low) cells, was analyzed by flow cytometry.

Cytotoxicity assay

The cytolytic activity of seVirus-T-cells was assessed by flow cytometry. Notably, only viable cells (>70%), sorted on a FACSAria, were used. CFSE-labeled PHA targets were pulsed with the appropriate viral peptides or peptide pools for 2 hours or o/n, respectively. Unpulsed and control peptide-pulsed targets were used as negative controls. Autologous and allogeneic targets (1.25×10^4) were mixed with seVirus-T-cells at a ratio 1:20. Of note, due to low numbers of A*02-sorted HAdV-specific T-cells, only 1.9×10^3 target cells were used. 4 h after incubation at 37°C, the cell suspension was transferred to Trucount^{TM} tubes and stained with DAPI (0.03 μg/ml). The absolute number of late apoptotic/necrotic targets (CFSE+/DAPI+) was analyzed. Thawed seHAdV-T-cells were cultured for 3 days before cytolytic acitivity was tested.

Ethics Statement

Cells from donors and patients were obtained upon approval from the local Ethics Committees of Tübingen and Vienna (EK Nr.514/2011) and (EK Nr.024/2011) and informed consent.

Statistical analysis

Fisher's exact test, p = 0.05 was used for IFN-γ - ELIspot data and students t test analysis was employed to determine the statistical significance (P) of all other findings. Data are shown as mean value with standard deviation and/or range.

Results

Prediction, identification and characterization of novel and known human ADV-epitopes

In order to identify new adenoviral epitopes for CD8$^+$ T-cell responses, we first predicted epitope candidates for the frequent HLA-types A*02, A*01, and A*24 using the SYFPEITHI software (www.syfpeithi.de). We chose two widespread adenoviral strains, Ad2 and Ad5, and focused on three proteins: protein II (hexon, major capsid protein), protein VIII, (minor capsid protein) [35], and E1A (an early antigen). We selected the top-scoring 2% of sequences for synthesis, and included published epitopes, resulting in 29 peptides for the HLA-A*02, 21 for HLA-A*01 and 21 for HLA-A*24 (Table S1 in File S1). All peptides were analyzed for their capacity to stimulate CD8$^+$ T-cells as defined by IFN-γ-ELIspot detection. To avoid overlooking HAdV-specific T-cells with very low frequency, PBMCs from at least 16 appropriate donors sharing the HLA allele presenting the peptide were stimulated with the peptide together with IL-2, and expanded for 13 days (Fig. 1A). Peptides were defined as immunodominant if the ELIspot response was specifically positive in more than 50% of appropriate, and negative in most inappropriate donors. These criteria were fulfilled for the novel E1A-based peptide LLD (A*02) as well as for the known hexon-peptides LTD (A*01), and TYF (A*24) which showed an IFN-γ response in 49/74, 68/73, and 44/58 cases, respectively (Fig. 1B, and Table S1 in File S1). All other known hexon-based peptides for YVL and TFY (both A*02) mediated either low responses or nonspecific recognition (Fig. 1C).

Applicability of multimers to detect very rare HAdV-specific T-cells in healthy donors

Using the LLD-based HLA-A*02 streptamer we assessed the functionality of this novel and of four other known epitopes complexed in multimers of HLA-types A*01, A*24, B*07 and B*35. Due to the very low frequency of HAdV-specific T-cells in freshly drawn blood, we cultured PBMCs for 6 to 12 days using HAdV-specific 9-mer peptides or 15-mer pepmixes and IL-15 as stimulants (Fig. 1D). After 12 days of expansion, A*02 streptamer-positive T-cells were reliably detectable in 5/5 HLA-A*02 positive donors, with frequencies ranging from 0.6 to 8.6% of CD8$^+$ T cells, representing an increase of 0.8 to 2 logs as compared to day 0 (Fig. 1E). The specificity of the new A*02-streptamer was confirmed by its failure to bind to CD4$^+$ T-cells in HLA-A*02 matched, and to CD8$^+$ T-cells in HLA-A*02 mismatched donors (data not shown). In addition, specific killing between 38% and 74% of A*02-multimer purified-T-cells could be achieved, if LLD peptide-loaded target cells were used with different peptide concentrations. No specific killing was observed when A*02-mismatched target cells were used (Figure 1F). Regarding the known epitopes, only 5/25 donors were determined positive with multimers on day 0 (range 0.06–0.2% of CD8$^+$ T-cells). On days 6 and 12, 12/13 and 25/25 of the matched donors were clearly positive, with a range from 0.09–2.1% to 0.64–28% of CD8$^+$ T cells (Fig. 1G), representing a 1–3 log increase in the frequency of multimer-positive T-cells.

To address cross reactivity, we tested whether common subgroup-C-derived HAdV-streptamers detect HAdV-specific T-cells specific for subgroups A–F. Therefore, PBMCs were expanded for 12 days with peptides derived from hexon proteins of different HAdV subgroups (A–F), followed by staining with subgroup-C-derived HAdV-streptamers. The subgroup-C-derived streptamers restricted to A*01 and B*07 did detect HAdV-specific T-cells from all six different subgroups. For the A*24- and B*35-subgroup-C-derived streptamers, HAdV-specific T-cells were neither detectable from subgroups A and B nor from A and F (Fig. 1H). Notably, the new E1A-derived A*02 peptide is not conserved in other subgroups, as determined by the basic local alignment search (blast), and can therefore not be employed to

Table 1. Patient characteristics.

Patient no.	Sex	Age at TX	Diagnosis	Donor	Source	Con-ditioning	GVHD prophylaxis	PCR-positive results in stool, first and last day	highest PCR-positive results in stool, copies/g	PCR-positive results in blood, first and last day	HAdV strain	Antiviral treatment	CD3+ >50/µl post TX, day	Detection of ADV-specific T cells during ADV-clearance, yes/no	Detection of ADV-specific T cells after ADV-clearance, yes/no	Status at month 6 post TX concerning ADV infection
1	w	19	T-ALL	FD, haplo, m T cell depletion	PBSC	Flu/VP16/ OKT3	mmf	day 102–272	5×10E7	day 109–110, 6×10E5	C	Cidofovir	between day 34–41	no	yes	died after Heart TX, no ADV infection
2	m	2	M Kostmann	MUD, m	BM	Flu/Thio/Mel/ ATG	CyA, mmf	day 21–260	2×10E7	not positive	C	Cidofovir	between day 14–21	no	yes	still alive, no ADV infection
3	w	3	MHC II Deficiency	MFD, f	BM	Flu/Thio/Mel/ ATG	CyA, mmf	day −15–75	1×10E10	day 13–27, 1×10E4	C	Cidofovir + Ribavirin	between day 13–20	no	yes	still alive, no ADV infection
4	w	8	NBL Rez.	FD, haplo, m T cell depletion	PBSC	Flu/Thio/Mel/ OKT3	CyA	day 106–252	1×10E6	not positive	C	none	between day 27–41	not determined	yes	still alive, no ADV infection
5	m	12	ALL Rez.	MUD, m	BM + Boost (day154)	TBI/VP16/ ATG	CyA, MTX	day 21–181	2×10E10	day 27–49, 1×10E3	A and C	Cidofovir	between day 28–34	not determined	yes	still alive, no ADV infection
6	m	5	Sept Granulomatose	MFD, f	BM	Flu/Thio/Mel/ ATG	CyA, mmf	day −11–92	2×10E5	not positive	C	none	between day 13–20	not determined	yes	still alive, no ADV infection
7	m	7	NBL IV	FD, haplo, f T cell depletion	PBSC	Flu/Thio/Mel/ OKT3	CyA	day 6–118	5×10E7	not positive	B and C	Cidofovir	between day 34–42	not determined	yes	still alive, no ADV infection
8	w	3	Hyper IGE Syndrom	MUD, f	BM	Flu/Thio/Mel/ ATG	CyA, mmf	day 5–13	1×10E4	not positive	C	Gancyclovir	between day 13–16	not determined	yes	still alive, no ADV infection
9	m	5	Fanconi, MDS	MFD, f	BM	FLU/BU/ATG/ Campath	CyA, mmf	day 11–281	9×10E6	not positive	A and C	Ribavirin	between day 14–18	not determined	yes	still alive, no ADV infection
10	m	6	C ALL Rez.	MUD, f	BM	TBI/VP16/ ATG		day 54–61	7×10E3	not positive	C	none	between day 19–22	not determined	yes	still alive, no ADV infection

Patient No. 2 had transient enteritic symptoms attributed to clostridium difficile infection;
Patient No. 10 had transient enteritic symptoms attributed to gut GVHD.
GVHD, graft-versus-host disease; ALL, acute lymphoblastic leukemia; Rel, relapse; Morbus Kostmann, MHC II, major histocompatibility complex class II, NBL rel, Neuroblastoma relapse; Sept, septic granulomatous disease; NBL IV, Neuroblastoma grade IV; IGE, immunoglobulin E; MDS, myelodysplastic syndrome; common ALL, FD, family donor; haplo, haploidentical; MUD, matched unrelated donor; MFD, matched family donor; m, male; f, female; PBSC, peripheral blood stem cells; BM, bone marrow; Flu, fludarabine; VP16, Etoposide; ThioMel, Thiotepa Melphalan ATG, antithymocyte globulin; TBI, total body irradiation; mmf, mycophenolate mofetil; CyA, cyclophosphamide A; PCR, polymerase chain reaction; HAdV, adenovirus.

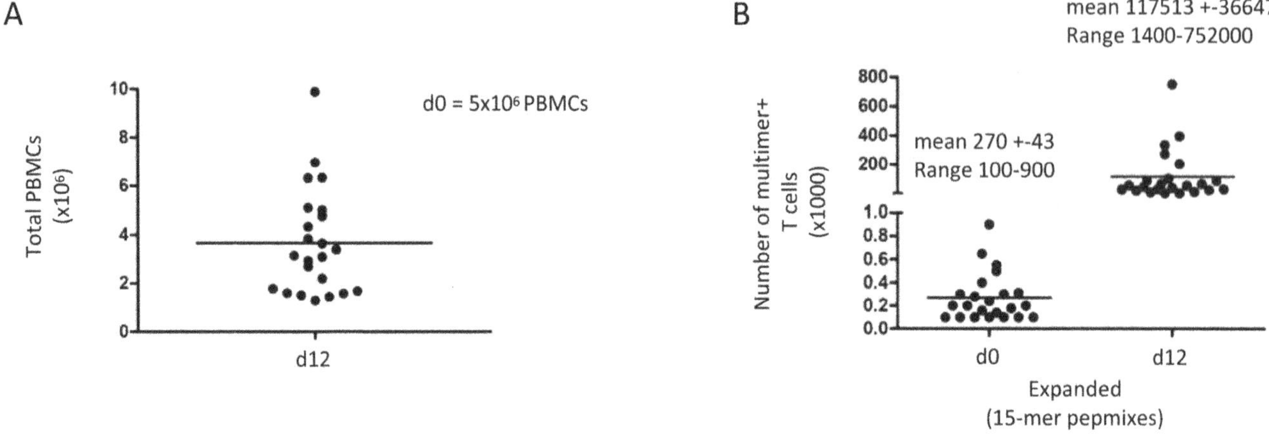

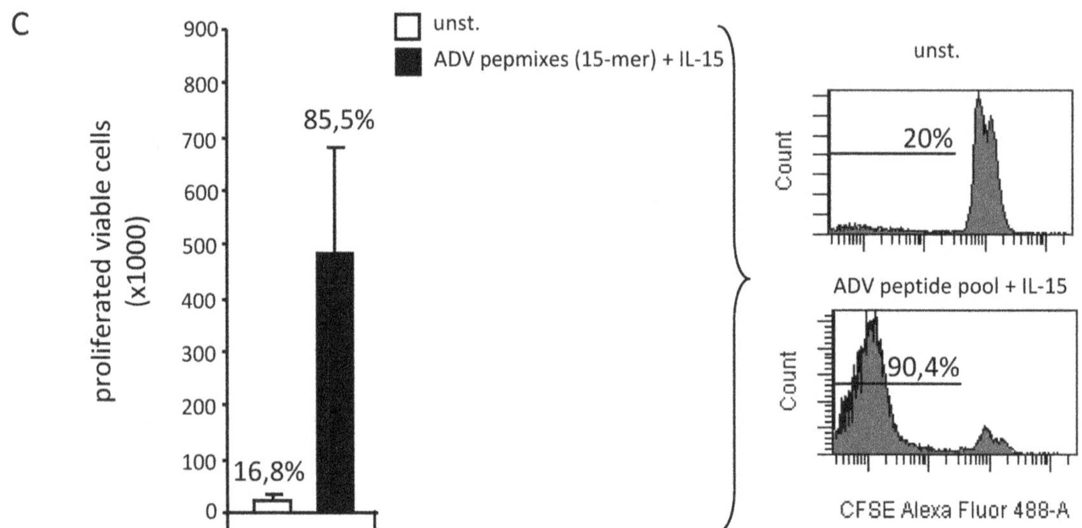

Figure 3. Generation and detailed phenotypic analysis of seHAdV-T-cells. PBMCs (5×10^6/12 well) were expanded for 12 days using the HAdV peptide pool and IL-15, as described in material and methods. A) The total number of PBMCs after expansion, and B) the absolute number of HAdV-multimer-specific T-cells at days 0 and 12, are shown from 24 donors, including mean +SEM and ranges. C) PBMCs (2.5×10^6/24 well) were CFSE-labeled without stimulation (unst.), or stimulated with the HAdV-peptide pool in the presence of IL-15, as described in Materials and Methods. A summarizing diagram + SEM of 3 donors shows cell number (x1000) (bars) and percentage (above bars) of viable proliferating cells after expansion including a representative histogram.

detect HAdV-specific T-cells from other subgroups (data not shown).

Beside HAdV, similar results with streptamers were seen for the detection of EBV and BKV-specific T-cells, before and after expansion (Figure A and B in Figure S1 in File S1). Whereas all 6 EBV-streptamers showed reliable staining results (Figure. A in Figure S1 in File S1) for BKV, only the B07-restricted streptamer (Figure B in Figure S1 in File S1) was functional. These data indicate that novel and known multimers, in combination with a short *in vitro* expansion period, is a reliable tool to monitor virus-specific T-cells.

In analogy to the multimer results, a short expansion period was also necessary to detect HAdV-, EBV- and BKV-specific T-cells when using the IFN-γ-CSA (Figure C – E in Figure S1 in File S1).

Reconstitution of HAdV-specific T-cells in the context of HAdV infection following HSCT

By applying the expansion protocol for diagnosis, we assessed whether the presence of $CD8^+$ and/or $CD4^+$ HAdV-specific T-cells in patients correlated with clearance of adenoviral load in stool and blood. All blood samples were from 10 patients positive for HAdV in stool (range 6×10^2–2×10^{10}copies/gram), 3 of them were also viremic (range 7×10^2–6×10^7 copies/ml). T-cell analyses performed in 2 patients with multimers and in 1 patient with the IFN-↖-CSA during HAdV-infection showed no detectable HAdV-specific T-cells (Fig. 2A and B). After clearance, however, samples from 9/9 patients stained with multimers (after expansion or magnetic selection) showed positive results. In 4/4 cases, $CD8^+$ and $CD4^+$ HAdV-specific T-cells were also detectable by the IFN-γ-CSA (Fig. 2A and B and Table 1). Of note, HAdV-specific T cells had been detectable in all respective donors prior to stem cell

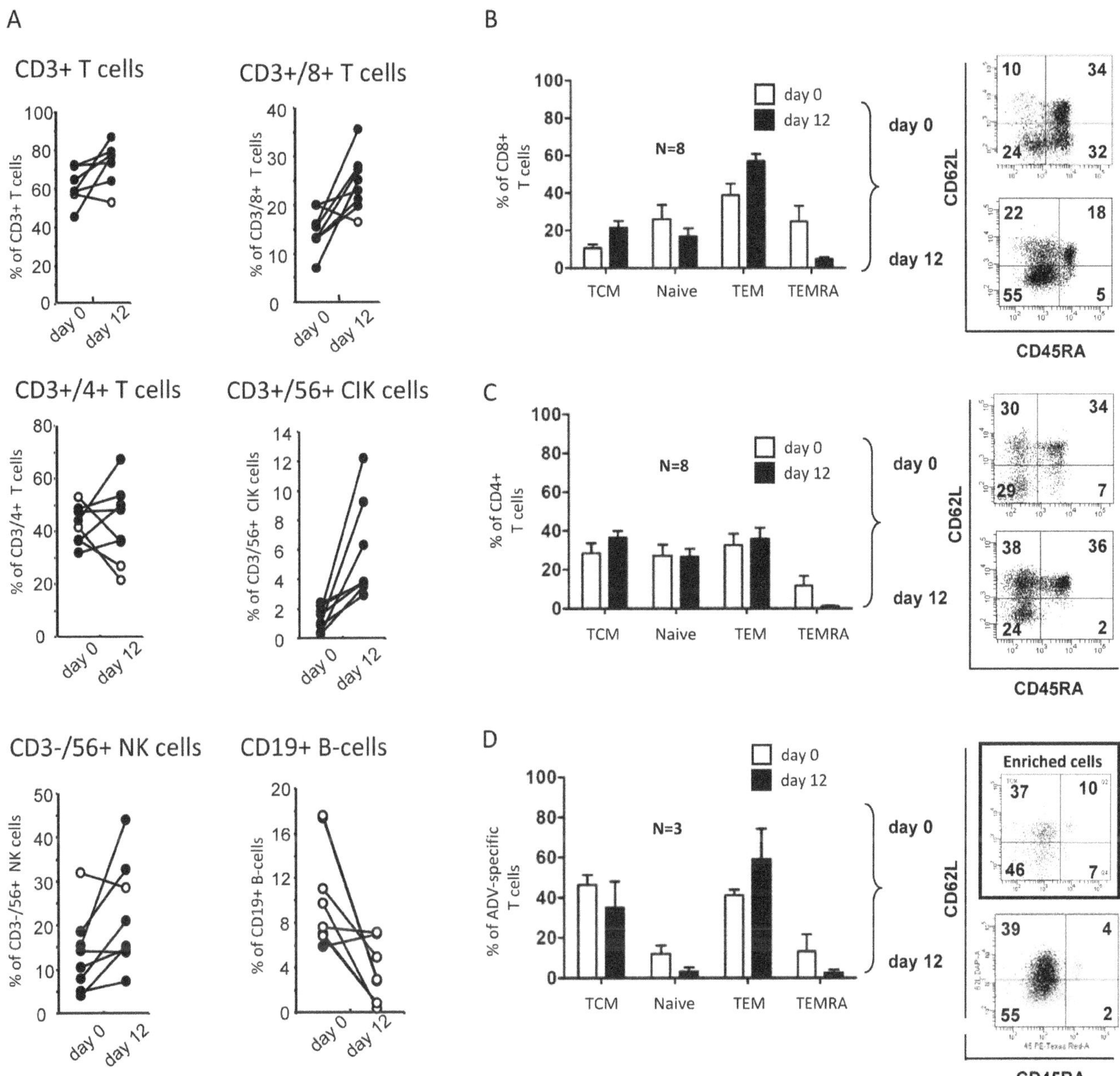

Figure 4. Phenotypic analysis of seHAdV-T-cells. A) Percentage values of different cell populations (as indicated, including cytokine-induced killer cells (CIK)) within PBMCs, before (day 0) and after expansion (day12) of 8 donors. Percentage values of TCM (upper left), Naïve (upper right), TEM (lower left) and TEMRA (lower right) T cell populations within CD8$^+$ (B), CD4$^+$ C), and HAdV-streptamer$^+$ T-cells D) on days 0 (white bars) and 12 (black bars). The graph shows mean+SEM of 8 (for CD4$^+$ and CD8$^+$ T-cells) and 3 (for HAdV-streptamer$^+$ T-cells) donors. Notably, for phenotypic analysis of HAdV-streptamer$^+$ T cells on day 0 (white bars), beads-based magnetic isolation was performed. Representative dot plots are shown.

donation (data not shown). More detailed analysis of patient 3 demonstrated that, shortly after viral clearance, multimer$^+$ HAdV-specific CD8$^+$ T-cells were clearly detectable at day 23 post HSCT and further increased during the following days (Fig. 2C). After 18 months, however, a clear population of HAdV-specific T-cells was only seen after short term cell expansion (Fig. 2C).

To determine the phenotype of CD8$^+$ HAdV-specific T-cells in patients who had cleared adenoviral infection several months before, multimer$^+$ HAdV-specific T-cells were magnetically enriched prior to analysis. HAdV-multimer$^+$ T-cells revealed clear populations of central memory T-cells (TCM) (median: 30%) and effector memory T-cells (TEMs) (median: 65%) emphasizing a prominent role of TCMs in maintaining long-term immunity in patients (Fig. 2D). Taken together, these results show that CD4$^+$ and CD8$^+$ HAdV-specific T-cells include high proportions of TCMs, and that their presence correlates with clearance of HAdV load in patients.

Generation and phenotypic characterization of seHAdV-T-cells for potential clinical use

Based on the protocol used for diagnosis (Fig. 1D), we generated seHAdV-T-cells (short-term expanded human adenovirus-specific T cells) with GMP-compliant adaptable peptide mixes and analyzed the absolute cell number and function in more detail.

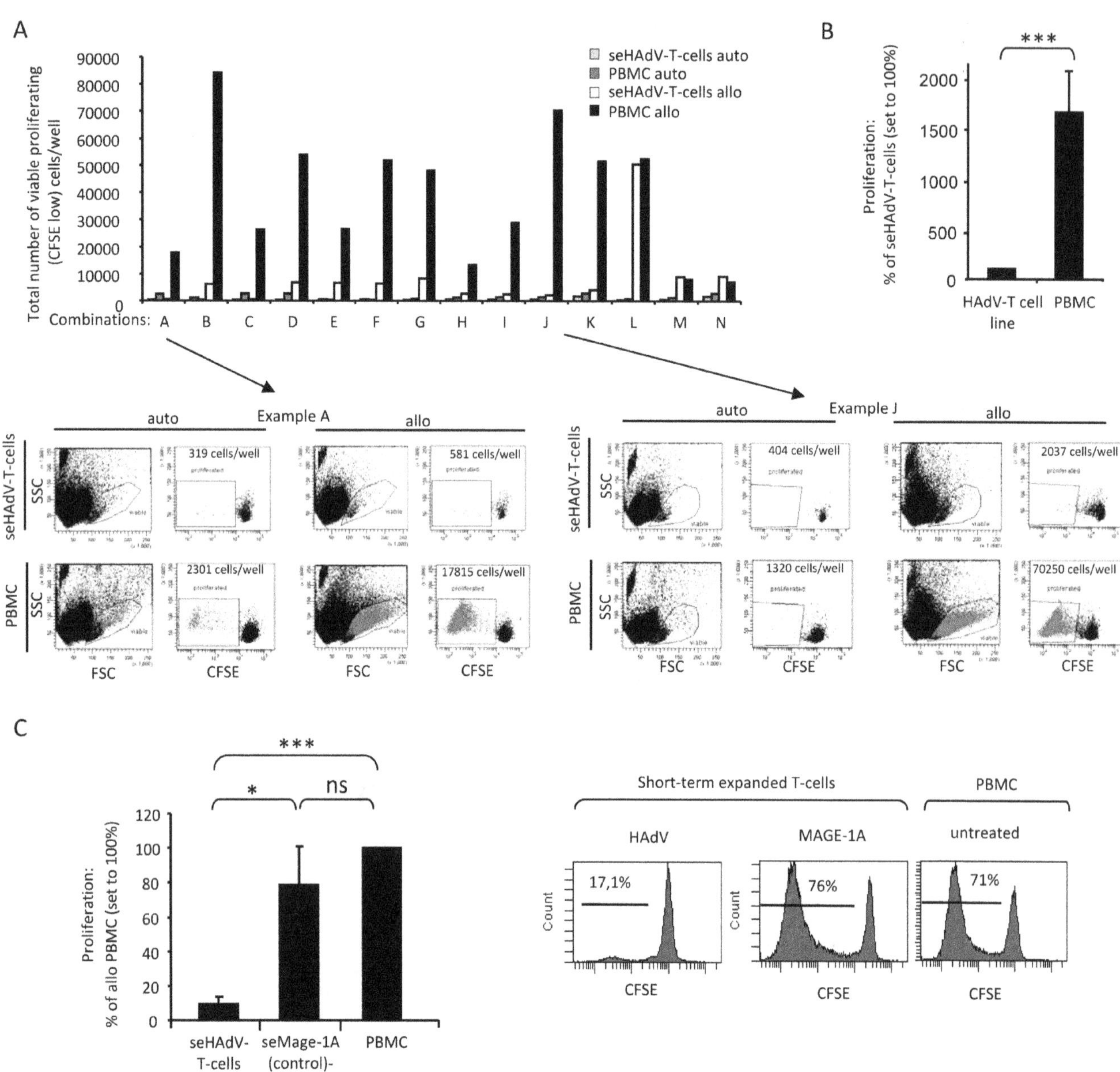

Figure 5. Alloreactive potential of PBMCs versus expanded control- and seHAdV-specific T-cells. CFSE-labeled autologous or allogeneic responder cells (PBMCs or seHAdV-T-cells) were mixed 1:1 with irradiated stimulator cells (PBMCs) and incubated for 7 to 8 days. A) The graph shows the total number of proliferated viable cells per 96 well plate of 14 different donor/recipient combinations A–N). Proliferation of seHAdV-T-cells or PBMCs in response to autologous (auto) or allogeneic (allo) irradiated PBMCs are shown. In addition, representative examples from donors A and J are given. B) A summarizing graph show mean + SEM from all combinations (except for L,M and N); The percentage of viable proliferating seHAdV-T-cells was set to 100% and calculated based on total cell number. C) seHAdV-T-cells or seMAGE-1A-T-cells (control) and PBMC were mixed with allogeneic irradiated stimulator PBMCs. A summarizing graph shows mean + SEM of 4 combinations. First, total cell number of viable proliferating (CFSE-low) seHAdV-, seMAGE-1A-T-cells and PBMCs/well are calculated. Based on these total cell number, the percentage values were analyzed and compared to allogeneic PBMCs, which was set to 100%. A representative histogram of one donor is shown, including percentage values of proliferated cells. Significance vs HAdV-T-cell line: o, p<=0.07; *, p<=0.01.***, p<=0.001.

Whereas the starting cell number of 5×10^6 PBMCs was slightly reduced to a median of 3.7×10^6 cells after 12 days of expansion (Fig. 3A), the total number of HAdV-streptamer$^+$ T-cells increased 435 fold from 270 to 117513 (Fig. 3B). For clinical use, the number of starting fresh/frozen PBMCs can be easily scaled up to 25×10^6 PBMCs (instead of 5×10^6),which should result in sufficiently high cell numbers for both treatment and quality control analyses.

To assess the percentage values and total cell numbers of viable proliferating seHAdV-T-cells after *in vitro* expansion in 24 well plates, PBMCs were labeled with CFSE prior to culture. Compared to unstimulated controls (total cell number (×1000): 21±13.8 or percentage value: 16.8), HAdV-peptide pool and IL-15-driven stimulation resulted in high numbers (×1000) (479,5±194) and percentage values (85.5%) of proliferating viable T-cells (Fig. 3C). But also the number of HAdV-streptamer$^+$ T-

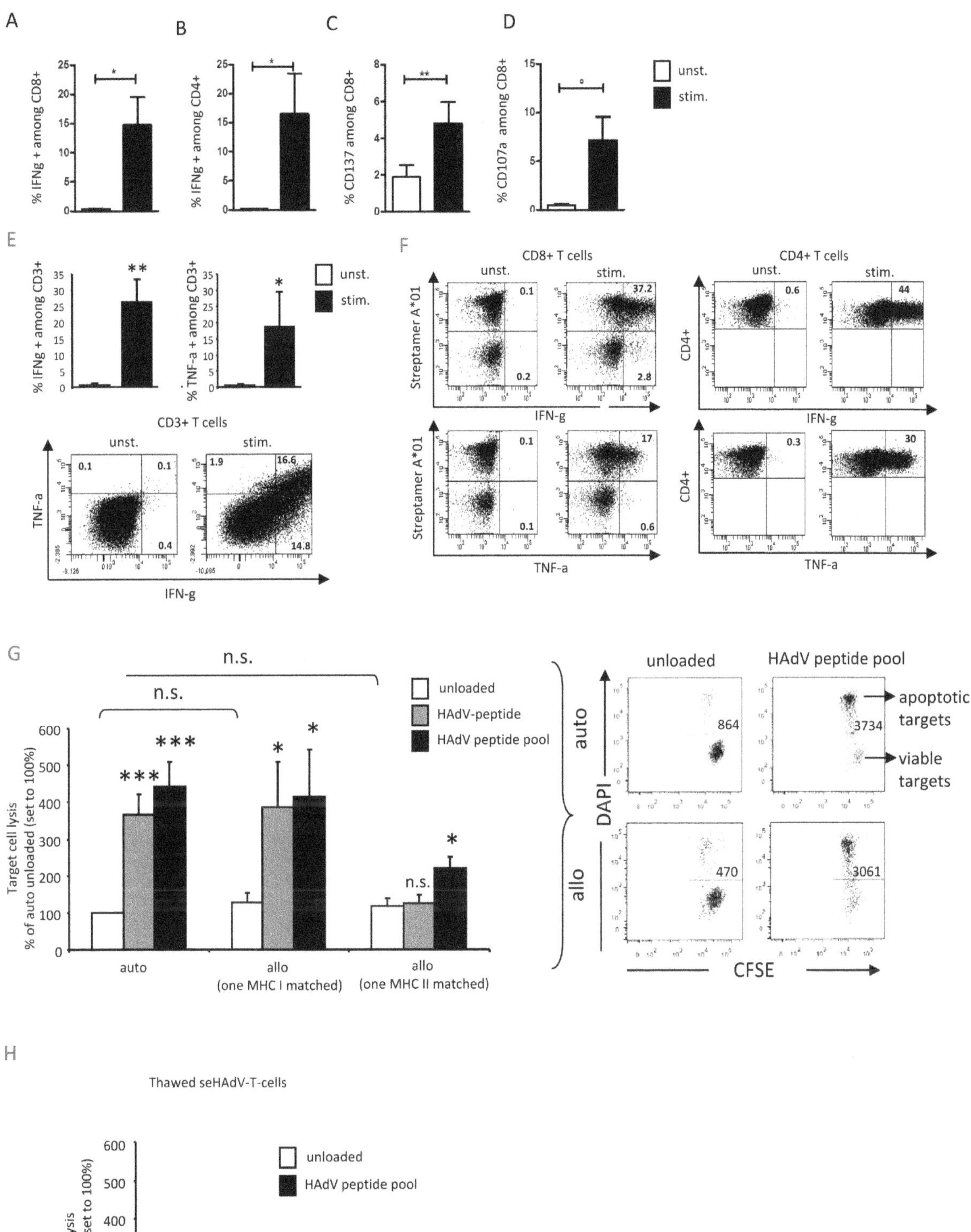

Figure 6. Functional and cytolytic activity of seHAdV-T-cells. seHAdV-T-cells were used for the cytotoxic assay. The percentage values of IFN-γ, CD137 and CD107a expressing seHAdV-T-cells among $CD4^+$ and/or $CD8^+$ are shown A–D) as indicated. E) The percentage values of IFN-γ and TNF-α among CD3+ cells are shown, including representative dot plots indicating simultaneous expression. F) Representative dot plots of IFN-γ and TNF-α-expressing $CD8^+$ T-cells including streptamer$^+$ T cells and $CD4^+$ T-cells. G) Specific lysis is shown of autologous and allogeneic PHA-blasts (target cells)

matched in only a single MHC I, or in only a single MHC II, unloaded (white bar), HAdV-peptide- (grey bar) or HAdV-peptide pool (black bar)-loaded, induced by seHAdV-T-cells. The total number of "dying" target cells/well was evaluated from each sample. Based on these, a summarizing graph shows the percentage of dying target cells related to unloaded autologous (auto) target cells which is set to 100%. Representative dot plots, indicating "dying" cells/well, are shown. H) Specific lysis of allogeneic, unloaded (white bar) or HAdV-peptide pool (black bar)-loaded target cells induced by post-thaw seHAdV-T-cells. Based on total cell number of dying cells, a summarizing graph shows the percentage of dying target cells related to unloaded target cells, which is set to 100%. Significance vs unloaded autologous targets: ns = not significant, *, p< = 0.01.*, p< = 0.001.**

cells/µl within the culture was high (mean: 33.2/µl) in HAdV-peptide pool- and IL-15 stimulated cells, whereas HAdV-specific cells were not detectable in unstimulated or control peptide(-MAGE-A1)-stimulated PBMCs (data not shown).

Phenotypic analysis revealed that, after expansion, 71%±3.8 were $CD3^+$ T-cells including 24%±2 $CD8^+$ T-cells and 42.4%±5.3 $CD4^+$ T-cells (Fig. 4A). Whereas the percentage of TCMs (21.6%±3.5) and TEMs (56.8%±3.9) was slightly increased in $CD8^+$ T-cells, no significant change was seen within $CD4^+$ T-cells (Fig. 4B and C). The percentage of TCMs within the $streptamer^+$ population was also not significantly altered (Fig. 4D), indicating that the expansion procedure did not lead to terminal cell differentiation. Of note, cultures supplemented with IL-15 showed highest numbers of $HAdV\text{-}multimer^+$ T-cells/µl (3.5-fold increase) compared to cultures stimulated in the absence of cytokines, and a 2-fold increase compared to IL-2 or IL-7 stimulation, but no detectable influence on their phenotype (data not shown).

Strongly reduced proliferative capacity of seHAdV-T-cells upon alloantigen stimulation

Next we tested the alloreactive potential of seHAdV-T-cells. In 11 out of 14 allogeneic-pairs, the mean proliferative response of allogeneic PBMCs was about 1.2 log higher compared to that of seHAdV-T-cells (Fig. 5A and B). Only 3 combinations showed comparable residual alloreactivity to allogeneic-PBMCs (combination: L, M, N) (Fig. 5A). Of note, a closer look at HAdV-$multimer^+$ T-cells within the culture revealed that they divided only once representing low if any alloreactivity (data not shown). In addition, we could show that the median alloreactive potential of control short-term expanded T-cells (stimulated with MAGE-1A and IL-15) was similar to that of PBMCs, and 0.9 log higher than that of seHAdV-T-cells (Fig. 5C). These results support our observation that the alloreactive potential of seHAdV-T-cells is strongly reduced after *in vitro* expansion.

seHAdV-T-cells are highly functional and specific, and fail to kill unpulsed-allogeneic target cells

The capacity of seHAdV-T-cells to express activation and cytotoxic markers, such as IFN-γ, CD137 and CD107a, was highly increased after restimulation with HAdV-pepmix-pulsed monocytes (Fig. 6A–D). Furthermore, seHAdV-T-cells produced both IFN-γ and TNF-α (Fig. 6E and F). The lysis of peptide or of peptide-pool-pulsed autologous target cells by seHAdV-T-cells was about 4-fold higher as compared to unpulsed targets (Fig. 6G). Similar lysis was seen when HAdV-pulsed-allogeneic target cells, matched in only one MHC class I or II antigen, were used (Fig. 6G). Unpulsed or control (CMV)-pulsed autologous or allogeneic targets were not recognized, which strongly supports their specificity and the loss of alloreactivity of seHAdV-T-cells (Fig. 6G and data not shown). This cytotoxic activity was also maintained in post-thaw seHAdV-T-cells (Fig. 6H).

Generation of short-term-expanded virus-specific T-cells against several viruses for potential clinical use

Our protocol to generate seHAdV-T-cells was adapted to expand also EBV-, CMV- and BKV-specific T-cells. Whereas the median absolute number of cells was not significantly altered after expansion, the total cell number of $streptamer^+$ T-cells was 1–2 log increased, irrespective of the type of virus-specific T-cells (Figure A, D, and G in Figure S2 in File S1). As seen for HAdV, the proportions of TCM and TEM of $CD4^+$ and $CD8^+$ virus-specific T-cell lines hardly changed during the expansion period (Figure B, E, and H in Figure S2 in File S1). Specific lysis by all cell lines was only observed for peptide-loaded autologous and allogeneic, but not for unloaded allogeneic target cells mismatched or matched in only 3 alleles. (Figure C, F, and J in Figure S2 in File S1).

Discussion

PCR screening for HAdV following allogeneic HSCT allows early detection of impending invasive HAdV-infections, and timely preemptive antiviral treatment [8,36]. Recently, it has been shown that the reconstitution of HAdV-specific T-cells plays a pivotal role in the clearance of HAdV infection [11,12,13,14]. Few groups suggested that combined monitoring of viral load and virus-specific immunity by ELIspot, tetramer staining or the IFN-γ-CSAs has a clinical impact on the therapeutic intervention for pediatric allogeneic HSCT patients [36,37,38,39]. One of the most sensitive and fastest tools to monitor virus-specific T cells are multimers. Therefore, efforts have been made over the past years to identify HAdV-derived MHC class I-restriced as well as MHC class II-restricted epitopes [14,27,40,41]. Nevertheless, the number of published class I epitopes remained rather low, and the focus has been on hexon, the main capsid protein of the virion. Our analyses of different proteins identified an immunodominant A*02-restricted HAdV subgroup C-specific epitope derived from the E1A protein. Based on this epitope, a functional multimer was produced that showed reliable staining results. To our knowledge, this is the first functional A*02-restricted multimer specific for HAdV. Other promising previously published A*02-restricted candidates failed to be useful for the production of functional multimers. Although in a pilot study the treatment of a single patient with pentamer+ CD8+ T-cells specific for HAdV was not successful [22], more studies will be necessary to determine whether polyclonal $CD4^+$ and $CD8^+$ HAdV-specific T-cells are necessary for successful immunotherapy.

However the detection of HAdV-specific T-cells is hampered by the low frequency of HAdV-specific T-cells in peripheral blood [14,17,18]. Even with the more sensitive ELIspot technique (procedure needing 3 days), false negative results cannot be excluded if uncultured PBMCs are used [29]. The prevalence of HAdV in the Caucasian population is supposed to be above 80% [32]. We demonstrated that in most cases a 6 day expansion period was sufficient to obtain clearly positive multimer-based results in 90% of donors. Similar results were seen when the IFN-γ-CSA instead of streptamers was used after expansion. Moreover, in addition to the generally known cross-reactivity of reactive T-cells between HAdV-subgroups [24], we could show that A*24 and B*35 streptamers are not able to recognize subgroup A- or subgroup A and F-derived HAdV-specific T-cells, respectively. This is a very important piece of information, if HAdV-multimers are supposed to be used for diagnosis or future multimer-based therapies.

So far, only one study including seven pediatric and six adult patients showed that, besides $CD4^+$ [7,12,13], also $CD8^+$ virus-specific T-cells [14] are detectable after HAdV clearance in patients after HSCT. We confirmed these results with additional 10 pediatric patients, using the IFN-γ-CSA or multimer analysis of expanded or magnetically selected cells. Out of 7 patients who were HAdV positive in stool and HAdV-negative in plasma, two had transient enteritic symptoms, which were attributed to *Clostridium difficile* infection and gut GvHD respectively, and five remained asymptomatic. HAdV-specific T-cells were detectable in all patients after clearance of infection. Of note, 3/10 patients who cleared HAdV infection, had received T-cell depleted grafts from haploidentical donors ($<10^5$ T-cells/kg BW). This may indicate that, even in the context of profound lymphopenia, viral antigen can trigger virus-specific immune responses. None of these patients reactivated HAdV infection within several months after HSCT, which could be due to the presence of residual HAdV-specific T-cells with characteristics of TCM and TEMs, as seen in all patients analyzed. It further strengthens the suggested important role of TCMs in mediating long-term protection [16,42]. Although the optimal time point for a T-cell immunotherapy in clinical practice is unknown, recent data suggest that the generation or isolation of virus-specific T-cells should occur within the first weeks after detection of a high viral load ($>10^6$ copies) in stool in order to allow prompt treatment in case of invasive HAdV infection [8,18,43,44].

Addressing these criteria, we used 5×10^5 fresh or frozen PBMCs (including 2.5 to 3.5×10^6 CD3+T cells) as starting material and managed to increase the number of HAdV-streptamer^+ T-cells 435-fold within 12 days. The slightly reduced cell number from 5 to 3.7×10^6 could be explained by the delayed stimulation with IL-15 and loss of unspecific T cells during the culture period. Of note, prophylactic cryo-preservation of PBMCs from appropriate donors prior to HSCT proved helpful to safe time. Culture of both fresh and frozen PBMCs resulted in high values of total proliferating cells (up to 85.5%) and at least 68.8±8%, if only highly proliferating cells were gated (data not shown). By using a similar but more strict gating strategy, an approach by Gerdemann et al., who also used peptide mixes but preferentially combined with IL-4 and IL-7, resulted in 52.4% of proliferating cells. In contrast to this work, natural killer (NK) and cytokine-induced killer (CIK) cells, which are assumed to be beneficial in the prevention and treatment of relapses[45,46], are still present after 12 days of expansion. Although our work shares certain features with the protocol by Gerdemann et al., it differs considerably with regard to the stimulation procedure itself, and consequently also with regard to the nature of expanded T-cells and focuses mainly on the safety of our seHAdV-T-cells, as mentioned above.

In our experiments, all seHAdV-T-cells were highly functional, and not only able to lyse antigen-pulsed autologous but also antigen-pulsed allogeneic target cells, if at least one MHC class I or II was matched, which, to our knowledge, had not been shown in that detail before and could be of high relevance for haploidentical or third party donors. For IL-4- and IL-7-driven expansion of HAdV-specific T-cells, at least a 16 day expansion period was necessary to obtain sufficient cytolytic activity [31]. In contrast to previous studies, the killing of MHC class I-matched HAdV-pulsed targets was much higher compared to MHC II-matched targets, indicating that mostly HAdV-specific $CD8^+$ T-cells are involved. This discrepancy might be explained by the use of 15mer instead of 30mer peptides, since the 30mer peptides were described to contain predominantly $CD4^+$ epitopes [29,47]. In addition, even post-thaw seHAdV-T-cells were able to kill partially matched allogeneic target cells albeit to a lower extend compared to fresh seHAdV-T-cells. This finding would enable the prophylactic generation and infusion on demand.

To address the potential risk of seHAdV-T-cells to induce GvHD, the percentage of residual unspecific T-cells - represented by non-proliferating T-cells during the culture period - was analyzed. Although about 15% of the seHAdV-T-cell population did not proliferate as indicated by their unchanged high CFSE load, MLRs showed that, in at least 11/14 donor/recipient pairs, the alloreactive potential of seHAdV-T-cells was reduced by 1.2 log compared to unmanipulated PBMCs. Only 1/14 cases (combination L) showed alloreactivity signals similar to those of the control PBMCs, although in the cytotoxic assay no significant alloreactivity was seen (data not shown). For the other two, the MLR might have failed since the alloreactivity of PBMCs was near the background level. However, residual alloreacivity in some combinations could also be explained by the fact that, in contrast to other studies [16,29] only one MHC allele was matched. Reduced or even absent alloreactivity of seHAdV-T-cells was further confirmed by comparison with control T-cells expanded with MAGE-A1-peptide pools, or by the failure to recognize and lyse allogeneic target cells. The fact that residual alloreactivity, despite expansion, can never be completely excluded, was also shown by other groups [16,18,29]. In addition, Chen et al. showed that the capacity of *in vitro* expanded alloreactive T-cells to survive and expand *in vivo* is limited [48]. This was also supported by Melenhorst et al. who showed no correlation between *in vitro* results and *in vivo* data concerning alloreactivity [49]. Clinical evidence supports that even a small number of virus-specific T-cells (like 10^3 to 10^4/kg body weight), which is easily achievable with our protocol, is sufficient to attain therapeutic efficacy, and infusion of such low lymphocyte numbers would further minimize the risk for GvHD [18]. By adapting our short-term expansion protocol, we were also able to generate high numbers of functional virus-specific T-cells directed against CMV, EBV, and BKV. Also these cells were able to lyse autologous and allogeneic peptide-loaded target cells, although, in some cases, significant lysis was hindered by the high intra-individual variability.

In conclusion, we optimized tools for diagnosis of HAdV-specific T-cells and underline the importance of $CD8^+$ HAdV-specific T-cells in the clearance of HAdV-load in patients. In addition, we were able to generate efficient virus-specific T-cells mainly against HAdV but also CMV, EBV, and BKV within 12 days. The usage of fresh or frozen PBMCs further enables an immunotherapy protocol within a short time span, with low cost and effort, and with the potential for broad clinical application.

Acknowledgments

The authors would like to thank Lothar Germeroth (IBA GmbH, Göttingen, Germany) for providing technical support and Thomas Weichhart (Clinical Division of Nephrology and Dialysis, Department of Internal Medicine III, Medical University of Vienna, Austria) and Maximilian Zeyda (Clinical Division of Endocrinology and Metabolism,

Department of Internal Medicine III, Medical University of Vienna, Austria) for carefully reading and discussing the manuscript.

Author Contributions

Conceived and designed the experiments: RG SS HGR G. Fritsch. Performed the experiments: RG CF SS JS GM JD. Analyzed the data: RG SS HGR G. Fritsch. Contributed reagents/materials/analysis tools: TL. Wrote the paper: RG. Provided RT-PCR data: G. Fischer. Provided data of HLA types: TL. Provided material and data of patients: SM AL. Assisted with manuscript writing: SS G. Fritsch JS SM BEV TL.

References

1. Lion T, Baumgartinger R, Watzinger F, Matthes-Martin S, Suda M, et al. (2003) Molecular monitoring of adenovirus in peripheral blood after allogeneic bone marrow transplantation permits early diagnosis of disseminated disease. Blood 102: 1114–1120.
2. Gooley TA, Chien JW, Pergam SA, Hingorani S, Sorror ML, et al. (2010) Reduced mortality after allogeneic hematopoietic-cell transplantation. N Engl J Med 363: 2091–2101.
3. Watcharananan SP, Kiertiburanakul S, Piyatuctsanawong W, Anurathapan U, Sungkanuparph S, et al. (2010) Cytomegalovirus, adenovirus, and polyomavirus co-infection among pediatric recipients of allogeneic stem cell transplantation: characteristics and outcome. Pediatr Transplant 14: 675–681.
4. George D, El-Mallawany NK, Jin Z, Geyer M, Della-Latta P, et al. (2012) Adenovirus infection in paediatric allogeneic stem cell transplantation recipients is a major independent factor for significantly increasing the risk of treatment related mortality. Br J Haematol 156: 99–108.
5. Schilham MW, Claas EC, van Zaane W, Heemskerk B, Vossen JM, et al. (2002) High levels of adenovirus DNA in serum correlate with fatal outcome of adenovirus infection in children after allogeneic stem-cell transplantation. Clin Infect Dis 35: 526–532.
6. Symeonidis N, Jakubowski A, Pierre-Louis S, Jaffe D, Pamer E, et al. (2007) Invasive adenoviral infections in T-cell-depleted allogeneic hematopoietic stem cell transplantation: high mortality in the era of cidofovir. Transpl Infect Dis 9: 108–113.
7. Myers GD, Krance RA, Weiss H, Kuehnle I, Demmler G, et al. (2005) Adenovirus infection rates in pediatric recipients of alternate donor allogeneic bone marrow transplants receiving either antithymocyte globulin (ATG) or alemtuzumab (Campath). Bone Marrow Transplant 36: 1001–1008.
8. Lion T, Kosulin K, Landlinger C, Rauch M, Preuner S, et al. (2010) Monitoring of adenovirus load in stool by real-time PCR permits early detection of impending invasive infection in patients after allogeneic stem cell transplantation. Leukemia 24: 706–714.
9. Hoffman JA, Shah AJ, Ross LA, Kapoor N (2001) Adenoviral infections and a prospective trial of cidofovir in pediatric hematopoietic stem cell transplantation. Biol Blood Marrow Transplant 7: 388–394.
10. Lankester AC, Heemskerk B, Claas EC, Schilham MW, Beersma MF, et al. (2004) Effect of ribavirin on the plasma viral DNA load in patients with disseminating adenovirus infection. Clin Infect Dis 38: 1521–1525.
11. Chakrabarti S, Mautner V, Osman H, Collingham KE, Fegan CD, et al. (2002) Adenovirus infections following allogeneic stem cell transplantation: incidence and outcome in relation to graft manipulation, immunosuppression, and immune recovery. Blood 100: 1619–1627.
12. Feuchtinger T, Lucke J, Hamprecht K, Richard C, Handgretinger R, et al. (2005) Detection of adenovirus-specific T cells in children with adenovirus infection after allogeneic stem cell transplantation. Br J Haematol 128: 503–509.
13. Heemskerk B, Lankester AC, van Vreeswijk T, Beersma MF, Claas EC, et al. (2005) Immune reconstitution and clearance of human adenovirus viremia in pediatric stem-cell recipients. J Infect Dis 191: 520–530.
14. Zandvliet ML, Falkenburg JH, van Liempt E, Veltrop-Duits LA, Lankester AC, et al. (2010) Combined CD8+ and CD4+ adenovirus hexon-specific T cells associated with viral clearance after stem cell transplantation as treatment for adenovirus infection. Haematologica 95: 1943–1951.
15. Einsele H, Roosnek E, Rufer N, Sinzger C, Riegler S, et al. (2002) Infusion of cytomegalovirus (CMV)-specific T cells for the treatment of CMV infection not responding to antiviral chemotherapy. Blood 99: 3916–3922.
16. Leen AM, Christin A, Myers GD, Liu H, Cruz CR, et al. (2009) Cytotoxic T lymphocyte therapy with donor T cells prevents and treats adenovirus and Epstein-Barr virus infections after haploidentical and matched unrelated stem cell transplantation. Blood 114: 4283–4292.
17. Leen AM, Myers GD, Sili U, Huls MH, Weiss H, et al. (2006) Monoculture-derived T lymphocytes specific for multiple viruses expand and produce clinically relevant effects in immunocompromised individuals. Nat Med 12: 1160–1166.
18. Feuchtinger T, Matthes-Martin S, Richard C, Lion T, Fuhrer M, et al. (2006) Safe adoptive transfer of virus-specific T-cell immunity for the treatment of systemic adenovirus infection after allogeneic stem cell transplantation. Br J Haematol 134: 64–76.
19. Cobbold M, Khan N, Pourgheysari B, Tauro S, McDonald D, et al. (2005) Adoptive transfer of cytomegalovirus-specific CTL to stem cell transplant patients after selection by HLA-peptide tetramers. J Exp Med 202: 379–386.
20. Feuchtinger T, Opherk K, Bethge WA, Topp MS, Schuster FR, et al. (2010) Adoptive transfer of pp65-specific T cells for the treatment of chemorefractory cytomegalovirus disease or reactivation after haploidentical and matched unrelated stem cell transplantation. Blood 116: 4360–4367.
21. Schmitt A, Tonn T, Busch DH, Grigoleit GU, Einsele H, et al. (2011) Adoptive transfer and selective reconstitution of streptamer-selected cytomegalovirus-specific CD8+ T cells leads to virus clearance in patients after allogeneic peripheral blood stem cell transplantation. Transfusion 51: 591–599.
22. Uhlin M, Gertow J, Uzunel M, Okas M, Berglund S, et al. (2012) Rapid Salvage Treatment With Virus-Specific T Cells for Therapy-Resistant Disease. Clin Infect Dis.
23. Jones MS 2nd, Harrach B, Ganac RD, Gozum MM, Dela Cruz WP, et al (2007) New adenovirus species found in a patient presenting with gastroenteritis. J Virol 81: 5978–5984.
24. Leen AM, Sili U, Vanin EF, Jewell AM, Xie W, et al. (2004) Conserved CTL epitopes on the adenovirus hexon protein expand subgroup cross-reactive and subgroup-specific CD8+ T cells. Blood 104: 2432–2440.
25. Zandvliet ML, van Liempt E, Jedema I, Kruithof S, Kester MG, et al. (2011) Simultaneous isolation of CD8(+) and CD4(+) T cells specific for multiple viruses for broad antiviral immune reconstitution after allogeneic stem cell transplantation. J Immunother 34: 307–319.
26. Zandvliet ML, Kester MG, van Liempt E, de Ru AH, van Veelen PA, et al. (2012) Efficiency and Mechanism of Antigen-specific CD8+ T-cell Activation Using Synthetic Long Peptides. J Immunother 35: 142–153.
27. Leen AM, Christin A, Khalil M, Weiss H, Gee AP, et al. (2008) Identification of hexon-specific CD4 and CD8 T-cell epitopes for vaccine and immunotherapy. J Virol 82: 546–554.
28. Schipper RF, van Els CA, D'Amaro J, Oudshoorn M (1996) Minimal phenotype panels. A method for achieving maximum population coverage with a minimum of HLA antigens. Hum Immunol 51: 95–98.
29. Comoli P, Basso S, Labirio M, Baldanti F, Maccario R, et al. (2008) T cell therapy of Epstein-Barr virus and adenovirus infections after hemopoietic stem cell transplant. Blood Cells Mol Dis 40: 68–70.
30. Sellar RS, Peggs KS (2012) The role of virus-specific adoptive T-cell therapy in hematopoietic transplantation. Cytotherapy 14: 391–400.
31. Gerdemann U, Keirnan JM, Katari UL, Yanagisawa R, Christin AS, et al. (2012) Rapidly Generated Multivirus-specific Cytotoxic T Lymphocytes for the Prophylaxis and Treatment of Viral Infections. Mol Ther 20: 1622–1632.
32. Garnett CT, Erdman D, Xu W, Gooding LR (2002) Prevalence and quantitation of species C adenovirus DNA in human mucosal lymphocytes. J Virol 76: 10608–10616.
33. Rammensee H, Bachmann J, Emmerich NP, Bachor OA, Stevanovic S (1999) SYFPEITHI: database for MHC ligands and peptide motifs. Immunogenetics 50: 213–219.
34. Dohnal AM, Graffi S, Witt V, Eichstill C, Wagner D, et al. (2009) Comparative evaluation of techniques for the manufacturing of dendritic cell-based cancer vaccines. J Cell Mol Med 13: 125–135.
35. Vellinga J, van den Wollenberg DJ, van der Heijdt S, Rabelink MJ, Hoeben RC (2005) The coiled-coil domain of the adenovirus type 5 protein IX is dispensable for capsid incorporation and thermostability. J Virol 79: 3206–3210.
36. Ohrmalm L, Lindblom A, Omar H, Norbeck O, Gustafson I, et al. (2011) Evaluation of a surveillance strategy for early detection of adenovirus by PCR of peripheral blood in hematopoietic SCT recipients: incidence and outcome. Bone Marrow Transplant 46: 267–272.
37. Abate D, Cesaro S, Cofano S, Fiscon M, Saldan A, et al. (2012) Diagnostic utility of human cytomegalovirus-specific T-cell response monitoring in predicting viremia in pediatric allogeneic stem-cell transplant patients. Transplantation 93: 536–542.
38. Gratama JW, Boeckh M, Nakamura R, Cornelissen JJ, Brooimans RA, et al. (2010) Immune monitoring with iTAg MHC Tetramers for prediction of recurrent or persistent cytomegalovirus infection or disease in allogeneic hematopoietic stem cell transplant recipients: a prospective multicenter study. Blood 116: 1655–1662.
39. Guerin-El Khourouj V, Dalle JH, Pedron B, Yakouben K, Bensoussan D, et al. (2011) Quantitative and qualitative CD4 T cell immune responses related to adenovirus DNAemia in hematopoietic stem cell transplantation. Biol Blood Marrow Transplant 17: 476–485.
40. Olive M, Eisenlohr L, Flomenberg N, Hsu S, Flomenberg P (2002) The adenovirus capsid protein hexon contains a highly conserved human CD4+ T-cell epitope. Hum Gene Ther 13: 1167–1178.
41. Serangeli C, Bicanic O, Scheible MH, Wernet D, Lang P, et al. (2010) Ex vivo detection of adenovirus specific CD4+ T-cell responses to HLA-DR-epitopes of the Hexon protein show a contracted specificity of T(HELPER) cells following stem cell transplantation. Virology 397: 277–284.
42. Stemberger C, Huster KM, Koffler M, Anderl F, Schiemann M, et al. (2007) A single naive CD8+ T cell precursor can develop into diverse effector and memory subsets. Immunity 27: 985–997.

43. Boeckh M, Nichols WG (2004) The impact of cytomegalovirus serostatus of donor and recipient before hematopoietic stem cell transplantation in the era of antiviral prophylaxis and preemptive therapy. Blood 103: 2003–2008.
44. Comoli P, Basso S, Zecca M, Pagliara D, Baldanti F, et al. (2007) Preemptive therapy of EBV-related lymphoproliferative disease after pediatric haploidentical stem cell transplantation. Am J Transplant 7: 1648–1655.
45. Miller JS, Soignier Y, Panoskaltsis-Mortari A, McNearney SA, Yun GH, et al. (2005) Successful adoptive transfer and in vivo expansion of human haploidentical NK cells in patients with cancer. Blood 105: 3051–3057.
46. Linn YC, Niam M, Chu S, Choong A, Yong HX, et al. (2012) The anti-tumour activity of allogeneic cytokine-induced killer cells in patients who relapse after allogeneic transplant for haematological malignancies. Bone Marrow Transplant 47: 957–966.
47. Veltrop-Duits LA, Heemskerk B, Sombroek CC, van Vreeswijk T, Gubbels S, et al. (2006) Human CD4+ T cells stimulated by conserved adenovirus 5 hexon peptides recognize cells infected with different species of human adenovirus. Eur J Immunol 36: 2410–2423.
48. Chen BJ, Deoliveira D, Cui X, Le NT, Son J, et al. (2007) Inability of memory T cells to induce graft-versus-host disease is a result of an abortive alloresponse. Blood 109: 3115–3123.
49. Melenhorst JJ, Leen AM, Bollard CM, Quigley MF, Price DA, et al. (2010) Allogeneic virus-specific T cells with HLA alloreactivity do not produce GVHD in human subjects. Blood 116: 4700–4702.

Pyruvate Kinase Deficiency in Sub-Saharan Africa: Identification of a Highly Frequent Missense Mutation (G829A;Glu277Lys) and Association with Malaria

Patrícia Machado[1], Licínio Manco[2], Cláudia Gomes[1], Cristina Mendes[1], Natércia Fernandes[3], Graça Salomé[3], Luis Sitoe[3], Sérgio Chibute[3], José Langa[4], Letícia Ribeiro[5], Juliana Miranda[6], Jorge Cano[7], João Pinto[1], António Amorim[8,9], Virgílio E. do Rosário[1], Ana Paula Arez[1]*

1 Centro de Malária e outras Doenças Tropicais, Unidade de Parasitologia Médica, Instituto de Higiene e Medicina Tropical, Universidade Nova de Lisboa, Lisboa, Portugal, **2** Centro de Investigação em Antropologia e Saúde (CIAS), Universidade de Coimbra, Coimbra, Portugal, **3** Faculdade de Medicina da Universidade Eduardo Mondlane, Maputo, Mozambique, **4** Banco de Sangue do Hospital Central de Maputo, Maputo, Mozambique, **5** Departmento de Hematologia, Centro Hospitalar de Coimbra, Coimbra, Portugal, **6** Hospital Pediátrico David Bernardino, Luanda, Angola, **7** Centro Nacional de Medicina Tropical, Instituto de Salud Carlos III, Madrid, Spain, **8** Instituto de Patologia e Imunologia Molecular da Universidade do Porto (IPATIMUP), Porto, Portugal, **9** Faculdade de Ciências da Universidade do Porto, Porto, Portugal

Abstract

Background: Pyruvate kinase (PK) deficiency, causing hemolytic anemia, has been associated to malaria protection and its prevalence in sub-Saharan Africa is not known so far. This work shows the results of a study undertaken to determine PK deficiency occurrence in some sub-Saharan African countries, as well as finding a prevalent PK variant underlying this deficiency.

Materials and Methods: Blood samples of individuals from four malaria endemic countries (Mozambique, Angola, Equatorial Guinea and Sao Tome and Principe) were analyzed in order to determine PK deficiency occurrence and detect any possible high frequent PK variant mutation. The association between this mutation and malaria was ascertained through association studies involving sample groups from individuals showing different malaria infection and outcome status.

Results: The percentage of individuals showing a reduced PK activity in Maputo was 4.1% and the missense mutation G829A (Glu277Lys) in the PKLR gene (only identified in three individuals worldwide to date) was identified in a high frequency. Heterozygous carrier frequency was between 6.7% and 2.6%. A significant association was not detected between either PK reduced activity or allele 829A frequency and malaria infection and outcome, although the variant was more frequent among individuals with uncomplicated malaria.

Conclusions: This was the first study on the occurrence of PK deficiency in several areas of Africa. A common PKLR mutation G829A (Glu277Lys) was identified. A global geographical co-distribution between malaria and high frequency of PK deficiency seems to occur suggesting that malaria may be a selective force raising the frequency of this 277Lys variant.

Editor: Georges Snounou, Université Pierre et Marie Curie, France

Funding: This study was supported by PEst-OE/SAU/LA0018/2011 - Proj. Estratégico LA0018 2011/2012 (http://cmdt.ihmt.unl.pt/index.php/pt/) and PTDC/SAU-MET/110323/2009, "Fundacão para a Ciência e Tecnologia/Ministério da Educação e Ciência", FCT/MEC (http://alfa.fct.mctes.pt/index.phtml.pt), Portugal. PM holds a FCT grant (SFRH/BD/28236/2006). IPATIMUP is an Associate Laboratory of the Portuguese Ministry of Education and Science, and is partially supported by Fundação para a Ciência e a Tecnologia. The funders had no role in study design, data collection and analysis, decision to publish, or preparation of the manuscript.

Competing Interests: The authors have declared that no competing interests exist.

* E-mail: aparez@ihmt.unl.pt

Introduction

Infectious diseases have been one of the major causes of mortality during most of human evolution. For many diseases, mortality and hence reproductive success are influenced by certain individual genotype. Consequently, some aspects of modern patterns of human genetic diversity should have been determined by diseases dating from prehistoric times [1]. The clearest example are provided by malaria, which even now affects 500 million people each year and kills some two million. The selective pressure that malaria has imposed to human populations has been reflected in dozens of molecular variants described as protective against the infection and disease [2–4]. Of these, the most well studied and widely accepted are probably the sickle cell allele (hemoglobin HbS allele), α and β thalassemias and glucose-6-phosphate (G6PD) deficiency (alleles A and A-), all showing an extensive overlap of geographical distribution and exceptionally high frequencies in malaria endemic regions.

Pyruvate kinase (PK) deficiency, caused by mutations in the pyruvate kinase, liver and RBC (PKLR) gene (chromosome 1q21) is one of the most recently described erythrocyte abnormalities associated to malaria. Evidences of its protective effect were obtained both in murine models [5] and in *Plasmodium falciparum in vitro* cultures using human PK-deficient blood [6,7]. Also, population studies showed that a selective pressure is shaping the PKLR genomic region in individuals from malaria endemic countries (Cape Verde, Angola and Mozambique), being malaria infection the most likely driving force [8,9].

PK catalyzes the conversion of phosphoenolpyruvate (PEP) into pyruvate with the synthesis of ATP in the last step of glycolysis. PEP and pyruvate are involved in a great deal of energetic and biosynthetic pathways and the regulation of PK activity has proven to be of great importance for the entire cellular metabolism [10]. PK deficiency, worldwide distributed, is the most common enzyme abnormality in the erythrocyte glycolytic pathway causing hereditary chronic nonspherocytic hemolytic anemia. It is transmitted as an autossomal recessive trait and clinical symptoms usually occur in homozygotes and in compound heterozygotes for two mutant alleles. The clinical phenotype is heterogeneous, ranging from a mild chronic hemolytic anemia to a severe anemia presenting at birth and requiring exchange transfusion [11].

High frequencies of PK deficiency have not yet been recorded in malaria endemic areas but a systematic analysis has never been performed. Considering the previous knowledge of co-distribution between malaria endemicity and protective polymorphisms, we questioned if a PK variant could be exceptionally prevalent in malaria endemic areas. Therefore, the aims of the present study were: i) to determine PK deficiency occurrence in sub-Saharan African countries, ii) to assess frequency of PK variants underlying this deficiency, iii) to investigate possible associations between PK deficiency and malaria infection.

Materials and Methods

Sampling

This study is based on the molecular analysis of six sets of blood samples collected in four sub-Saharan African areas – Mozambique, Angola, Equatorial Guinea and Sao Tome and Principe (see Figure 1) - and in a malaria non-endemic area – Portugal (Europe).

In this study, 296 unrelated whole blood samples from individuals who attended to the Central Hospital of Maputo (Mozambique) between September and December 2008 were analyzed: 144 from children (6 months to 14 years-old) who presented to the Emergency Services of the Pediatric Department with some kind of complaint, and 152 from healthy blood donor adults (16 to 65 years-old) who presented to the Blood Bank. In order to increase the sample size of the set with a malaria outcome characterization, an additional group of 151 DNA samples extracted from blood samples collected from 3 months to 15 years-old children in Mozambique [9] was also genotyped.

In the Pediatric Department, blood was collected by venous puncture after the clinician examination but before the administration of any anti-malarial drug and/or blood transfusion. The registration of symptoms, axillary temperature and hemoglobin level was done for all individuals. Children who had received a blood transfusion in the last six months were excluded from the study. Anemic and *Plasmodium* infection status were considered at collection time. In the Blood Bank, the blood samples were randomly collected from blood donors. In the admission, a solubility test for rapid detection of hemoglobin S (adapted from Loh [12]) was performed in order to exclude allele S carriers. After blood collection in a tube, a blood spot in a filter paper was prepared from each sample for later subsequent DNA extraction by a standard phenol-chloroform method.

In addition to these samples from Mozambique, a set of 343 DNA samples from malaria-infected and non-infected unrelated individuals, which were already available from other studies, were also analyzed: 164 from Angola [9], 38 from Equatorial Guinea [13] and 67 from Sao Tome and Principe [14]. Finally, 74 samples from non-infected Portuguese individuals from all age groups were used as control samples [8]. Overall, 790 samples were analyzed.

Ethics statement

Regarding the survey in Mozambique, the human isolates collection was approved by local Ethical Committee (Comité Nacional de Bioética para a Saúde, Health Ministry of Mozambique, IRB 00002657, ref. 226/CNBS/08) and IHMT (Conselho de Ética do Instituto de Higiene e Medicina Tropical, CEIHMT, 14-2011-PN). A detailed work plan, questionnaires and informed consent forms were submitted to the Ethical Committees of the participant institutions in the study, which approved the survey. Each individual and parent/tutor of the children was informed of the nature and aims of the study and was told that participation was voluntary; written informed consent was obtained from each person (or parent/tutor). Blood sample collection followed strict requirements set by the Ethical Committees: blood samples from children who attended to the Pediatric Department were the remaining volume of the samples previously collected for the medical diagnosis; in the Blood Bank, during the blood donation, a small volume was put aside in a tube. In this way, no extra blood collection was needed and the patient, blood donor and the routine health services were not significantly disturbed. All ethical aspects related with the other sets of samples collected in previous studies, are described in the respective reports [8,9,13,14].

Plasmodium infection and malaria outcome groups

In the Central Hospital of Maputo, the rapid test OptiMAL-IT (DiaMed, Switzerland) was used for malaria diagnosis in all the patients with suspicion of malaria infection, and a blood smear was prepared for microscopic visualization to confirm diagnosis; later, all samples were amplified by Polymerase Chain Reaction (PCR), using *Plasmodium* species specific primers [15].

Malaria outcome was defined as follows: (i) Severe Malaria (SM): positive PCR for any species of *Plasmodium*, fever (i.e. axillary temperature $\geq$37,5°C), hemoglobin level of Hb$\leq$5 g/dL and/or any of these symptoms: coma, prostration or convulsions; (ii) Uncomplicated Malaria (UM): positive PCR for any *Plasmodium* species, fever and hemoglobin level of Hb>5 g/dL; and (iii) Asymptomatic Infection (AI): positive PCR for any *Plasmodium* species in the absence of fever (i.e. axillary temperature <37,5°C) or other symptoms of clinical illness; (iv) No infection (NI): negative PCR and absence of fever or other symptoms of clinical illness.

Based on malaria infection and symptoms data, the 144 samples from the Pediatric Department of Central Hospital of Maputo collected in 2008 were organized in the following malaria outcome groups: SM (18 samples); UM (27 samples) and NI (99 samples). The 152 samples from the Blood Bank were organized in the following groups: AI (4 samples) and NI (148 samples). Outcome groups were also defined using the same criteria for the set of isolates from Angola (43 SM, 43 UM, 37 AI and 41 NI) and for the set of isolates previously collected in Mozambique (52 SM, 97 UM and 2 NI), both described in Machado *et al.* [9]. In total, we had 611 samples with malaria infection and outcome characterization - 459 samples from children (113 SM, 167 UM, 37 AI and 142 NI) and 152 samples from adults (4 AI and 148 NI).

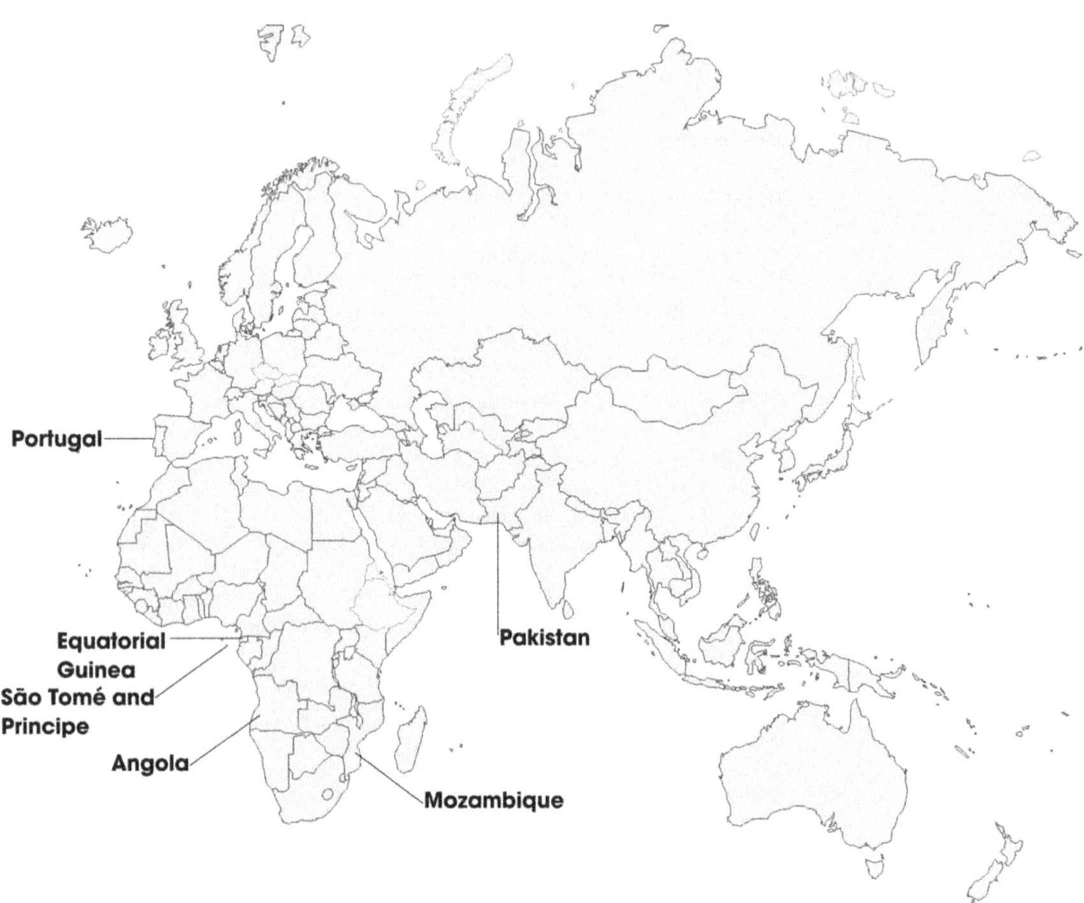

Figure 1. Geographic location of the countries Mozambique, Angola, Sao Tome and Principe, Equatorial Guinea (Africa), Pakistan (Asia) and Portugal (Europe).

Determination of PK activity

PK activity was measured in lyzed erythrocytes from all the 296 fresh blood samples (after plasma and buffy coat strict removal) collected in Mozambique in 2008, with an enzymatic assay adapted from Beutler [16], according to the instructions of the kit "Determination of pyruvate kinase (EC 2.7.1.40) in erythrocytes hemolysate or serum/heparinized plasma" (Instruchemie, The Netherlands). The enzymatic reactions were running at room temperature. A PK-deficient and a normal control were used in each assay to validate the activity values and to classify the samples within the following phenotypes: normal, intermediate or deficient activity.

Identification of a PK variant underlying PK-reduced activity

Samples with a PK activity value less than or equal to 75% of the normal control sample activity were analyzed by the Single Strand Conformational Polymorphism (SSCP) method (described in Manco *et al.* [17]) in order to find a mutation associated with this phenotype. The promoter region and eleven exons of the PKLR gene were amplified with specific primers (see Table S1, supporting information) and run in an acrylamide-bisacrylamide gel (10%), together with a wild-type amplicon, to detect differences in migration patterns caused by an alteration in DNA chain composition (exon 2 was not analyzed since it is specific for the hepatic isoenzyme). The amplification conditions were: initial denaturation at 94°C for 5 minutes, followed by 35 cycles of 94°C for 45 seconds, a specific annealing temperature for 45 seconds (see Table S1), and 72°C for 1 minute, with a final extension at 72°C for 5 minutes. The samples with a different migration pattern were further analyzed by automatic DNA sequencing (Macrogen Inc., Korea). The exon 7, in which a mutation was identified, was then amplified in all samples from all groups by PCR with the specific primers and conditions indicated in Table S1 and the amplicons were sequenced (Macrogen Inc., Korea).

Statistical analysis

The association between alleles and malaria outcome groups was assessed by Pearson's chi-square tests and Fisher's exact test, this latter considered when there were a few cases in each comparison group (less than five), using the Simple Interactive Statistical Analysis software (SISA) [18]. Odds ratios (OR) and 95% confidence intervals (CI) were also estimated using SISA. Arlequin 3.1 software [19] was used to determine allele frequencies, population pairwise F_{ST} (to test for differentiation between populations), expected and observed values of heterozygosity and to perform Hardy–Weinberg equilibrium tests. Prediction of the possible impact of the amino acid substitution on the structure and function of the human PK protein was performed with the Polyphen software [20]. Finally, PyMol software [21] was used for the 3D structure simulation of the wild type and mutant variants.

Results

PK deficiency screening in Maputo, Mozambique

Ninety-eight from the 144 samples collected in the Pediatric Department (68%) in Mozambique in 2008 were from children with a hemoglobin concentration <9 g/dL (considered anemic) and 41 samples (28.5%) were infected with *P. falciparum*. Nineteen of the infected individuals were also anemic. Four (2.6%) of the 152 samples from the adult blood donors in Blood Bank showed an asymptomatic infection with *P. falciparum* (see Table 1)

From the 296 samples set, 12 (4.1%) presented PK activity values between 39% and 75% of the normal control activity (established in an average of 3.2 U/g Hb) (see Table 2): 8 from the Blood Bank (5.3%) and 4 from the Pediatrics (2.8%). They were all classified as intermediate activity phenotype. From the 98 samples with a hemoglobin level <9 g/dl (Pediatric Department), only 3 (3.1%) had a PK reduced activity.

Identification of a PK variant underlying PK-reduced activity

A migration pattern alteration was observed in the amplicon of exon 7 of 5 out of 12 samples with low activity (41.7%) by SSCP (see Figure 2): 4 from blood donors and 1 from Pediatrics. Sequencing of these 5 amplicons revealed a G>A substitution in all of them, being in homozygosis (A/A) in one sample. This is a non-synonymous mutation located in the nucleotide 829 of the PK mRNA sequence originating an alteration of the amino acid 277 of the PK protein: a glutamic acid (Glu, coded by GAG) is replaced by a lysine (Lys, coded by AAG). When this mutation was searched in all the other 284 samples with normal activity, it was detected in heterozygosis in 16 samples: 7 from children and 9 from blood donors. Overall, 21 samples (7.1%) had the 829A allele that displayed a frequency of 3.7%.

No association was found between the 829A allele and anemia (2.7–9 g/dL Hb). Conversely, a strong association was found between the allele 829A and PK deficient activity: $\chi^2 = 14.38$ (P<0.00), OR = 5.58 (95% CI: 2.07–15.03). Of the 6 samples with the lowest PK activity values (between 39% and 47% of the normal activity), 5 had the mutation. All the 6 other samples with an activity between 47% and 75% of the normal activity were wild type.

As visualized in the 3D PK structure simulation (see Figure 3), this 277 residue is exposed, showing a peripheral position. The prediction of the substitution Glu277Lys effect on the structure and function of the human protein PK was "Possibly Damaging" (score of 0.90) supporting the previous OR result and suggesting that this mutation is likely to be non-functional.

Searching the mutation G829A in other African malaria endemic areas

The mutation G829A was found in the other three African countries, always in heterozygosis: in 11 samples from Angola (6.7%), 1 sample from Equatorial Guinea (2.6%) and 2 samples from Sao Tome and Principe (3.0%). Allele 829A frequencies were 3.4%, 1.3% and 1.5%, respectively. In the Mozambican group from 2005, the frequency of individuals heterozygous for 829A was 5.3%, giving an allele frequency of 2.6%. The mutation was not found in the control group from Portugal. Considering all the Mozambican 447 samples, a frequency of carrier individuals of 5.8% and 829A allele frequency of 3.0% were estimated.

The observed genotype frequencies (829GG, 829AG and 829AA) were according to Hardy-Weinberg expectations for all populations (P = 0.40 in Mozambique; P = 1.00 in Angola, Equatorial Guinea and Sao Tome and Principe). Estimates of F_{ST} were non-significant between all pairs of African populations ($F_{ST} \leq 0.00$ for all) (P = 1.00 for Mozambique vs. Angola; P = 0.50 for Mozambique vs. Equatorial Guinea; P = 0.30 for Mozambique vs. Sao Tome and Principe; P = 0.51 for Angola vs. Equatorial Guinea; P = 0.35 for Angola vs. Sao Tome and Principe; and P = 1.00 for Equatorial Guinea vs. Sao Tome and Principe).

Association among PK-reduced activity, the mutation G829A and malaria infection/outcome

Six-hundred and eleven DNA samples belonging to individuals characterized for their infection and malaria disease outcome status were analyzed: 459 samples from children (113 SM, 167 UM, 37 AI and 142 NI) from Angola and Mozambique and 152 samples from adults (4 AI and 148 NI), from Mozambique. No significant differentiation between samples from Angola and Mozambique were observed, so all samples together were considered for this analysis.

Allele 829A frequencies were as follows (see Table 3): in children, 3.1% in SM, 3.3% in UM, 2.7% in AI and 2.5% in NI; in adults 4.4% in NI. In terms of malaria infection in children, allele A frequencies were 3.2% in infected and 2.5% in non-infected. In adults, this analysis in terms of infection was not considered due to the low number of infected individuals. Although the mutation frequency was higher in uncomplicated (UM) than in severe malaria (SM) group, no significant association was observed between 829A allele and disease outcome ($\chi^2 = 0.02$, P = 1.00; OR = 1.07, 95% CI: 0.41–2.80). No significant association was found either between 829A allele and infection ($\chi^2 = 0.33$, P = 0.57; OR = 1.29, 95% CI: 0.54–3.08) or between PK deficient activity (low enzyme activity) and infection (P = 0.30), though 11 from the 12 samples with PK reduced activity were non-infected.

Table 1. PK activity, anemia and *Plasmodium* infection status in the sample set from Maputo, Mozambique (2008).

	Pediatrics	Blood Bank	Total
Age Group	Children (6 months–14 years old); with some complaint	Adults (16–65 years old); healthy blood donors	6 months–65 years old
Nr of samples	144	152	296
Low PK activity (39–75% of control)	4 (2.8%)	8 (5.3%)	12 (4.1%)
Anemia (Hb<9 g/dL)	98 (68.1%)	n.d.	n.d.
***Plasmodium* infection**	41 (28.5%)	4 (2.6%)	45 (15.2%)
Anemia+Infection	19 (13.2%)	n.d.	n.d.

n.d.: not determined.

Table 2. Samples with a reduced PK activity (between 39 and 75% of the normal control) and respective infection status and malaria outcome and 829 locus genotype.

					PK Activity U/g Hb				
#	Sample	Assay	Activity	Average	Control N	Average/Control N	Control DEF	Inf/Malaria outcome	829G/A
1	**BS_128**	1	1.69	**1.69**	3.48	**0.49**	0.85	NI	GG
2	**BS_176**	1	1.88						
	BS_176	2	1.93	**1.91**	3.48	**0.55**	0.85	NI	GG
3	**BS_197**	1	1.56						
	BS_197	2	1.34	**1.45**	3.48	**0.42**	0.85	NI	**GA**
4	**BS_199**	1	1.73						
	BS_199	2	0.99	**1.36**	3.48	**0.39**	0.85	NI	**GA**
5	**BS_212**	1	1.85						
	BS_212	2	1.43	**1.64**	3.48	**0.47**	0.85	NI	**GA**
6	**BS_220**	1	1.35						
	BS_220	2	1.52	**1.44**	3.48	**0.41**	0.85	NI	GG
7	**BS_230**	1	1.46						
	BS_230	2	1.59	**1.53**	3.48	**0.44**	0.85	NI	**AA**
8	**BS_327**	1	1.74						
	BS_327	2	1.96	**1.85**	3.48	**0.53**	0.85	NI	GG
9	**N_1159**	1	1.93						
	N_1159	2	2.27	**2.10**	2.91	**0.72**	0.73	NI	GG
10	**N_1391**	1	2.19	**2.19**	2.91	**0.75**	0.73	NI	GG
11	**N_1464**	1	1.69	**1.69**	2.91	**0.58**	0.73	NI	GG
12	**O_2341**	1	1.35	**1.35**	2.91	**0.46**	0.73	SM	**GA**

BS: samples collected in the Blood Bank; O and N: samples collected in the Department of Pediatrics; Inf/Malaria outcome: infection status and malaria outcome; 829G/A: 829 genotype; NI: non-infected; SM: severe malaria.

Discussion

This is the first study aimed at determining PK deficiency occurrence as well as at studying a potential widespread PKLR mutation in the African continent.

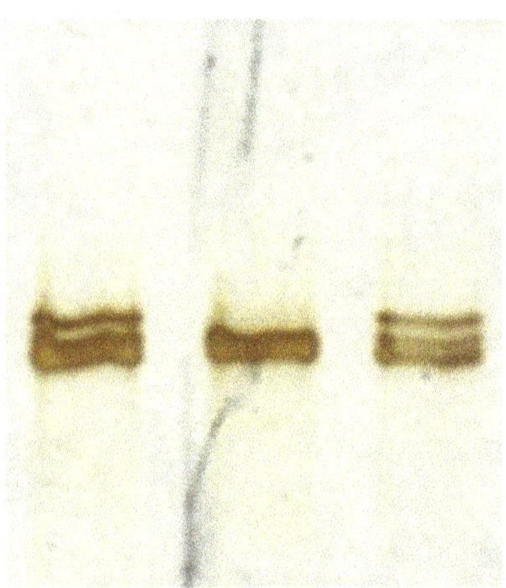

Figure 2. SSCP results showing a migration pattern alteration in the exon 7 amplicons caused by the G829A substitution (10% acrylamide-bisacrylamide gel) - samples at the extremes (wild type isolate in the middle).

In the first instance, PK deficiency was studied in samples from Maputo, Mozambique, measuring PK activity in anemic individuals, as this is described as a symptom of the disease. However, anemia was neither associated to PK reduced activity nor 829A allele. The overall prevalence rate of PK reduced activity was 4.1% in the study population (5.3% from blood donors and 2.8% from children). Although children samples were, most of them, clinical cases with a considerable anemic status, a higher PK deficiency prevalence was not found in these samples and no association was detected between PK low activity and anemia. In this regard, a study carried in 2002 revealed that 74% of the children under five and 50% of the women in reproductive age from Mozambique was anemic [22], showing that anemia is not a proper indicator of erythrocyte deficiencies in developing countries.

The missense mutation G829A (Glu277Lys) was identified in 41.7% of Mozambican PK deficient isolates with a strong association with reduced activity phenotype. This mutation was then searched in additional Mozambican samples and other sub-Saharan regions and the 829A allele was detected in all of them at allele frequencies between 1.3% (in Equatorial Guinea) and 3.4% (in Angola). The allele 829A was not present in the Portuguese samples. Although two African groups could be established according to these frequencies (Angola and Mozambique with higher frequencies vs. Equatorial Guinea and Sao Tome and Principe with lower frequencies), F_{ST} values were not significantly different between them. These differences may be explained by sample size bias (447 samples from Mozambique and 164 from

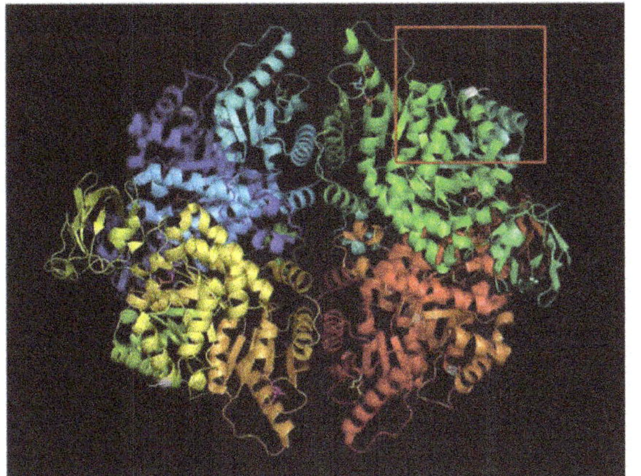

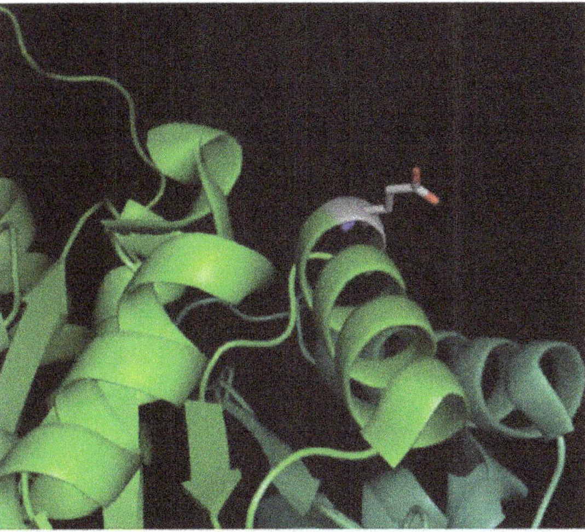

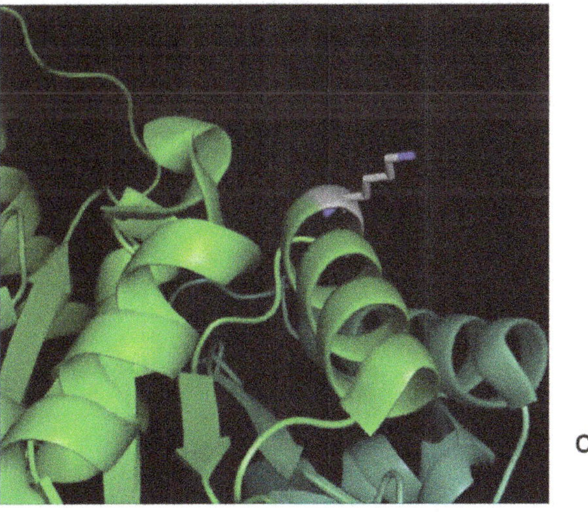

Figure 3. Location of the amino acid 277 in the PK protein and simulation of the 3D wild type 277Glu and mutant 277Lys PK variants structure with the software PyMol. a) Peripheral position of the amino acid 277 (domain A); b) Wild type variant 277Glu; c) Mutant variant 277Lys.

Angola were processed against 38 from Equatorial Guinea and 64 from Sao Tome and Principe) or design bias (isolates from Mozambique and Angola were obtained in hospital-based studies, whereas the others were collected in households by active search). In addition, genetic substructure among geographic regions cannot be excluded as a hypothesis for this disparity. Differences in malaria selective pressure are not a probable cause, since it has probably been similar in all these regions in the past.

Prevalence of PK deficiency seems to vary greatly among ethnic groups and geographic regions, as well as the mutations in the PKLR gene. Some authors have estimated a prevalence of 1:20 000 in the general white population [23]. In Europe, an incidence of 3.3 per million has been reported in the north of England [24], and a prevalence of 0.24% and 1.1% have been described in Spain [25] and Turkey [26], respectively. In Asia, the frequency of PK deficiency among the Hong Kong Chinese population was <0.1% [27] whilst among the south Iranian population was 1.9% [28]. In Saudi Arabia, a prevalence of 3.12% was registered in newborns [29]. These studies were all based in PK activity measurements. The estimated mutant allele frequencies of common variants generally vary between 0.2 and 0.8% [23] with the highest heterozygous prevalence described so far in Saudi Arabia (6%) [28,30] and Hong Kong (3.4%) [31]. However, these last allele frequencies were not calculated from mutation genotyping but only estimated from the Beutler's screening qualitative procedure and enzyme assay [16], which result in less reliable estimates of heterozygosity. Moreover, consanguinity is extremely high in Saudi Arabia, exceeding 80% in some regions [29], which tends to bias the results.

The PK deficiency recorded in Mozambique (4.1%) and 829GA heterozygous prevalence (2.6–6.7%) determined from unrelated individuals from sub-Saharan populations is, to our knowledge, the highest estimated worldwide so far. We initially hypothesized that this would be the result of a strong malaria pressure, but a significant association between both PK low activity and 829A and malaria infection and outcome was not found. However, only 12 samples were available for testing a possible effect of low enzyme activity on severity of malaria and 20 samples for testing a possible effect of 829A allele meaning that larger numbers are required to formally conclude. Moreover, since this was a cross-sectional study, infection and malaria outcome groups were established according to a malaria phenotype in a specific time point (the collection day), that may not accurately reflect the true individual phenotype. Nevertheless, there was higher mutation prevalence in the uncomplicated malaria group supporting that further analysis is essential to complete the present study.

The Glu277Lys mutation here identified has been previously reported in the PKLR mutation database [32] and has recently been described [30] in only two individuals: one from the Mandenka ethnic group (one of the largest ethnic groups in West Africa) and other from the Brahui ethnic group from Pakistan, showing that is also present in Middle East. Since the haplotypes that include this mutation in these two individuals are different, it was suggested that it has arisen separately. In Pakistan, as in sub-Saharan countries, malaria continues to be a major public health problem. Both *P. falciparum* and *Plasmodium vivax* are widely distributed and the estimated number of annual malaria episodes in this country is 1.5 million [33].

The simulation of this Glu277Lys substitution on the human PK protein suggested that this mutation is likely to be non-functional. This residue is extremely well conserved and the result complies with the prediction from SIFT from a previous work [30]. Probably, the charge change (Glu is negatively whereas Lys is positively charged) at an exposed site alters the enzyme action. Considering this result together with the knowledge about PK deficiency that clinical symptoms usually occur in homozygotes for a mutant PKLR allele, it was surprising to find that the 829AA genotype belonged to a healthy blood donor without anemia

Table 3. Allele 829A frequencies in infection and malaria outcome groups.

	CHILDREN[1]			ADULTS[2]		
Infection/Clinical group	**Samples**	**829A carriers**	**829A frequency**	**Samples**	**829A carriers**	**829A frequency**
SM	113	7 (6.2%)	3.1%	0	0 (0%)	0 (0%)
UM	167	11 (6.6%)	3.3%	0	0 (0%)	0 (0%)
AI	37	2 (5.4%)	2.7%	4	0 (0%)	0 (0%)
NI	142	7 (4.9%)	2.5%	148	13[3] (8.8%)	4.7%
INF (SM+UM+AI)	317	20 (6.3%)	3.2%	4	0 (0%)	0 (0%)
TOTAL	459	27 (5.9%)	2.9%	152	13 (8.6%)	4.6%

[1]Samples from children well characterized for infection and malaria outcome status from Maputo, Mozambique (collected within this study and in a previous one [9]) and from Angola (collected previously [9]) who attended to the Pediatrics Department.
[2]Samples from adult blood donors from Maputo, Mozambique (collected within this study).
[3]Including one 829AA homozygote (the only one identified in the study).
SM: severe malaria; UM: uncomplicated malaria; AI: asymptomatic infection; NI: non-infected; INF: infected.

symptoms, with a PK activity of 0.44 with regard to the normal control. In this case we were expecting an activity similar to the deficient control sample (0.8 U/g Hb). However, the results obtained regarding PK activity must carefully be considered since the range of values obtained in Mozambique was narrow, far below the values expected with the use of the kit and generally obtained in other labs (about 3.7–8.2 U/g Hb at 25°C and about 7.4–16.4 U/g Hb at 37°C), with a thin gap between normal and reduced activity. This can be explained by the lower room temperature in the lab (about 20°C), when compared to those generally maintained in this procedure (25°C or 37°C). Yet, the procedure was efficient since it was possible to identify samples with reduced activity. Actually, there was no direct relation between the genotype and phenotype: although a significant association between 829A and a reduction in the enzyme activity was found out (and the samples with the lowest activity were those ones with the 829A allele), the phenotype of allele A carriers was highly variable with a large number of individuals within normal PK activity range. A previous study emphasizes the difficulty in predicting the consequences of mutations simply from the location and the nature of the target residues [10]: the clinical manifestations of a genetic disease reflect the interactions of a variety of physiological and environmental factors, including genetic background, concomitant functional polymorphisms of other enzymes, posttranslational or epigenetic modifications, ineffective erythropoiesis and differences in splenic function, and do not solely depend on the molecular properties of the altered molecule.

To conclude, a geographical co-distribution between malaria and PK-deficiency seems to occur: the Middle East and sub-Saharan Africa are the regions with the highest PK deficiency prevalence described so far, as determined in the present study. These are regions with a strong malaria pressure, suggesting that malaria may be an agent of contribute to the selection of PK deficiency variants in these regions. Conversely, the prevalence of PK deficiency is extremely low in the general white populations. Moreover, some of the genes that confer resistance to malaria are among the most variable genes in the human genome [4] and this is the case for PKLR gene, which presents more than 180 mutations and 8 polymorphic sites [11].

Additional studies with a larger sampling effort including longitudinal malaria clinical history characterization and a search of the variant 277Lys in other malaria endemic regions will be conducted to clarify the results in this survey.

Acknowledgments

Authors would like to express their gratitude to Dra. Umbelina Rebelo, Dra. Celeste Bento and Dr. Luís Relvas from the Hematology Department, Centro Hospitalar de Coimbra, as well as to Dra. Isabel Abergaria and the technicians from the Clinical Chemistry Lab, Instituto Nacional de Saúde Dr. Ricardo Jorge (Portugal) for all their help concerning the methodologies and protocols for PK assays. The authors also want to thank to João Rodrigues for doing the 3D structure simulation of the PK variants with PyMol software. Deep appreciation for the contribution of D. Violeta and Sábado from the Pediatric Lab and all the technicians from the Blood Bank (Central Hospital of Maputo, Mozambique) for collecting blood samples and to all volunteers that agreed in participate in the present study. Very special thanks to Natacha, Antónia, Dida and Juliana, Filipa and Pedro for their unconditional support during the stay at Mozambique.

Author Contributions

Conceived and designed the experiments: APA. Performed the experiments: PM CG CM LM. Analyzed the data: PM APA. Contributed reagents/materials/analysis tools: APA LM AA. Wrote the paper: PM APA. Did the field work at Mozambique (2008): PM GS JL LS NF SC. Processed the biological material and data collection in Mozambique, Angola, Sao Tome and Principe, Equatorial Guinea and Portugal, respectively: NF JM JP JC AA. Contributed with a critical review of the paper: AA CM JC JP LM LR SC VdR.

References

1. Jobling MA, Hurles ME, Tyler-Smith C (2004) Human evolutionary genetics: origins, peoples and disease. Garland Science, New York.
2. Verra F, Mangano VD, Modiano D (2009) Genetics of susceptibility to *Plasmodium falciparum*: from classical malaria resistance genes towards genome-wide association studies. Parasite Immunol 31: 234–253.
3. Allison AC (2009) Genetic control of resistance to human malaria. Curr Opin Immunol 21: 499–505.
4. Hedrick PW (2011) Population genetics of malaria resistance in humans. Heredity 107: 283–304.
5. Min-Oo G, Fortin A, Tam MF, Nantel A, Stevenson MM, et al. (2003) Pyruvate kinase deficiency in mice protects against malaria. Nat Genet 35: 357–362.

6. Ayi K, Min-Oo G, Serghides L, Crockett M, Kirby-Allen M, et al. (2008) Pyruvate kinase deficiency and malaria. N Engl J Med 358: 1805–1810.
7. Durand PM, Coetzer TL (2008) Pyruvate kinase deficiency protects against malaria in humans. Haematologica 93: 939–940.
8. Alves J, Machado P, Silva J, Gonçalves N, Ribeiro L, et al. (2010) Analysis of malaria associated genetic traits in Cabo Verde, a melting pot of European and sub Saharan settlers. Blood Cells Mol Dis 44: 62–68.
9. Machado P, Pereira R, Rocha AM, Manco L, Fernandes N, et al. (2010) Malaria: looking for selection signatures in the human PKLR gene region. Br J Haematol 149: 775–784.
10. Valentini G, Chiarelli LR, Fortin R, Dolzan M, Galizzi A, et al. (2002) Structure and function of human erythrocyte pyruvate kinase. Molecular basis of nonspherocytic hemolytic anemia. J Biol Chem 277: 23807–23814.
11. Zanella A, Fermo E, Bianchi P, Chiarelli LR, Valentini G (2007) Pyruvate kinase deficiency: the genotype-phenotype association. Blood Rev 21: 217–231.
12. Loh WP (1968) A new solubility test for rapid detection of haemoglobin. J Indiana State Med Assoc 61: 1651–1652.
13. Mendes C, Dias F, Figueiredo J, Mora VG, Cano J, et al. (2011) Duffy negative antigen is no longer a barrier to *Plasmodium vivax* - molecular evidences from the African West Coast (Angola and Equatorial Guinea). PLoS Negl Trop Dis 5: e1192.
14. Pinto J, Sousa CA, Gil V, Ferreira C, Gonçalves L, et al. (2000) Malaria in São Tomé and Príncipe: parasite prevalences and vector densities. Acta Trop 76: 185–193.
15. Snounou G, Viriyakosol S, Jarra W, Thaithong S, Brown KN (1993) Identification of the four human malaria parasite species in field samples by the polymerase chain reaction and detection of a high prevalence of mixed infections. Mol Biochem Parasitol 58: 283–292.
16. Beutler E (1984) Red Cell Metabolism: A Manual of Biochemical Methods. Grune & Stratton, Philadelphia, PA.
17. Manco L, Ribeiro ML, Almeida H, Freitas O, Abade A, et al. (1999) PK-LR gene mutations in pyruvate kinase deficient Portuguese patients. Br J Haematol 105: 591–595.
18. Simple Interactive Statistical Analysis software, SISA. Available: http://www.quantitativeskills.com/sisa/. Accessed 2012 Jun 29.
19. Excoffier L, Laval G, Schneider S (2005) Arlequin (version 3.0): an integrated software package for population genetics data analysis. Evol Bioinform Online 1: 47–50. Available: http://cmpg.unibe.ch/software/arlequin3/. Accessed 2012 Jun 29.
20. Polyphen software. Available: http://genetics.bwh.harvard.edu/php/. Accessed 2012 9 Aug 9.
21. The PyMOL Molecular Graphics System, Version 1.2r3pre, Schrödinger, LLC. Available: http://www.pymol.org/. Accessed 2012 Jun 29.
22. Ministério da Saúde, Direcção Geral da Saúde, República de Moçambique (2002) Moçambique: Investir na Nutrição é Reduzir a Pobreza. Análise das Consequências dos Problemas Nutricionais nas Crianças e Mulheres. Maputo.
23. Beutler E, Gelbart T (2000) Estimating the prevalence of pyruvate kinase deficiency from the gene frequency in the general white population. Blood 95: 3585–3588.
24. Carey PJ, Chandler J, Hendrick A, Reid MM, Saunders PW, et al. (2000) Prevalence of pyruvate kinase deficiency in northern European population in the north of England. Northern Region Haematologists Group. Blood 96: 4005–4006.
25. García SC, Moragón AC, López-Fernández ME (1979) Frequency of glutathione reductase, pyruvate kinase and glucose-6-phosphate dehydrogenase deficiency in a Spanish population. Hum Hered 29: 310–313.
26. Akin H, Baykal-Erkiliç A, Aksu A, Yücel G, Gümüşlü S (1997) Prevalence of erythrocyte pyruvate kinase deficiency and normal values of enzyme in a Turkish population. Hum Hered 47: 42–46.
27. Feng CS, Tsang SS, Mak YT (1993) Prevalence of pyruvate kinase deficiency among the Chinese: determination by the quantitative assay. Am J Hematol 43: 271–273.
28. Yavarian M, Karimi M, Shahriary M, Afrasiabi AR (2008) Prevalence of pyruvate kinase deficiency among the south Iranian population: quantitative assay and molecular analysis. Blood Cells Mol Dis 40: 308–311.
29. Abu-Melha AM, Ahmed MA, Knox-Macaulay H, Al-Sowayan SA, el-Yahia A (1991) Erythrocyte pyruvate kinase deficiency in newborns of eastern Saudi Arabia. Acta Haematol 85: 192–194.
30. Berghout J, Higgins S, Loucoubar C, Sakuntabhai A, Kain KC, et al. (2012) Genetic diversity in human erythrocyte pyruvate kinase. Genes Immun 13: 98–102.
31. Fung RH, Keung YK, Chung GS (1969) Screening of pyruvate kinase deficiency and G6PD deficiency in Chinese newborn in Hong Kong. Arch Dis Child 44: 373–376.
32. University Medical Center. (2007) PKLR Mutation Database. Laboratory for Red Blood Cell Research: Ultrecht. Available: http://www.pklrmutationdatabase.com/. Accessed 2012 Jun 29.
33. WHO EMRO (2011) World Health Organization, Regional Office of the Eastern Mediterranean, Epidemiological Situation, Country Profiles. Available: http://www.emro.who.int/rbm/CountryProfiles-pak.htm. Accessed 2012 Jun 29.

13

Systematic Review of Evidence-Based Guidelines on Medication Therapy for Upper Respiratory Tract Infection in Children with AGREE Instrument

Linan Zeng[1,2,3], Lingli Zhang[1,2,3]*, Zhiqiang Hu[1,4], Emily A. Ehle[5], Yuan Chen[1,2,3], Lili Liu[1,4], Min Chen[1,4]

1 Department of Pharmacy, West China Second University Hospital, Sichuan University, Sichuan, China, **2** Key Laboratory of Birth Defects and Related Diseases of Women and Children, Sichuan University, Ministry of Education, Sichuan, China, **3** Evidence-Based Pharmacy Centre, West China Second University Hospital, Sichuan University, Sichuan, China, **4** West China School of Pharmacy, Sichuan University, Sichuan, China, **5** Department of Pharmacy, The Nebraska Medical Centre, Omaha, Nebraska, United States of America

Abstract

Objectives: To summarize recommendations of existing guidelines on the treatment of upper respiratory tract infections (URTIs) in children, and to assess the methodological quality of these guidelines.

Methods: We searched seven databases and web sites of relevant academic agencies. Evidence-based guidelines on pediatric URTIs were included. AGREE II was used to assess the quality of these guidelines. Two researchers selected guidelines independently and extracted information on publication years, institutions, target populations, recommendations, quality of evidence, and strength of recommendations. We compared the similarities and differences of recommendations and their strength. We also analyzed the reasons for variation.

Results: Thirteen guidelines meeting our inclusion criteria were included. Huge differences existed among these 13 guidelines concerning the categorization of evidence and recommendations. Nearly all of these guidelines lacked the sufficient involvement of stake holders. Further, the applicability of these guidelines still needs to be improved. In terms of recommendations, penicillin and amoxicillin were suggested for group A streptococcal pharyngitis. Amoxicillin and amoxicillin-clavulanate were recommended for acute bacterial rhinosinusitis (ABRS). An observation of 2–3 days prior to antibiotic therapy initiation for mild acute otitis media (AOM) was recommended with amoxicillin as the suggested first choice agent. Direct evidence to support strong recommendations on the therapy for influenza is still lacking. In addition, the antimicrobial durations for pharyngitis and ABRS were still controversial. No consensus was reached for the onset of antibiotics for ABRS in children.

Conclusions: Future guidelines should use a consistent grading system for the quality of evidence and strength of recommendations. More effort needs to be paid to seek the preference of stake holders and to improve the applicability of guidelines. Further, there are still areas in pediatric URTIs that need more research.

Editor: Oliver Schildgen, Kliniken der Stadt Köln gGmbH, Germany

Funding: This work was supported by the National Natural Science Foundation of China (Project Number: 81373381). The funders had no role in study design, data collection and analysis, decision to publish, or preparation of the manuscript.

Competing Interests: The authors have declared that no competing interests exist.

* E-mail: zhlingli@sina.com

Introduction

Acute respiratory infections (ARIs) are classified as upper respiratory tract infections (URTIs) or lower respiratory tract infections (LRTIs) [1]. URTIs include the common cold, laryngitis, pharyngitis/tonsillitis, acute rhinitis, acute rhinosinusitis and acute otitis media (AOM) [2]. URTIs in children are a frequent illness accounting for a high proportion of doctor office visits [3,4]. A national survey report from the UK showed the consultation rates of URTIs were 3,103 and 1,002 per 10,000 person years at risk in children aged 0–4 and 5–15 years, respectively [5].

A proliferation of clinical guidelines published in peer-reviewed journals has been seen due to the high morbidity of URTIs. It is important that these guidelines provide appropriate guidance for the treatment of URTIs. Nevertheless, the growing number of guidelines has been accompanied with a growing concern about variance and conflicts among guideline recommendations and the quality of guidelines [18].To date, there have been no systematic attempts to compare recommendations from available guidelines for the treatment of children with URTIs.

The aim of this study is to assess the quality of evidence-based guidelines for drug therapy of URTIs in children and to compare the recommendations of the existing evidence-based guidelines. Special attention was devoted to areas of disagreement and discussion with an ultimate aim to improve the clinical practice in treatment of URTIs for children. Such an assessment is important as it may explain some of the variability in guideline recommen-

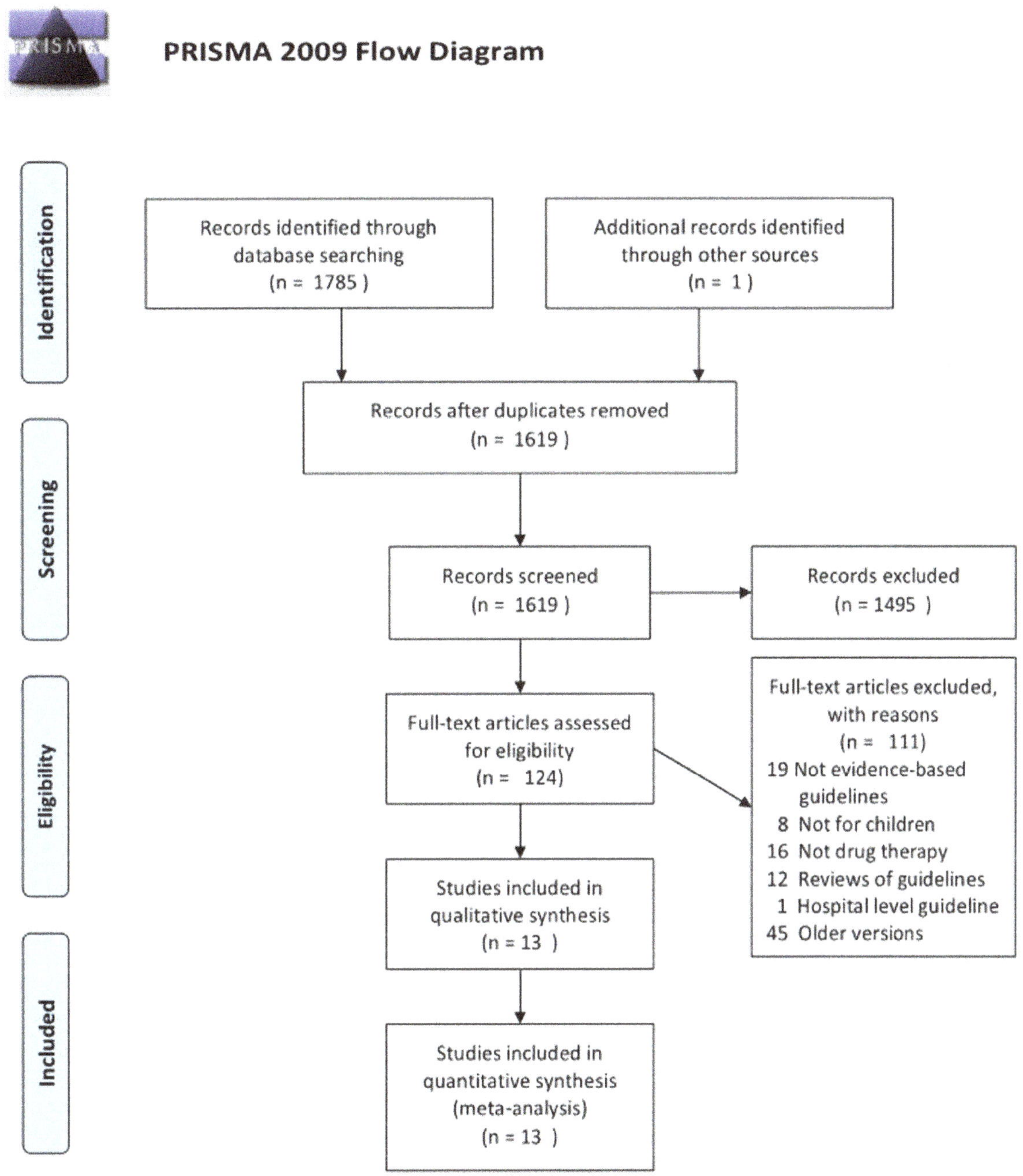

PRISMA 2009 Flow Diagram

Identification

Records identified through database searching (n = 1785)

Additional records identified through other sources (n = 1)

Records after duplicates removed (n = 1619)

Screening

Records screened (n = 1619)

Records excluded (n = 1495)

Eligibility

Full-text articles assessed for eligibility (n = 124)

Full-text articles excluded, with reasons (n = 111)
19 Not evidence-based guidelines
8 Not for children
16 Not drug therapy
12 Reviews of guidelines
1 Hospital level guideline
45 Older versions

Studies included in qualitative synthesis (n = 13)

Included

Studies included in quantitative synthesis (meta-analysis) (n = 13)

Figure 1. Summary of guideline search and review process.

dations and may assist health care providers in choosing among available guidelines.

Methods

Data Sources

We searched Pubmed, Guidelines International Network (GIN), U.S. National Guideline Clearinghouse (NGC) and four Chinese databases: Chinese Biomedical Literature Database (CBM), China Knowledge Resource Integrated Database (CNKI), VIP Database and Wanfang Database for evidence-based guidelines (until March 2013) using the following items: respiratory tract infections, common cold, laryngitis, pharyngitis, tonsillitis, rhinitis, rhinosinusitis, otitis media, middle ear inflammation, influenza, grippe as Medical Subject Headings (MeSH) or keywords. The searches were limited to guidelines published in English or Chinese. We also searched guidelines at web sites of academic agencies, such as American Academy of Pediatrics (AAP) and Infectious Diseases Society of America (IDSA). Retrieved references were considered if they met our inclusion criteria.

Guideline Selection

Inclusion criteria. Types: evidence-based guideline with systematic literature review and grading system for quality of evidence and/or strength of recommendation [6].

Table 1. Characteristics of 13 Evidence-Based Guidelines.

Guidelines by Medical Condition	Country	Institution[1]	Target Population	Conflicts of Interest[2]	Method to Formulate Recommendations	Quality of Evidence[3]	Strength of Recommendations[4]	Reference
Pharyngitis								
Shulman 2012	America	IDSA	Adult and child	SCI	Consensus development based on evidence	GRADE	GRADE	[8]
Rhinosinusitis								
Blomgren 2005	Finland	FSP	Adult and child	FPO	Consensus development based on evidence	Grading system from Evidence-based Medicine Working Group (A–D)	NA	[9]
Esposito 2008	Italy	SIP	child	EI	Consensus development based on evidence	Self designed grading system in accordance with the Italian National Guidelines Plan(I–VI)	Self designed grading system in accordance with the Italian National Guidelines Plan (A–E)	[10]
Chow 2012	America	IDSA	Adult and child	SCI	GRADE	GRADE	GRADE	[11]
Wald 2013	America	AAP	child	SCI	BRIDGE-Wiz[5]	Self designed grading system in accordance with the AAP policy statement (A–D,X)	Self designed grading system in accordance with the AAP policy statement "Classifying Recommendations for Clinical Practice Guidelines" (Strong recommendation, recommendation, option)	[12]
Influenza								
Bellamy 2006	–	WHO	Adult and child	SCI	GRADE	GRADE	GRADE	[13]
Bautista 2009	–	WHO	Adult and child	SCI	Consensus development based on evidence	GRADE	GRADE	[14]
Harper 2009	America	IDSA	Adult and child	SCI	Consensus development based on evidence	CTFPHE	CTFPHE	[15]
Morciano 2009	Italy	SNLG	Adult and child	FPO	Based on systematic review of available evidence	Self designed grading system in accordance with the Italian National Guidelines Plan(I–VI)	Self designed grading system in accordance with the Italian National Guidelines Plan (A–E)	[16]
Otitis media								
Bain 2003	England	SIGN	child	EI	Based on systematic review of available evidence	SIGN	SIGN	[17]
Takahashi 2012	Japan	JOS	child	NA	Based on available data	Grading system from Japan Stroke Society (I–IV)	Grading system from the US Preventive Services Task Force report (A–E)	[18]
Lieberthal 2013	America	AAP	child	SCI	Consensus development based on evidence	Self designed grading system in accordance with the AAP policy statement (A–D,X)	Self designed grading system in accordance with the AAP policy statement "Classifying Recommendations for Clinical Practice Guidelines" (Strong recommendation, recommendation, option)	[19]

Table 1. Cont.

Guidelines by Medical Condition	Country	Institution[1]	Target Population	Conflicts of Interest[2]	Method to Formulate Recommendations	Quality of Evidence[3]	Strength of Recommendations[4]	Reference
URTIs[6]								
Snellman 2013	America	ISCI	Adult and child	EI	Based on evidence summaries	Self designed grading system In transition to GRADE (High, Moderate, Low)	NA	[20]

Notes:
[1]IDSA, Infectious Diseases Society of America; FSP, The Finnish Society of Otorhinolaryngology; SIP, Italian Society of pediatrics; AAP, American Academy of Pediatrics; WHO, World Health Organization; SNLG, Italian National Guidelines System; SIGN, Scottish Intercollegiate Guidelines Network; JOS, Japan Otological Society; ICSI, Institute for Clinical Systems Improvement; UMHS,University of Michigan Health System.
[2]EI, editorial independence declared; FPO, funding by external public organization reported; SCI, statement about conflicts of interest of group members present.
[3]GRADE, Grading of Recommendations Assessment, Development and Evaluation; CTFPHE, Canadian Task Force on the Periodic Health Examination.
[4]NA: Not available.
[5]An interactive software tool that leads guideline development through a series o f questions that are intended to create a more actionable set of key action statements.
[6]URTIs refer to guidelines which include multiple diseases in URTIs.

Diseases: URTIs including rhinosinusitis, pharyngitis, laryngitis, rhinitis, otitis media, tonsillitis, common cold and influenza.

Patients: children ages 0–18 years old

Interventions: drug therapy

Exclusion criteria. Types: guideline of hospital level; old version of guideline

Diseases: non-infectious upper respiratory diseases

Interventions: vaccines

Guideline Quality Assessment

Appraisal of guidelines with the AGREE instrument. Quality of evidence-based guidelines was assessed by using AGREE II from the following domains: scope and purpose, stakeholder involvement, rigor of development, clarity of presentation, applicability, editorial independence and overall guideline assessment. Each of the AGREE II items and the two global rating items were rated on a 7-point scale (1-strongly disagree to 7-strongly agree). A score was assigned depending on the completeness and quality of reporting. Domain scores were calculated by summing up all the scores of the individual items in a domain and by scaling the total as a percentage of the maximum possible score for that domain. The scaled domain score was calculated as: (obtained score-minimum possible score)/(maximum possible score-minimum possible score) [7].

Appraisal of agreement between reviewers. We used the intraclass correlation coefficient (ICC) as a measure of agreement between reviewers. The ICC was applied to each guideline. Calculations were carried out by using SPSS 13.0.

Data Extraction

Two researchers selected guidelines independently and extracted the following information: publication years, institutions, target populations, recommendations, quality of evidence, and strength of recommendations. We compared the similarities and differences of recommendations and their strength and analyzed the reasons for variation.

Results

Guideline Search and Review Process

A total of 1,785 citations and abstracts were identified in the initial searches. Finally, 13 guidelines meeting our inclusion criteria were included, covering a period from 2005 to 2013 (Figure 1). These 13 guidelines focused on drug therapy for pharyngitis, rhinosinusitis, otitis media and influenza. For the remaining URTIs (laryngitis, tonsillitis, rhinitis), no guidelines for children were found.

Characteristics and Quality of Guidelines

Half of the 13 guidelines are from America developed by the American Academy of Pediatrics (AAP) and the Infectious Diseases Society of America (IDSA). Five guidelines are developed specially for children, while the rest are for both adults and children. All guidelines, except one, announced the conflict of interests and none were founded by industrial partners. All guidelines stated the formulation of recommendations was based on evidence. However, there is a huge variation in the grading systems of evidence quality and recommendation strength used (Table 1).

Comparison of the Categorization of Evidence and Recommendations of the 13 Guidelines (Table 2)

There were huge differences among 13 guidelines concerning the categorization of evidence and recommendations. Eight

Table 2. Comparison of the categorization of evidence and recommendations of 13 guidelines.

Levels	CTFPHE	SIGN	GRADE	Self designed grading system In transition to GRADE[2]	Grading system from Evidence-based Medicine Working Group	Grading system from AAP	Grading system from Japan Stroke Society	Grading system from Italian National Guidelines System
Quality of evidence								
1	**I**: Evidence from ≥1 properly RCT[1]	**1^{++}**:High quality meta-analyses, SR of RCTs, RCTs with a very low risk of bias.	**High quality**: Further research is very unlikely to change our confidence in the estimate of effect.	**High Quality Evidence:** Further research is very unlikely to change our confidence in the estimate of effect.	**A:**Several relevant, high-quality scientific studies with homogeneous results	**A:**Well-designed RCTs or DS on relevant population	**Ia**: Meta-analysis (with homogeneity) of RCTs	**I**: multiple RCTs and/ or SR of randomized studies
		1^{+}: Well conducted meta-analyses, SR, RCTs with a low risk of bias.					**Ib**: At least one RCT	
		1^{-}: Meta-analyses, SR, RCTs with a high risk of bias						
2	**II**: Evidence from ≥1 well-designed clinical trial, without randomization; from cohort or case-controlled analytic studies; from multiple time-series; from dramatic results from uncontrolled experiments	**2^{++}**:High quality SR of case control or cohort studies; High quality case control or cohort studies with a very low risk of confounding or bias and a high probability that the relationship is causal.	**Moderate quality**: Further research is likely to have an important impact on our confidence in the estimate of effect and may change the estimate.	**Moderate Quality Evidence**: Further research is likely to have an important impact on our confidence in the estimate of effect and may change the estimate.	**B:**At least 1 relevant, high-quality study or several adequate studies	**B:**RCT or DS with minor limitations; overwhelmingly consistent evidence from OS	**IIa**: At least one well-designed, controlled study but without randomization.	**II**: one single adequate randomized trial
		2^{+}: Well conducted case control or cohort studies with a low risk of confounding or bias and a moderate probability that the relationship is causal.					**IIb**: At least one well-designed, quasi-experimental study.	
		2^{-}:Case control or cohort studies with a high risk of confounding or bias and a significant risk that the relationship is not causal						
3	**III:** Evidence from opinions of respected authorities, based on clinical experience, descriptive studies, or reports of expert committees	**3:**Non-analytic studies, eg case reports, case series.	**Low quality**: Further research is very likely to have an important impact on our confidence in the estimate of effect and is likely to change the estimate.	**Low Quality Evidence:** Further research is very likely to have an important impact on our confidence in the estimate of effect and is likely to change the estimate or any estimate of effect is very uncertain.	**C:**At least 1 adequate scientific study	**C:**OS	**III**: At least one well-designed, non-experimental descriptive study	**III**: non-randomized cohort, concurrent or historical studies, or their meta-analysis

Table 2. Cont.

Levels	CTFPHE	SIGN	GRADE	Self designed grading system In transition to GRADE[2]	Grading system from Evidence-based Medicine Working Group	Grading system from AAP	Grading system from Japan Stroke Society	Grading system from Italian National Guidelines System
4		**4:** Expert opinion	**Very low quality:** Any estimate of effect is very uncertain.		**D:**Expert panel evaluation or other information	**D:**Expert opinion, case reports, or reasoning from first principles	**IV:**Expert committee reports, opinions and/or experience of Respected authorities	**IV:**retrospective case-control studies
5						X: Exceptional situations in which validating studies cannot be performed and there is a clear preponderance of benefit or harm.		**V**: non-controlled case-series studies
6								**VI**: Expert opinion or opinions from panels as indicated in guidelines or consensus conferences
Strength of recommen-dation								
1	**A:** Good evidence to support a recommen-dation for or against use	**A:** rated as 1^{++} or 1^{+},and directly applicable to the target population	**strong recommendation:** the desirable effects of an intervention clearly outweigh the undesirable effects, or clearly do not	NA	NA	**Strong Recommendation:** quality of evidence is excellent benefits strongly outweigh the harms	**Strongly recommended:** strong evidence is available, benefits substantially outweigh harms.	**A:** the specified strongly recommended and based on good quality scientific evidence
2	**B:** Moderate evidence to support a recommenda-tion for or against use	**B:** rated as 2^{++},and directly applicable to the target population; or Extrapolated evidence from studies rated as 1^{++} or 1^{+}	**weak recommendation:** the trade-offs are less certain–either because of low quality evidence or because evidence suggests that desirable and undesirable effects are closely balanced			Recommendation: quality of evidence is not as strong; benefits exceed the harms	Recommended: fair evidence is available, benefits outweigh harms.	**B:** There are doubts as to whether the particular procedure should be always be recommended, but should be carefully considered.
3	**C:** Poor evidence to support a recommen-dation	**C:** Evidence level 3 or 4; or Extrapolated evidence from studies rated as 2^{+}				**Option:** suspect evidence or well-done studies but little clear advantage to one approach vs another	**No recommendation made:** fair evidence is available, but the balance of benefits and harms is close.	**C:** There is substantial uncertainty concerning the procedure or intervention.

Table 2. Cont.

Levels	CTFPHE	SIGN	GRADE	Self designed grading system In transition to GRADE[2]	Grading system from Evidence-based Medicine Working Group	Grading system from AAP	Grading system from Japan Stroke Society	Grading system from Italian National Guidelines System
4						**No recommendation:** lack of evidence and an unclear balance between benefits and harms.	**Recommended against:** harms outweigh benefits.	**D:** the specified procedure is not recommended
5							**Insufficient evidence** to determine the balance of benefits and harms.	**E:** the specified procedure is strongly advised against.

Notes:
[1]RCT: randomized controlled trials; DS: diagnostic studies; OS: Observational studies.
[2]All existing ICSI Evidence Grading System incorporating GRADE methodology and all new literature considered by the work group for this revision has been assessed using GRADE methodology.

different grading systems were used, two of which failed to give strength of recommendations. Four guidelines used GRADE [21–25]. One guideline used SIGN [26] and one used CTFPHE [27]. Seven guidelines used other grading systems. The variation in terms of grading system may decrease the comparability of guidelines and confuse readers.

Evaluation of the AGREE Domains of Guidelines Analyzed (Table 3)

Scope and purpose. This domain evaluates the overall objectives, expected benefit or outcomes, and target population of guidelines. The medium score for this domain was 90.28% (76.39%–97.22%), indicating that most guidelines satisfied criteria of this domain.

Stake holder involvement. This domain evaluates the degree of relevant professional group involvement and whether the views and preferences of the target population have been considered and the definition of target users has been clearly presented. The overall score in this domain was low with a medium of 61.11% (33.33%–83.33%). Most of the guidelines involved relevant professionals in the development process and declared the target population. However, the guideline developers did not seek the preference of target populations sufficiently resulting in a decrease in score of this domain.

Rigour of development. This domain addresses the method of evidence search, grading, summarizing and the formulation of recommendations. The medium score for this domain was 76.04% (32.81%–91.15%), with 1 guideline scoring <50%. This guideline failed to demonstrate the link between evidence and recommendations. It was not reviewed externally before its publication either.

Clarity of presentation. This domain evaluates presentation and format of guidelines. The medium score was 95.83% (90.28%–98.61%), indicating that all guidelines satisfied criteria of this domain.

Applicability. This domain evaluates the consideration of facilitators or barriers to its implementation, as well as monitoring criteria. The medium score of this domain was 56.25% (10.42%–83.22%), the lowest of all domains. Four of 13 guidelines scored ≤ 50%. Most guidelines failed to consider the applicability sufficiently in guideline development.

Editorial independence. This domain addresses founding issues and competing interests of guideline development members. The medium score was 81.25% (8.33%–97.92%), with 3 guidelines scoring<50%.

Agreement among reviewers. Table 3 summarizes the degree of agreement for 13 guidelines by ICC. The ICC values indicate overall agreement between reviewers was excellent (80%) for 8 of 13 guidelines and substantial (70%) for the other 5 guidelines.

Recommendations

Recommendations towards drug therapy of Group A streptococcal pharyngitis for children (Table 4). Recommendations on antibiotics from IDSA and ISCI are consensus. The first choice was penicillin or amoxicillin. For penicillin-allergic patients, cephalosporins, clindamycin, or macrolides were recommended. Only IDSA, however, gave a recommendation on the duration of antibiotics (10 days). In terms of adjunctive therapy, IDSA suggested nonsteroidal anti-inflammatory drugs (NSAIDs) as adjunct to an appropriate antibiotic for treatment of moderate to severe symptoms or control fever. Aspirin should be avoided in children due to the risk of Reye's syndrome [28].

Recommendations towards drug therapy of acute bacterial rhinosinusitis (ABRS)/sinusitis for children

Table 3. Quality Assessment by AGREE II of 13 Evidence-based Guidelines.

Guidelines by Medical Condition, y	Scores,%						Agreement among reviewers for AGREE instrument items	Overall Assessment[1]
	Domain 1 Scope and Purpose	Domain 2 Stakeholder Involvement	Domain 3 Rigour of Development	Domain 4 Clarity of Presentation	Domain 5 Applicability	Domain 6 Editorial Independence		
Pharyngitis								
Shulman 2012	94.44	63.89	91.15	95.83	39.58	97.92	0.89	Y
Rhinosinusitis								
Blomgren 2005	86.11	55.56	32.81	94.44	10.42	16.67	0.91	YM
Esposito 2008	90.28	33.33	72.92	98.61	34.38	83.33	0.89	YM
Chow 2012	90.28	63.89	72.40	98.61	83.33	87.50	0.91	Y
Wald 2013	94.44	79.17	81.77	94.44	56.25	89.58	0.76	Y
Influenza								
Bellamy 2006	86.11	56.94	84.38	95.83	60.42	81.25	0.78	Y(3Y,1YM)
Bautista 2009	93.06	61.11	72.40	95.83	55.21	77.08	0.83	Y(3Y,1YM)
Harper 2009	95.83	61.11	78.65	94.44	58.33	89.58	0.92	Y
Morciano 2009	76.39	45.83	70.31	95.83	54.17	58.33	0.84	Y(3Y,1YM)
Otitis media								
Takahashi 2012	86.11	77.78	61.98	90.28	25.00	8.33	0.83	YM
Lieberthal 2013	93.06	61.11	90.10	94.44	70.83	72.92	0.84	Y(3Y,1YM)
Bain 2003	84.72	62.50	76.04	95.83	66.67	62.50	0.76	Y(3Y,1YM)
URTI[2]								
Snellman 2013	97.22	83.33	83.33	94.44	72.92	95.83	0.77	Y(3Y,1YM)
Medium (range)	90.28 (76.39–97.22)	61.11 (33.33–83.33)	76.04 (32.81–91.15)	95.83 (90.28–98.61)	56.25 (10.42–83.33)	81.25 (8.33–97.92)	/	/

Notes:
[1]Y: Yes; YM: Yes, with modifications; N: No.
[2]URTIs refer to guidelines which include multiple diseases in URTIs.

Table 4. Main Therapeutic Options on Group A Streptococcal Pharyngitis for Children According to Guidelines.

Therapy recommended	Shulman 2012,IDSA	Snellman 2013,ISCI
Target of population	Children >3 years	Children
Antibiotics		
Onset of antibiotics	Diagnosis of pharyngitis	Culture positive cases of group A streptococcal pharyngitis
Type of antibiotics		
First-line	Penicillin, amoxicillin (strong, high)	Penicillin, amoxicillin
Second-line (penicillin allergy)	A first-generation cephalosporin[1], clindamycin, clarithromycin, azithromycin (strong, moderate)	Cephalosprins[1], macrolides, clindamycin, amoxicillin-clavulanate (2 low quality studies; 1 high quality study)
Duration	10 days[2]	-
Adjunctive drugs		
NSAIDs[3]	For treatment of moderate to severe symptoms or control fever (high, strong)	-
Corticosteroids	NR[4] (moderate, weak)	-

Notes:
[1]The first-generation cephalosporins can be used for patients who are not anaphylactically sensitive.
[2]Azithromycin should be given for 5 days.
[3]NSAIDs: nonsteroidal anti-inflammatory drug.
[4]NR: not recommended.

(Table 5). All of the 5 guidelines supported the use of antibiotics in pediatric ABRS. However, AAP emphasized the onset of antibiotics should be in cases of severe onset or worsening course, while the other four recommended antibiotics for all clinical diagnosed ABRS. Guidelines from FSP and SIP recommended amoxicillin as first-line choice due to the low risk of treatment failure [10]. IDSA, however, suggested amoxicillin-clavulanate rather than amoxicillin as empiric antimicrobial therapy, considering the increasing prevalence of H. influenza among URTI of children and the high prevalence of β-lactamase-producing respiratory pathogens in ABRS [29,30]. For children with risk factors, amoxicillin-clavulanate was recommended. For non-type 1 hypertension, both ISCI and IDSA recommended doxycycline as an alternative for older children. Nevertheless, a variance appeared in terms of antibiotics for type 1 hypertension patients. ISCI and IDSA suggested levofloxacin, while AAP recommended cephalosporins based on recent studies which indicated the risk of a serious allergic reaction to cephalosporinsin patients with penicillin or amoxicillin allergy appeared to be nil [31–33]. The duration of antibiotic therapy is still controversial (3–28) [34]. In addition, all guidelines consistently deprecated decongestants, antihistamine and systemic corticosteroids (not local corticosteroids) in pediatric ABRS.

Recommendations towards drug therapy of influenza (Table 6). H1N1: Both IDSA and WHO recommended antivirals for confirmed or highly suspected H1N1 infection. However, IDSA recommended zanamivir rather than oseltamivir, while WHO recommended oseltamivir for children (>1 year) who have severe or progressive clinical illness.

H3N2: Only IDSA released a guideline on the treatment of H3N2 and recommended oseltamivir or zanamivir for laboratory-confirmed or highly suspectedH3N2. IDSA also warned that adamantanes should not be used.

H5N1: The recommendations on use of antiviral drugs for H5N1 were based predominantly on studies of infection with human influenza rather than clinical trials on treatment of H5N1 patients. Both WHO and IDSA placed a high value on the prevention of death and relatively low values on adverse reactions, development of resistance, and costs of treatment. Oseltamivir and zanamivir were recommended as first-line therapy and amantadine was recommended when neuraminidase inhibitors were not available.

Influenza-like syndrome: The SNLG did not recommend the routine use of amantadine, rimantadine, oseltamivir or zanamivir for influenza-like syndrome because of their side effects, the emerging resistance phenomena, and the irrelevance of the outcomes considered in the selected studies. Instead, SNLG recommended the use of oseltamivir in the post-exposure prophylaxis in non-vaccinated institutionalized patients.

Recommendations towards drug therapy of acute otitis media (Table 7). SIGN, JOS and AAP all recommended an observation of 2–3 days before antibiotic therapy for mild AOM. AAP recommended amoxicillin as the first choice and an antibiotic with additional β-lactamase for children with risk factors. SIGN and JOS recommend amoxicillin, amoxicillin-clavulanic, cephalosporins and macrolides with a statement that cephalosporins and macrolides can be used but less safe than amoxicillin [35]. Duration of antimicrobial therapy is still controversial [36]. SIGN recommended a 5 day course according to British National Formulary, while AAP recommended a 5 to 10 day course based on the age of children [35,37]. Further, only SIGN evaluated the efficacy and safety of adjunctive therapies [38].

Discussions

Variation of Evidence and Recommendation Grading System

CTFPHE was first published in 1979 by Canadian Ministry of Health. The quality of evidence is based on the study design and the strength of recommendation depends on sufficiency of evidence. CTFPHE was the first grading system developed and is the foundation of many other grading systems. However, the CTFPHE still has some drawbacks [27]. For instance, a lack of strong relevance between quality of evidence and strength of recommendation and lack of consideration of results exist consistently among studies [39]. Consequently, many other

Table 5. Main Therapeutic Options on Acute Bacterial Rhinosinusitis(ABRS)/Sinusitis for Children According to Guidelines.

Therapy recommended	Blomgren 2005, FSO	Esposito 2008, SIP	Chow 2012, IDSA	Wald 2013, AAP	Snellman 2013, ISCI
Target of population	Children >1 year	Children >1 year	Children	Children aged 1–18 years	Children
Antibiotics					
Onset of antibiotics	Clinical diagnosis of ABRS (B)	Clinical diagnosis of ABRS (I,A)	Clinical diagnosis of ABRS (strong, moderate)	Severe onset or worsening course ABRS (B, strong recommendation)	Clinical diagnosis of ABRS (high quality)
Types of antibiotics					
First-line	Amoxicillin	**Mild:** Amoxicillin (IV,B)	Amoxicillin-clavulanate (Strong, moderate)	Amoxicillin or amoxicillin- clavulanate (B, Recommendation).	Amoxicillin-clavulanate (high dose may consider in children <2 years) (Guideline).
Second-line					
With risk factors[1]	-	**Mild:** Amoxicillin-clavulanic or cefaclor (IV, B) **Severe:** ceftriaxone, amoxicillin-clavulanic, ampicillin-sulbactam (IV, B)	Amoxicillin-clavulanate (weak, moderate) or third-generation oral cephalosporin+clindamycin (weak, moderate).	Amoxicillin-clavulanate	-
Hypersensitivity					
Non-type I	-	-	Third-generation oral cephalosporin+clindamycin (weak, moderate), doxycycline (>8 years)	Cefdinr, cefuroxime, cefpodoxime	Doxycycline (for older children), Levofoxacin
Type I	-	-	Levofloxacin (weak, low).	Cefdinir, cefuroxime, cefpodoxime, or cefixime +clindamycin	
Durations	7days	**Mild**: 10–14 days (IV,B) **Severe**: 14–21 days (IV,B)	10–14 days (weak, low-moderate).	10–28 days	3–14 days (Low quality evidence)
Adjunctive drugs					
Corticosteroids	Recommended to allergic patients	NR (II,A)	Recommended to allergic patients (weak, moderate)	-	Recommended for recurrent or allergic patients (high quality evidence).
Decongestants	NR[2]	NR (II,A)	NR(strong, low-moderate)	-	NR
Antihistamines	NR	NR (II,A)	NR(Strong, low-moderate)	-	NR

Notes:
[1]Risk factors include: previous receive of antibiotic therapy; attendance at school, local or systematic diseases that favor infections due to antibiotic-resistant pathogens; from geographic regions with high endemic rates of invasive penicillin-nonsusceptible (PNS) S. pneumonia; severe infection; age<2; recent hospitalization; immunocompromised.
[2]NR: not recommended.

organizations developed their own grading systems [40,41]. SIGN grading system developed by the Scottish Intercollegiate Guidelines Network is one of the most-widely used systems [26]. However, it still failed to consider the consistency and indirectness of study results. In 2000, GRADE working group was founded based on organizations from 19 countries including WHO. The aim of this group is to develop a consolidated grading system for quality of evidence and strength of recommendation. In 2004, the first edition of this grading system was published and was recognized by more than 30 organizations including WHO and Cochrane Collaboration. Although the 13 guidelines included in our study were published after 2005, only four of them use the GRADE system. We suggest further guidelines use a comparable uniform grading system to evaluate the quality of evidence and strength of recommendations.

Quality of Guidelines

The potential benefits of guidelines are only as good as the quality of the guidelines themselves. Appropriate methodologies and rigorous strategies in the guideline development process are important for the successful implementation of the resulting recommendations [7]. For these 13 guidelines, two domains are the main problems which decrease the quality and reliability of guidelines. The first is a failure to seek patients' views and preferences or fail to report this information. Many methods can be used to consider patients' expectations such as: formal consultations with patients, participation of patients on guideline development group or external review group, or a literature review of patients' values. However, these processes were seldom performed or described in guideline development or the final reports of guidelines. This problem is also found in other disease guidelines [42,43,44]. The second problem is a lack of consideration of applicability of guidelines. How to facilitate the application of guidelines is as important as how to develop a high quality guideline.

Table 6. Main Therapeutic Options on Influenza for Children According to Guidelines.

Therapy recommended	H1N1		H3N2	H5N1		Influenza-like syndrome
	Harper 2009, IDSA	**Bautista 2009, WHO**	**Harper 2009, IDSA**	**Bellamy 2006, WHO**	**Harper 2009, IDSA**	**Morciano 2009, SNLG**
Target of population	Children>1 year	Children (≤12) and Adolescents(13–18 years)	Children >1 year	Children	Children >1 year	Children
Antivirals						
Onset of antivirals	Laboratory-confirmed or highly suspected infection (A, II)	Confirmed or strongly suspected infection (Low, Strong)	Laboratory-confirmed or highly suspected infection (A, II)	Confirmed or strongly suspected infection	Laboratory-confirmed or highly suspected infection (A, II)	Post-exposure prophylaxis in non-vaccinated institutionalized patients
Choose of antivirals	Zanamivir, adamantine (rimantadine) (A, II)	**Pandemic H1N1 with severe or progressive clinical illness:** oseltamivir (Low, strong) **Uncomplicated pandemic H1N1:** oseltamivir, zanamivir(Low,strong)	Oseltamivir, zanamivir (A-II)	Oseltamivir (strong, very low), zanamivir (≥7 years) (weak, very low).	Oseltamivir, zanamivir (A-II)	Oseltamivir (C/I)
Antibiotics						
				Severe community-acquired pneumonia: follow guidelines (strong) **Mechanical ventilation:** recommend treatment or prevention of ventilator associated or hospital acquired pneumonia (strong)		**Non-complicated:** NR[1](E/I) **Influenza-like syndrome-related sore throat:** NR, unless symptoms are complicated by bacterial infections(D/I)
NSAIs						
		Aspirin: NR (strong, regulatory warning)				Paracetamol, ibuprofen (B/I)

Notes:
[1]NR: not recommended.

The facilitators and barriers that may impact the application of guidelines should be considered when developing the guideline. Also, there is a need to consider how to disseminate and implement the guideline effectively using additional materials such as a quick reference guide, educational tools and patient leaflets. These factors are important but often ignored by guideline developers. Studies on the effectiveness of clinical guideline implementation strategies showed that successful guideline implementation strategies should be multifaceted, and actively engage clinicians throughout the process [45,46]. Thus, future guidelines should pay more attention to the implementation process of guidelines.

Factors Contributing to Inconsistencies of Guidelines

Although an important level of consensus appears throughout the various guidelines, there are still some conflicts in recommendations for drug choice and durations of therapy. There are three main reasons contributing to the variances. First, the geographic difference leads to the variance of pathogens and its drug resistance. Second, the recommendations of guidelines were based on different evidence. Recent studies may overturn the results of previous studies. Thus, the timely updated guidelines are more reliable. Third, the expectation and preference of guideline developers and patients may influence the final recommendation. Therefore, a local guideline is more useful for health professionals if there is a conflict among guidelines.

Suggestions for Future Research

The durations of antimicrobial therapy for rhinosinustis and acute otitis media are still controversial. More studies are needed to compare the different durations of antibiotics in children. In addition, the antivirials for influenza also lack direct evidence. Many recommendations are based on indirect evidence. Thus, more clinical trials or prospective observational studies are needed.

Conclusions

Future guidelines should use a consistent grading system for quality of evidence and strength of recommendations and seek the preference of stake holders to improve the applicability of guidelines. Further, there are still some areas in pediatric URTI that need more research.

Table 7. Main Therapeutic Options on Acute Otitis Media (AOM) for Children According to Guidelines.

Therapy recommended	Bain 2003, SIGN	Takahashi 2012, JOS	Lieberthal 2013, AAP
Target of population	Children	Children <15 years	Children aged 6 months-12years
Antibiotics			
Onset of antibiotics	**Mild**: observation for 3 days without use of antimicrobial agents (1+,B)	**Mild**: observation for 3 days without use of antimicrobial agents (A)	**Mild AOM in children (>2 years)** antibiotic therapy or observation for 2–3 days (B, Recommendation) **Mild bilateral AOM in children (6–23 months):** antibiotic therapy (B, Recommendation). **Mild unilateral AOM in children (6–23 months):** antibiotic therapy or observation for 2–3 days (B, Recommendation). **Severe:** antibiotic therapy (B, Strong Recommendation).
Types of antibiotics	Amoxicillin, amoxicillin-clavulanic, cefaclor, cotrimoxazole, trimethoprim, erythromycin (1+,B)	Amoxicillin, amoxicillin-clavulanate, ampicillin, cefditoren, ceftriaxone (A)	**First-line**[1]: amoxicillin (B,Recommendation). **Second-line**[2]: an antibiotic with additional β-lactamase (C, Recommendation).
Duration	5 days (1+, B).	-	<2 years: 10 days; 2–5 years: 7 days; >6 years: 5–7 days
Adjunctive			
decongestants	NR[3] (1++, A)	-	-
antihistamines	NR (1++, A)	-	-
paracetamol	Recommended for analgesia[4] (1+, D)	-	-

Notes:
[1]The child does not received amoxicillin in the past 30days or does not have concurrent purulent conjunctivitis or the child is not allergic to penicillin.
[2]The child has received amoxicillin in the last 30 days or has concurrent purulent conjunctivitis, or has a history of recurrent AOM unresponsive to amoxicillin.
[3]NR: Not Recommended.
[4]Parents should give paracetamol for analgesia but should be advised of the potential danger of overuse.

Acknowledgments

We thank all the anonymous reviewers for invaluable comments on earlier manuscript drafts.

Author Contributions

Conceived and designed the experiments: L. Zhang. Performed the experiments: L. Zeng ZH YC LL MC. Analyzed the data: L. Zeng ZH. Wrote the paper: L. Zeng. Revised the language of the paper: EAE.

References

1. Jamison DT, Breman JG, Measham AR, Alleyne G, Claeson M, et al. (2006) Disease Control Priorities in Developing Countries. Acute Respiratory Infections in Children. 2nd edition. Washington (DC): Wold Bank and Oxford University Press. Chapter 25.
2. National Institute for Health and Clinical Excellence (2008) Respiratory Tract Infection-Antibiotic Prescribing: Prescribing of Antibiotics for Self-Limiting Respiratory Tract Infections in Adults and Children in Primary Care. (Clinical guideline 69.) London: National Institute for Health and Clinical Excellence. Available at:http://www.ncbi.nlm.nih.gov/books/NBK53632/Accessed 2014 Jan12.
3. Clucas DB, Carville KS, Connors C, Currie BJ, Carapetis JR, et al. (2008) Disease burden and health-care clinic attendances for young children in remote Aboriginalcommunities of northern Australia. WHO 86: 275–281.
4. Liao P, Ku M, Lue K, Sun H (2011) Respiratory tract infection is the major cause of the ambulatory visits in children. IJP 37: 43.
5. McCormick A, Fleming D, Charlton J, Royal College of General Practitioners (1995) Morbidity statistics from general practice Fourth national study 1991–1992. Available at:http://www.herc.ox.ac.uk/icohde/datasets/190. Accessed 2014 January 12.
6. Lim W, Arnold DM, Bachanova V, Haspel RL, Rosovsky RP, et al. (2008) Evidence-Based Guidelines-An Introduction. ASH Education Program Book 2008: 26–30.
7. AGREE Next Steps Consortium (2009). The AGREE II Instrument. Available: http://www.agreetrust.org Accessed 2014.1.12.
8. Shulman ST, Bisno AL, Clegg HW, Gerber MA, Kaplan EL et al. (2012) Clinical practice guideline for the diagnosis and management of group A streptococcal pharyngitis: 2012 update by the Infectious Diseases Society of America. Clin Infect Dis 55: e86–e102.
9. Blomgren K, Alho OP, Ertama L, Huovinen P, Korppi M, et al.(2005) Acute sinusitis: Finnish clinical practice guidelines. Scand J Infect Dis 37: 245.
10. Esposito S, Principi N (2008) Guidelines for the diagnosis and treatment of acute and subacute rhinosinusitis in children. J Antimicrob Chemoth 20: 147–157.
11. Chow AW, Benninger MS, Brook I, Brozek JL, Goldstein EJC, et al. (2012) IDSA clinical practice guideline for acute bacterial rhinosinusitis in children and adults. Clin Infect Dis 54: e72–e112.
12. Wald ER, Applegate KE, Bordley C, Darrow DH, Glode MP, et al. (2013) Clinical practice guideline for the diagnosis and management of acute bacterial sinusitis in children aged 1 to 18 years. Pediatrics 132: e262–e280.
13. Schünemann HJ, Hill SR, Kakad M, Bellamy R, Uyeki TM, et al. (2007) WHO rapid advice guidelines on pharmacological management of humans infected with avian influenza A (H5N1) virus. WHO. Lancet Infect Dis 7: 21–31.
14. World Health Organization (2010) WHO Guidelines for Pharmacological Management of Pandemic Influenza A (H1N1) 2009 and other Influenza Viruses. Revised February 2010. Available at: http://www.who.int/csr/resources/publications/swineflu/h1n1_use_antivirals_20090820/en/. Accessed 2014 January 12.
15. Harper SA, Bradley JS, Englund JA, File TM, Gravenstein S, et al. (2009) Seasonal influenza in adults and children–diagnosis, treatment, chemoprophylaxis, and institutional outbreak management: clinical practice guidelines of the Infectious Diseases Society of America. Clin Infect Dis 48: 1003–1032.
16. Morciano C, Vitale A, Masi S, Sagliocca L, Sampaolo L, et al. (2009) Italian evidence-based guidelines for the management of influenza-like syndrome in adults and children. Annali dell'Istituto superiore di sanità 45: 185–192.
17. Scottish Intercollegiate Guidelines Network (2003) Diagnosis and management of childhood otitis media in primary care. Available at: http://www.sign.ac.uk/guidelines/fulltext/66/section5.html. Accessed 2014 January 12.
18. Subcommittee of Clinical Practice Guideline for Diagnosis and Management of Acute Otitis Media in Children (2012) Clinical practice guidelines for the diagnosis and management of acute otitis media (AOM) in children in Japan. Auris Nasus Larynx http://www.ncbi.nlm.nih.gov/pubmed/?term=Clinical%20practice%20guidelines%20for%20the%20diagnosis%20and%20management%20of%20acute%20otitis%20media%20(AOM)%20in%20children%20in%20Japan39: 1–8.
19. Lieberthal AS, Carroll AE, Chonmaitree T, Ganiats TG, Hoberman A, et al. (2013) The Diagnosis and Management of Acute Otitis Media. Pediatrics 131: e964-e999.
20. Snellman L, Adams W, Anderson G, Godfrey A, Gravley A, et al. Institute for Clinical Systems Improvement. (2013) Diagnosis and Treatment of Respiratory Illness in Children and Adults. Available at: http://bit.ly/RespIll. Accessed 2014 Jan. 12.
21. Guyatt GH, Oxman AD, Vist GE, Kunz R, Falck-Ytter Y, et al. (2008) Rating quality of evidence and strength of recommendations: GRADE: an emerging consensus on rating quality of evidence and strength of recommendations. BMJ 336: 924–926.

22. Guyatt GH, Oxman AD, Kunz R, Vist GE, Falck-Ytter Y, et al. (2008) Rating Quality of Evidence and Strength of Recommendations: What is "quality of evidence" and why is it important to clinicians? BMJ 336: 995–998.
23. Schünemann HJ, Oxman AD, Brozek J, Glasziou P, Jaeschke R, et al. (2008) Rating Quality of Evidence and Strength of Recommendations: GRADE: Grading quality of evidence and strength of recommendations for diagnostic tests and strategies. BMJ 336: 1106–1110.
24. Guyatt GH, Oxman AD, Kunz R, Jaeschke R, Helfand M, et al. (2008) Rating quality of evidence and strength of recommendations: Incorporating considerations of resources use into grading recommendations. BMJ: 336: 1170–1173.
25. Guyatt GH, Oxman AD, Kunz R, Falck-Ytter Y, Vist GE, et al. (2008) Rating quality of evidence and strength of recommendations: Going from evidence to recommendations. BMJ 336: 1049–1051.
26. Harbour R, Miller J (2001) A new system for grading recommendations in evidence based guidelines. BMJ 323: 334–336.
27. Canadian Task Force on the Periodic Health Examination: The periodic health examination. (1979) CMAJ 121: 1193–1254.
28. Schrör K (2007) Aspirin and Reye Syndrome. Pediatr Drugs 9: 195–204.
29. Coker TR, Chan LS, Newberry SJ, Limbos MA, Suttorp MJ, et al. (2010) Diagnosis, microbial epidemiology, and antibiotic treatment of acute otitis media in children. JAMA 304: 2161–2169.
30. Tristram S, Jacobs MR, Appelbaum PC (2007) Antimicrobial resistance in Haemophilus influenzae. Clin microbiol rev 20: 368–389.
31. DePestel DD, Benninger MS, Danziger L, LaPlante KL, May C, et al. (2008) Cephalosporin use in treatment of patients with penicillin allergies. JAPhA 48: 530–540.
32. Pichichero ME (2005) A review of evidence supporting the American Academy of Pediatrics recommendation for prescribing cephalosporin antibiotics for penicillin-allergic patients. Pediatrics 115: 1048–1057.
33. Pichichero ME, Casey JR (2007) Safe use of selected cephalosporins in penicillin-allergic patients: a meta-analysis. Otolaryng Head Neck 136: 340–347.
34. American Academy of Pediatrics, Subcommittee on Management of Sinusitisand Committee on Quality Improvement (2001) Clinical practice guideline: management of sinusitis. Pediatrics 108: 798–808.
35. Marcy M, Takata G, Shekelle P, Mason W, Wachsman L, et al. Management of acute otitis media. Available: http://hstat.nlm.nih.gov/hq/Hquest/db/local.epc.er.erta15/screen/TocDisplay/s/55230/action/Toc.Accessed 2014.1.12.
36. Kozyrskyj A, Klassen TP, Moffatt M, Harvey K (2002). Short course antibiotics for acute otitis media. Cochrane Database Syst Rev. 2010 Sep 8;(9):CD001095. doi: 10.1002/14651858.CD001095.pub2.
37. Cohen R, Levy C, Boucherat M, Langue J, Autret E, et al. (2000) Five vs. ten days of antibiotic therapy for acute otitis media in young children. Pediatr Infect Dis J 19: 458–463.
38. Flynn C, Griffin G, Tudiver F (2002) Decongestants and antihistamines for acute otitis media in children. Cochrane DB Syst Rev(Online):CD001727.
39. Atkins D, Eccles M, Flottorp S, Guyatt GH, Henry D, et al. (2004) Systems for grading the quality of evidence and the strength of recommendations I: critical appraisal of existing approaches The GRADE Working Group. BMC Health Services Research 4: 38.
40. Agency for Health Care Policy and Research (1992) Acute pain management: operative or medical procedures and trauma. Available at: http://archive.ahrq.gov/clinic/medtep/acute.htm. Accessed 2014 January 12.
41. Eccles M, Clapp Z, Grimshaw J, Adams PC, Higgins B, et al. (1996) North of England evidence based guidelines development project: methods of guideline development. BMJ 312: 760–762.
42. Vecchio AL, Giannattasio A, Duggan C, De Masi S, Ortisi MT, et al. (2011) Evaluation of the quality of guidelines for acute gastroenteritis in children with the AGREE instrument. J Pediatr Gastr Nutr 52: 183–189.
43. Ferket BS, Colkesen EB, Visser JJ, Spronk S, Kraaijenhagen RA, et al. (2010) Systematic review of guidelines on cardiovascular risk assessment: which recommendations should clinicians follow for a cardiovascular health check? Arch Intern Med 170: 27–40.
44. Burda BU, Norris SL, Holmer HK, Ogden LA, Smith M (2011) Quality varies across clinical practice guidelines for mammography screening in women aged 40–49 years as assessed by AGREE and AMSTAR instruments. J Clin Epidemiol 64: 968–976.
45. Prior M, Guerin M, Grimmer-Somers K (2008) The effectiveness of clinical guideline implementation strategies–a synthesis of systematic review findings. J Eval Clin Pract 14: 888–897.
46. Solberg LI (2000) Guideline implementation: what the literature doesn't tell us. Joint Commission Journal on Quality and Patient Safety 26: 525–537.

14

Rapid Antigen Group A Streptococcus Test to Diagnose Pharyngitis

Emily H. Stewart[1¶], Brian Davis[2¶], B. Lee Clemans-Taylor[3], Benjamin Littenberg[4], Carlos A. Estrada[5,6*], Robert M. Centor[3]

1 Walter Reed National Military Medical Center, Bethesda, Maryland, United States of America, 2 University of Texas Southwestern Medical Center, Dallas, Texas, United States of America, 3 The University of Alabama at Birmingham, Huntsville Campus, Huntsville, Alabama, United States of America, 4 University of Vermont, Burlington, Vermont, United States of America, 5 University of Alabama at Birmingham, Birmingham, Alabama, United States of America, 6 Birmingham Veterans Affairs Medical Center and Veterans Affairs Quality Scholar Program, Birmingham, Alabama, United States of America

Abstract

Background: Pharyngitis management guidelines include estimates of the test characteristics of rapid antigen streptococcus tests (RAST) using a non-systematic approach.

Objective: To examine the sensitivity and specificity, and sources of variability, of RAST for diagnosing group A streptococcal (GAS) pharyngitis.

Data Sources: MEDLINE, Cochrane Reviews, Centre for Reviews and Dissemination, Scopus, SciELO, CINAHL, guidelines, 2000–2012.

Study Selection: Culture as reference standard, all languages.

Data Extraction and Synthesis: Study characteristics, quality.

Main Outcome(s) and Measure(s): Sensitivity, specificity.

Results: We included 59 studies encompassing 55,766 patients. Forty three studies (18,464 patients) fulfilled the higher quality definition (at least 50 patients, prospective data collection, and no significant biases) and 16 (35,634 patients) did not. For the higher quality immunochromatographic methods in children (10,325 patients), heterogeneity was high for sensitivity (inconsistency [I^2] 88%) and specificity (I^2 86%). For enzyme immunoassay in children (342 patients), the pooled sensitivity was 86% (95% CI, 79–92%) and the pooled specificity was 92% (95% CI, 88–95%). For the higher quality immunochromatographic methods in the adult population (1,216 patients), the pooled sensitivity was 91% (95% CI, 87 to 94%) and the pooled specificity was 93% (95% CI, 92 to 95%); however, heterogeneity was modest for sensitivity (I^2 61%) and specificity (I^2 72%). For enzyme immunoassay in the adult population (333 patients), the pooled sensitivity was 86% (95% CI, 81–91%) and the pooled specificity was 97% (95% CI, 96 to 99%); however, heterogeneity was high for sensitivity and specificity (both, I^2 88%).

Conclusions: RAST immunochromatographic methods appear to be very sensitive and highly specific to diagnose group A streptococcal pharyngitis among adults but not in children. We could not identify sources of variability among higher quality studies. The present systematic review provides the best evidence for the wide range of sensitivity included in current guidelines.

Editor: Sean D. Reid, Wake Forest University School of Medicine, United States of America

Funding: RMC received funding from Justin Rogers Foundation. The funders had no role in study design, data collection and analysis, decision to publish, or preparation of the manuscript.

Competing Interests: RMC has received funding from the Justin Rogers Foundation.

* Email: cestrada@uab.edu

¶ These authors are co-first authors on this work.

Introduction

Rapid antigen testing to detect group A Streptococcal (GAS) infection provides important information for the antibiotic decision making for patients presenting with acute pharyngitis. Pharyngitis accounts for over 13 million office visits annually in the United States [1], highlighting the importance of these decisions. Patients with GAS pharyngitis can develop either suppurative or non-suppurative complications. Given the importance of chronic rheumatic fever in the 1950s, preventing acute rheumatic fever became the main focus of treating pharyngitis at the time. While the incidence of acute rheumatic fever has decreased, the focus in patients with acute pharyngitis is on treating GAS infections to decrease suppurative complications (especially peritonsillar abscess), decrease person-to-person spread, and to shorten symptom duration.

The Infectious Diseases Society of America (IDSA) guideline [2] on streptococcal pharyngitis recommends using a rapid test in patients with a modest probability of GAS infection, treating those with a positive rapid test and withholding antibiotics in rapid test negative patients. The guideline recommends culturing rapid test negative children and treating patients having positive cultures; the guideline does not recommend culturing the rapid test negative adults given the lower prevalence and significantly reduced chance of non-suppurative complications of the disease in the adult population [2], unless the clinician wishes to increase diagnostic sensitivity.

The IDSA guidelines and reviews have documented excellent specificity of rapid antigen streptococcal testing; however, the sensitivity estimate varies from 70% to 95% [3–6]. These reports did not apply a systematic approach to make these estimates. A systematic review published in Spanish [7] did not examine potential sources of heterogeneity.

The present study explores the variability of sensitivity and specificity using a systematic approach; the goal of this systematic review was to identify accurate, unbiased estimates of rapid antigen streptococcus test (RAST) characteristics for children, adults, and RAST variety.

Materials and Methods

We performed a systemic review and meta-analysis of the performance of various rapid antigen streptococcus tests to diagnose Group A streptococcal pharyngitis in adult and pediatric populations using standard guidelines for diagnostic studies [8]. We also used the Preferred Reporting Items for Systematic reviews and Meta-Analyses for reporting [9]. We limited our study to more recent publications because the technology of rapid antigen testing has improved over the years and to exclude tests no longer used.

Data Sources and Searches

In preparation for identifying search terms, a professional medical librarian (BLCT) searched the National Library of Medicine's MEDLINE electronic database from January 2000 to April 2012 using PubMed, limiting the search to the English language only and meta-analyses or systematic reviews. We then ran preliminary test searches to identify all possible terms necessary to design a comprehensive and systematic search strategy. Finally, we used medical subject headings (MeSH terms) and text words to search for three main concept areas: target condition, index test, and test characteristics (see Methods S1). The three main concepts were combined using AND as the Boolean operator. In addition, we supplemented the search with the PubMed/MEDLINE's Clinical Queries feature to combine the target condition with the diagnosis/broad automatic filter. We completed the first search on April 11, 2012 and repeated the same search strategy on October 26, 2012 to update the search and expand the scope by including non-English citations.

We also checked online through PubMed/MEDLINE and hand searched several major infectious disease, clinical microbiology, and pediatric textbooks for updates to current guidelines on the use of rapid antigen detection tests in the diagnosis of group a beta-hemolytic streptococcus including the Infectious Diseases Society of America (IDSA), American Heart Association, American Academy of Pediatrics, the American College of Physicians (ACP), the Centers for Disease Control, and the American Academy of Family Physicians. In addition, we searched the electronic sources Cochrane Reviews, Centre for Reviews and Dissemination [10], UpToDate, DynaMed, and Essential Evidence Plus; we also reviewed references from personal files (RMC, one of the authors). We also reviewed references from cost-effectiveness studies.

We did not include data from package inserts of commercially available RAST as study characteristics were not included [11]. Finally, we searched the electronic sources Scopus [12], SciELO (Scientific Electronic Library Online) [13], and CINAHL (Cumulative Index to Nursing and Allied Health Literature) on December 6, 2012 for studies published after 2000 without language limits.

Study Selection

Two of the authors independently reviewed the titles of the initial search results and excluded titles that were not relevant, non-English, lacking a RAST, review articles, studies that lacked culture as reference standard, or other reasons (ex: duplicate publications, non-human studies, case reports, letters to the editor, no data reported). Discrepancies were included in the second review. A third author reviewed all excluded titles (CAE). In the second review, two authors independently read the titles and abstracts for the same exclusion criteria; a third author resolved conflicts. In the third review, one author read the articles and another confirmed the excluded articles (a third author resolved conflicts during this step). We excluded articles that did not use a culture reference standard.

Data Extraction and Quality Assessment

We recorded country of study, funding source, index test location (point-of-care or laboratory), number of swabs for the reference test (one or two), culture medium, age of population, setting (outpatient clinic, student health, emergency room), inclusion and exclusion criteria, and study design (prospective, retrospective). We constructed 2×2 contingency tables (true positives, false positives, false negatives, true negatives) from the published data for the main study results and for any subgroups reported. We excluded articles where a 2×2 contingency table could not be calculated from the published data. We used the Quality Assessment of Diagnostic Accuracy Studies (QUADAS) checklist to assess methodological quality of the studies [14]. Each of two authors abstracted data for half of the studies selected; at the end, the other author reviewed the abstracted data for independent verification.

Data Synthesis and Analysis

Based on the 2×2 contingency table, we computed prevalence, sensitivity, and specificity for each study and each subgroup.

We examined heterogeneity with graphical methods using coupled forest plots of sensitivity and specificity and hierarchical summary receiver-operating characteristic (HSROC) curves [8,15–17]. The HSROC uses a random-effects model and accounts for the relationship between sensitivity and specificity in each study. The HSROC analyses provide estimates of uncertainty that includes a 95% confidence region (for the summary estimate) and a 95% prediction region (for a forecast of the sensitivity and specificity in a future study) [18]. Wider prediction regions suggest significant heterogeneity [8,17]. The summary ROC may also identify a threshold effect, suggested by a shoulder-like appearance of the curve, that could explain heterogeneity between studies [8].

We also used the inconsistency (I^2) value to examine heterogeneity and regarded values as low, moderate, or high heterogeneity for values of 25%, 50%, or 75% (respectively). However, a recent review noted limitations of the I^2 as it does not account for the correlation between sensitivity and specificity, does not account for variation explained by threshold effects, and overestimates heterogeneity [17]. We include pooled estimates of sensitivity and specificity in the results section when values were deemed homogeneous enough or for illustration purposes.

We explored heterogeneity, a-priori, by examining studies of highest quality, defined as those with at least 50 patients, prospective data collection, and three items of the QUADAS methodological quality criteria [14]: "Did the whole sample or a random selection of the sample, receive verification using a reference standard for diagnosis?" (partial verification avoided), "Did patients receive the same reference standard regardless of the index test results?" (differential verification avoided), and "Was the reference standard independent of the index test (i.e.: the index test did not form part of the reference standard)?" (incorporation bias avoided). We did not require blinding of the reference standard or the index test to define a study as high quality.

We examined publication bias with the Deeks' funnel plots and tested asymmetry with linear regression of log diagnostic odds ratios (DOR) on the inverse root of the effective sample size [19]. In the absence of publication bias, studies of smaller sample size would have a wider distribution of results (in diagnostic test studies, DOR) due to random variation as compared to studies with larger sample size that would have a narrower distribution of results. A non-vertical line with a p value$<$0.10 for the slope of the coefficient indicates asymmetry and suggests publication bias. The Deeks' funnel plot method [19] overcomes limitations of other methodologies.

We also explored heterogeneity post-hoc. The purpose of these analyses was to identify study sub-groups with sufficient clinical and statistical homogeneity to calculate summary estimates of sensitivity and specificity. We limited the exploratory analyses to the highest quality studies as defined above. We analyzed age groups separately, exclusive pediatric population vs. other, as the clinical features and epidemiology are different. We also analyzed separately by index test methodology (immuno-chromatographic, enzyme immunoassay, optical immune-assay). Finally, we explored sponsorship (commercial vs. none or none reported), location of performance of the index test (laboratory vs. point-of-care or not reported), risk score (Centor or McIassac), location of care (outpatient vs. emergency room), publication year (2000–2005 vs. 2006–2012), prevalence (by tertiles), and region (USA/Canada vs. Europe vs. other). We also performed meta-regression to estimate the independent contribution of the variables listed above that may explain heterogeneity [20].

We used STATA 11.2 software (College Station, Texas, USA) and the midas [20] and metandi [18] modules for statistical analyses.

Results

Study selection

Figure 1 displays the overall summary of the evidence search; we could not retrieve three studies for full article review [21–23]. Our searches identified all 24 studies included in the systematic review published in Spanish [7]. We included 58 studies that examined 55,766 patients [24–81]. One study [28] utilized two designs, hence 59 studies are mentioned in the rest of the manuscript. The overall prevalence of GAS infection was 28.2% (15,254/54,098 patients) (range 3.7% to 66.6%); we did not include one study [28] in the prevalence calculation as only patients with positive cultures were reported (n = 1,688).

Characteristics of Included Studies

The Table S1 in File S1 displays the overall study characteristics. The study design was prospective in all but eight (11.9%) studies [39,40,50–52,55,63,66], most were in the pediatric population (n = 35, 59.3%). The setting was solely in outpatient areas (n = 37, 62.7%) or emergency room settings (n = 19, 32.2%). Point of care testing was done in 27 studies (45.6%). Commercial funding was acknowledged in 16 studies (27.2%) [33,36,41,48,49,57–61,64,68,70,71,78,80]. The Table S2 in File S1 displays the main study characteristics for each study.

Quality of Included Studies (Risk of Bias)

The overall quality of the studies using the QUADAS criteria is shown in Figure 2; in 48 (81.4%) studies partial verification bias was avoided, in 47 (79.7%) studies differential verification bias was avoided, and in 47 (79.7%) studies incorporation bias was avoided (Figure 2). The quality assessment for each study is shown in the Table S3 in File S1. The funnel plot shown in Figure S1 in File S2 was asymmetric and the regression line was not vertical, suggesting the presence of publication bias (p$<$0.001). In the absence of publication bias, studies of smaller sample size would have a wider distribution of results due to random variation as compared to studies with larger sample size.

Analyses – Quantitative, Qualitative, and Heterogeneity

The operating test characteristics of the studies are shown in the Table S4 in File S1. The sensitivity ranged from 44% to 100%. The specificity ranged from 69% to 100%.

We explored heterogeneity a-priori by examining studies of highest quality (those with at least 50 patients, prospective data collection, and no verification or differential verification or incorporation biases). Of the 59 studies, 43 (72.9%; 18,464 patients) fulfilled the higher quality definition [24–29,31–34,36–38,41–46,48,49,53,54,56,57,59–62,64,65,67–71,73,75–79,81] and 16 (27.1%; 35,634 patients) did not [28,30,35,39,40,47,50,51,58,63,66,72,74,80]. The coupled forest plots for sensitivity and specificity and HSROC are shown for higher quality studies (Figure S2 in File S2, Figure S4 in File S2) and lower quality studies (Figure S3 in File S2, Figure S4 in File S2). Both, higher and lower quality studies were highly heterogeneous as demonstrated by high inconsistency values and confidence intervals in the forest plots and wide prediction regions in the HSROC. Also, the summary ROCs have a shoulder-like appearance, suggesting a threshold effect for both higher and lower quality studies.

Exploratory Analyses- Higher Quality Studies – Pediatrics and Adults Strata

Among the higher quality studies, immunochromatographic methods were described in 34 strata (28 pediatric, six adults), in five enzyme immunoassay strata (three pediatric, two adults), and in four optical immunoassay methods (three pediatric, one adult). The summary of diagnostic accuracy estimates for studies of higher methodological quality is shown in Table 1.

Pediatrics -Immunochromatographic Methods

The prevalence of GAS infection in the 28 pediatrics strata was 29.7% (3,062/10,325 patients) (range 11.0% to 66.6%). The studies were of high methodological quality, four studies met all 14

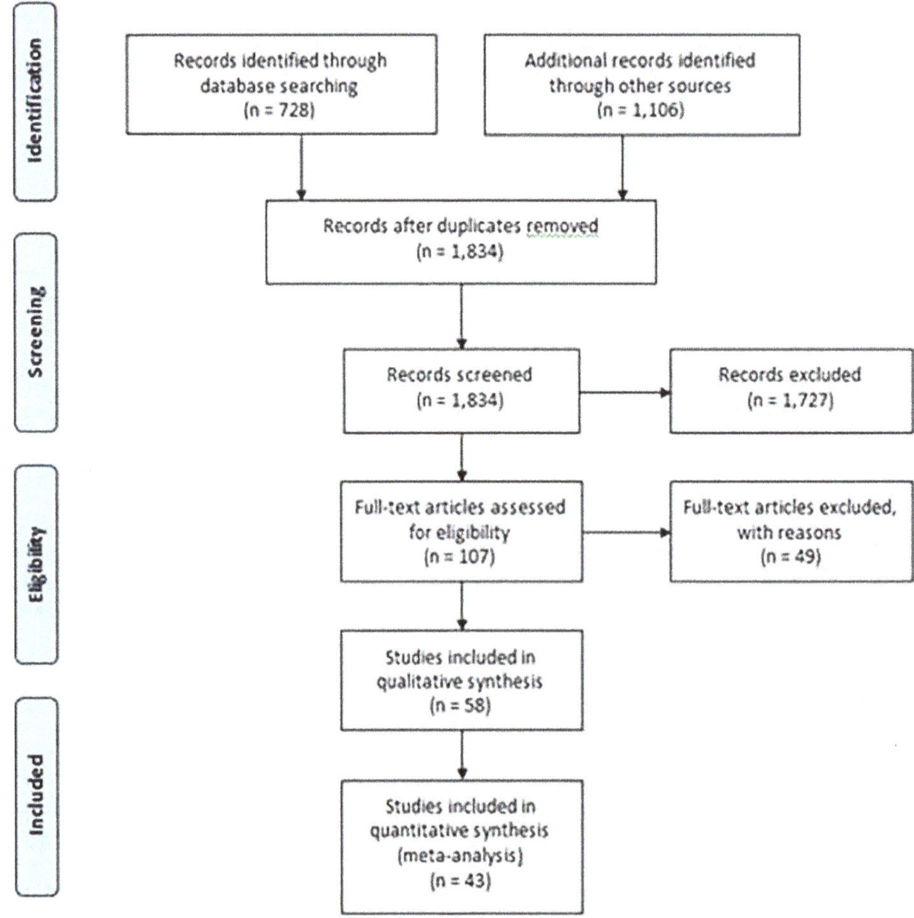

Figure 1. PRISMA Flow Diagram.

criteria [36,48,49,78], nine met 13 criteria [26,31,34,37,38,41, 43,46,65], three met 12 criteria [25,32,71], and two met 10 criteria [24,57] (Table S3 in File S1).

The coupled forest plots for sensitivity and specificity shows high heterogeneity (I^2 = 88% for sensitivity and I^2 = 86% for specificity; Figure 3, Table 1). As mentioned in the Methods section, we explored additional variables that may explain heterogeneity. In three of the 28 strata, the testing was performed in the laboratory. None of the 28 strata reported Centor or McIssac score. Supplementary figures show HSROC subgroups, no single variable yielded homogenous groups, sponsorship (Figure S5 in File S2), location of care (Figure S6 in File S2), publication year (Figure S7 in File S2), prevalence (Figure S8 in File S2), and region (Figure S9 in File S2). The sensitivity and specificity of the studies remained heterogeneous (large prediction regions) regardless of sponsorship, studies conducted in emergency rooms, studies published more contemporarily, studies with higher GAS infection prevalence, and studies conducted in North America and Europe. Meta-regression showed that in the univariate analyses all strata mentioned above but prevalence of GAS infection by tertile were significant predictors for heterogeneity for both sensitivity and specificity. However, in the joint model, outpatient setting (p = 0.03) and prevalence of GAS infection by tertile prevalence of GAS (p = 0.05) were the only significant variables (data not shown).

Among the 28 high quality studies in the pediatrics strata and immunochromatographic methods, the sensitivity was over 90% in 14 strata (n = 3,362 patients; prevalence of GAS infection, median 32% [Q1–Q3, 28–33%]) [34,37,38,43,46,48,57,65,71], between 80–90% in eight strata (n = 4,277 patients; prevalence of GAS infection, median 25% [Q1–Q3, 24–36%]) [24,25,32,34,36,49], and less than 80% in six strata (n = 2,685 patients; prevalence of GAS infection, median 25% [Q1–Q3, 21–29%]) [26,31,36,41,78].

Among the 28 high quality studies in the pediatrics strata and immunochromatographic methods, the specificity was over 95% in 17 strata (n = 7,451 patients; prevalence of GAS infection, median 29% [Q1–Q3, 25–33%]) [25,26,32,34,36,37,41,49,65, 71,78], >90–95% in eight strata (n = 2,340 patients; prevalence of GAS infection, median 32% [Q1–Q3, 22–36%]) [26,34,36,38, 46,48,57], 80–90% in two strata (n = 323 patients; prevalence of GAS, 25–26%) [24,31], and less than 80% in one strata (n = 211 patients; prevalence of GAS infection, 34%) [43].

Pediatrics - Enzyme Immunoassay and Optical Immunoassay Methods

The prevalence of GAS infection in the 3 enzyme immunoassay pediatric strata was 36.3% (124/342 patients) (range 33.3% to 38.5%). The coupled forest plots for sensitivity and specificity shows no or little heterogeneity (I^2 = 0% for sensitivity and I^2 = 55% for specificity; Figure 4, top panels; Table 1). The pooled sensitivity was 86% (95% CI, 79–92%) and the pooled specificity was 92% (95% CI, 88–95%).

The prevalence of GAS infection in the 3 optical immunoassay pediatric strata was 29.7% (977/3,294 patients) (range 28.7% to

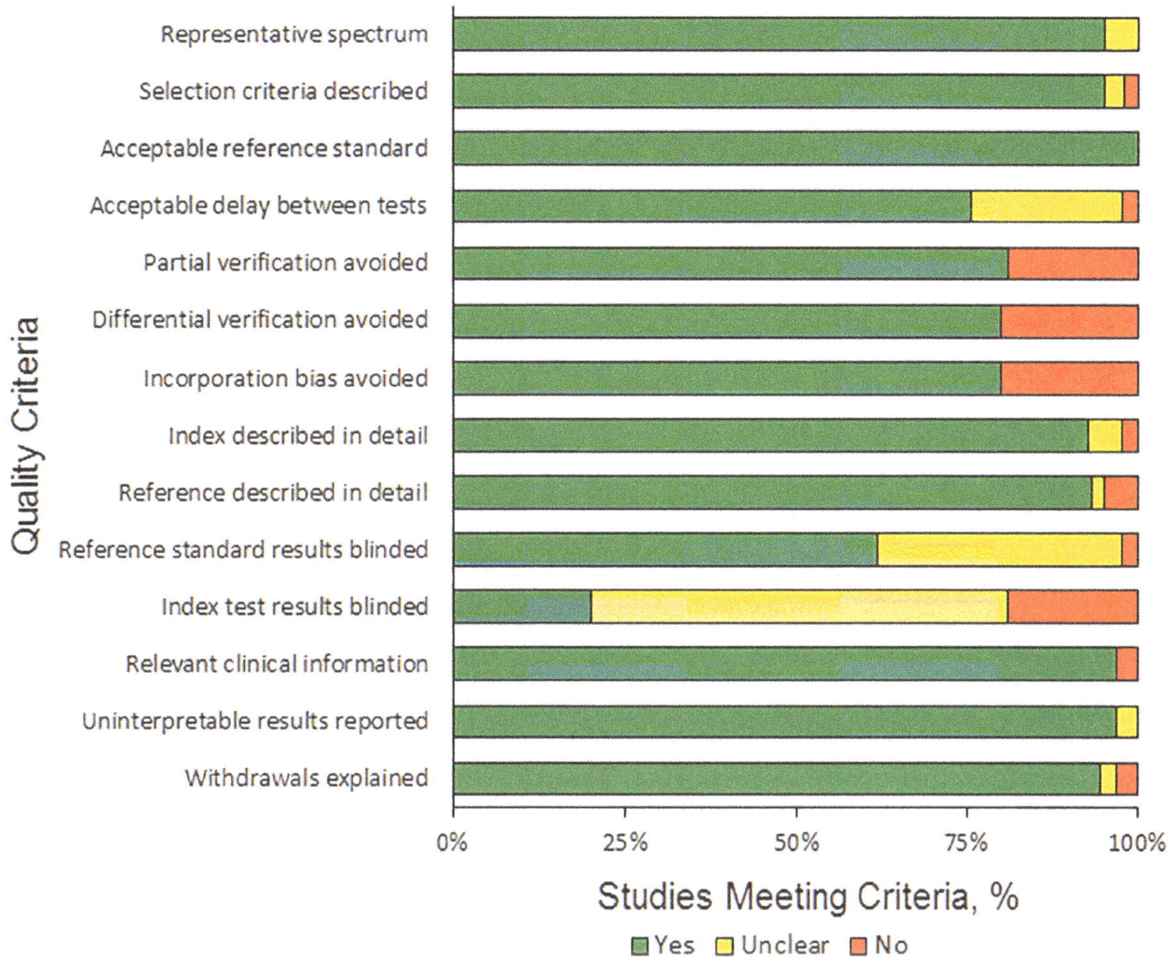

Figure 2. Quality Assessment of Diagnostic Accuracy Studies (QUADAS) assessments of the quality of included studies.

33.3%). The coupled forest plots for sensitivity and specificity shows moderate to high heterogeneity ($I^2 = 67\%$ for sensitivity and $I^2 = 90\%$ for specificity; Figure 4; bottom panels, Table 1). The pooled sensitivity was 80% (95% CI, 77–82%) and the pooled specificity was 93% (95% CI, 92–94%).

Adults - Immunochromatographic Methods

The prevalence of GAS infection in the 6 adults strata was 21.3% (259/1,216 patients) (range 16.1% to 25.7%). The coupled forest plots for sensitivity and specificity shows modest heterogeneity ($I^2 = 61\%$ for sensitivity and $I^2 = 72\%$ for specificity; Figure 5; top panels, Table 1). The pooled sensitivity was 91% (95% CI, 87–94%) and the pooled specificity was 93% (95% CI, 92 to 95%). One outlier study [75] met 12 quality criteria (Table S3 in File S1) and enrolled 100 patients presenting to an emergency room in Istanbul [75]. Another outlier study, [29] met nine quality criteria (Table S3 in File S1) and enrolled 148 patients presenting to two primary care settings in Boston (Massachusetts).

Adults - Enzyme immunoassay and Optical Immunoassay Methods

The prevalence of GAS infection in the 2 EIA adult strata was 21.9% (73/333 patients). The coupled forest plots for sensitivity and specificity shows high heterogeneity ($I^2 = 88\%$ for sensitivity and $I^2 = 88\%$ for specificity; Figure 5; bottom panels, Table 1). The pooled sensitivity was 86% (95% CI, 81–91%) and the pooled specificity was 97% (95% CI, 96 to 99%).

The prevalence of GAS infection in the single OIA adult strata was 40.7% (33/81 patients), Table 1.

Discussion

In this systematic review of rapid antigen strep testing, the number of patients included in studies that met high methodological quality criteria was significantly smaller than the number of patients included in lower quality studies (18,464 vs. 35,634, respectively). We also observed publication bias. We could not identify important sources of the high heterogeneity of sensitivity and specificity estimates among higher quality studies using immunochromatographic methods in children (10,325 patients). For higher quality studies using enzyme immunoassay in children (342 patients), the pooled sensitivity was 86% and the pooled specificity was 92% (studies had no or little heterogeneity). In children, immunochromatographic and enzyme immunoassay methods outperform optical immunoassay methods. For the higher quality immunochromatographic methods in the adult population (1,216 patients), the pooled sensitivity was 91% and the pooled specificity was 93%; however, heterogeneity was modest for sensitivity and specificity.

Table 1. Summary of diagnostic accuracy estimates, higher study methodological quality*.

Type of test	Pediatrics	Adults
Immunochromatographic		
Number of patients	10,325	1,216
Number of strata	28	6
Sensitivity, %	86 (85–87)	91 (87–94)
Specificity, %	96 (95–96)	93 (92–95)
Inconsistency (I^2)		
- Sensitivity	88%	61%
- Specificity	86%	72%
Enzyme Immunoassay (EIA)		
Number of patients	342	333
Number of strata	3	2
Sensitivity, %	86 (79–92)	86 (81–91)
Specificity, %	92 (88–95)	97 (96–99)
Inconsistency (I^2)		
- Sensitivity	0%	88%
- Specificity	55%	88%
Optical immunoassay (OIA)		
Number of patients	3,294	81
Number of strata	3	1
Sensitivity, %	80 (77–82)	94 (80–99)
Specificity, %	93 (92–94)	69 (54–81)
Inconsistency (I^2)		
- Sensitivity	67%	-
- Specificity	90%	-

*Numbers in parenthesis are 95% confidence intervals.

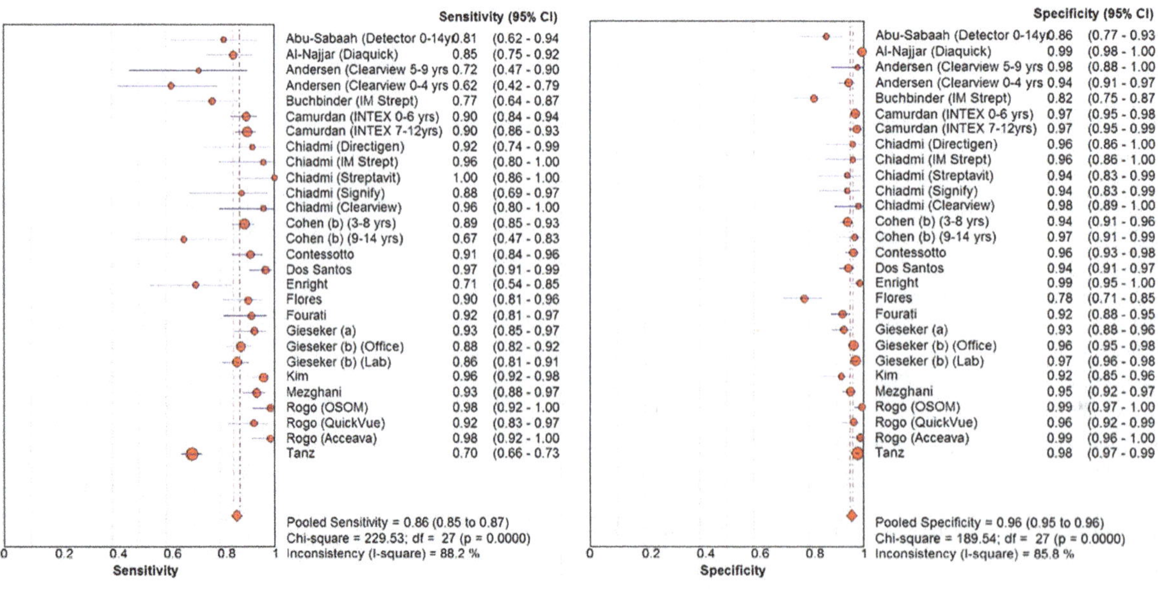

Figure 3. Pediatric strata, forest plots for immunochromatographic methods, higher study methodological quality.

Enzyme immunoassay

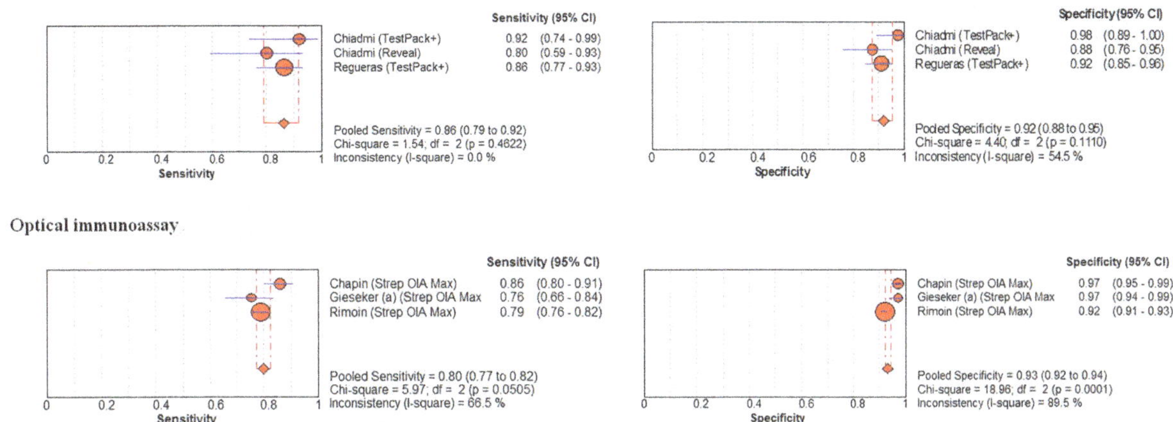

Figure 4. Pediatric strata, forest plots for enzyme immunoassay (EIA, top panels) and optical immunoassay (OIA, bottom panels) methods to diagnose group A streptococcal pharyngitis, higher study methodological quality.

The appropriate diagnosis and management of pharyngitis patients continues to provoke controversy. The controversy exists not just between "experts" but also between guideline panels. Matthys and colleagues reviewed 10 guidelines from both North America and Europe [82]. These guidelines took three different approaches to pharyngitis patients. Some European countries consider pharyngitis a self-limited problem with only rare complications. They eschew testing or antibiotic treatment.

Some guidelines recommend either rapid antigen strep testing or empiric treatment of patients more likely to have GAS pharyngitis, with neither testing nor treatment for patients very unlikely to have GAS infection [82]. Other guidelines aim to limit antibiotic use, and "require" a positive rapid antigen strep test prior to prescribing antibiotics [2].

The debate between the first strategy and the other two strategies rests on a disagreement over the benefits of treating GAS pharyngitis. The debate between the remaining two strategies depends on our estimates of the sensitivity of rapid antigen strep testing and the implications of not treating patients with false negative rapid strep tests.

The profound heterogeneity of the test characteristics among the most studied method, immunochromatographic, represents the major finding of our analysis. When an analysis reveals this degree of heterogeneity then one cannot reliably assign a point estimate to either sensitivity or specificity. Although the pooled estimate of sensitivity (85%; 95% CI 84 to 87%) reported in the systematic review published in Spanish [7] is remarkably similar to the one provided for immunochromatographic methods shown in Table 1 of our study, none can be used as a reliable point estimate given the large heterogeneity observed. While we observed no or little heterogeneity of enzyme immunoassay methods in children,

Immunochromatographic

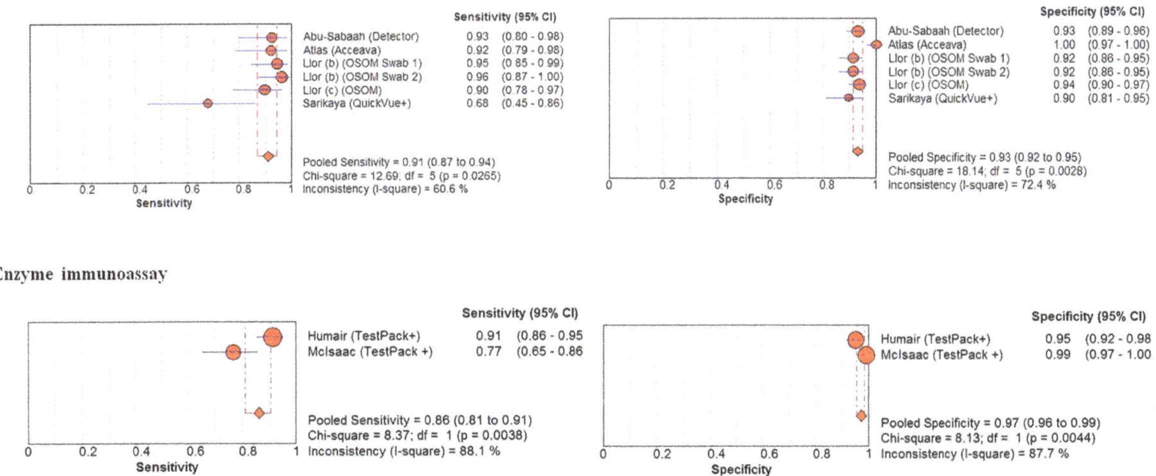

Figure 5. Adult strata, forest plots for immunochromatographic (top panels), enzyme immunoassay (EIA, middle panels) and optical immunoassay (OIA, bottom panels) methods to diagnose group A streptococcal pharyngitis, higher study methodological quality.

we caution the reader given the relatively small sample size in this group.

Why do these studies show such great heterogeneity for most of the groups? We can only speculate that several factors influence this finding. First, we have a mixture of practical studies in routine clinical settings and research studies with specially trained study personnel. Second, the tests have significant technical variances, as they use different methods to determine the presence of the group A antigen; hence, we could not examine a threshold effect. Finally, evidence suggests the high variability in sensitivity based on clinical spectrum, inoculum size, technical training, and personnel conducting the tests [83–85]; the nature of reporting of the studies reviewed precluded further exploration. In our pre-specified approach, we were not able to identify the source of such heterogeneity. Standardization of tests across manufacturers would better define the sensitivity of the RAST. Our finding of great heterogeneity means that we do not have strong confidence in the estimate of sensitivity.

We do not expect this analysis to resolve the ongoing debates about relying on rapid antigen strep testing to make treatment decisions. However, physician decision makers would appreciate accurate estimates of the test characteristics of any test that we use. This study provides estimates of the test characteristics; however, the consistency of performance leaves a broad range of confidence.

Our study has limitations. We could not retrieve three studies for full article review [21–23] and we observed publication bias.

Conclusion

In conclusion, RAST immunochromatographic methods appear to be very sensitive and highly specific to diagnose group A streptococcal pharyngitis among adults but not in children. Using the best evidence, we could not identify important sources of variability of sensitivity and specificity. The present systematic review provides the best evidence for the wide range of sensitivity included in current guidelines.

Supporting Information

File S1 Contains the following files: **Table S1.** Study Characteristics, Overall (n = 59). **Table S2.** Study Characteristics. **Table S3.** Quality assessment using QUADAS criteria. **Table S4.** Operating Test Characteristics.

File S2 Contains the following files: **Figure S1.** Funnel plot for rapid antigen tests diagnostic odds ratio. EES = Effective Sample Size. The non-vertical regression line suggests publication bias. The non-vertical regression line suggests publication bias (the results of the studies do not fall into the "funnel" depicted in blue). In the absence of publication bias, studies of smaller sample size would have a wider distribution of Diagnostic Odds Ratios; represented as a wider distribution at the base, which is absent from the plot. **Figure S2.** Forest plots sensitivities and specificities from test accuracy studies of rapid antigen tests to diagnose group A streptococcal pharyngitis for higher study methodological quality. Study test characteristics are sensitivity (left panel) and specificity (right panel). Circles represent the sensitivity or specificity and are proportional to study sample size. Blue lines represent 95% confidence intervals. Diamonds represent pooled estimates of sensitivity or specificity, red lines correspond to their respective 95% confidence intervals. **Figure S3.** Forest plots sensitivities and specificities from test accuracy studies of rapid antigen tests to diagnose group A streptococcal pharyngitis for lower study methodological quality. Study test characteristics are sensitivity (left panel) and specificity (right panel). Circles represent the sensitivity or specificity and are proportional to study sample size. Blue lines represent 95% confidence intervals. Diamonds represent pooled estimates of sensitivity or specificity, red lines correspond to their respective 95% confidence intervals. **Figure S4.** Hierarchical summary receiver-operating characteristic curve plots of rapid antigen tests to diagnose group A streptococcal pharyngitis by study methodological quality. **Figure S5.** Pediatric strata, immunochromatographic methods, higher quality studies. HSROC by sponsorship. **Figure S6.** Pediatric strata, immunochromatographic methods, higher quality studies. HSROC by location of care. **Figure S7.** Pediatric strata, immunochromatographic methods, higher quality studies. HSROC by publication year. **Figure S8.** Pediatric strata, immunochromatographic methods, higher quality studies. HSROC by prevalence. **Figure S9.** Pediatric strata, immunochromatographic methods, higher quality studies. HSROC by region.

Acknowledgments

Drs. Stewart and Davis contributed equally to the study conception, design, and overall conduction of the study and both qualify as first authors. Drs. Stewart and Davis were medical students at the time of the study and now are at Walter Reed National Military Medical Center (Dr. Stewart) and University of Texas Southwestern Medical Center (Dr. Davis).

The contents of this article are solely the responsibility of the authors and do not necessarily represent the official views of the Department of Veterans Affairs. Presented in part at the Southern Society of General Internal Medicine, New Orleans, February 22–23, 2013, and at the Society of General Internal Medicine National Meeting, Denver, Colorado, April 24–27, 2013.

Author Contributions

Conceived and designed the experiments: EHS BD BLCT RMC BL CAE. Performed the experiments: EHS BD. Analyzed the data: RMC BL CAE. Contributed reagents/materials/analysis tools: EHS BD BLCT RMC BL CAE. Contributed to the writing of the manuscript: EHS BD BLCT RMC BL CAE.

References

1. Ambulatory Health Care Data (2010) National Ambulatory Medical Care Survey: Summary Tables. Centers for Disease Control and Prevention. Available at: http://www.cdc.gov/nchs/ahcd/web_tables.htm#2010. Accessed October 13, 2014.
2. Shulman ST, Bisno AL, Clegg HW, Gerber MA, Kaplan EL, et al. (2012) Clinical practice guideline for the diagnosis and management of group A streptococcal pharyngitis: 2012 update by the Infectious Diseases Society of America. Clin Infect Dis 55: 1279–1282.
3. Gerber MA, Shulman ST (2004) Rapid diagnosis of pharyngitis caused by group A streptococci. Clin Microbiol Rev 17: 571–580.
4. Hillner BE, Centor RM (1987) What a difference a day makes: a decision analysis of adult streptococcal pharyngitis. J Gen Intern Med 2: 244–250.
5. Neuner JM, Hamel MB, Phillips RS, Bona K, Aronson MD (2003) Diagnosis and management of adults with pharyngitis. A cost-effectiveness analysis. Ann Intern Med 139: 113–122.
6. Wessels MR (2011) Clinical practice. Streptococcal pharyngitis. N Engl J Med 364: 648–655.
7. Ruiz-Aragon J, Rodriguez Lopez R, Molina Linde JM (2010) [Evaluation of rapid methods for detecting Streptococcus pyogenes. Systematic review and meta-analysis]. An Pediatr (Barc) 72: 391–402.

8. Leeflang MM, Deeks JJ, Gatsonis C, Bossuyt PM, Cochrane Diagnostic Test Accuracy Working G (2008) Systematic reviews of diagnostic test accuracy. Ann Intern Med 149: 889–897.
9. Moher D, Liberati A, Tetzlaff J, Altman DG, Group P (2009) Preferred reporting items for systematic reviews and meta-analyses: the PRISMA statement. PLoS Med 6: e1000097.
10. Centre for Reviews and Dissemination. University of York. National Institute for Health Research (NHS). Available at: http://www.crd.york.ac.uk/CRDWeb/. Accessed October 13, 2014.
11. Patel T, Brown E, Davis B, Clemans-Taylor BL, Centor RM, et al. (2014) What does industry tell us about test characteristics? The rapid antigen streptococcus test. J Invest Med 62: 584–585.
12. Scopus. Elsevier B.V. Available at URL: http://www.info.sciverse.com/scopus. Accessed October 13, 2014.
13. Scientific Electronic Library Online (SciELO). Available at URL: http://www.scielo.org/php/index.php. Accessed October 13, 2014.
14. Whiting P, Rutjes AW, Dinnes J, Reitsma J, Bossuyt PM, et al. (2004) Development and validation of methods for assessing the quality of diagnostic accuracy studies. Health Technol Assess 8: iii, 1–234.
15. Rutter CM, Gatsonis CA (2001) A hierarchical regression approach to meta-analysis of diagnostic test accuracy evaluations. Stat Med 20: 2865–2884.
16. Macaskill P (2004) Empirical Bayes estimates generated in a hierarchical summary ROC analysis agreed closely with those of a full Bayesian analysis. J Clin Epidemiol 57: 925–932.
17. Bossuyt P, Davenport C, Deeks J, Hyde C, Leeflang M, et al. (2013) Chapter 11:Interpreting results and drawing conclusions. In: Deeks JJ, Bossuyt PM, Gatsonis C (editors), Cochrane Handbook for Systematic Reviews of Diagnostic Test Accuracy Version 0.9. The Cochrane Collaboration, 2013. Available at URL: http://srdta.cochrane.org/. Accessed October 13, 2014.
18. Harbord RM, Whiting P (2009) metandi: Meta-analysis of diagnostic accuracy using hierarchical logistic regression. Stata Journal 9: 211–229.
19. Deeks JJ, Macaskill P, Irwig L (2005) The performance of tests of publication bias and other sample size effects in systematic reviews of diagnostic test accuracy was assessed. J Clin Epidemiol 58: 882–893.
20. Dwamena B (2007) MIDAS: Stata module for meta-analytical integration of diagnostic test accuracy studies. Boston College Department of Economics, 2007. Available at: http://ideas.repec.org/c/boc/bocode/s456880.html. Accessed October 13, 2014.
21. Shaheen BH, Hamdan AT (2006) Rapid identification of streptococcal pharyngitis Qatar Med J 15: 37–39.
22. Faverge B, Marie-Cosenza S, Bietrix M, Attou D, Bensekhria S, et al. (2004) [Use in hospital of a rapid diagnosis test of group A streptococcal pharyngotonsillitis in children]. Arch Pediatr 11: 862–863.
23. Bischoff A (2007) [Diagnosis of streptococcal tonsillitis. Rapid test prevents treatment error]. MMW Fortschritte der Medizin 149: 17.
24. Abu-Sabaah AH, Ghazi HO (2006) Better diagnosis and treatment of throat infections caused by group A beta-haemolytic streptococci. Br J Biomed Sci 63: 155–158.
25. Al-Najjar FY, Uduman SA (2008) Clinical utility of a new rapid test for the detection of group A Streptococcus and discriminate use of antibiotics for bacterial pharyngitis in an outpatient setting. Int J Infect Dis 12: 308–311.
26. Andersen JB, Dahm TL, Nielsen CT, Frimodt-Moller N (2003) [Diagnosis of streptococcal tonsillitis in the pediatric department with the help of antigen detection test]. Ugeskr Laeger 165: 2291–2295.
27. Araujo Filho BC, Imamura R, Sennes LU, Sakae FA (2005) Role of rapid antigen detection test for the diagnosis of group A beta-hemolytic streptococcus in patients with pharyngotonsillitis. Braz J Otorhinolaryngol 71: 168–171.
28. Armengol CE, Schlager TA, Hendley JO (2004) Sensitivity of a rapid antigen detection test for group A streptococci in a private pediatric office setting: answering the Red Book's request for validation. Pediatrics 113: 924–926.
29. Atlas SJ, McDermott SM, Mannone C, Barry MJ (2005) The role of point of care testing for patients with acute pharyngitis. J Gen Intern Med 20: 759–761.
30. Ayanruoh S, Waseem M, Quee F, Humphrey A, Reynolds T (2009) Impact of rapid streptococcal test on antibiotic use in a pediatric emergency department. Pediatr Emerg Care 25: 748–750.
31. Buchbinder N, Benzdira A, Belgaid A, Dufour D, Paon JC, et al. (2007) [Streptococcal pharyngitis in the pediatric emergency department: value and impact of rapid antigen detection test]. Arch Pediatr 14: 1057–1061.
32. Camurdan AD, Camurdan OM, Ok I, Sahin F, Ilhan MN, et al. (2008) Diagnostic value of rapid antigen detection test for streptococcal pharyngitis in a pediatric population. Int J Pediatr Otorhinolaryngol 72: 1203–1206.
33. Chapin KC, Blake P, Wilson CD (2002) Performance characteristics and utilization of rapid antigen test, DNA probe, and culture for detection of group a streptococci in an acute care clinic. J Clin Microbiol 40: 4207–4210.
34. Chiadmi F, Schlatter J, Mounkassa B, Ovetchkine P, Vermerie N (2004) [Fast diagnostic tests in the management of group A beta-heamolytic streptococcal pharyngitis]. Ann Biol Clin (Paris) 62: 573–577.
35. Cohen R, Levy C, Ovetchkine P, Boucherat M, Weil-Olivier C, et al. (2004) Evaluation of streptococcal clinical scores, rapid antigen detection tests and cultures for childhood pharyngitis. Eur J Pediatr 163: 281–282.
36. Cohen JF, Chalumeau M, Levy C, Bidet P, Thollot F, et al. (2012) Spectrum and inoculum size effect of a rapid antigen detection test for group A streptococcus in children with pharyngitis. PLoS One 7: e39085.
37. Contessotto Spadetto C, Camara Simon M, Aviles Ingles MJ, Ojeda Escuriet JM, Cascales Barcelo I, et al. (2000) [Rational use of antibiotics in pediatrics: impact of a rapid test for detection of beta-haemolytic group A streptococci in acute pharyngotonsillitis]. An Esp Pediatr 52: 212–219.
38. dos Santos AG, Berezin EN (2005) [Comparative analysis of clinical and laboratory methods for diagnosing streptococcal sore throat]. J Pediatr (Rio J) 81: 23–28.
39. Dimatteo LA, Lowenstein SR, Brimhall B, Reiquam W, Gonzales R (2001) The relationship between the clinical features of pharyngitis and the sensitivity of a rapid antigen test: evidence of spectrum bias. Ann Emerg Med 38: 648–652.
40. Edmonson MB, Farwell KR (2005) Relationship between the clinical likelihood of group a streptococcal pharyngitis and the sensitivity of a rapid antigen-detection test in a pediatric practice. Pediatrics 115: 280–285.
41. Enright K, Kalima P, Taheri S (2011) Should a near-patient test be part of the management of pharyngitis in the pediatric emergency department? Pediatr Emerg Care 27: 1148–1150.
42. Ezike EN, Rongkavilit C, Fairfax MR, Thomas RL, Asmar BI (2005) Effect of using 2 throat swabs vs 1 throat swab on detection of group A streptococcus by a rapid antigen detection test. Arch Pediatr Adolesc Med 159: 486–490.
43. Flores Mateo G, Conejero J, Grenzner Martinel E, Baba Z, Dicono S, et al. (2010) [Early diagnosis of streptococcal pharyngitis in paediatric practice: Validity of a rapid antigen detection test]. Aten Primaria 42: 356–361.
44. Fontes MJ, Bottrel FB, Fonseca MT, Lasmar LB, Diamante R, et al. (2007) Early diagnosis of streptococcal pharyngotonsillitis: assessment by latex particle agglutination test. J Pediatr (Rio J) 83: 465–470.
45. Forward KR, Haldane D, Webster D, Mills C, Brine C, et al. (2006) A comparison between the Strep A Rapid Test Device and conventional culture for the diagnosis of streptococcal pharyngitis. Can J Infect Dis Med Microbiol 17: 221–223.
46. Fourati S, Smaoui H, Jegiurim H, Berriche I, Taghorti R, et al. (2009) [Use of the rapid antigen detection test in group A streptococci pharyngitis diagnosis in Tunis, Tunisia]. Bull Soc Pathol Exot 102: 175–176.
47. Fox JW, Marcon MJ, Bonsu BK (2006) Diagnosis of streptococcal pharyngitis by detection of Streptococcus pyogenes in posterior pharyngeal versus oral cavity specimens. J Clin Microbiol 44: 2593–2594.
48. Gieseker KE, Mackenzie T, Roe MH, Todd JK (2002) Comparison of two rapid Streptococcus pyogenes diagnostic tests with a rigorous culture standard. Pediatr Infect Dis J 21: 922–927.
49. Gieseker KE, Roe MH, MacKenzie T, Todd JK (2003) Evaluating the American Academy of Pediatrics diagnostic standard for Streptococcus pyogenes pharyngitis: backup culture versus repeat rapid antigen testing. Pediatrics 111: e666–670.
50. Gurol Y, Akan H, Izbirak G, Tekkanat ZT, Gunduz TS, et al. (2010) The sensitivity and the specifity of rapid antigen test in streptococcal upper respiratory tract infections. Int J Pediatr Otorhinolaryngol 74: 591–593.
51. Hall MC, Kieke B, Gonzales R, Belongia EA (2004) Spectrum bias of a rapid antigen detection test for group A beta-hemolytic streptococcal pharyngitis in a pediatric population. Pediatrics 114: 182–186.
52. Hinfey P, Nicholls BH, Garcia F, Ripper J, Cameron Y, et al. (2010) Sensitivity of a rapid antigen detection test for the diagnosis of group a streptoccal pharyngitis in the emergency department. J Emerg Med 56: S132.
53. Humair JP, Revaz SA, Bovier P, Stalder H (2006) Management of acute pharyngitis in adults: reliability of rapid streptococcal tests and clinical findings. Arch Intern Med 166: 640–644.
54. Johansson L, Mansson NO (2003) Rapid test, throat culture and clinical assessment in the diagnosis of tonsillitis. Fam Pract 20: 108–111.
55. Kawakami S, Ono Y, Yanagawa Y, Miyazawa Y (2003) [Basic and clinical evaluation of the new rapid diagnostic kit for detecting group A streptococci with the immunochromatographical method]. Rinsho Biseibutshu Jinsoku Shindan Kenkyukai Shi 14: 9–16.
56. Keahey L, Bulloch B, Jacobson R, Tenenbein M, Kabani A (2002) Diagnostic accuracy of a rapid antigen test for GABHS performed by nurses in a pediatric ED. Am J Emerg Med 20: 128–130.
57. Kim S (2009) The evaluation of SD Bioline Strep A rapid antigen test in acute pharyngitis in pediatric clinics. Korean J Lab Med 29: 320–323.
58. Lindbaek M, Hoiby EA, Lermark G, Steinsholt IM, Hjortdahl P (2004) Which is the best method to trace group A streptococci in sore throat patients: culture or GAS antigen test? Scand J Prim Health Care 22: 233–238.
59. Llor C, Hernandez Anadon S, Gomez Bertomeu FF, Santamaria Puig JM, Calvino Dominguez O, et al. (2008) [Validation of a rapid antigenic test in the diagnosis of pharyngitis caused by group a beta-haemolytic Streptococcus]. Aten Primaria 40: 489–494.
60. Llor C, Calvino O, Hernandez S, Crispi S, Perez-Bauer M, et al. (2009) Repetition of the rapid antigen test in initially negative supposed streptococcal pharyngitis is not necessary in adults. Int J Clin Pract 63: 1340–1344.
61. Llor C, Madurell J, Balague-Corbella M, Gomez M, Cots JM (2011) Impact on antibiotic prescription of rapid antigen detection testing in acute pharyngitis in adults: a randomised clinical trial. Br J Gen Pract 61: e244–251.
62. Maltezou HC, Tsagris V, Antoniadou A, Galani L, Douros C, et al. (2008) Evaluation of a rapid antigen detection test in the diagnosis of streptococcal pharyngitis in children and its impact on antibiotic prescription. J Antimicrob Chemother 62: 1407–1412.

63. Mayes T, Pichichero ME (2001) Are follow-up throat cultures necessary when rapid antigen detection tests are negative for group A streptococci? Clin Pediatr (Phila) 40: 191–195.
64. McIsaac WJ, Kellner JD, Aufricht P, Vanjaka A, Low DE (2004) Empirical validation of guidelines for the management of pharyngitis in children and adults. JAMA 291: 1587–1595.
65. Mezghani Maalej S, Rekik M, Boudaouara M, Jardak N, Turki S, et al. (2010) [Childhood pharyngitis in Sfax (Tunisia): epidemiology and utility of a rapid streptococcal test]. Med Mal Infect 40: 226–231.
66. Mirza A, Wludyka P, Chiu TT, Rathore MH (2007) Throat culture is necessary after negative rapid antigen detection tests. Clin Pediatr (Phila) 46: 241–246.
67. Nerbrand C, Jasir A, Schalen C (2002) Are current rapid detection tests for Group A Streptococci sensitive enough? Evaluation of 2 commercial kits. Scand J Infect Dis 34: 797–799.
68. Parviainen M, Koskela M, Ikäheimo I, Kelo E, Sirola H, et al. (2011) A novel strep A test for a rapid test reader compared with standard culture method and a commercial antigen assay. Eur Infect Dis 5: 143–145.
69. Regueras De Lorenzo G, Santos Rodriguez PM, Villa Bajo L, Perez Guirado A, Arbesu Fernandez E, et al. (2012) [Use of the rapid antigen technique in the diagnosis of Streptococcus pyogenes pharyngotonsillitis]. An Pediatr (Barc) 77: 193–199.
70. Rimoin AW, Walker CL, Hamza HS, Elminawi N, Ghafar HA, et al. (2010) The utility of rapid antigen detection testing for the diagnosis of streptococcal pharyngitis in low-resource settings. Int J Infect Dis 14: e1048–1053.
71. Rogo T, Schwartz RH, Ascher DP (2011) Comparison of the Inverness Medical Acceava Strep A test with the Genzyme OSOM and Quidel QuickVue Strep A tests. Clin Pediatr (Phila) 50: 294–296.
72. Roosevelt GE, Kulkarni MS, Shulman ST (2001) Critical evaluation of a CLIA-waived streptococcal antigen detection test in the emergency department. Ann Emerg Med 37: 377–381.
73. Rosenberg P, McIsaac W, Macintosh D, Kroll M (2002) Diagnosing streptococcal pharyngitis in the emergency department: Is a sore throat score approach better than rapid streptococcal antigen testing? Cjem 4: 178–184.
74. Santos O, Weckx LL, Pignatari AC, Pignatari SS (2003) Detection of Group A beta-hemolytic Streptococcus employing three different detection methods: culture, rapid antigen detecting test, and molecular assay. Braz J Infect Dis 7: 297–300.
75. Sarikaya S, Aktas C, Ay D, Cetin A, Celikmen F (2010) Sensitivity and specificity of rapid antigen detection testing for diagnosing pharyngitis in the emergency department. Ear Nose Throat J 89: 180–182.
76. Schmuziger N, Schneider S, Frei R (2003) [Reliability and general practice value of 2 rapid Streptococcus A tests]. HNO 51: 806–812.
77. Sheeler RD, Houston MS, Radke S, Dale JC, Adamson SC (2002) Accuracy of rapid strep testing in patients who have had recent streptococcal pharyngitis. J Am Board Fam Pract 15: 261–265.
78. Tanz RR, Gerber MA, Kabat W, Rippe J, Seshadri R, et al. (2009) Performance of a rapid antigen-detection test and throat culture in community pediatric offices: implications for management of pharyngitis. Pediatrics 123: 437–444.
79. Uhl JR, Adamson SC, Vetter EA, Schleck CD, Harmsen WS, et al. (2003) Comparison of LightCycler PCR, rapid antigen immunoassay, and culture for detection of group A streptococci from throat swabs. J Clin Microbiol 41: 242–249.
80. Van Limbergen J, Kalima P, Taheri S, Beattie TF (2006) Streptococcus A in paediatric accident and emergency: are rapid streptococcal tests and clinical examination of any help? Emerg Med J 23: 32–34.
81. Wong MC, Chung CH (2002) Group A streptococcal infection in patients presenting with a sore throat at an accident and emergency department: prospective observational study. Hong Kong Med J 8: 92–98.
82. Matthys J, De Meyere M, van Driel ML, De Sutter A (2007) Differences among international pharyngitis guidelines: not just academic. Ann Fam Med 5: 436–443.
83. Cohen JF, Chalumeau M, Levy C, Bidet P, Benani M, et al. (2013) Effect of clinical spectrum, inoculum size and physician characteristics on sensitivity of a rapid antigen detection test for group A streptococcal pharyngitis. Eur J Clin Microbiol Infect Dis 32: 787–793.
84. Fox JW, Cohen DM, Marcon MJ, Cotton WH, Bonsu BK (2006) Performance of rapid streptococcal antigen testing varies by personnel. J Clin Microbiol 44: 3918–3922.
85. Toepfner N, Henneke P, Berner R, Hufnagel M (2013) Impact of technical training on rapid antigen detection tests (RADT) in group A streptococcal tonsillopharyngitis. Eur J Clin Microbiol Infect Dis 32: 609–611.

15

Viral Etiology of Respiratory Tract Infections in Children at the Pediatric Hospital in Ouagadougou (Burkina Faso)

Solange Ouédraogo[1], Blaise Traoré[1], Zah Ange Brice Nene Bi[1], Firmin Tiandama Yonli[1], Donatien Kima[1], Pierre Bonané[1], Lassané Congo[1], Rasmata Ouédraogo Traoré[1], Diarra Yé[1], Christophe Marguet[2], Jean-Christophe Plantier[3], Astrid Vabret[4], Marie Gueudin[3]*

1 Charles de Gaulle Pediatric University Hospital, Ouagadougou, Burkina Faso, **2** Respiratory Diseases, Allergy and CF Unit, Paediatric Department, Rouen University Hospital Charles Nicolle, EA3830, Inserm CIC204, Rouen, France, **3** Laboratory of Virology, GRAM EA 2656 Rouen University Hospital Charles Nicolle, Rouen, France, **4** Laboratory of Human and Molecular Virology, Caen University Hospital Clemenceau, Caen, France

Abstract

Background: Acute respiratory infections (ARIs) are a major cause of morbidity and mortality in children in Africa. The circulation of viruses classically implicated in ARIs is poorly known in Burkina Faso. The aim of this study was to identify the respiratory viruses present in children admitted to or consulting at the pediatric hospital in Ouagadougou.

Methods: From July 2010 to July 2011, we tested nasal aspirates of 209 children with upper or lower respiratory infection for main respiratory viruses (respiratory syncytial virus (RSV), metapneumovirus, adenovirus, parainfluenza viruses 1, 2 and 3, influenza A, B and C, rhinovirus/enterovirus), by immunofluorescence locally in Ouagadougou, and by PCR in France. Bacteria have also been investigated in 97 samples.

Results: 153 children (73.2%) carried at least one virus and 175 viruses were detected. Rhinoviruses/enteroviruses were most frequently detected (rhinovirus n = 88; enterovirus n = 38) and were found to circulate throughout the year. An epidemic of RSV infections (n = 25) was identified in September/October, followed by an epidemic of influenza virus (n = 13), mostly H1N1pdm09. This epidemic occurred during the period of the year in which nighttime temperatures and humidity were at their lowest. Other viruses tested were detected only sporadically. Twenty-two viral co-infections were observed. Bacteria were detected in 29/97 samples with 22 viral/bacterial co-infections.

Conclusions: This study, the first of its type in Burkina Faso, warrants further investigation to confirm the seasonality of RSV infection and to improve local diagnosis of influenza. The long-term objective is to optimize therapeutic management of infected children.

Editor: Pierre Roques, CEA, France

Funding: Sanofi Pasteur funded this study in its entirety. The funder approved the study design but had no role in data collection and analysis, decision to publish, or preparation of the manuscript.

Competing Interests: This study was funded by Sanofi Pasteur. An agreement was signed with the university hospital of Rouen which managed the funds.

* Email: Marie.Gueudin@chu-rouen.fr

Introduction

Respiratory viruses are ubiquitous, but most epidemiological knowledge relates to developed countries. In contrast, the burden of acute respiratory infections (ARIs) is particularly heavy among children in developing countries, with high mortality and hospital admission rates. The number of deaths related to ARIs has been estimated at 1.9 million children aged less than 5 years, 70% of whom live in Africa or South-East Asia [1]. In Burkina Faso (West Africa), ARIs are also a major cause of child admissions to hospital [2] with a 17.6% mortality rate in children aged under 5 years [3]. For a long time now, *Streptococcus pneumonia*, *Haemophilus influenza* and *Staphylococcus aureus* have been considered as the sole causal agents of severe ARIs in developing countries, and guidelines recommend prescribing antibiotics. Conversely, detection of viruses by molecular methods has provided evidence that a growing number of respiratory viruses are potent pathogenic agents for the respiratory tract. Thus, respiratory syncytial virus (RSV), human metapneumovirus (hMPV), rhinoviruses, parainfluenza (PIVs) and influenza viruses are currently recognized as common ARI etiologies in young children in developed countries [4,5]. The etiology of ARI is complex and emphasized by the demonstration of viral, bacterial or mixed co-infections in the respiratory tracts [5,6,7].

However, in developing countries and especially in Africa, studies on virus-related ARIs are limited to very few countries. Nevertheless, the results of these studies confirm epidemiological data reported in developed countries and underline the fact that viruses also cause frequent upper or lower airway infections. Early diagnosis facilitates early management and is recognized as one way to combat ARIs [8]. In fact, lack of sensitivity and specificity of symptoms prevents differentiation between influenza or any other viral infection and malaria [9,10]. The recommended early and easy use of antibiotics is not effective in viral ARIs, and can only prevent occurrence of bacterial super infection. In this context, viral diagnosis can prevent use of unnecessary costly antibiotics or antimalarial treatments.

To our knowledge, no specific data concerning the circulation of these viruses is currently available for Burkina Faso, even for influenza virus, which is the most documented virus internationally [11].

We carried out a prospective study, over a period of one year at Charles de Gaulle pediatric University Hospital in Ouagadougou (Burkina Faso). The aim was to determine the microbiological agents of these respiratory diseases using rapid detection of antigens by immunofluorescence, multiplex molecular tests, and bacterial cultures on nasopharyngeal samples. We aimed to improve our knowledge on the circulation of viruses and the type of ARIs that they cause.

Materials and Methods

Patients

This prospective study was conducted at Charles de Gaulle pediatric hospital in Ouagadougou, between July 1st 2010 and June 30th 2011. Inclusion criteria were as follows: Children aged under three years attending or hospitalized with an upper or lower airway infection. Upper respiratory infections were defined as congestive otitis, rhinitis associated with fever, and a hoarse cough suggesting tracheitis or laryngitis. Lower respiratory infection were defined as acute febrile respiratory distress, acute bronchiolitis, acute coughing or wheezing, febrile chest sounds suggesting pneumonia, bronchiolitis, asthma exacerbation. Oral parental consent was obtained to use a part of the nasopharyngeal aspiration for PCRs and clinical data were collected. In French law, the right to use the end of the samples is written in the code of public health: Code de la santé publique - Article L1211-2. The ethics committee in Burkina Faso was not consulted as it was recent when the study started.

Detection of viruses

At the hospital laboratory in Ouagadougou, antigens for RSV, hMPV, influenza virus A and B, parainfluenza type 1, 2, and 3, and adenovirus were detected by direct immunofluorescence assay (DFA) from nasopharyngeal aspiration (NPA) samples, employing commercial monoclonal antibodies conjugated with fluorescein isothiocyanate (Imagen, Oxoid, UK). A positive result was indicated by DFA, if a technician noted presence of at least one cell showing a typical fluorescence pattern, provided that at least 20 respiratory cells were available in the sample. All the samples were frozen at −80°C and further analyzed by molecular methods at the virology laboratory of Caen University Hospital. Nucleic acids were extracted with a Qiasymphony kit (Qiasymphony Virus/Bacteria Minikit, Qiagen, Courtaboeuf, France), and RT-PCR was carried out for detection of RSV, hMPV, influenza A and B viruses (RSV/hMPV r-gene, Influenza A/B r-gene, Argène Biomérieux) and rhinovirus/enterovirus and influenza C virus (in-house multiplex RT-PCR) [12]. Viral subtyping was carried out according to the National Reference Center for Influenza techniques (Institut Pasteur, Paris, France).

Bacterial growths

Bacteriological examinations were carried out only on 97 samples collected between the end of March and end of June 2011. NPA cultures were performed for growth of common and potentially pathogenic aerobic bacteria: *Streptococcus pneumoniae, Haemophilus influenzae, Moraxella catharralis, Staphylococcus aureus*, and *Klebsiella pneumonia*.

Climatic data

Burkina Faso has a tropical Sudanian-Sahelian climate with two opposite seasons: a rainy season, with 300 to 1200 mm of precipitation, and a dry season characterized by the Harmattan, a hot dry wind loaded with dust and originating in the Sahara Desert. The data used were obtained from the meteorological archives of Ouagadougou Airport *(source http://rp5.ru/archive.php?wmo_id = 65503&lang = fr)*. From daily data available, we calculated mean monthly values for temperature and humidity at 6 AM and 12 noon.

Statistical analysis

MedCalc software was used for the comparison of rates realized in Table 1. A P value of 0.05 was considered statistically significant. For the climatic data, mean monthly values for humidity and temperature for the months with or without detection of RSV or influenza A virus were compared using t-test after verification of the equality of variances by a F-test.

Results

Two hundred and nine children (boys: 58.4%) were included in this study. They were all aged less than three years, and 60.8% of them were less than 1 year old. Seventy-three children (34.9%) attended outpatient consultation, and 136 (65.1%) were admitted to hospital. Respiratory symptoms are described in Table 1.

One hundred and fifty-three children (73.2%) carried at least one virus (table 1). Children with positive results were mostly identified by RT-PCR (n = 149, 71.3%), and only 21 (10%) were detected by DFA. Positive results by DFA were as follows: adenovirus (n = 3), parainfluenza virus 1 (n = 2), parainfluenza virus 2 (n = 1), parainfluenza virus 3 (n = 5), and RSV (n = 10). RT-PCR detected: rhinovirus (n = 88; 59.1%), enterovirus (n = 38; 25.5%), RSV (n = 24; 16.1%), influenza (n = 13, including one case of influenza C; 8.7%), and one case of hMPV. Co-infections were detected in 14 samples (9.4%). Only one discordant result was observed for one sample, which was positive for RSV by DFA and negative by PCR. Among the viruses tested, only influenza B was never detected. Twenty-two (14.4%) viral co-infections were observed involving mainly rhinovirus or enteroviruses. Ninety eight (72.1%) of the inpatients carried at least one virus and 55 (75.3%) of the outpatients.

Bacterial cultures were carried out for 97 samples. Eighteen (18.6%) were negative for Bacteria and Viruses, 50 (51.5%) were positive for one or more viruses, 7 (7.2%) were positive for one or more bacteria and 22 (22.7%) were positive with a viral/bacterial co-infection. *Staphylococcus aureus, Klebsiella pneumonia*, and *Streptococcus pneumonia* were isolated in 14 cases (42.4%), 10 cases (30.3%), and 9 cases (27.7%) respectively.

Twenty-two viral/bacterial co-infections were diagnosed, 20 of which involved an enterovirus and/or a rhinovirus. The remaining two viral/bacterial co-infections associated *Staphylococcus aureus*/ PIV-3 and *Staphylococcus aureus*/adenovirus. Four bacterial co-infections were detected: *Staphylococcus aureus/Klebsiella pneumoniae* (n = 2) and *Staphylococcus aureus/Streptococcus pneumoniae* (n = 2). Rhinovirus was also detected in three of these four cases. 76 of the 97 children (78.4%) were hospitalized and 26 (34.2%) of them were infected with a Bacteria.

Table 1. Respiratory viruses detected either by direct immunofluorescence or RT-PCR and the associated final diagnosis (in some cases, more than one), * significant difference ($p = 0.0006$) with the group where no virus was detected.

Virus and viral co-infection	N (%) results		Children under 1 year old	Children admitted to hospital	Pneumonia	Bronchiolitis	Bronchitis/Asthma	Laryngitis	Nasopharyngitis/Otitis
None	56	26.8%	37	38	8	6	26	3	28
Adenovirus only	2	1.0%	1	2		1	2		1
Adenovirus + Rhinovirus	1	0.5%	1	1					1
Influenza A only	8	3.8%	4	3	2		3	1	4
Influenza A + Enterovirus	1	0.5%	0	0					1
Influenza A + Rhinovirus	2	1.0%	2	2		2	1		1
Influenza A + Rhinovirus + Enterovirus	1	0.5%	0	0					1
Influenza C + Rhinovirus	1	0.5%	1	1		1			
Parainfluenza 1 + Rhinovirus	1	0.5%	0	0					1
Parainfluenza 1 + RSV	1	0.5%	1	0			1		1
Parainfluenza 2	1	0.5%	1	1			1		
Parainfluenza 3 + Enterovirus	4	1.9%	2	3	1	1	3		2
Parainfluenza 3 + Rhinovirus	1	0.5%	0	1		1			
RSV only	19	9.1%	14	14	6	10*	8		5
RSV + Rhinovirus	3	1.4%	2	3	1	2	1		
RSV + Enterovirus	2	1.0%	2	2		2	2		
Metapneumovirus	1	0.5%	1	0		1	1		
Enterovirus only	26	12.4%	12	18	3	2	11	1	18
Rhinovirus only	74	35.4%	43	44	8	11	35	3	37
Rhinovirus + Enterovirus	4	1.9%	3	3	1	2	1		3
Total	**209**	**100.0%**	**127**	**136**	**30**	**42**	**96**	**8**	**104**

Monthly distribution and weekly detailed circulation of viruses (Figure 1 and Table 2), showed two successive winter epidemics. A RSV epidemic (24 RSV A, 1 RSV B) occurred between mid-September and end of October, with six co-infections including five rhinoviruses/enteroviruses. Nineteen of the 25 children infected with RSV were hospitalized which correspond to 14% of all the inpatients and 8% of the outpatients without significant difference ($p = 0.2517$). Children with RSV had significantly more bronchiolitis than the others ($p = 0.0006$) (table 1). RSV was found in the samples of 16 of the 70 children (22.9%) under the age of 6 months and in 9 of the 139 children above 6 months (6.5%) with significant difference ($p = 0.0012$).

This epidemic of RSV infection was followed by an epidemic of influenza A infection (H1N1pdm09, n = 8 and H3N2, n = 4) from mid-December to mid-February. These viruses were frequently associated with a rhinovirus or enterovirus (38.4%). Six children were hospitalized.

One hundred and nineteen children (56.9%) had a rhinovirus or an enterovirus which was detected during the year, with higher rates of rhinoviruses in April, May and June 2011. Rhinovirus and enterovirus were detected in 56.6% of the inpatients and 57.5% of the outpatients without significant difference ($p = 0,8353$). Of the 97 samples that underwent both bacteriological and virological investigation, 44 were positive for only enterovirus or human rhinovirus. A total of 56.5% of these children were under the age of 1 year and 39% were hospitalized.

Three adenovirus infections were detected at the end of February and five infections with parainfluenza virus 3 from March to June 2011. Only one of the three children infected with adenovirus was co-infected with a rhinovirus. The five children infected with parainfluenza virus 3 were co-infected with a rhinovirus or enterovirus and four of the five children were hospitalized.

An effect of climate has often been put forward as an explanation for the circulation patterns of respiratory viruses. A comparison of our findings for influenza and RSV with the available climatic data (Figure 2) showed that the influenza epidemic coincided with the period in which nighttime temperature ($p = 0.0007$) and relative humidity ($p = 0.0343$) were lowest. No significant climatic data were related to RSV epidemic.

Discussion

The epidemiology of respiratory virus infections is unknown in Burkina Faso, although suspected considering previous studies conducted in neighboring countries [13,14]. Firstly, this study provides evidence of the role of viruses in upper and lower airway diseases in this country. Our findings highlight the fact that three quarters of infants or young children with any respiratory symptoms carry at least one virus. This rate of detection concords with previous studies in developed and African countries [15,16,17,18]. Most of the viruses were identified by molecular diagnosis, and direct immunofluorescence yield was low but concordant with previous work [19], achieving only 10% of positive results. One discrepancy has been observed with a sample positive by DFA and negative by PCR without possible control. It has been verified that the exclusion of this sample would not have changed the statistical conclusions of the study. RSV must be considered as a main etiologic agent even if rhinoviruses or enteroviruses were most frequently detected. RSV is well known for being one of the main agents associated with upper or lower airway infections in infants, and it has been demonstrated that RSV causes more severe diseases than other respiratory viruses [6]. Although it is a universal virus, data on RSV circulation are still limited in Africa. In a previous review, *Stensballe et al.* suggested that RSV outbreaks begin on the southern coast and move northward from January to July [20]. In our study, the RSV outbreak in Burkina Faso was observed during the fall. This was consistent with data on RSV epidemics occurring in the fall or winter in neighboring countries like Senegal [13], Nigeria [21] and Cameroon [17]. In Ghana [14], another neighboring country to the south, RSV circulation was however observed throughout the year with a peak rate in summer. The influence of the climate remains difficult to demonstrate, and the various climates associated with RSV epidemics tend to prove the lack of impact of climate on their onset. In Burkina Faso, the peak for RSV infections coincided with the dry season, as reported in Nigeria and South Africa [21]. In contrast, RSV epidemics occur during

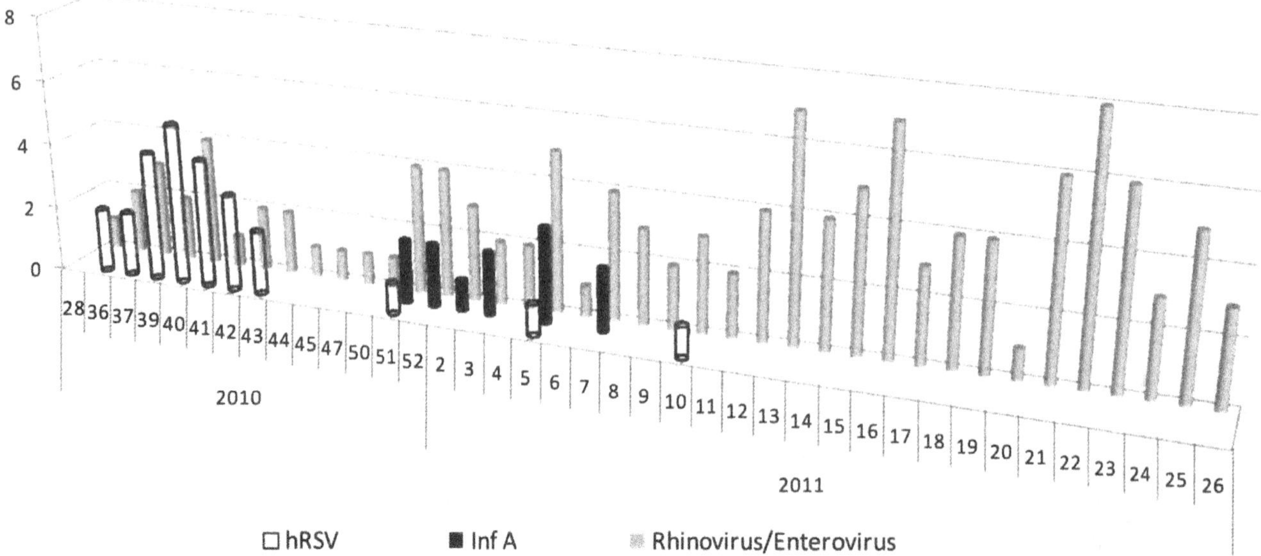

Figure 1. Weekly distribution of the three main detected viruses.

Table 2. Monthly distribution of viruses.

Year/Month	AdV	Inf A	Inf C	hRSV	hMPV	PIV 1	PIV 2	PIV 3	RhV	EnV	Total	
2010/07									1		1	0.6%
2010/09				6					5		11	6.3%
2010/10				16	1				5	6	28	15.9%
2010/11									3		3	1.7%
2010/12		4		1		1			7	2	15	8.5%
2011/01		3							6	3	12	6.8%
2011/02	2	5		1					6	6	20	11.4%
2011/03				1		1		2	10	4	18	10.2%
2011/04	1							1	14	8	24	13.6%
2011/05								1	14	4	19	10.8%
2011/06			1				1	1	17	5	25	14.2%
	3	12	1	25	1	2	1	5	88	38	176	
	1.7%	6.8%	0.6%	14.2%	0.6%	1.1%	0.6%	2.8%	50.0%	21.6%		

the rainy season in Mozambique [21] and Ghana [14]. Lastly in Kenya the duration of RSV seasons was long, but there were no clear climate patterns that appeared to coincide with changes in RSV circulation [19,22].

The second main finding of our study was the high rate of picornaviruses, and more than half of this population carried rhinoviruses or enteroviruses. The technique that we used for virus detection was not based on sequencing, and discrimination between the two species cannot be guaranteed. Nevertheless, it is clear that these viruses circulated throughout the year and were mainly isolated alone, although they are implicated in all but one viral co-infections. This high rate underlines the major involvement of these viruses in respiratory tract infections, as previously reported elsewhere in the world [23]. Picornaviruses are not the focus of the rare epidemiological studies conducted in Africa. They also appear to be the most frequent viruses identified in Cameroon, and Kenya [24], and a recent molecular study [25] detected all three (A, B and C) strains of rhinovirus in up to 35% of samples collected, as previously described in developing countries.

The bacteriological examinations were carried out during only 3 months, which is an important limitation for data analysis. During this period more than one quarter of this young population had a bacteria/virus co-infection. These co-infections associated an enterovirus or a rhinovirus with common potentially pathogenic bacteria encountered in childhood. When co-infections are identified, the respective contribution of each microbiological agent in the pathogenesis of respiratory tract infections remains unclear. Among the virus/virus co-infections, RSV was clearly identified as the most virulent agent, and its pathogenic effect predominated rhinovirus [6]. It is more difficult however to assess the respective pathogenic effect of bacteria or viruses detected simultaneously. Positive nasopharyngeal bacterial culture is a weak predictor of upper airway infections since healthy individuals often carry pathogenic bacteria. The presence of bacteria does not allow to conclude or to exclude to an isolated bacterial infection in upper airway infections. Conversely, Rhinovirus was detected as the sole causal agent in severe acute respiratory distress [24] and pneumonia [26] in Kenya and South Africa, respectively. This latter is in contrast with the better outcome attributed to Rhinovirus in developed countries [23], which is not necessarily associated with more severe disease.

Clinical diagnoses involving life-threatening infections such as malaria and meningitis were mentioned in the data collected. However, laboratory confirmation of these diagnoses was not part of our study and it was not possible to further analyze these cases.

Lastly, influenza A appeared as the fourth most prevalent virus in Ouagadougou, and was detected from mid December to the end of February. This result has not been compared with the Global Influenza Surveillance and Response System database, as no data on influenza epidemics was available from Burkina Faso for this season. This winter epidemic period of influenza A infection does not match that reported for neighboring countries. Nevertheless, this influenza epidemic occurred during the coldest period of the year, when relative humidity was low. This agreed with recent reports, showing that survival of the influenza virus in the external environment is related to low relative humidity and temperature [27,28,29]. No influenza B virus was identified in this study, contrasting with the high rates observed in neighboring countries over the same period. As our study mainly included very young children, for whom influenza virus was not reported as a major pathogenic agent [6], the likelihood of detecting either influenza A or B was reduced. Moreover, we are not able to rule out a concomitant circulation of influenza B in older populations.

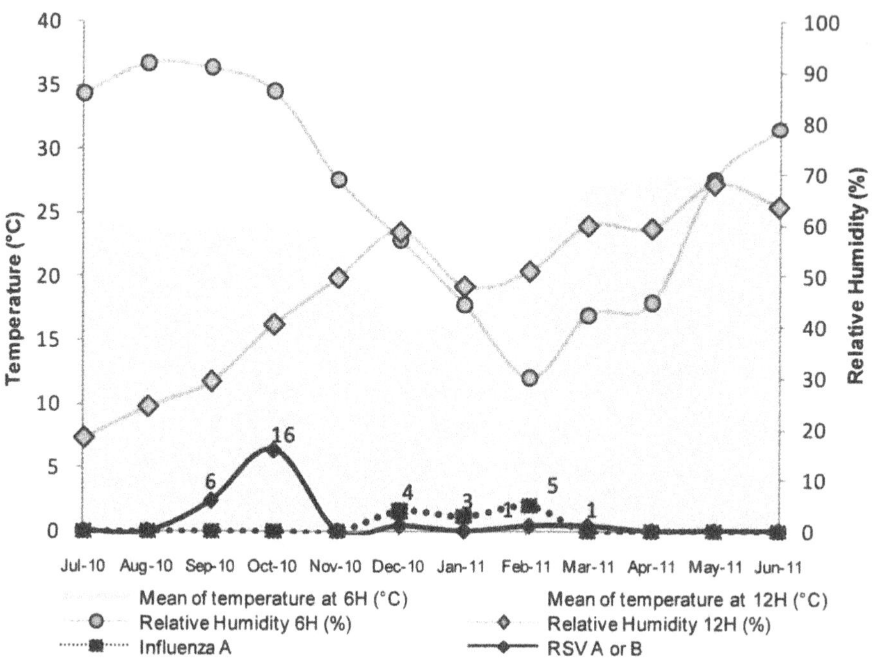

Figure 2. Progression of the epidemics of RSV and influenza virus infections related to temperature and relative humidity values recorded at 6 AM and 12 noon.

Our study is the first of its type in Burkina Faso and warrants follow-up to confirm the seasonality of RSV infection and the period during which this virus circulates. The results presented here assess the involvement of the most frequent pathogenic viruses in upper and lower respiratory tract infections in young children from Burkina Faso. Our findings raise the question of sparing antibiotics by introducing routine detection of viruses. Such a strategy would be supported by the weak mortality attributed to RSV, which is the most aggressive viral agent in Africa [21]. However, the expensive cost of multiplex PCR testing prevents feasibility in routine practice. The less costly direct immunofluorescence assay has shown very low yield in this study, and consequently can not be recommended as an alternative routine test. Further studies are warranted to achieve the best strategy for management of childhood respiratory tract infections in Burkina Faso. More extensive research on the etiological agents of ARIs can only be beneficial, facilitating early adoption of appropriate treatment strategies.

Acknowledgments

The authors are grateful to Nikki-Sabourin-Gibbs, Rouen University Hospital, for editing the manuscript. We also thank Mrs Krystyna Astier for her constant support of the cooperation between the university hospitals of Rouen and Ouagadougou.

Author Contributions

Conceived and designed the experiments: MG SO CM RO DY. Performed the experiments: RO AV BT ZABNB FTY. Analyzed the data: MG SO. Contributed reagents/materials/analysis tools: DK PB LC. Wrote the paper: SO MG CM JCP.

References

1. Williams BG, Gouws E, Boschi-Pinto C, Bryce J, Dye C (2002) Estimates of world-wide distribution of child deaths from acute respiratory infections. Lancet Infect Dis 2: 25–32.
2. Tall FR, Valian A, Curtis V, Traore A, Nacro B, et al. (1994) [Acute respiratory infections in pediatric hospital at Bobo-Dioulasso (Burkina Faso)]. Arch Pediatr 1: 249–254.
3. Liu L, Johnson HL, Cousens S, Perin J, Scott S, et al. (2012) Global, regional, and national causes of child mortality: an updated systematic analysis for 2010 with time trends since 2000. Lancet 379: 2151–2161.
4. Tregoning JS, Schwarze J (2010) Respiratory viral infections in infants: causes, clinical symptoms, virology, and immunology. Clin Microbiol Rev 23: 74–98.
5. Ruuskanen O, Lahti E, Jennings LC, Murdoch DR (2011) Viral pneumonia. Lancet 377: 1264–1275.
6. Marguet C, Lubrano M, Gueudin M, Le Roux P, Deschildre A, et al. (2009) In very young infants severity of acute bronchiolitis depends on carried viruses. PLoS One 4: e4596.
7. Kouni S, Karakitsos P, Chranioti A, Theodoridou M, Chrousos G, et al. (2012) Evaluation of viral co-infections in hospitalized and non-hospitalized children with respiratory infections using microarrays. Clin Microbiol Infect.
8. Simoes EAF, Cherian T, Chow J, Shahid-Salles SA, Laxminarayan R, et al. (2006) Acute Respiratory Infections in Children.
9. Ho A, Fox R, Seaton RA, MacConnachie A, Peters E, et al. (2010) Hospitalised adult patients with Suspected 2009 H1N1 Infection at Regional Infectious Diseases Units in Scotland–most had alternative final diagnoses. J Infect 60: 83–85.
10. Lillie PJ, Duncan CJ, Sheehy SH, Meyer J, O'Hara GA, et al. (2012) Distinguishing malaria and influenza: early clinical features in controlled human experimental infection studies. Travel Med Infect Dis 10: 192–196.
11. Gessner BD, Shindo N, Briand S (2011) Seasonal influenza epidemiology in sub-Saharan Africa: a systematic review. Lancet Infect Dis 11: 223–235.
12. Bellau-Pujol S, Vabret A, Legrand L, Dina J, Gouarin S, et al. (2005) Development of three multiplex RT-PCR assays for the detection of 12 respiratory RNA viruses. J Virol Methods 126: 53–63.
13. Niang MN, Diop OM, Sarr FD, Goudiaby D, Malou-Sompy H, et al. (2010) Viral etiology of respiratory infections in children under 5 years old living in tropical rural areas of Senegal: The EVIRA project. J Med Virol 82: 866–872.
14. Kwofie TB, Anane YA, Nkrumah B, Annan A, Nguah SB, et al. (2012) Respiratory viruses in children hospitalized for acute lower respiratory tract infection in Ghana. Virol J 9: 78.
15. Laurent C, Dugue AE, Brouard J, Nimal D, Dina J, et al. (2012) Viral epidemiology and severity of respiratory infections in infants in 2009: a prospective study. Pediatr Infect Dis J 31: 827–831.

16. Marcone DN, Ellis A, Videla C, Ekstrom J, Ricarte C, et al. (2013) Viral etiology of acute respiratory infections in hospitalized and outpatient children in Buenos Aires, Argentina. Pediatr Infect Dis J 32: e105–110.
17. Njouom R, Yekwa EL, Cappy P, Vabret A, Boisier P, et al. (2012) Viral etiology of influenza-like illnesses in Cameroon, January-December 2009. J Infect Dis 206 Suppl 1: S29–35.
18. D'Acremont V, Kilowoko M, Kyungu E, Philipina S, Sangu W, et al. (2014) Beyond malaria–causes of fever in outpatient Tanzanian children. N Engl J Med 370: 809–817.
19. Okiro EA, Ngama M, Bett A, Nokes DJ (2012) The incidence and clinical burden of respiratory syncytial virus disease identified through hospital outpatient presentations in Kenyan children. PLoS One 7: e52520.
20. Stensballe LG, Devasundaram JK, Simoes EA (2003) Respiratory syncytial virus epidemics: the ups and downs of a seasonal virus. Pediatr Infect Dis J 22: S21–32.
21. Robertson SE, Roca A, Alonso P, Simoes EA, Kartasasmita CB, et al. (2004) Respiratory syncytial virus infection: denominator-based studies in Indonesia, Mozambique, Nigeria and South Africa. Bull World Health Organ 82: 914–922.
22. Haynes AK, Manangan AP, Iwane MK, Sturm-Ramirez K, Homaira N, et al. (2013) Respiratory syncytial virus circulation in seven countries with Global Disease Detection Regional Centers. J Infect Dis 208 Suppl 3: S246–254.
23. Debiaggi M, Canducci F, Ceresola ER, Clementi M (2012) The role of infections and coinfections with newly identified and emerging respiratory viruses in children. Virol J 9: 247.
24. Feikin DR, Njenga MK, Bigogo G, Aura B, Aol G, et al. (2013) Viral and bacterial causes of severe acute respiratory illness among children aged less than 5 years in a high malaria prevalence area of western Kenya, 2007–2010. Pediatr Infect Dis J 32: e14–19.
25. Onyango CO, Welch SR, Munywoki PK, Agoti CN, Bett A, et al. (2012) Molecular epidemiology of human rhinovirus infections in Kilifi, coastal Kenya. J Med Virol 84: 823–831.
26. Pretorius MA, Madhi SA, Cohen C, Naidoo D, Groome M, et al. (2012) Respiratory viral coinfections identified by a 10-plex real-time reverse-transcription polymerase chain reaction assay in patients hospitalized with severe acute respiratory illness–South Africa, 2009–2010. J Infect Dis 206 Suppl 1: S159–165.
27. Azziz Baumgartner E, Dao CN, Nasreen S, Bhuiyan MU, Mah EMS, et al. (2012) Seasonality, timing, and climate drivers of influenza activity worldwide. J Infect Dis 206: 838–846.
28. Lowen AC, Mubareka S, Steel J, Palese P (2007) Influenza virus transmission is dependent on relative humidity and temperature. PLoS Pathog 3: 1470–1476.
29. Tamerius J, Nelson MI, Zhou SZ, Viboud C, Miller MA, et al. (2011) Global influenza seasonality: reconciling patterns across temperate and tropical regions. Environ Health Perspect 119: 439–445.

16

Missed Opportunities for Early Access to Care of HIV-Infected Infants in Burkina Faso

Malik Coulibaly[1]*, Nicolas Meda[1,2], Caroline Yonaba[3], Sylvie Ouedraogo[4], Malika Congo[5], Mamoudou Barry[6], Elisabeth Thio[1], Issa Siribié[1], Fla Koueta[4], Diarra Ye[4], Ludovic Kam[3], Stéphane Blanche[7], Phillipe Van De Perre[8], Valériane Leroy[9], for the MONOD Study Group ANRS 12206¶

1 Projet MONOD ANRS 12206, Centre de Recherche Internationale pour la Santé, Site ANRS Burkina, Université de Ouagadougou, Ouagadougou, Burkina Faso, **2** Centre Muraz, Bobo Dioulasso, Burkina Faso, **3** Service de Pédiatrie, CHU Yalgado Ouédraogo, Ouagadougou, Burkina Faso, **4** Service de Pédiatrie Médicale, CHU Charles de Gaulle, Ouagadougou, Burkina Faso, **5** Laboratoire de Bactériologie - Virologie CHU Yalgado Ouédraogo, Ouagadougou, Burkina Faso, **6** Service de laboratoire, CHU Charles de Gaulle, Ouagadougou, Burkina Faso, **7** Groupe hospitalier Necker- Enfants malades, Paris, France, **8** Inserm U1058, Université Montpellier 1, Montpellier, France, **9** Inserm, U897, Institut de Santé Publique, Epidémiologie et Développement (ISPED), Université de Bordeaux, Bordeaux, France

Abstract

Objective: The World Health Organization (WHO) has recommended a universal antiretroviral therapy (ART) for all HIV-infected children before the age of two since 2010, but this implies an early identification of these infants. We described the Prevention of Mother-to-Child HIV Transmission (PMTCT) cascade, the staffing and the quality of infrastructures in pediatric HIV care facilities, in Ouagadougou, Burkina Faso.

Methods: We conducted a cross-sectional survey in 2011 in all health care facilities involved in PMTCT and pediatric HIV care in Ouagadougou. We assessed them according to their coverage in pediatric HIV care and WHO standards, through a desk review of medical registers and a semi-structured questionnaire administered to health-care workers (HCW).

Results: In 2011, there was no offer of care in primary health care facilities for HIV-infected children in Ouagadougou. Six district hospitals and two university hospitals provided pediatric HIV care. Among the 67 592 pregnant women attending antenatal clinics in 2011, 85.9% were tested for HIV. The prevalence of HIV was 1.8% (95% Confidence Interval: 1.7%–1.9%). Among the 1 064 HIV-infected pregnant women attending antenatal clinics, 41.4% received a mother-to-child HIV transmission prevention intervention. Among the HIV-exposed infants, 313 (29.4%) had an early infant HIV test, and 306 (97.8%) of these infants tested received their result within a four-month period. Among the 40 children initially tested HIV-infected, 33 (82.5%) were referred to a health care facility, 3 (9.0%) were false positive, and 27 (90.0%) were initiated on ART. Although health care facilities were adequately supplied with HIV drugs, they were hindered by operational challenges such as shortage of infrastructures, laboratory reagents, and trained HCW.

Conclusions: The PMTCT cascade revealed bottle necks in PMTCT intervention and HIV early infant diagnosis. The staffing in HIV care and quality of health care infrastructures were also insufficient in 2011 in Ouagadougou.

Editor: Julian W. Tang, Alberta Provincial Laboratory for Public Health/University of Alberta, Canada

Funding: The study was supported in part by the MONOD ANRS 12206 project granted by the European and Developing Countries Clinical Trial Partnership (EDCTP), the CRP-santé in Luxembourg and the French ANRS-Inserm. Dr. Malik Coulibaly is a fellow PhD candidate of the Doctoral School of Society, Politics and Public Health, Bordeaux, France funded by the MONOD consortium. The content of this publication is solely the responsibility of the authors and does not necessarily represent the official views of any of the institutions mentioned above. The funders had no role in study design, data collection and analysis, decision to publish, or preparation of the manuscript.

Competing Interests: The authors have declared that no competing interests exist.

* Email: coulmalik@yahoo.fr

¶ Membership of the MONOD Study Group ANRS 12206 is provided in Appendix S1.

Introduction

Despite the efficacy of Prevention of Mother-To-Child- HIV Transmission (PMTCT), Human Immunodeficiency Virus (HIV) pediatric infection still occurs in Africa because of the lack of operational access to this intervention. Without any intervention, mortality of HIV infected children can reach up to 35% before the first birthday and up to 52% before the second birthday [1,2], and the untreated survivors would need substantial care [3]. However early antiretroviral treatment routinely started before 12 weeks of age significantly increases infant survival by 76%, reduces morbidity and enhances immunological benefits [4,5,6,7]. The 2010 World Health Organization (WHO) revised guidelines recommend early antiretroviral treatment in all HIV infected children less than two years of age, regardless of their immune status [8]. These guidelines also recommend a routine Early Infant Diagnosis (EID) from six-weeks of age of all HIV-exposed children. EID requires sophisticated technology before 18 months of age because of the persistence of maternal antibodies in infants [9]. In addition, the uptake at each step in the EID cascade highlights that even with the highest reported level of uptake, nearly half of HIV-infected infants may not successfully complete the cumulative cascade [10]. In sub-Saharan Africa, HIV-exposed infants continue to suffer from insufficient access to EID and antiretroviral therapy. In 2010, a survey was conducted in Burkina Faso, Ghana and Côte d'Ivoire, to identify the major challenges regarding HIV prophylaxis for children in West Africa [11]. The results of this survey indicated that only a small proportion of HIV-exposed newborns received antiretroviral prophylaxis. Scaling-up management of early pediatric HIV infection remains challenging in West African countries in 2011. But there is a need to increase the PMTCT coverage and to trace the children born in the setting of the PMTCT programs [12]. It is crucial to identify the barriers at the national level. Burkina Faso is a West-African developing country where HIV prevalence was about 1.0% in 2010 [13]. HIV EID in children born to HIV-infected mothers is organized in cascade from the district health care facilities, towards district hospital laboratories, to the university hospital laboratories. There are few data on the full PMTCT cascade coverage and postnatal services in regard to infants born to HIV-infected mothers. Problems are related to resource management, and lack of assessment of sites.

We described the access to pediatric HIV diagnosis and care in Ouagadougou, the capital of Burkina Faso. We also assessed the health care facilities regarding the conformance of staff and infrastructures with WHO standards for the care of HIV infected infants in Ouagadougou in 2010–2011.

Methods

Access to HIV care for infants in Burkina Faso

Burkina Faso is administratively divided into 13 regions, 45 provinces and 351 rural and urban municipalities. In 2011, the public health system was organized around four types of hospitals: district, confessional, regional, and university hospitals. Besides the public health facilities, Burkina Faso had also a large number of private health care facilities and traditional healers [14].

The "big" Ouagadougou equated the Center region with a population of 2 136 582 inhabitants in 2011, of whom 39.7% were children less than 15 years of age [14]. The Center region was the most populous and urbanized of the 13 administrative regions of Burkina Faso, with a land area of 2 869 square kilometers [15]. We identified in this region two university hospitals, five district hospitals, one confessional hospital, eight hospitals without surgical units, and 81 primary health care facilities [16]. According to the 2010 health and demographic survey, the HIV prevalence in Ouagadougou was estimated at 2.1% (95% CI: 1.5–2.7) in 2010 [13].

PMTCT services are integrated in the national health system. All pregnant women who come for antenatal care in a health care facility are expected to be counseled for HIV testing. In case of consent, HIV screening is performed on-site using rapid HIV antibody tests, with a simultaneous HIV result delivery. The pregnant women who attend antenatal consultation with a documented positive result are also tested for the sake control, unless that they are already treated with antiretroviral drugs. In any case, there were included in the PMTCT cascade.

In Burkina Faso, the option A of PMTCT was still recommended in 2011 and HIV-infected pregnant women were eligible to antiretroviral treatment on the basis of CD4 count. Pregnant women with more than 350 cells/mm^3 CD4 count were prescribed zidovudine at 28 weeks gestation in antepartum. In intrapartum, at onset of labor, a single dose of nevirapine and the first dose of zidovudine/lamivudine were given. In postpartum, a daily zidovudine/lamivudine was given for seven days. Whenever the pregnant women's CD4 count was inferior or equal to 350 cells/mm^3 a triple antiretroviral therapy was started as soon as diagnosed, and continued for life. Infants received a daily nevirapine dose from birth up to one week after the complete cessation of breastfeeding. When mothers were not breastfeeding or were on antiretroviral drugs, infants were given *a* daily nevirapine dose up to six weeks of age. Infant breastfeeding was the most recommended feeding option.

After delivery, HIV-infected mothers and their children were advised to go to the nearest health care facility for a postnatal visit and an EID preformed since six weeks of age. This EID was based on a first deoxyribonucleic acid polymerase chain reaction (DNA PCR) test on a Dried Blood Spot (DBS) and was scheduled once a month. The DBS were sent for processing by the corresponding district hospital to one of the three laboratories in Ouagadougou region (the university hospital Yalgado Ouédraogo, the university hospital Charles de Gaulle, and the Saint Camille hospital). All HIV tests results were sent back to the health care facilities via the corresponding district hospitals. In case of a first positive DBS result, a second DNA PCR test is performed on a blood sample to confirm HIV infection [17].

Context and study design

The study was conducted in the implementation phase of the MONOD ANRS 12206 clinical trial (ClinicalTrial.gov registry n°NCT01127204), which was approved by the national ethics committee and the Burkina Faso Ministry of Health. The study was conducted in the capital of the country (Ouagadougou). Health professionals who were interviewed and parents of children who were enrolled for treatment provided a clear written consent. The ethics committee approved the consent procedure. The informed consent was waived for the use of aggregate register data.

The ANRS 12206 MONOD trial is a randomized controlled trial whose aim is to assess a simplified once daily antiretroviral treatment in virologically suppressed HIV infected children initially treated with a triple therapy containing lopinavir/ritonavir before the age of two (Appendix S1).

We undertook a cross-sectional survey from January 2011 to January 2012, to evaluate the performance of PMTCT cascade, and the conformance of infrastructures and staff in health care facilities with pediatric HIV services in Ouagadougou.

Study site and population

We included all the health care facilities providing PMTCT services, infant HIV diagnosis and antiretroviral treatments in Ouagadougou. We first used their 2011 aggregate data to document the PMTCT cascade. Then, in each health care facility, we interviewed all the heads of the various services: health districts, health care facilities, PMTCT services, laboratories, pharmacies, pediatric services, statistics and epidemiology surveillance division, and human resource services.

Data collection

We used 2010 and 2011 Ministry of Health statistical yearbook, as the reference figures [14,16]. We designed a semi-structured questionnaire with three sections according to the staff targeted: pediatric, laboratory and pharmacy services. Two medical epidemiologists, one midwife and one sociologist carried out the desk review and interviewed the selected health professionals. The questionnaire reviewed variables related to PMTCT statistics (cascade of HIV care from antenatal services to EID of HIV-exposed children at six weeks of age and antiretroviral treatment care for HIV-infected children), infrastructures, laboratory reagents, essential drug management and health professionals staffing (doctors, nurses, pharmacists, and laboratory technicians). The staff interviews helped to check registers and identify difficulties faced in providing early HIV infant diagnosis and treatment, and possible solutions.

In 2011, there were 103 health care facilities providing PMTCT services in Ouagadougou and we collected data from all of them. In each health care facility, there was a statistics manager who was in charge of collecting data monthly in a register provided by the Ministry of Health. Pregnant women received for antenatal consultation were recorded in a register that was later used by the statistics manager. A report was then sent to the district head of statistics and epidemiology surveillance division, who compiled the different health care facility reports with Excel software. In our study, we monthly recorded data in term of aggregate number of the different variables related to the PMTCT cascade, from the health care facility registers as well as the district registers, for comparison. In case of discrepancies, we monitored the data recording process to correct the errors. Finally, we were able to document individual data for the HIV-infected children diagnosed and transferred to HIV pediatric care for antiretroviral treatment in the MONOD trial.

For drug management, we checked the registers where the drug management was recorded to determine the availability of drugs and stock-outs. We checked the availability of antiretroviral drugs needed for the national guideline treatment: zidovudine or stavudine or abacavir, lamivudine or emtricitabine, nevirapine or efavirenz, and lopinavir/ritonavir. For opportunistic infection treatment and prophylaxis, we checked the availability of the following drugs: cotrimoxazole, nistatine, miconazole, amphotericine B, ciprofloxacine, ceftriaxone, acyclovir, and anti-tuberculosis drugs.

Finally, we checked the laboratory reagent management and availability with the responsible of laboratories in the corresponding registers.

To document the PMTCT cascade, we used the Ministry of Health method to estimate the expected number of pregnancies, based on the expected number of births multiplied by 1.10 [14]. The expected number of births is equal to the number of women of childbearing age multiplied by the corrected fertility rate of the Center region, equal to 0.1247. The logic of multiplying the expected number of births by 1.10 to obtain the number of expected pregnancies comes from a study of Sedgh et al. who found that 10% of pregnancies end in abortions in Western Africa [18].

Essential infrastructure requirement for health care centers

In 2008, WHO published an operational manual for HIV high prevalence resource constraint settings, to assess health care facilities serving HIV infected people [19].

The WHO defines health care facility's space, design, power supply, water, hygiene and sanitation, and equipment requirements to be able to deliver quality HIV prevention, care and treatment services. We assessed health care facilities using the following WHO criteria: space, privacy and confidentiality, infection control (tuberculosis infection and HIV infection), safe water supply and hygiene (sanitation, hand washing and other hygiene practices, waste management, latrine/toilet, and cleaning), communications, power, and fire safety. The standards require using color-coded waste containers and fire extinguishers. Space requirement is at least 9 m^2 for consultation room, 2.25 m^2 for counseling room, 9 m^2 for laboratory specimen analysis room, and 9 m^2 for pharmacy room [19].

We checked the space available in pediatric consultation ward, laboratory, and pharmacy rooms. This criteria was classified as conform if the available space was superior or equal to that required by the WHO standards. We also checked other qualitative criteria such as the availability of power supply, infection control and the respect of privacy and confidentiality by health professionals. The conformance was good if all the criteria were met. For laboratory tests, we assessed the capacity for performing the required tests in hospitals, without neither shortages of laboratory reagents nor failure of medical devices.

Finally, the conformance was good if antiretroviral drugs and drugs for opportunistic infection treatment and prophylaxis were available to treat HIV infected children with a regimen recommended by the national guidelines.

Statistical analysis

The prevalence of HIV infected pregnant women was calculated by dividing the number of HIV infected pregnant women by the total number of pregnant women screened for HIV infection. The 95% confidence intervals were determined according to the following formula: $(P - Z_{1-\frac{\alpha}{2}}\sqrt{\frac{P(1-P)}{n}} + \frac{1}{2n}, P + Z_{1-\frac{\alpha}{2}}\sqrt{\frac{P(1-P)}{n}} + \frac{1}{2n})$ [20] where p = prevalence, n = sample size. We described the coverage of pediatric HIV services and the flow from HIV-exposed children to access to ART, of HIV-infected children. The cascade of care was compiled on Microsoft Excel software using proportions. All the proportions of the PMTCT cascade were calculated by dividing the total number of favorable cases by the number of eligible cases with their 95% confidence intervals according to the formula previously mentioned.

Results

From the 103 health care facilities providing PMTCT services in Ouagadougou in 2011, 127 health professionals were interviewed: 7 (5.5%) pediatricians, 5 (3.9%) general practitioners, 10 (7.9%) pharmacists, 5 (3.9%) nurse-epidemiologists, 75 (59.1%) nurses, 7 (5.5%) midwives, 9 (7.1%) pharmacist assistants, 5 (3.9%) laboratory technicians, 2 (1.6%) biologists, and 2 (1.6%) human resource managers.

Staffing in pediatric HIV health services

In 2010, there was no HIV treatment for HIV-infected children in primary health care facilities in Ouagadougou. All pediatric HIV care was provided by the six district hospitals, and two university hospitals. In these hospitals, a total of 225 health professionals were directly involved in pediatric HIV infection care, and among them 40% worked in the two university hospitals (Table 1). Overall, 10.7% were pediatricians, 4.4% general practitioners, 19.1% nurses, 5.8% counselors, 8.9% pharmacists, and 29.8% laboratory technicians. Six of the eight hospitals had at least one pediatrician.

In 2010, the total population of children less than 15 years old in the whole region was estimated at 811 115 [16]. With an HIV prevalence of 0.26% in children less than 15 years old [11], we estimated the number of HIV infected children less than 15 to be about 2 109 (811 115×0.26%) in Ouagadougou. With 24 pediatricians in this area (10.7% of the overall staff dedicated to pediatric HIV care), one pediatrician was responsible for 33 797 (811 115/24) children less than 15 years age of whom 88 (2 109/24) were HIV infected.

Table 1. Staff involved in HIV pediatric care per health district or university hospitals, and qualification, in Ouagadougou, in 2010.

	Pediatricians	General practitioners	Pharmacists	Laboratory technicians	Psychologist/ counselors	Nurses	Others	Total
District hospitals	8	9	6	38	6	30	36	133
Mean per hospital	1.6	1.8	1.2	7.6	1.2	6	7.2	26.6
University hospital	16	1	14	29	7	13	12	92
Mean per hospital	8	0.5	7	14.5	3.5	6.5	6	46

Others: pharmacy assistants and laboratory assistants.

When evaluating the conformance of health staff requirements of the WHO standards in the health district hospitals [19], the staff is overall insufficient: general practitioners are less than 1/10 000, and pharmacists are less than 1/20 000 in all the five health districts of Ouagadougou. We had more than 1/4000 nurses in four health districts. Overall, both physician and pharmacist staff were scarce.

PMTCT cascade

In 2011, out of the 76 935 expected pregnancies in the Center region, 67 592 attended at least one antenatal consultation (87.8%). Among the pregnant women attending antenatal consultation, 58 036 accepted to be HIV-tested (85.9%) and the HIV prevalence was 1.8% (95% CI: 1.7%–1.9%). Furthermore, 441 out of the 1 064 HIV-infected pregnant women (41.4%) benefitted from a PMTCT intervention (option A). Then, only 313 (29.4%) HIV-exposed infants (0–18 months) had an HIV virologic test on a DBS, and 306 (97.8%) among these infants tested received their results, usually within a month, but sometimes within a four-month period. Still among the infants tested, 40 children were initially identified as HIV-infected, and 33 (82.5%) out the infants tested, were referred to the MONOD study sites before the age of two for an HIV test confirmation using a deoxyribonucleic acid polymerase chain reaction (DNA PCR). With three children identified as false positive (9%) and 30 (91%) confirmed to be HIV-infected, the HIV prevalence was estimated to be 9.6% (95% CI: 6.3%–12.9%). Finally, 27 children (90.0%) were enrolled in the MONOD ANRS 12206 trial and treated with a triple lopinavir/ritonavir based therapy (Table 2). Their median age at diagnosis was 13 months [IQR: 7–19].

Seven children (17.5%) were not referred for HIV care. One of them died before his laboratory result was released. The six remaining did not come back for their laboratory results and we were not able to contact them because of missing telephone numbers or addresses in the health care facility registers.

Among the six (18.2%) children who were referred to MONOD clinical sites, but were not enrolled in the trial to start an antiretroviral therapy, two died before being able to initiate treatment because of their advanced stage of HIV disease. One was lost to-follow-up after his father refusal to consent for treatment, and three were finally controlled as HIV-negative and not eligible for antiretroviral treatment.

Infrastructures

The conformance of infrastructures was globally gauged "not conform" because of two criteria: safe waste management and fire safety. Indeed, none of the health care facilities had either segregate color-coded waste containers or fire extinguishers.

Essential laboratory tests and apparatus

The availability of essential laboratory tests was checked in health care facilities (Table 3). The lack of some of the laboratory tests was associated to either a failure/lack of the corresponding laboratory apparatus or a reagent shortage. The table 4 displays the reasons for the laboratory non conformance. In addition, lack of apparatus maintenance has been underlined in all the health care facilities.

Essential drugs

The availability of essential antiretroviral drugs was quite good in 2010, and the conformance was judged to be good in spite of few shortages which did not affect the treatment of HIV-infected patient according to national guidelines. A shortage of seven days

Table 2. The PMTCT cascade until HIV pediatric care in Ouagadougou, 2011.

Designation	Number	Percentage (%)	Confidence Interval 95%
Pregnant women expected	76 935	100%	-
Pregnant women attending antenatal consultation	67 592	87.8 (100%)	[87.6–88.0]
Pregnant women having been counseled for HIV testing	60 156	89.0	[88.8–89.2]
Pregnant women having been HIV-tested	58 036	85.9 (100%) (96.5% of the counseled women)	[85.6–86.1]
HIV-infected pregnant women	1 064	1.8 (100%)	[1.7–1.9]
Pregnant women exposed to PMTCT intervention	441	41.4	[38.4–44.4]
HIV-exposed infants having been HIV-tested using DBS	313	29.4 (100%)	[26.6–32.2]
DBS tests results returned	306	97.8	[96.0–99.6]
Infants identified as HIV-infected on the first DBS test (100%)	40	12.8	[8.9–16.6]
HIV-infected infants referred to pediatric care	33	82.5	[71.9–95.5]
Infants confirmed as HIV-infected on the second test (DNA PCR on blood sample)	30	9.6 (100%)	[6.3–12.9]
HIV-infected infants initiated on antiretroviral therapy	27	90.0	[79.2–100.0]

100% is the reference number.
DNA PCR = deoxyribonucleic acid polymerase chain reaction.
DBS = dried blood spot.

was observed for lopinavir/ritonavir, lamivudine and abacavir in Charles de Gaulle university hospital in 2010. In addition, Bogodogo district hospital noticed a shortage of 30 days for the combination lamivudine + nevirapine + stavudine (triomune junior). The drugs for opportunistic infections were available and conform to WHO standards, but they were not free of charge for HIV-infected patients in 2010, except anti-tuberculosis drugs and cotrimoxazole.

Discussion

This cross-sectional survey assessed for the first time the staff, the infrastructures and the PMTCT cascade from prenatal PMTCT up to pediatric HIV care, in all health care facilities providing pediatric HIV care services in Ouagadougou. We documented that only 40% of HIV-infected women received a PMTCT intervention and less than a third of HIV-exposed children were tested during the postnatal period. Moreover, it provides a description of the health care system in this country, useful to understand some of the weaknesses of the system when it comes to the issue of EID in all HIV exposed children, and their access to antiretroviral therapy.

There are several drawbacks in our observations. Firstly, the incompleteness of the data collected may be the source of information bias in this study. Our study method was partially based on desk review, where we checked the statistics in the available registers. Unfortunately, we could not get all the information related to our objectives. For instance, it had not been possible to routinely determine the duration of laboratory reagent shortage. Secondly, we were not able to really link one-to-one the PMTCT with the postnatal data, and we assumed that each HIV-pregnant woman was supposed to give one alive pregnancy outcome, without taking into account multiple pregnancy outcomes or stillbirth. Furthermore, some of the infants tested in 2011, had their mothers attend their first antenatal consultation in the preceding years, and some of the pregnant women tracked in 2011 will give birth in 2012 as well, resulting in a kind of compensation allowing the PMTCT and EID coverage estimates. Consequently, we feel that these figures were accurate enough to understand the overall patient flow throughout the health care system services. Thirdly, the conformance of health care services was determined with respect to the WHO standards, ideally suitable for district hospitals [19]. These standards might not be suitable when applied to university hospitals, where a higher standard of care is expected. Lastly, in terms of representativeness, our results showed a similar proportion of antenatal consultations among pregnant women in Ouagadougou, compared to the rest of the country (88%) [14]. As a matter of fact, Ouagadougou had a greater number of private health facilities compared to the rest of the country [14], and their statistics were

Table 3. Conformance of Ouagadougou hospitals according to WHO standards, in 2010.

WHO criteria of conformance	District hospital	University hospital
	N=6	N=2
	# conform/N	# conform/N
Infrastructure		
Room space >9 m^2	6/6	2/2
Power (electricity) available	6/6	2/2
Tap water available	6/6	2/2
Tuberculosis infection control (ventilated waiting rooms, cough control, good patient flow)	6/6	2/2
HIV infection control (injection safety, appropriate use and disposal of sharps, personal protective equipment for staff, post exposure prophylaxis available)	6/6	2/2
Waste management (3 color-containers available)	0/6	0/2
Privacy of patient's test protected	6/6	2/2
Communication (land line available)	6/6	2/2
Fire extinguisher available	0/6	0/2
Conclusion	**Not conform**	**Not conform**
Laboratory test available		
Rapid HIV antibody test	4/6	2/2
DBS	6/6	2/2
CD4 count	1/6	1/2
Hemoglobin determination	5/6	2/2
Serum alanin aminotransferase	4/6	2/2
Serum creatinin & blood urea nitrogen	4/6	2/2
Bilirubin determination	4/6	2/2
Lactic acid	5/6	2/2
Blood sugar	4/6	2/2
Tuberculosis diagnostics	6/6	2/2
Pregnancy test	6/6	2/2
Urine dipstick for sugar and protein	6/6	2/2
Conclusion	**Not conform**	**Not conform**
Drugs available		
Antiretroviral drugs	6/6	2/2
Opportunistic infection drugs	6/6	2/2
Conclusion	**Conform**	**Conform**
Staff		
One general practitioner for 10 000	0/6	Not applicable*
One pharmacist for 20 000	0/6	Not applicable*
One nurse for 4 000	4/6	Not applicable*
Conclusion	**Not conform**	**Not applicable**

*The university hospitals are located in the center region, but patients are referred from the whole country.

not included in our figures. As a result, the number of antenatal consultations was lower than that was really carried out in Ouagadougou. However, in our study, we considered all pregnant women who were on PMTCT antiretroviral protocol with the hypothesis that their children would be referred to the public system if they were found to be HIV-infected.

Our study helped to identify major challenges facing EID and antiretroviral treatment access for children in Burkina Faso. A survey conducted in Burkina Faso, Ghana and Côte d'Ivoire, from January 2010 to February 2011 had already reported the lack of access to child PMTCT prophylaxis [11]. Our results confirm that in the urban setting of Ouagadougou. The level of missed opportunities was so high that it was difficult to cover sufficiently with PMTCT intervention, the mother-infant couple, estimated at 59%, as well as to offer EID to all HIV-exposed children, reaching 71%. We also conclude that these missed opportunities should be greater at the national level considering the fact that the health

Table 4. Reasons for Ouagadougou laboratory non conformance in 2010.

	District hospitals N = 6		University hospitals N = 2	
Laboratory tests non available	**Lack or apparatus failure**	**Reagent shortage**	**Lack or apparatus failure**	**Reagent shortage**
Rapid HIV antibody test	Non applicable	2	Non applicable	0
CD4 count	5	5	1	0
Hemoglobin determination	1	0	0	0
Serum alanin aminotransferase	1	1	0	0
Serum creatinin & blood urea nitrogen	1	1	0	0
Bilirubin determination	1	1	0	0
Lactic acid	1	0	0	0
Blood sugar	1	1	0	0

care system would be more complex and thus weaker at the rural level in comparison to the urban one.

Some factors could explain these missed opportunities and could be separately addressed. Firstly, the low awareness of HIV prevention and care services in the community could explain the non-attendance of EID services or the rejection of these services by families. In Burkina Faso, only 20.1% of the population attended the secondary school in 2008/2009 [21] and therefore we think that substantial efforts should be developed to make them aware of the benefit of PMTCT services. In addition, men should also be targeted in education, because they are likely to be reluctant to carrying out HIV screening, and they can greatly support their wives in using PMTCT services [22,23].

Secondly, we highlighted the lack of adequate quantitative and qualitative health care workers (HCW) to cover the needs. At the six-week postnatal visit for instance, due to the fact that nurses were not all trained to perform DBS, the DBS could only be performed one day in a month. Mothers who would like have their infant HIV-tested could only return on this unique day, leading to a high attrition rate because of the inadequate offer of this simple service.

Thirdly, the inaccessibility to EID services is also related to the health system organization, as the current DBS sample circuit and transportation is too complicated and should be simplified. Indeed, the need to go through each district hospital while the final laboratory test is performed in each university laboratory hospital should be considered. It would be more efficient to perform the DBS directly in the health care facilities, to limit the lost to follow-up rate. In the neighboring country of Côte d'Ivoire, we had a similar problem of low coverage rate of EID, favored by the civil war, with only 24% of the HIV exposed children early diagnosed in 2010 [24]. In comparison, a study carried out in 2008, showed that DNA polymerase chain reaction testing in routine was 35.2% for children hospitalized in Malawi, but their age was not specified [25].

Similarly, the low PMTCT intervention coverage is related to problems in the health service organization. When a pregnant woman attends antenatal consultation in a health care facility, she is counseled and screened for HIV with a rapid HIV antibody test. In case of HIV infection, she is referred to the referent district hospital in order to carry out the other tests such as CD4 count, before visiting a doctor who would prescribe an option A antiretroviral treatment, mainly based on nevirapine. Then, she is later sent back in the former health care facility, to pursue her antenatal follow-up. Although not documented, we assume that some pregnant women could not reach the district hospitals, thus increasing the number of lost to follow-up. This could explain why a lot of pregnant women attend antenatal consultation but do not benefit from PMTCT intervention, when they are HIV-infected.

Fourthly, there are also laboratory related challenges, with the need to offer routine services while the HIV-prevalence is still low, leading to frequent laboratory reagent shortages. Thairu et al. also confirmed our results about maintenance and reagent stock management, in their study in Burkina Faso and Zimbabwe [26]. A frequently-cited barrier to expansion of EID programs is the cost of the required laboratory assays.

Thus, substantial sequential barriers explain the low PMTCT and EID complete cascade coverage, and the lack of personnel and infrastructure requirements. A review reported that even with the highest reported levels of uptake, nearly half of HIV-infected infants may not complete the cascade successfully [10].

Additionally, we raise the overall problem of the EID strategy performances. In settings with low HIV prevalence or well performing PMTCT program, vertical transmission rates may be as low as 2% at six weeks and the positive predictive value of a single test will be approximately 50%, meaning that only half of infants who are tested positive are truly infected [27,28]. For this reason, a confirmatory test is essential, especially in the context of a low HIV prevalence country such as Burkina Faso. Indeed, in our study, the high rate of false positive DBS (9%) highly affects the positive predictive value of the national HIV screening strategy. Acknowledging this, the test confirmation is a priority and laboratories should implement reliable quality control system and constantly work on maintaining high quality standards of EID.

Antiretroviral access for HIV-infected children looked good in our study when compared to the estimates of the Ethiopian study, where only 8.4% of positive babies had access to antiretroviral treatment [29]. But, it is important to point out the contribution of the Monod trial implementation in our results, which set up a network whose aim was to improve the coverage of pediatric antiretroviral therapy beyond the EID.

A shortage of some antiretroviral drugs was observed in two health care facilities for several days, as a result of delays in reporting. In effect, antiretroviral drugs are provided by the Ministry of Health division for HIV/AIDS (Comité Ministériel de Lutte contre le Sida), and they required periodic reports, before delivery. Hence, a delay in providing a report will ultimately end in a delay in drug supply.

Moreover, while all antiretroviral drugs were free of charge in Burkina Faso in 2010, the opportunistic infection drugs are charged to families. It has already been reported that having to pay for HIV treatment and laboratory tests, increases the risk of lost to follow-up [30].

When analyzing the conformance of health centers with respect to the PMTCT cascade, we can point out that the infrastructure requirements are almost met, and that the absence of fire extinguishers and segregate color-codes waste containers, did not affect antenatal consultation rate which is quite good in a developing country setting such as this. However, the non conformance to laboratory test requirements explained why we observed an attrition of the cascade at the number of children tested for HIV infection. The conformance of pharmacies was found to be good and consequently two-third of HIV infected children were treated. The missed opportunity for treatment was related to communication and pregnant women HIV testing circuit problem.

Globally, the causes of non conformance at the district and university hospitals are almost similar because they are public centers (except Saint Camille hospital), run by the Ministry of Health. The causes could be a lack of resources, or a mismanagement of the available resources.

The problem could be alleviated by improving the communication process between the peripheral health services and the national procurement system. The community awareness should also be improved and contextualized to the socio-cultural needs of the region.

Moreover, training in a large scale on DBS practicing and in HIV care among HCW would be useful and promote task shifting activities [31,32,33]. Finally, characteristics of the health care facilities could be determinant in improving the pediatric HIV care in Africa as reported in the HEART project [34]: characteristics associated with favorable children enrolment in care are nutritional support, linkages with associations of people living with HIV, access to EID and integration of PMTCT services. Applying the South African strategies to improve antiretroviral treatment in the province of KwaZulu-Natal could be beneficial. In addition to training all the staff in contact with mothers and children, they carried out campaigns aimed at increasing HIV testing during immunization and clinics, routinely testing of HIV in children with tuberculosis and malnutrition, and systematically testing for HIV, all children admitted at hospital [35]. However, in Burkina Faso, as the HIV prevalence is lower than that of South Africa, it would be more efficient to start the systematic HIV diagnosis by screening first the children with rapid HIV antibody tests. Expanding these characteristics to improve pediatric HIV treatment in Burkina Faso, warrants further evaluation for improving the scaling up of pediatric HIV care. Finally, as it was reported in South Africa, it is possible to improve the identification of HIV-infected children and ensure a prompt start on ART when needed with relatively simple measures, limited staffing and budgets [35].

Despite an overall good access to prenatal services in Ouagadougou in 2011, there are still many missed opportunities for both the prevention of mother-to-child transmission and the early access to diagnosis and antiretroviral therapy for HIV-infected children before two years of life. The government should look forward to improving the awareness and education among the population, training health care workers for HIV diagnosis and care, facilitating the access to EID and making health care facilities more attractive to families. In addition, the DBS circuit should be simplified to avoid lost to follow-up. Early access to EID and to antiretroviral therapy will require political willingness and leadership to address these health system barriers in Burkina Faso.

Acknowledgments

We acknowledge the Head of Ministry of Health division for AIDS (Comité Ministériel de Lutte contre le Sida), in Burkina Faso, Dr Marie-Joseph Sanou, the regional Director of Health, Dr Amédée Prosper Djiguemdé and all heads of health care facilities in Ouagadougou and their staff for their contribution to data collection. We are grateful to the French GIP ESTHER for its assistance to HIV infected children in Burkina Faso. We would like to give special thanks to Pr Louis Rachid Salmi for his helpful suggestion on using WHO standards.

Author Contributions

Conceived and designed the experiments: M. Coulibaly NM VL PV SB DY LK CY SO MB IS ET M. Congo. Performed the experiments: M. Coulibaly IS ET. Analyzed the data: M. Coulibaly IS VL. Contributed reagents/materials/analysis tools: CY M. Congo MB NM VL PV. Wrote the paper: M. Coulibaly VL SB PV NM FK. Edit the manuscript: VL SB PV ET MB LK CY SO IS DY FK M. Congo.

References

1. Newell ML, Brahmbhatt H, Ghys PD (2004) Child mortality and HIV infection in Africa: a review. AIDS 18 Suppl 2: S27–34.
2. Newell ML, Coovadia H, Cortina-Borja M, Rollins N, Gaillard P, et al. (2004) Mortality of infected and uninfected infants born to HIV-infected mothers in Africa: a pooled analysis. Lancet 364: 1236–1243.
3. Desmonde S, Coffie P, Aka E, Amani-Bosse C, Messou E, et al. (2011) Severe morbidity and mortality in untreated HIV-infected children in a paediatric care programme in Abidjan, Cote d'Ivoire, 2004–2009. BMC Infect Dis 11: 182.
4. Goetghebuer T, Le Chenadec J, Haelterman E, Galli L, Dollfus C, et al. (2012) Short- and long-term immunological and virological outcome in HIV-infected infants according to the age at antiretroviral treatment initiation. Clin Infect Dis 54: 878–881.
5. Prendergast AJ, Penazzato M, Cotton M, Musoke P, Mulenga V, et al. (2012) Treatment of young children with HIV infection: using evidence to inform policymakers. PLoS Med 9: e1001273.
6. Prendergast A, Mphatswe W, Tudor-Williams G, Rakgotho M, Pillay V, et al. (2008) Early virological suppression with three-class antiretroviral therapy in HIV-infected African infants. AIDS 22: 1333–1343.
7. Violari A, Cotton MF, Gibb DM, Babiker AG, Steyn J, et al. (2008) Early antiretroviral therapy and mortality among HIV-infected infants. N Engl J Med 359: 2233–2244.
8. WHO (2010) Antiretroviral therapy for HIV infection in infants and children: Towards universal access. Recommendations for a public health approach. 2010 revision.
9. Nielsen K, Bryson YJ (2000) Diagnosis of HIV infection in children. Pediatr Clin North Am 47: 39–63.
10. Ciaranello AL, Park JE, Ramirez-Avila L, Freedberg KA, Walensky RP, et al. (2011) Early infant HIV-1 diagnosis programs in resource-limited settings: opportunities for improved outcomes and more cost-effective interventions. BMC Med 9: 59.
11. Tchidjou HK, Maria Martino A, Goli LP, Diop Ly M, Zekeng L, et al. (2012) Paediatric HIV infection in Western Africa: the long way to the standard of care. J Trop Pediatr 58: 451–456.
12. Ndondoki C, Brou H, Timite-Konan M, Oga M, Amani-Bosse C, et al. (2013) Universal HIV screening at postnatal points of care: which public health approach for early infant diagnosis in Cote d'Ivoire? PLoS One 8: e67996.

13. Ministère de l'Economie et des Finances Burkina Faso (2011) Enquête Démographique et de Santé et à indicateurs Multiples (EDSBF-MICS IV) 2010. Ouagadougou, Burkina Faso. 50 p. Available: www.measuredhs.com/pubs/pdf/PR9/PR9.pdf. Accessed 2012 September 12.
14. Ministère de la Santé Burkina Faso (2012) Annuaire statistique 2011. Ouagadougou, Burkina Faso. 244 p. Available: http://www.sante.gov.bf/phocadownload/Annuaire_statistique_2011.pdf. Accessed 2013 May 27.
15. Institut National de la Statistique et de la Démographie Burkina Faso (2011) La région du centre en chiffres. Ouagadougou, Burkina Faso. 7 p. Available: http://www.insd.bf/n/contenu/statistiques_regions/regions_en_chiffres_en_2011/reg_chif_c_2011.pdf. Accessed 2014 August 4.
16. Ministère de la Santé Burkina Faso (2011) Annaire statistique 2010. Ouagadougou, Burkina Faso. 204p. Availaible: http://www.sante.gov.bf/phocadownload/Publications_statistiques/Annuaire/annuaire_statistique_sante_2010.pdf. Accessed: 2014 October 5.
17. Ministère de la Santé Comité Ministériel de Lutte contre le SIDA Burkina Faso (2008) Normes et protocoles de prise en charge médicale des personnes vivant avec le VIH au Burkina Faso. Ouagadougou.
18. Sedgh G, Henshaw S, Singh S, Ahman E, Shah IH (2007) Induced abortion: estimated rates and trends worldwide. Lancet 370: 1338–1345.
19. WHO (2008) Operations Manual for Delivery of HIV Prevention, Care and Treatment at Primary Health Centres in High-Prevalence, Resource-Constrained Settings. Geneva, Switzerland. 392 p.
20. Forthofer RN, Lee ES, Hernandez M (2007) Biostatistics: A guide to Design, Analysis, and Discovery: Elsevier. 502 p.
21. Institut National de la Statistique et de la Démographie Burkina Faso (2013) Tableau 05.34: Evolution du taux brut de scolarisation de l'ensemble du secondaire (en %). Ouagadougou, Burkina Faso. Available: http://www.insd.bf/n/contenu/tableaux/T0534.htm. Accessed 2013 May 27.
22. Desgrees-Du-Lou A, Brou H, Djohan G, Becquet R, Ekouevi DK, et al. (2009) Beneficial effects of offering prenatal HIV counselling and testing on developing a HIV preventive attitude among couples. Abidjan, 2002–2005. AIDS Behav 13: 348–355.
23. Brou H, Djohan G, Becquet R, Allou G, Ekouevi DK, et al. (2008) Sexual prevention of HIV within the couple after prenatal HIV-testing in West Africa. AIDS Care 20: 413–418.
24. Folquet-Amonissani M, Dainguy M. E, Amani-Bossé C, Elian-Kouakou J, Méa-Assandé V, et al. Early infant diagnosis and access to pediatric HIV care: barriers and challenges in Abidjan, Ivory Coast in 2011; 2012; Washington DC, USA.
25. Van Rompaey S, Kimfuta J, Kimbondo P, Monn C, Buve A (2011) Operational assessment of access to ART in rural Africa: the example of Kisantu in Democratic Republic of the Congo. AIDS Care 23: 686–693.
26. Thairu L, Katzenstein D, Israelski D (2011) Operational challenges in delivering CD4 diagnostics in sub-Saharan Africa. AIDS Care 23: 814–821.
27. WHO (2010) WHO recommendations on the diagnosis of HIV infection in infants and children. Geneva, Switzerland. 64 p.
28. WHO (2014) March 2014 supplement to the 2013 consolidated guidelines on the use of antiretroviral drugs for treating and preventing HIV infection recommendations for a public health approch. Geneva, Swetzerland. 128 p.
29. Nigatu T, Woldegebriel Y (2011) Analysis of the prevention of mother-to-child transmission (PMTCT) service utilization in Ethiopia: 2006–2010. Reprod Health 8: 6.
30. Leroy V, Malateste K, Rabie H, Lumbiganon P, Ayaya S, et al. (2013) Outcomes of antiretroviral therapy in children in Asia and Africa: a comparative analysis of the IeDEA pediatric multiregional collaboration. J Acquir Immune Defic Syndr 62: 208–219.
31. Zachariah R, Ford N, Philips M, Lynch S, Massaquoi M, et al. (2009) Task shifting in HIV/AIDS: opportunities, challenges and proposed actions for sub-Saharan Africa. Trans R Soc Trop Med Hyg 103: 549–558.
32. Creek T, Tanuri A, Smith M, Seipone K, Smit M, et al. (2008) Early diagnosis of human immunodeficiency virus in infants using polymerase chain reaction on dried blood spots in Botswana's national program for prevention of mother-to-child transmission. Pediatr Infect Dis J 27: 22–26.
33. Oga MA, Ndondoki C, Brou H, Salmon A, Bosse-Amani C, et al. (2011) Attitudes and practices of health care workers toward routine HIV testing of infants in Cote d'Ivoire: the PEDI-TEST ANRS 12165 Project. J Acquir Immune Defic Syndr 57 Suppl 1: S16–21.
34. Adjorlolo-Johnson G, Wahl Uheling A, Ramachandran S, Strasser S, Kouakou J, et al. (2013) Scaling up pediatric HIV care and treatment in Africa: clinical site characteristics associated with favorable service utilization. J Acquir Immune Defic Syndr 62: e7–e13.
35. Bland RM, Ndirangu J, Newell ML (2013) Maximising opportunities for increased antiretroviral treatment in children in an existing HIV programme in rural South Africa. BMJ 346: f550.

The Predictive Value of the NICE "Red Traffic Lights" in Acutely Ill Children

Evelien Kerkhof[1], Monica Lakhanpaul[2], Samiran Ray[3], Jan Y. Verbakel[4], Ann Van den Bruel[5], Matthew Thompson[5], Marjolein Y. Berger[6], Henriette A. Moll[1], Rianne Oostenbrink[1]*, for the European Research Network on recognising serious InfEctions (ERNIE) members¶

1 Erasmus MC-Sophia Children's Hospital, Department of General Pediatrics, Rotterdam, The Netherlands, 2 Department of General and Adolescent Pediatrics, University College London, Institute of Child Health, London, United Kingdom, 3 Pediatric Intensive Care Unit, Great Ormond Street Hospital, London, United Kingdom, 4 Department of General Practice, Katholieke Universiteit Leuven, Leuven, Belgium, 5 Department of Primary Care Health Sciences, University of Oxford, Radcliffe Observatory Quarter, Oxford, United Kingdom, 6 Department of General Practice, University Groningen, University Medical Centre Groningen, Groningen, The Netherlands

Abstract

Objective: Early recognition and treatment of febrile children with serious infections (SI) improves prognosis, however, early detection can be difficult. We aimed to validate the predictive rule-in value of the National Institute for Health and Clinical Excellence (NICE) most severe alarming signs or symptoms to identify SI in children.

Design, Setting and Participants: The 16 most severe ("red") features of the NICE traffic light system were validated in seven different primary care and emergency department settings, including 6,260 children presenting with acute illness.

Main Outcome Measures: We focussed on the individual predictive value of single red features for SI and their combinations. Results were presented as positive likelihood ratios, sensitivities and specificities. We categorised "general" and "disease-specific" red features. Changes in pre-test probability versus post-test probability for SI were visualised in Fagan nomograms.

Results: Almost all red features had rule-in value for SI, but only four individual red features substantially raised the probability of SI in more than one dataset: "does not wake/stay awake", "reduced skin turgor", "non-blanching rash", and "focal neurological signs". The presence of ≥3 red features improved prediction of SI but still lacked strong rule-in value as likelihood ratios were below 5.

Conclusions: The rule-in value of the most severe alarming signs or symptoms of the NICE traffic light system for identifying children with SI was limited, even when multiple red features were present. Our study highlights the importance of assessing the predictive value of alarming signs in clinical guidelines prior to widespread implementation in routine practice.

Editor: Soren Gantt, University of British Columbia, Canada

Funding: EK is supported by ZonMW, a Dutch organisation for health research and development; RO is supported by an unrestricted grant of the Europe Container Terminals B.V and by a fellowship award of European Society of Pediatric Infectious Diseases. The funders had no role in study design, data collection and analysis, decision to publish, or preparation of the manuscript.

Competing Interests: ML was the clinical director leading the NICE fever guideline; we believe this improved the clinical contents of the study.

* E-mail: r.oostenbrink@erasmusmc.nl

¶ Authors who wrote the paper on behalf of the (ERNIE) is provided in the Acknowledgments.

Introduction

Fever is one of the most common symptoms among children presenting to ambulatory care.[1–3] The majority of children presenting with an acute illness to ambulatory care will have self-limiting viral infections, with only a small proportion having a serious infection (SI).[1,4–6] Early recognition and treatment of children with SI are related to better prognosis,[7,8] however identification of SI at first presentation can be difficult.

The National Institute for Health and Clinical Excellence (NICE) 2013 guideline for the management of children with feverish illness provides comprehensive guidance on the assessment, investigation and management of children presenting at different settings, including primary care and pediatric specialty settings.[6,9] One of the key elements of the guideline is a "traffic light" system for the diagnostic assessment of children under five years of age presenting with a feverish illness. This evidence and consensus-based system includes clinical features identified from existing scoring systems for acutely ill children,[10–13] and disease-specific signs and symptoms. Children with the most alarming (or "red") features are considered at higher risk of SI, for whom subsequent management includes invasive investigations, treatment, and hospital admission.

As one of the few evidence-based guidelines for children with fever [14,15] and the only for both primary and secondary care, the NICE febrile child guideline has been implemented in many settings in not only the United Kingdom but also in other countries. Recently, two studies reported low specificities for the approach that any abnormal amber or red feature would indicate possible SI.[16,17] This could be due to the inclusion of amber features, whose association with SI may be weaker.

In this study we aimed to determine the predictive ("rule-in") value of the red features of the NICE traffic light system, both for the individual red features as their combinations for identifying children with SI in various acute pediatric settings in Europe.

Methods

Identification of datasets

We used data on seven independent cohorts [4,18–23] collected by collaborators of the European Research Network on recognising serious InfEctions (ERNIE) group.[24] Data were prospectively collected at first contact using standardised (site-specific) documentation of patient characteristics, except for Monteny et al [19] where data was collected using structured clinical proformas separate from the consultation. All datasets were cohort studies of children in various age ranges (0–16 years), presenting to ambulatory care settings (i.e. general or family practice, pediatric outpatient clinic, pediatric assessment unit or emergency department) with an acute illness or infection.

Two datasets based on primary care settings were considered as low prevalence settings of SI (<5%) and five datasets based on emergency care settings as high prevalence settings (>5%).[25] More details on the original cohorts have been published elsewhere ([4,18–23]).

Ethical approval

This research conforms to the Helsinki Declaration and to local legislation. The original study authors have all agreed to share their data, and had obtained ethical approval from their local research ethics committees for the initial data collection, prior to this study.

Processing of included datasets

Key characteristics of each dataset are shown in table 1. We selected children under the age of five years with an acute illness based on general symptoms [4,21,22] or specifically on the presence of fever [18–20,23], as this is the target group of the NICE guideline (table 1).

The NICE traffic light system includes 16 red features, which are categorised into 5 main domains: Colour (1 red feature), Activity (4 red features), Respiratory (3 red features), Hydration (1 red feature), and Other (7 red features).[6,9] When study variables were not entirely identical to the red features in the NICE febrile child guideline, we identified proxies where possible. Identification and handling of variables has been described earlier [17], a full list of all approximations is described in table S1. When a red feature was not recorded in the dataset and no suitable proxy was identified, this item was excluded from that specific dataset. Table S2 outlines the unrecorded and missing data from each dataset separately.

Missing values were not imputed because the necessary missing-at-random assumption was likely to be incorrect. We considered red features that were "not documented" in individual patient records as "absent", given that the red feature or its proxy was recorded in that particular dataset.[17]

The translation, recoding and data-checking were performed by two authors (EK, JV) and the results of each step were discussed with all primary study authors.[17]

Outcome measures

Serious infections (SI) were defined as sepsis (including bacteremia), meningitis, pneumonia, osteomyelitis, cellulitis, and complicated urinary tract infections. [25] Serious infections (SI) were not only based on clinical diagnosis, but reference standard test criteria were used to determine final diagnoses of SI. Detailed description on these reference standard test criteria are available in the original study papers.[4,18–23] Assessment of the diagnoses to ensure comparability of outcomes was discussed with the lead investigator of each study as described earlier.[17]

Statistical analysis

The individual red features were analysed in every dataset separately. Additionally, results were categorised as "general" red features (items 1–7 and 9–10) and "disease-specific" red features (items 8 and 11–16).

We assessed the rule-in value for SI for each red feature separately by calculating positive likelihood ratios (LR+). Red features were considered to have rule-in value if they raised the probability of illness with a positive likelihood ratio of more than 5.0.[25] The univariable association between each individual red feature and the presence of SI was tested by Chi-square analysis. Likelihood ratios, sensitivity and specificity were measured for the presence of ≥1 RTL, ≥2 RTLs and ≥3 RTLs. The sensitivity and specificity for "general" and "disease-specific" red features were plotted in receiver operating characteristic (ROC) space.

The incremental diagnostic value for up to more than four red features compared to one red feature was evaluated by logistic regression analyses with forward selection (Wald test, p-value <0.05).

We visualised the change in pre-test probability versus post-test probability for SI in a Fagan nomogram.[26]

No overall pooled likelihood ratios were calculated because of the substantial clinical heterogeneity between datasets (differences in setting, inclusion criteria, immunisation schedules and definition of serious infection).[17] All analyses were done with SPSS software (version 20.0, SPSS Inc, Chicago).

Results

Included datasets

We selected 6,260 children under five years of age of seven pre-existing datasets (n = 6,260/10,812, 58%) for diagnostic studies in children with an acute illness (table 1). Children were included based on fever,[19,20,23] acute illness,[4,18] acute infection,[21] and referral for meningeal signs.[22] Children with various severities of co-morbidity were excluded in five studies,[4,19–23], one study excluded children if the acute episode was caused by an exacerbation of a chronic condition[4] and one study excluded children who required immediate resuscitation [18] (table 1). All studies included sepsis, meningitis, pneumonia and complicated urinary tract infections in their outcome definition. Osteomyelitis and cellulitis were explicitly mentioned in five and three datasets, respectively.

The median age of the selected children ranged from 0.8 years to 1.9 years. The prevalence of SI ranged from 1.2% to 4.1% in two datasets from general practice [4,19] and from 9.3% to 40.2% in five datasets from emergency departments and a pediatric assessment unit [18,20–23].

Red traffic lights included in the datasets

Data on all red features included in domains "Colour" and "Hydration" were available in all datasets. The red features "no response to social cues", and "weak, high-pitched or continuous

Table 1. Characteristics of datasets with children <5 years of age suspected of acute illness*.

Dataset	Setting	Country	Inclusion Criteria	Exclusion Criteria	n/ original study population (%)	Prevalence Serious Infection % (CI)	Median Age (IQR)
1. Bleeker et al. 2007[23]	ED	NL	Children aged 1–36 months with fever (T>38) at emergency department, no clear focus identified after evaluation GP or history by pediatrician	Chronic disease, Immunodeficiency	595/595 (100)	23.0 (19.6–26.4)	0.8 (0.3–1.4)
2. Brent et al. 2011[18]	ED	UK	All children presenting with a medical problem to the pediatric emergency-care unit whatever their age	Children who required immediate resuscitation. Comorbidity and chronic illness	494/2777 (18)	9.3 (6.7–11.9)	1.5 (0.9–2.7)
3. Oostenbrink et al. 2004[22]	ED	NL	Children aged 1 month-16 years, meningeal signs at GP, pediatrician or self-referred with neck pain	Comorbidity, ventriculoperitoneal drain	423/593 (71)	40.2 (35.5–44.9)	1.1 (0.5–2.7)
4. Roukema et al. 2008[20]	ED	NL	Children aged 1 month-16 years with fever (T>38) at emergency department, without meningeal irritation	Chronic disease, Immunodeficiency	1459/1750 (83)	11.7 (10.1–13.4)	1.4 (0.7–2.6)
5. Thompson et al. 2009[21]	PAU	UK	Children aged 3 months-16 years with suspected acute infection	Children with diseases liable to cause repeated serious bacterial infection, and infections resulting from penetrating trauma	434/700 (62)	37.1 (32.5-41.7)	1.6 (0.9–2.7)
6. Monteny et al. 2008[19]	GP	NL	Children aged 3 months-6 years, contacting a GP cooperative after hours with fever as the presenting symptom	Language barriers, no repeated inclusion within the last two weeks	487/506 (96)	4.1 (2.3-5.9)	1.7 (0.9–3.0)
7. Van den Bruel et al. 2007[4]	GP/AP/ ED	BE	Non-referred children ≤16 years with acute illness for max 5 days	Traumatic or neurological illness, intoxication, psychiatric or behavioural problems without somatic cause or an exacerbation of a chronic condition. No repeated inclusion of same infant within 5 days. Exclusion of physicians if the assumption of consecutive inclusion was probably violated	2368/3891 (60)	1.2 (0.8–1.6)	1.9 (0.9–3.2)

*Using temperature >38.0°C or general symptoms of acute illness.
GP = General Practice; AP = Ambulatory Pediatric Care; ED = Emergency Department; PAU = Pediatric Assessment Unit; BE = Belgium; NL = the Netherlands; UK = United Kingdom; CI = Confidence Interval IQR= interquartile range.

cry" of domain "Activity" were not recorded in two [20,23], and one dataset [18], respectively. Other red features in this domain were available in all datasets. Red features related to the "Respiratory" domain were not recorded in four ("grunting") [4,21–23], one ("tachypnoea") [22], and two ("chest indrawing") [22,23], datasets respectively. "Disease-specific" red features (items 8 and 11–16) were recorded less frequently in all datasets but in particular in low prevalence settings (range missing values 0–50%), see table S2).

Performance of individual red traffic lights

Table 2 shows positive and negative likelihood ratios of the 16 individual red features for each dataset separately. All red features with high rule-in value (LR+ >5) are highlighted in bold.

Four of all 16 red features did not achieve high rule-in value (LR+ <5) including two red features which were not available in the datasets or were not reaching significance ($p<0.05$) when present.

The one red feature which provided high rule-in value in two datasets from both low and higher prevalence settings, was "does not wake or if roused does not stay awake" (LR+5.9 (95% CI 3.5–10.0) and LR+7.8, 95% CI 4.4–13.6, respectively). The red features "reduced skin turgor", "non-blanching rash", and "focal neurological signs" showed high rule-in value in two high prevalence settings each (range LR+5.0-9.7)[18,20,22]. The red features "pale/mottled/ashen/blue", "appears ill to a healthcare professional", "weak, high-pitched or continuous cry", "tachypnoea", "moderate or severe chest indrawing", and "age 0–3 months & temperature ≥38°C" showed high rule-in value in one low prevalence setting (range LR+5.9-83.6)[4]. High rule-in value for the red features "grunting" and "bulging fontanelle", was observed in one high prevalence dataset (range LR+7.8–11.3).[20] In two high prevalence settings for none of the red features high rule-in value was observed.[21,23]

Performance of multiple red traffic lights

The association between SI and the number of positive red features with the performance measures of positive likelihood ratios, sensitivity and specificity is shown in table 3. We measured the maximum predictive value of multiple red features by logistic regression analysis and the slope of the ROC-curve. We noted a significant increase of rule-in value with the number of positive red features in most datasets (range LR+2.1 – 10.0 when ≥3 red features), with the exception of Monteny et al.[19] (p-value <0.05). This was also observed in the increased values of specificity when more red features were present. The presence of 4 or more red features did not contribute to discriminative value compared to up to 3 red features. The proportion of children having ≥3 red features ranged from 2% to 50% and did not differ between low and high prevalence settings. "General" red features were almost entirely responsible for the total ROC-area (table 3). We did not test disease-specific red features on disease-specific outcome measures due to the small numbers of these events. In figure 1 we visualised the change in pre-test to post-test probability for SI when three or more (general or disease-specific) red features were present in a Fagan nomogram.[27] For example, the 9% pre-test probability of having a SI for a child in the Brent et al dataset increases to 28% (95% CI 17–42%) post-test probability when having three or more red features, but decreases only to 7% (95% CI 6–9%) if less than three red features were present.

Discussion

Main findings

This is the first study on broadly validating the diagnostic performance of the individual red features and their combinations of the NICE febrile child guideline in acutely ill children in various settings in Europe. Although we observed rule-in value for almost all individual red features in at least one dataset, only four red features raised the probability of SI with a positive likelihood ratio of more than 5.0 in more than one setting: "does not wake or if roused does not stay awake", "reduced skin turgor", "non-blanching rash", and "focal neurological signs". Children with more than one red feature had an increased risk of SI, however, more than three red features did not further increase disease probability.

Comparison with other studies

To our knowledge there are three previous studies that estimated the predictive value of any amber or red feature for the detection of SI, but they did not evaluate the individual features of the NICE traffic light system separately. De et al.[16] found that the NICE traffic light system failed to identify a substantial proportion of children with serious bacterial infections. Combining the amber and red feature categories resulted in a sensitivity of 85.8% and specificity of 28.5% for the detection of any serious bacterial infections. Within the original data of Thompson et al. the diagnostic value of vital signs and the NICE traffic light system for identifying children with SI was assessed in a pediatric assessment unit.[21] They stated that the presence of one or more amber and red features was 85% sensitive, but only 29% specific in identifying serious or intermediate infections.[21] However, this original study was performed in children up to 16 years of age in contrast to this present study limited to children up to 5 years of age. Finally, a previous study assessing the diagnostic value of any abnormal amber or red feature (not considering combinations) of the NICE traffic light system to rule-out SI, had sensitivity of 97–100% in low and intermediate prevalence settings and 87–99% in high prevalence settings.[17] The results of all three validation studies suggest possible clinical value for ruling-out SI using both amber and red features, but at the expense of a large group of children testing false positive. However, up to 15% of children with a serious infection will be missed. Alternatively, the presence of any amber or red feature does not allow ruling-in SI considering the very low specificity. In low prevalence settings, alarming signs are preferably highly sensitive to correctly rule-out SI in order to limit incorrect referral.[24] In high prevalence settings specificity is more important because a high rate of false positive children could result in high admission rates and unnecessary investigations.[24] Unfortunately there was too much heterogeneity in our datasets to stratify according to prevalence.

Clinical and research implications

With decreasing incidence of SI, clinicians may increasingly rely on alarming symptoms described in (inter)national clinical guidelines. Broad validation could support the wider adoption of the NICE guideline in various settings in Europe and other high-income countries. Although the traffic light system of the NICE febrile child guideline is mostly based on systematic literature reviews and consensus, only four red features achieved high rule-in value in more than one dataset and none of them across all settings. Moreover, in at least as many datasets these four red features did not achieved high rule-in value and therefore hampers strong conclusions.

Table 2. Likelihood ratios individual red traffic lights.

Dataset	LR (CI)	prevalence	COLOUR: Pale/ mottled/ ashen/ blue	ACTIVITY: No response to social cues	ACTIVITY: Ill appearance	ACTIVITY: Does not (stay) wake	ACTIVITY: Weak/ high/ continuous cry	RESPIRATORY: Grunting	RESPIRATORY: Tachypnoea	RESPIRATORY: Chest indrawings	HYDRATION: Reduced skin turgor	OTHER: Age <3 m & temp ≥38°C	OTHER: Non-blanching rash	OTHER: Bulging fontanelle	OTHER: Neck stiffness	OTHER: Status epilepticus	OTHER: Focal neurologic signs	OTHER: Focal seizures
			positive likelihood ratio (LR+) and negative likelihood ratio (LR-)															
Bleeker et al.[23]	LR +	High	2.3 (1.5–3.4)*	-	1.4 (1.2–1.7)*	2.6 (1.0–6.9)*	1.1 (0.9–1.3)	-	3.0 (1.9–4.6)*	-	1.9 (1.3–2.8)*	1.5 (1.1–2.1)*	-	1.8 (0.7–4.4)	-	-	-	-
(n = 595)	LR -		0.9 (0.8–0.9)	-	0.7 (0.6–0.9)	1.0 (0.9–1.0)	0.9 (0.8–1.1)		0.8 (0.8–0.9)		0.9 (0.8–1.0)	0.9 (0.8–1.0)	-	1.0 (0.9–1.0)	-	-	-	-
Brent et al.[18]	LR +	High	2.6 (1.8–3.8)*	1.6 (0.4–7.0)	2.7 (2.0–3.6)*	1.4 (0.2–11.1)	-	**7.8 (2.2–28.0)***	2.9 (1.7–4.9)*	4.9 (2.2–10.8)*	**9.7(0.6–153.1)***	1.9 (0.6–6.5)	**	**	**	**	**	**
(n = 494)	LR -		0.7 (0.5–0.9)	1.0 (0.9–1.0)	0.5 (0.4–0.7)	1.0 (1.0–1.0)	-	0.9 (0.8–1.0)	0.8 (0.6–0.9)	0.9 (0.7–1.0)	1.0 (0.9–1.0)	1.0 (0.9–1.0)	**	**	**	**	**	**
Oostenbrink et al. [22]	LR +	High	1.9 (1.0–3.5)*	1.9 (1.4–2.5)*	3.0 (0.8–11.7)	**7.8 (4.4–13.6)***	1.1 (0.7–1.8)	-	-	-	**7.4 (1.7–33.5)***	1.6 (0.9–2.9)	**7.2 (3.3–15.9)***	2.7 (1.6–4.4)*	1.8 (1.6–2.0)*	-	**7.4 (2.6–21.4)***	**
(n = 423)	LR -		0.9 (0.9–1.0)	0.8 (0.7–0.9)	1.0 (0.9–1.0)	0.6 (0.6–0.7)	1.0 (0.9–1.1)	-	-	-	0.9 (0.9–1.0)	0.9 (0.9–1.0)	0.8 (0.8–0.9)	0.8 (0.8–0.9)	0.2 (0.1–0.3)	-	0.9 (0.8–0.9)	**
Roukema et al. [20]	LR +	High	1.5 (0.2–12.8)	-	2.7 (1.6–4.5)*	2.8 (1.2–6.5)*	2.9 (1.4–6.3)*	2.9 (1.6–5.3)*	2.6 (1.4–4.7)*	1.2 (0.7–2.1)	1.9 (0.2–16.8)	1.8 (1.0–3.3)*	**7.5 (1.5–37.0)***	**11.3(1.9–67.1)***	4.8 (1.9–12.2)*	**	**5.0 (2.5–10.2)***	1.5 (0.2–12.8)
(n = 1459)	LR -		1.0 (1.0–1.0)	-	0.9 (0.9–1.0)	1.0 (1.0–1.0)	1.0 (0.9–1.0)	0.9 (0.9–1.0)	1.0 (0.9–1.0)	1.0 (0.9–1.0)	1.0 (1.0–1.0)	1.0 (0.9–1.0)	1.0 (1.0–1.0)	1.0 (1.0–1.0)	1.0 (1.0–1.0)	**	0.9 (0.9–1.0)	1.0 (1.0–1.0)
Thompson et al.[21]	LR +	High	1.3 (1.0–1.6)	2.4 (0.9–6.2)	**	1.5 (0.9–2.5)	1.5 (1.1–2 .1)*	-	4.7 (1.5–14.4)*	1.5 (1.0–2.3)	2.0 (0.8–4.9)	**	1.7 (0.9–3.4)	-	**	-	-	-
(n = 434)	LR -		0.9 (0.8–1.0)	1.0 (0.9–1.0)	**	0.9 (0.9–1.0)	0.9 (0.8–1.0)	-	0.9 (0.9–1.0)	0.9 (0.8–1.0)	1.0 (0.9–1.0)	**	1.0 (0.9–1.0)	-	**	-	-	-
Monteny et al.[19]	LR +	Low	1.7 (1.1–2.5)*	1.4 (0.9–2.1)	1.7 (0.6–4.9)	1.8 (1.0–3.2)	0.8 (0.5–1.4)	1.5 (1.2–1.8)*	**	**	0.8 (0.1–5.4)	**	0.4 (0.1–2.8)	**	1.8 (1.1–2.9)*	-	-	-
(n = 487)	LR -		0.7 (0.4–1.1)	0.7 (0.5–1.2)	0.9 (0.8–1.1)	0.8 (0.5–1.1)	1.2 (0.8–1.7)	0.4 (0.1–1.0)	**	**	1.0 (0.9–1.1)	**	1.1 (1.0–1.2)	**	0.7 (0.4–1.1)	-	-	-
Van den Bruel et al.[4]	LR +	Low	**83.6 (12.2–572.4)***	3.2 (1.9–5.3)*	**6.6 (4.5–10.0)***	**5.9 (3.5–10.0)***	**7.0 (4.1–11.8)***	-	**7.3 (4.1–12.9)***	**8.0 (4.9–13.1)***	2.2 (0.3–15.5)	**9.3 (2.3–38.1)***	**	-	**	-	-	-
(n = 2368)	LR -		0.9 (0.8–1.0)	0.7 (0.5–1.0)	0.5 (0.4–0.8)	0.7 (0.5–0.9)	0.7 (0.5–0.9)	-	0.7 (0.6–0.9)	0.6 (0.5–0.9)	1.0 (0.9–1.1)	0.9 (0.8–1.0)	**	-	**	-	-	-

'General' red traffic lights: Pale/ mottled/ ashen/ blue; No response to social cues; Ill appearance; Does not (stay) wake; Weak/ high/ continuous cry; Grunting; Tachypnoea; Reduced skin turgor; Age <3 m & temp ≥38°C.
'Disease specific' red traffic lights: Chest indrawings; Non-blanching rash; Bulging fontanelle; Neck stiffness; Status epilepticus; Focal neurologic signs; Focal seizures.
CI: confidence interval.
*P-value <0.05 (Chi-square analysis).
**Red traffic light not positive in non SI- and/or SI population.
-Not recorded.

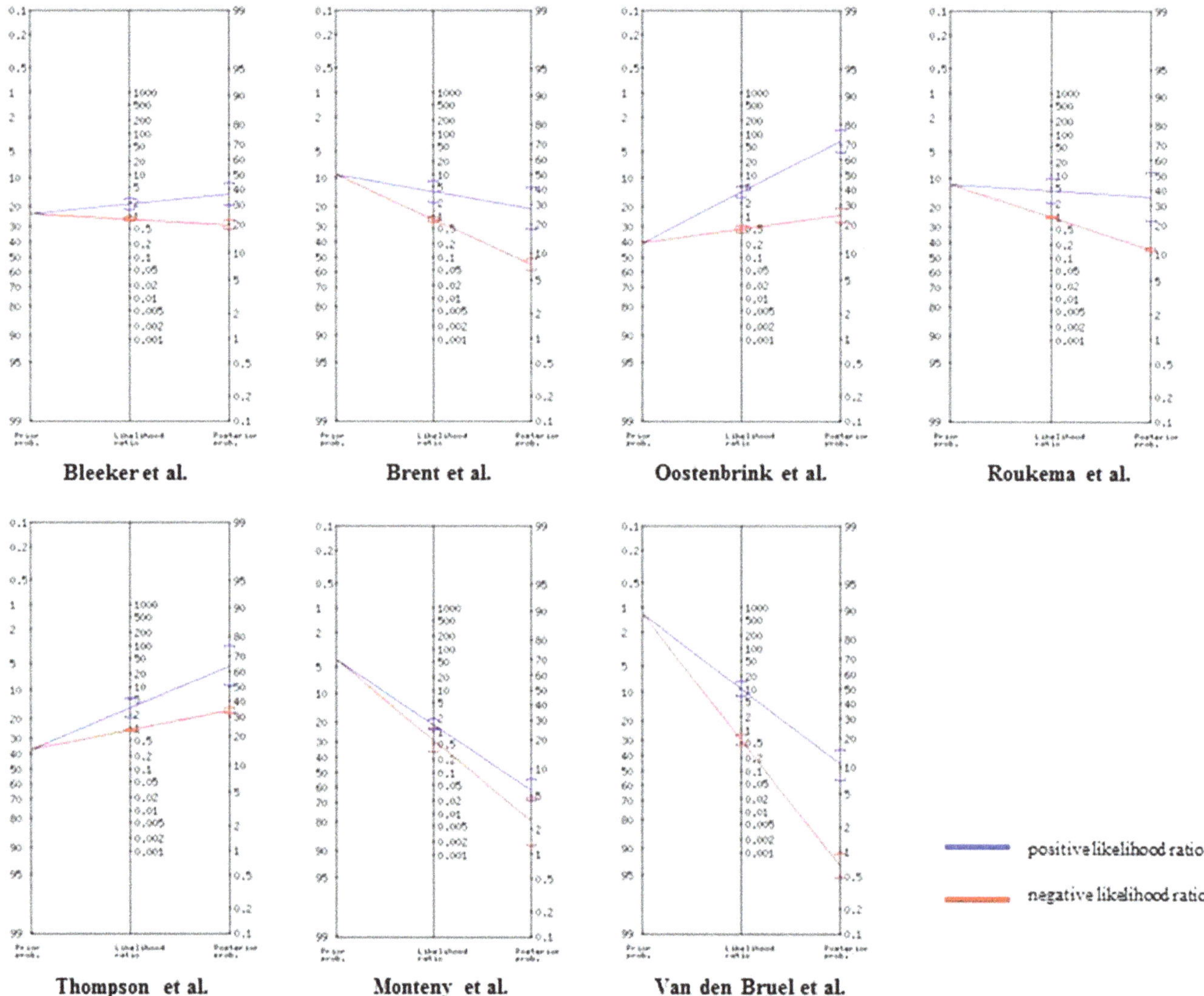

Figure 1. Calculation of post-test pobability for serious infections if ≥3 red traffic lights present using Fagan nomogram.

The rule-in value of several other red features was not confirmed in multiple settings either, questioning their inclusion in this setting-independent traffic light system.

Our observations of varying rule-in values of red features in the 7 databases did not support the development of one prediction model including the most important red features. However, we consistently observed an association between 3 or more red features and SI but combinations of red features will never be able to definitely rule-in a SI without uncertainty. This could be due to dilution of their accuracy by the inclusion of aspecific red features or because of the interaction between different red features.

The relatively lower recording of "disease-specific" features hampered our analyses, in particular in low prevalence settings. This may in part have been caused by the fact that it is more difficult to identify proxies for such features, in contrast to more general features.

The main findings in our study corresponds with the limited performance of the Yale Observation Scale, on which the NICE traffic light system is partly based.[17,25] In the revised 2013 guideline[9] two red features were deleted of the previous 2007 protocol[6] or transferred to amber features: "Age 3–6m & temperature ≥39°C" and "bile-stained vomiting". This is supported by our findings that we did not find rule-in value for the former but only had one dataset available for the latter which showed high rule-in value though. Next, as disease specific red features are strongly related to specific but rare diseases, their positive documentation rate is already expected to be low. Although these disease specific red features may be relevant for one specific outcome, it is difficult to evaluate these in the general population of fever with a broad differential diagnosis. However, achieving complete certainty with clinical features is not the goal here. Rather, red features should lift the probability of SI over a certain decision threshold: either to refer, request additional testing or start empiric treatment. As we do not know at what specific risk thresholds we (intuitively) undertake action, clinical interpretation of post-test probabilities as expressed in Fagan nomograms (figure 1) remains difficult. As diagnosis assessment is a dynamic process and may be influenced by evolution of symptoms in time, repeated assessment of deviating red features in those with only one or two features in particular, may improve the evaluation of SI.

Finally, the NICE traffic light system could also be improved by taking more recent evidence into account, such as on peripheral circulation, parental concern [25] or urine analysis [16].

Table 3. Likelihood ratios and ROC-areas of combinations of multiple red traffic lights.

		BLEEKER et al.[23]	BRENT et al.[18]	OOSTENBRINK et al.[22]	ROUKEMA et al.[20]	THOMPSON et al.[21]	MONTENY et al.[19]	VAN DEN BRUEL et al.[4]
		N_{total} = 595 SI = 137;23.0%	N_{total} = 494 SI = 46;9.3%	N_{total} = 423 SI = 170;40.2%	N_{total} = 1,459 SI = 171;11.7%	N_{total} = 434 SI = 161;37.1%	N_{total} = 487 SI = 20;4.1%	N_{total} = 2,368 SI = 28;1.2%
Number red features	LR +/- (CI)							
≥1 RTL	Likelihood ratio +	1.18 (1.10–1.27)*	1.94 (1.57–2.39)*	1.39 (1.27–1.51)*	1.75 (1.39–2.20)*	1.28 (1.12–1.46)*	1.08 (1.05–1.12)	3.33 (2.76–4.02)*
	Likelihood ratio -	0.41 (0.24–0.70)	0.42 (0.26–0.69)	0.13 (0.06–0.28)	0.81 (0.72–0.91)	0.59 (0.43–0.80)	-	0.24 (0.12–0.53)
≥2 RTLs	Likelihood ratio +	1.49 (1.25–1.79)*	3.70 (2.68–5.12)*	2.36 (1.94–2.87)*	3.40 (2.24–5.16)*	1.75 (1.31–2.33)*	1.25 (1.07–1.46)	6.38 (4.82–8.44)*
	Likelihood ratio -	0.68 (0.55–0.84)	0.49 (0.35–0.69)	0.35 (0.26–0.46)	0.88 (0.82–0.94)	0.78 (0.67–0.89)	0.36 (0.10–1.35)	0.36 (0.21–0.62)
≥3 RTLs	Likelihood ratio +	2.10 (1.50–2.93)*	3.90 (2.15–7.08)	4.65 (3.29–6.58)*	4.14 (2.02–8.50)	2.97 (1.66–5.31)*	1.44 (1.07–1.95)	10.0 (6.43–15.45)*
	Likelihood ratio -	0.81 (0.72–0.91)	0.79 (0.67–0.94)	0.47 (0.39–0.57)	0.95 (0.91–1.00)	0.88 (0.81–0.95)	0.58 (0.30–1.15)	0.56 (0.40–0.79)
	Sens/Spec (CI)							
≥1 RTL	Sensitivity	0.91 (0.84-0.94)	0.74 (0.60-0.84)	0.96 (0.92-0.98)	0.36 (0.29-0.43)	0.76 (0.69-0.82)	1.00 (0.84-1.00)	0.82 (0.64-0.92)
	Specificity	0.23 (0.20-0.27)	0.62 (0.57-0.66)	0.31 (0.25-0.37)	0.80 (0.77-0.82)	0.40 (0.35-0.46)	0.07 (0.05-0.10)	0.75 (0.74-0.77)
≥2 RTLs	Sensitivity	0.58 (0.50-0.66)	0.59 (0.44-0.72)	0.76 (0.70-0.82)	0.16 (0.12-0.23)	0.40 (0.33-0.48)	0.90 (0.70-0.97)	0.68 (0.49-0.82)
	Specificity	0.61 (0.56-0.65)	0.84 (0.81-0.87)	0.68 (0.62-0.73)	0.95 (0.94-0.96)	0.77 (0.72-0.82)	0.28 (0.24-0.32)	0.89 (0.88-0.91)
≥3 RTLs	Sensitivity	0.31 (0.24-0.39)	0.26 (0.16-0.40)	0.59 (0.51-0.66)	0.06 (0.03-0.11)	0.17 (0.12-0.24)	0.70 (0.48-0.85)	0.46 (0.30-0.64)
	Specificity	0.85 (0.82-0.88)	0.93 (0.91-0.95)	0.87 (0.83-0.91)	0.98 (0.98-0.99)	0.94 (0.91-0.96)	0.51 (0.47-0.56)	0.95 (0.94-0.96)
	ROC-area (CI)							
All red features		0.64 (0.59–0.70)	0.73 (0.65–0.82)	0.79 (0.74–0.84)	0.59 (0.54–0.63)	0.63 (0.57–0.68)	0.65 (0.53–0.77)	0.84 (0.75–0.93)
General#		0.64 (0.59–0.70)	0.73 (0.65–0.81)	0.69 (0.64–0.75)	0.59 (0.54–0.64)	0.60 (0.55–0.66)	0.65 (0.54–0.76)	0.82 (0.72–0.91)
Disease spec.^		0.51 (0.46–0.57)	0.56 (0.47–0.66)	0.77 (0.72–0.81)	0.53 (0.48–0.58)	0.56 (0.50–0.62)	0.56 (0.43–0.69)	0.69 (0.57–0.81)

*P-value <0.05 (added value of e.g. ≥3 RTLs above ≥2 RTLs, by logistic regression analysis).
LR: likelihood ratio (positive and negative).
Sens: sensitiviteit; Spec: specificiteit; CI: confidence interval.
#1. Colour: pale / mottled/ ashen/ blue; 2. No response to social cues; 3. Ill appearance; 4. Does not (stay) awake; 5. Weak/ high pitched/ continuous cry; 6. Grunting; 7. Tachypnoea; 9. Reduced skin turgor; 10. Age <3 m & temp ≥38°C;
^8. Chest indrawing 11. Non-blanching rash; 12. Bulging fontanelle; 13. Neck stiffness; 14. Status epilepticus; 15. Focal neurologic symptoms; 16. Focal seizures.

Strengths and limitations

We assessed the NICE red traffic lights in 6,260 children from seven existing datasets with various pediatric populations and settings including two low prevalence primary care settings, which are usually underrepresented in diagnostic studies in this area.[24] In addition, we validated the red features separately to identify their individual predictive value.

Despite the large amount of data, not all red features had been recorded in all datasets, necessitating the use of proxy variables.[17] Furthermore, differences in population characteristics (table 1), such as age distribution or prevalence of specific diagnoses within the group of SI, prevented the calculation of overall diagnostic performance measures.

Furthermore, by assuming missing red features as not present and more complete documentation of red features in ill children, we may have overestimated our likelihood ratios by increasing the contrast between children with and without SI.

However, the variability in variables and case-mix reflects clinical practice and therefore will strengthen generalizability of our results.

Conclusion

Our results support rule-in value of several individual red features from the NICE febrile child guideline in specific settings, although not consistent. However most features had little rule-in value across multiple settings. The NICE red traffic lights, even when three or more features are present, seem to have limited value for ruling-in serious infections. Our results underline the importance to widely validate the predictive value of individual and combinations of multiple red features in clinical guidelines, prior to widespread dissemination and adoption.

Acknowledgments

The authors wrote the paper on behalf of the European Research Network on Recognising Serious Infection (ERNIE). The principal investigators are: Marjolein Berger, Frank Buntinx, Bert Aertgeerts, Monica Lakhanpaul, David Mant, Henriette Moll, Rianne Oostenbrink, Richard Stevens, Matthew Thompson, Ann Van den Bruel and Jan Verbakel. We gratefully acknowledge the members of the ERNIE group for the collaboration and their advice on the message of the manuscript. We want to thank the emergency-personnel of all ambulatory care settings for their participation and careful collection of the required data. We acknowledge the researchers Sacha Bleeker, Andrew Brent, Samiran Ray, Jolt Roukema, Matthew Thompson, Miriam Monteny and Ann Van den Bruel for the data acquisition and contribution of the original studies.

Disclaimer: for this study we selected children with an acute illness from seven cohorts collected by the collaboration of the European Research Network on recognising serious InfEctions(ERNIE) group.[4,18,19,20–23]

Author Contributions

Conceived and designed the experiments: EK ML SR HAM RO. Performed the experiments: EK ML SR JV AVDB MT MYB HAM RO. Analyzed the data: EK RO. Contributed reagents/materials/analysis tools: ML JV AVDB MT MYB HAM RO. Wrote the paper: EK RO. Reviewed and revised the manuscript: EK ML SR JV AVDB MT MYB HAM RO. Translation, synopsis and recoding of the datasets: EK SR JV. Participated in recoding and data checking and in discussion about each step of the results: ML SR JV AVDB MT MYB HAM RO.

References

1. Armon K, MacFaul R, Hemingway P, Werneke U, Stephenson T (2004) The impact of presenting problem based guidelines for children with medical problems in an accident and emergency department. Arch Dis Child 89: 159–164.
2. Bruijnzeels MA, Foets M, van der Wouden JC, van den Heuvel WJ, Prins A (1998) Everyday symptoms in childhood: occurrence and general practitioner consultation rates. Br J Gen Pract 48: 880–884.
3. Moll van Charante EP, van Steenwijk-Opdam PC, Bindels PJ (2007) Out-of-hours demand for GP care and emergency services: patients' choices and referrals by general practitioners and ambulance services. BMC Fam Pract 8: 46.
4. Van den Bruel A, Aertgeerts B, Bruyninckx R, Aerts M, Buntinx F (2007) Signs and symptoms for diagnosis of serious infections in children: a prospective study in primary care. Br J Gen Pract 57: 538–546.
5. Craig JC, Williams GJ, Jones M, Codarini M, Macaskill P, et al. (2010) The accuracy of clinical symptoms and signs for the diagnosis of serious bacterial infection in young febrile children: prospective cohort study of 15 781 febrile illnesses. BMJ 340: c1594.
6. National Institute for Health and Clinical Excellence (2007) Feverish illness in children - Assessment and initial management in children younger than 5 years. London: National Institute for Health and Clinical Excellence.
7. Inwald DP, Tasker RC, Peters MJ, Nadel S, Paediatric Intensive Care Society Study G (2009) Emergency management of children with severe sepsis in the United Kingdom: the results of the Paediatric Intensive Care Society sepsis audit. Arch Dis Child 94: 348–353.
8. Kumar A (2009) Optimizing antimicrobial therapy in sepsis and septic shock.Crit Care Clin 25: 733–751, viii.
9. Chen SM, Chang HM, Hung TW, Chao YH, Tsai JD, et al. (2013) Diagnostic performance of procalcitonin for hospitalised children with acute pyelonephritis presenting to the paediatric emergency department. Emerg Med J 30: 406–410.
10. McCarthy PL, Sharpe MR, Spiesel SZ, Dolan TF, Forsyth BW, et al. (1982) Observation scales to identify serious illness in febrile children. Pediatrics 70: 802–809.
11. Teach SJ, Fleisher GR (1995) Efficacy of an observation scale in detecting bacteremia in febrile children three to thirty-six months of age, treated as outpatients. Occult Bacteremia Study Group. J Pediatr 126: 877–881.
12. McCarthy PL, Lembo RM, Baron MA, Fink HD, Cicchetti DV (1985) Predictive value of abnormal physical examination findings in ill-appearing and well-appearing febrile children. Pediatrics 76: 167–171.
13. Baker MD, Avner JR, Bell LM (1990) Failure of infant observation scales in detecting serious illness in febrile, 4- to 8-week-old infants. Pediatrics 85: 1040–1043.
14. Berger MY, Boomsma LJ, Albeda FW, Dijkstra RH, Graafmans TA, et al. (2008) Guideline Children with fever [NHG-standaard Kinderen met koorts]. Dutch College of General Practitioners [Nederlands Huisartsen Genootschap].
15. Chiappini E, Principi N, Longhi R, Tovo PA, Becherucci P, et al. (2009) Management of fever in children: summary of the Italian Pediatric Society guidelines. Clin Ther 31: 1826–1843.
16. De S, Williams GJ, Hayen A, Macaskill P, McCaskill M, et al. (2013) Accuracy of the "traffic light" clinical decision rule for serious bacterial infections in young children with fever: a retrospective cohort study. BMJ 346: f866.
17. Verbakel JY, Van den Bruel A, Thompson M, Stevens R, Aertgeerts B, et al. (2013) How well do clinical prediction rules perform in identifying serious infections in acutely ill children across an international network of ambulatory care datasets? BMC Med 11: 10.
18. Brent AJ, Lakhanpaul M, Thompson M, Collier J, Ray S, et al. (2011) Risk score to stratify children with suspected serious bacterial infection: Observational cohort study. Arch Dis Child 96: 361–367.
19. Monteny M, Berger MY, van der Wouden JC, Broekman BJ, Koes BW (2008) Triage of febrile children at a GP cooperative: determinants of a consultation. Br J Gen Pract 58: 242–247.
20. Roukema J, Steyerberg EW, van der Lei J, Moll HA (2008) Randomized trial of a clinical decision support system: impact on the management of children with fever without apparent source. J Am Med Inform Assoc 15: 107–113.
21. Thompson M, Coad N, Harnden A, Mayon-White R, Perera R, et al. (2009) How well do vital signs identify children with serious infections in paediatric emergency care? Arch Dis Child 94: 888–893.
22. Oostenbrink R, Moons KG, Derksen-Lubsen AG, Grobbee DE, Moll HA (2004) A diagnostic decision rule for management of children with meningeal signs. Eur J Epidemiol 19: 109–116.
23. Bleeker SE, Derksen-Lubsen G, Grobbee DE, Donders AR, Moons KG, et al. (2007) Validating and updating a prediction rule for serious bacterial infection in patients with fever without source. Acta Paediatr 96: 100–104.
24. Oostenbrink R, Thompson M, Steyerberg EW, ERNIE members (2012) Barriers to translating diagnostic research in febrile children to clinical practice: a systematic review. Arch Dis Child 97: 667–672.

Safety and Effectiveness of Combination Antiretroviral Therapy during the First Year of Treatment in HIV-1 Infected Rwandan Children: A Prospective Study

Philippe R. Mutwa[1,2]*, Kimberly R. Boer[2,6], Brenda Asiimwe-Kateera[2], Diane Tuyishimire[7], Narcisse Muganga[1], Joep M. A. Lange[2], Janneke van de Wijgert[2,3,4], Anita Asiimwe[8], Peter Reiss[2], Sibyl P. M. Geelen[2,5]

1 Kigali University Teaching Hospital, Department of Pediatrics, Kigali, Rwanda, **2** Department of Global Health and Amsterdam Institute for Global Health and Development, Academic Medical Center, Amsterdam, The Netherlands, **3** Institute of Infection and Global Health, University of Liverpool, Liverpool, United of Kingdom, **4** Rinda Ubuzima, Kigali, Rwanda, **5** Wilhelmina Children's Hospital, University Medical Centre Utrecht, Utrecht, The Netherlands, **6** Biomedical Research, Epidemiology Unit, Royal Tropical Institute, Amsterdam, The Netherlands, **7** Outpatients Clinic, Treatment and Research on HIV/AIDS Centre, Kigali, Rwanda, **8** Ministry of Health of Rwanda, Kigali, Rwanda

Abstract

Background: With increased availability of paediatric combination antiretroviral therapy (cART) in resource limited settings, cART outcomes and factors associated with outcomes should be assessed.

Methods: HIV-infected children <15 years of age, initiating cART in Kigali, Rwanda, were followed for 18 months. Prospective clinical and laboratory assessments included weight-for-age (WAZ) and height-for-age (HAZ) z-scores, complete blood cell count, liver transaminases, creatinine and lipid profiles, CD4 T-cell count/percent, and plasma HIV-1 RNA concentration. Clinical success was defined as WAZ and WAZ >−2, immunological success as CD4 cells ≥500/mm^3 and ≥25% for respectively children over 5 years and under 5 years, and virological success as a plasma HIV-1 RNA concentration <40 copies/mL.

Results: Between March 2008 and December 2009, 123 HIV-infected children were included. The median (interquartile (IQR) age at cART initiation was 7.4 (3.2, 11.5) years; 40% were <5 years and 54% were female. Mean (95% confidence interval (95%CI)) HAZ and WAZ at baseline were −2.01 (−2.23, −1.80) and −1.73 (−1.95, −1.50) respectively and rose to −1.75 (−1.98, −1.51) and −1.17 (−1.38, −0.96) after 12 months of cART. The median (IQR) CD4 T-cell values for children <5 and ≥5 years of age were 20% (13, 28) and 337 (236, 484) cells/mm^{3}respectively, and increased to 36% (28, 41) and 620 (375, 880) cells/mm^3. After 12 months of cART, 24% of children had a detectable viral load, including 16% with virological failure (HIV-RNA>1000 c/mL). Older age at cART initiation, poor adherence, and exposure to antiretrovirals around birth were associated with virological failure. A third (33%) of children had side effects (by self-report or clinical assessment), but only 9% experienced a severe side effect requiring a cART regimen change.

Conclusions: cART in Rwandan HIV-infected children was successful but success might be improved further by initiating cART as early as possible, optimizing adherence and optimizing management of side effects.

Editor: Rashida A. Ferrand, London School of Hygiene and Tropical Medicine, United Kingdom

Funding: This work was funded by Infectious Diseases Network for Treatment and Research in Africa. An African-Dutch partnership programme, funded by The Netherlands-African partnership for Capacity development and Clinical interventions against Poverty-related diseases (NACCAP). The funders had no role in study design, data collection and analysis, decision to publish, or preparation of the manuscript.

Competing Interests: The authors have declared that no competing interests exist.

* Email: mutwaph@gmail.com

Introduction

There is strong evidence that combination antiretroviral therapy (cART) reduces morbidity and mortality, promotes normal growth and development, and improves quality of life in children infected by HIV [1,2,3,4,5,6]. However, cART effectiveness depends on durable suppression of viral replication. Ongoing HIV replication leads to chronic inflammation, and when cART is not used appropriately this can lead to HIV drug resistance and treatment failure, which limits future treatment options [7,8]. Data from low and middle-income countries (LMIC) have demonstrated good cART effectiveness and tolerability in most children, but some children remain underweight and stunted or do not improve their CD4 T-cell count or viral load after several years of treatment [9,10,11]. Advanced disease at cART initiation was found to be associated with poor outcomes [9,12,13,14], indicating that earlier treatment may improve effectiveness of cART. Initiation of cART in children is guided by pediatric clinical staging and age-dependent CD4 values.

In Rwanda the national ART guidelines were recently revised to promote an earlier start of cART in children and adolescents, and a roll out of pediatric care and treatment centers throughout the country was achieved [15]. As a result, the number of HIV-infected children on cART in Rwanda has rapidly increased from 468 in 2005 to an estimated 8,032 in 2013 [16]. The main objectives of this study were to prospectively document responses to cART in the first year of treatment in a cohort of HIV-infected Rwandan children, and to determine the incidence and severity of side effects of cART.

Methods

Ethical considerations

The Rwanda National Ethics Committee (RNEC) and the Medical Ethics Review Committee of the University Medical Center of Utrecht, the Netherlands, approved the study protocol. In accordance with the RNEC guidelines written informed consent was obtained from primary caregivers of all children. In addition, verbal assent was obtained from children between 7 and 12 years of age, and written assent from children age 12 or older. The Rwandan national guidelines for disclosure to children recommend to inform children at 7 years of age of their HIV status.

Study design, population and period

In this longitudinal prospective cohort study, HIV-infected cART-naïve children below 15 years of age who initiated cART between March 2008 and December 2009 were followed by the study team for a minimum of 9 and a maximum of 18 months. Study participation ended after 18 months of follow-up or in September 2010, when funding for the study ended. All children continued to be followed in routine HIV care at a public clinic after their study participation ended. The study was conducted at the Treatment and Research AIDS Center (TRACplus) Outpatient Clinic in Kigali, Rwanda. During the study period, the TRACplus clinic was providing HIV care and treatment to 686 HIV-infected children. Among these children, 444 (65%) were already on cART before the study period, 174 became eligible for treatment. With the strategy to scale up pediatric treatment services, 51 children were transferred to clinics closer to their homes, hence they were not enrolled for the study. One hundred and twenty three (18%) children were enrolled. These children were usually referred from Kigali University Teaching Hospital (which is adjacent to the TRACplus clinic), nearby district hospitals, or health centers providing Prevention of Mother to Child HIV Transmission (PMTCT) services; a few children were diagnosed at the TRACplus facility itself. All children below the age of 15 years who initiated cART at the TRACplus clinic during the study period were given the opportunity to enroll in the study.

cART guidelines and regimens

At the time of study initiation, the 2007 Rwandan ART guidelines (based on the 2006 WHO ART guidelines) were operational, which recommended cART initiation in children and adolescents less than 15 years of age if they were classified as WHO pediatric clinical stage III or IV, or had a severe immunodeficiency based on age-dependent CD4 values: CD4 $<1500/mm^3$ or $<25\%$ if ≤ 11 months; $<750/mm^3$ or $<20\%$ if 12–35 months; $<15\%$ or $<350/mm^3$ if 36–59 months; and $<350/mm^3$ if ≥ 5 years of age [17,18]. Children enrolled in the study received cART, cotrimoxazole prophylaxis, and free medication for all acute illnesses during the length of the study. They were initiated on a first-line cART regimen consisting of two nucleoside reverse transcriptase inhibitors (NRTIs) and a non-nucleoside reverse transcriptase inhibitor (NNRTI). A cART regimen was defined as nevirapine-based, efavirenz-based or protease-inhibitor (PI)-based. The Rwandan ART guidelines were revised in 2009, and from then onwards, children known to have been exposed to nevirapine in the context of PMTCT were initiated on a first-line regimen with two NRTIs and a protease inhibitor (PI) [19]. For the purposes of this study, a treatment switch was defined as modifying the regimen to another regimen, within the first-line (including modification from one NRTI to another) or from first-line to second-line. Children would typically switch from a nevirapine-containing regimen to an efavirenz-containing regimen if side effects occurred due to nevirapine, or if they developed tuberculosis. A treatment switch from one NRTI to another NRTI could be due to national ART guidelines changes, side effects, or stock outs. A modification from a first line (NNRTI-containing) regimen to a second line (PI-containing) regimen was indicated in case of virological failure.

Clinic procedures

By the time a child and caregiver were approached for study participation, the decision to start cART had already been taken by a committee of clinicians and social workers as per routine clinic procedures. Children who subsequently also consented to study participation initiated cART at study enrollment. At this enrollment visit, primary caregivers and children were counseled and interviewed by study staff. The face-to-face interviews included questions about socio-demographics (including orphan status and guardianship), HIV infection history, and variables deemed of importance in the context of cART adherence (see below). In accordance with the national ART guidelines, a clinical assessment was conducted at enrollment and at 2, 4, 8 and 12 weeks after enrollment, and subsequently every three months if the child was clinically doing well, until a maximum of 18 months of follow up was reached or the end of the study (whichever came earlier). Children had additional visits to the clinic in case of unforeseen problems (e.g. infections, or presumed adverse effects of cART). The study was conducted within the public health sector; clinic visits combined routine follow-up procedures and additional study-related procedures such as close laboratory monitoring including CD4 and viral load as well as treatment adverse effect assessment. The study was designed in such a way that no extra visits were needed for the sake of the study. For the study a reimbursement of transport fees was given to the parents per visit for the equivalent of 5 USD. The assessment included a physical examination with measurement of height and weight, pediatric WHO clinical staging, clinical symptoms, and targeted evaluations of side-effects using a standardized checklist. A general physical exam was also conducted and clinician findings were recorded on a standardized CRF covering each body system. In addition to the clinical and laboratory evaluations targeting side effects (see below), side effects were also assessed by standardized face-to-face interview at each study visit. In addition, participants were asked if they had any other symptoms that had not yet been covered in the interview.

Laboratory testing

All laboratory tests were performed at the National Reference Laboratory (NRL) in Kigali, Rwanda. Blood was drawn by venipuncture: a complete blood cell count and liver transaminases [Alanine Amino Transferase (AST) and Aspartate Amino Transferase (AST)] were determined by Cobas Integra 400 plus (Roche Diagnostics, Indianapolis IN, USA) at enrollment and at 1, 3, 6, 12, and 18 months follow-up. CD4 T-cell counts and percentages were determined at enrollment and at 3, 6, 12 and 18 months follow-up by flow-cytometric measurement using a FACS Calibur (Becton Dickinson, San Jose, CA, USA). Plasma HIV-1 RNA concentration (Roche Cobas AmpliPrep/Cobas TaqMan HIV-1, Roche Molecular Systems, France, with a lower limit of detection of 40 copies/mL), creatinine (Cobas Integra 400 plus, Roche Diagnostics, Indianapolis IN, USA) and a lipid profile (low-density lipoprotein, high-density lipoprotein and triglycerides, Human Humastar 180, Human GmbH, Wiesbaden Germany) were determined at enrollment and at months 6, 12 and 18. Children with virological failure (see definition below) and children with plasma HIV-RNA concentrations between 40 and 1000 copies/mL were scheduled for additional HIV-1 RNA testing within 6 months.

Adherence assessments

Caregivers and children, if age appropriate, received adherence counseling before enrollment and then at each follow-up visit. Caregivers were requested to return all medication containers and any unused medications at the next scheduled visit. For adherence monitoring, the caregivers were asked questions by face-to-face interviewing using a structured questionnaire; adherence assessment was conducted at every clinic and pharmacy follow-up visit.

They were asked how many doses of the prescribed medication the child had missed during the previous 30 days and at what time points this occurred, and reasons for non-adherence, both child-related (e.g. refusal, spitting, or vomiting) or caregiver-related (e.g. forgetting). They were also asked questions about the socio-economic status of the household (level of caregivers' education, household income), and distance to the clinic. Children were categorized as non-adherent if having taken less than 95% of the prescribed medication in the last 30 days. In addition, study nurses and pharmacy staff counted pills dispensed and returned unused, assuming that all other pills were used.

Statistical analysis

All statistical analyses were performed using STATA Version 12 (Copyright 1984–2007 StataCorp TX USA). All statistical analyses were assessed for statistical significance at the $p<0.05$ level. Descriptive statistics are presented as proportions for categorical data and means with standard deviations (SD) and medians with IQR for parametric and non-parametric continuous data, respectively.

Study endpoints. The primary objective of this study was to determine the proportion of children achieving good clinical, immunological, and virological outcomes in the first year of cART as well as predictors of these outcomes. Good clinical outcome was defined as weight-for-age (WAZ) or height-for-age (HAZ)≥ -2 z-score. WAZ and HAZ were calculated using Epinfo version 3.5.1 (Centers for Disease Control and Prevention, Atlanta, GA). Immunological success was defined as achievement of CD4 cells $\geq 500/mm^3$ for children above 5 years of age and a CD4 percentage $\geq 25\%$ for children under 5 years of age. Virological success was defined as an HIV-1 RNA concentration <40 copies/mL per study time point. Children were categorized as WHO clinical stage I–IV throughout the study according to the WHO pediatric clinical classification system [18].

A secondary objective of the study was to document the occurrence and severity of side effects at any time point as well as predictors of the occurrence of side effects. Self-reported side effects and clinical findings were categorized into 5 main groups: gastro-intestinal, neurological, skin/mucosal, respiratory, and other. The severity of each side effect was assessed using the US National Institute of Allergy and Infectious Diseases Division of AIDS Table for Grading the Severity of Adult and Pediatric Adverse Events (DAIDS-AE) [20]. Grade 1 (mild) was defined as symptoms causing no or minimal interference with usual social and functional activities; grade 2 (moderate) as symptoms causing greater than minimal interference with usual social and functional activities; grade 3 (severe) as symptoms causing inability to perform usual social and functional activities; and grade 4 (potentially life-threatening) as symptoms causing inability to perform basic self-care functions or medical or operative intervention indicated to prevent permanent impairment, persistent disability, or death. Side effects were classified as transient if they were recorded at one or multiple time-points but eventually disappeared without any changes to cART regimen and without treatment of the side effects. They were classified as persistent when they required cART regimen changes or treatment of the side effect. Children were considered to have severe anemia if hemoglobin was <7.5 g/dl, and severe liver abnormality if ALT and/or AST was >5 times the normal values.

Another secondary objective of the study was to assess adherence over time and predictors of adherence. Children were categorized as poorly adherent if they had taken less than 95% of the prescribed medication, based on either self-report or pill counts, or if the caregiver had missed a scheduled pharmacy appointments for ≥ 2 consecutive days, as only a 15- or 30-day supply of medication was provided at each clinic visit. Adherence assessment was conducted at every visit and was measured for the last 30 days preceding the clinic visit.

Statistical modeling. Due to repeated measurements of the outcome, generalizing estimating equation (GEE) models were used to determine outcome changes over time, assuming an exchangeable correlation, (where the correlation is the same for all outcomes within a subject; which is best suited for longitudinal studies in which the same subjects are followed over time). The associations between outcomes and different explanatory variables were evaluated using bivariable GEE models (due to sample size limitations, only one explanatory factor was added at a time). In the WAZ and HAZ models, these explanatory variables included age group, CD4 count, gender, PMTCT exposure and adherence at visits 3, 6 and 9. In the models with positive immunological response as the outcome, children of all ages were combined into one model by combining percentages $\geq 25\%$ for children below 5 years and absolute CD4 T-cell counts ≥ 500 cell/mm^3 for children older than 5 years of age as positive outcomes. Explanatory variables included age group, CD4 count, WHO stage, gender, PMTCT exposure and adherence during the previous 3 or 6 months. In the models with virological success as the outcome, the same explanatory variables were tested as in the immunological success models, but also distance to the TRACplus clinic, orphan status, caregiver education, viral load at initiation and history of treatment switches. Furthermore, adherence over the last 6 months was used (instead of the last 3 months in all other models) because viral load was only measured once every 6 months. In the models with adherence over time as the outcome, explanatory variables included cART regimen, gender, caregiver's educational level, orphan status, and distance to the TRACplus clinic. The proportions of children with side effects were calculated per time point. From the literature, the most relevant predictors associated with side effects were considered gender and age [21]. Using Kaplan–Meier survival analysis, gender and age were analyzed for all side effects jointly and for each group separately.

Results

Baseline characteristics

One hundred and twenty three children were enrolled in the study (figure 1). The median (IQR) age at cART initiation was 7.4 years (3.2, 11.5); 40% of children were below 5 years of age and 54% were female (Table 1). Twenty-five (20%) children were diagnosed with HIV during PMTCT follow-up services, 58 (47%) children when they presented with clinical symptoms, and 40 (33%) children after their parents or siblings were diagnosed with HIV or were suspected to have died of HIV-related diseases. More than a quarter of the children (26%) were orphaned and cared for by other family members or living in an orphanage.

More children were stunted than underweight, with a mean (SD) HAZ and WAZ of −2.01 (1.2) and −1.73 (1.3), respectively. The median (IQR) CD4 T-cell values for children <5 years and ≥ 5 years of age were 20 (13, 28) percent and 337 (236, 484) cells/ mm^3 respectively. The median (IQR) plasma HIV-1 RNA concentration was 283,000 copies/mL (59,800, 1,100,000) for children less than 5 years of age and 90,600 copies/mL (12,800, 268,000) for those ≥5 years. The initial cART regimens are described in Table 1.

Study follow-up and clinical outcomes

Due to termination of funding in September 2010, not all children could be followed for 18 months; 116 children had been followed for 9 months; 104 for 12 months and 72 children for 18 months. The longitudinal analysis includes all data up to 12 months. One child (14 years old) presenting with WHO clinical stage 4 and a CD4 T-cell count of 2 cells/mm^3 died one month after cART initiation. He developed high fever, respiratory distress and increased lymphadenopathy, and the presumed cause of death was immune reconstitution inflammatory syndrome (IRIS). Two children were diagnosed with tuberculosis (one after 1 month on cART and the second child after 4 months of cART); no other children developed opportunistic infections during follow-up. One child was lost to follow-up, and one child moved and was transferred to another treatment center. At the time of the current analysis 98% of children were alive.

Table 2 summarizes anthropometric and biological parameters over time. Mean WAZ (GEE odds ratio (OR): 1.05 (95% confidence interval (CI): 1.03, 1.06; p-value <0.001)) and HAZ (GEE OR: 1.02 (95% CI: 1.01, 1.03; p-value <0.001)) improved significantly during the 12 months. At 12 months of follow-up, the proportion of children who were underweight had decreased from 42% to 20% (GEE OR: 0.90 (95% CI: 0.87, 0.94; p-value <0.001)) and the proportion of children who were stunted decreased from 51% to 41% (GEE OR: 0.96 (95% CI: 0.95, 0.99; p-value<0.001)). The median (range) ALT and AST concentrations at baseline were 19.5 (15.0, 25.0) and 39.0 (29.0,

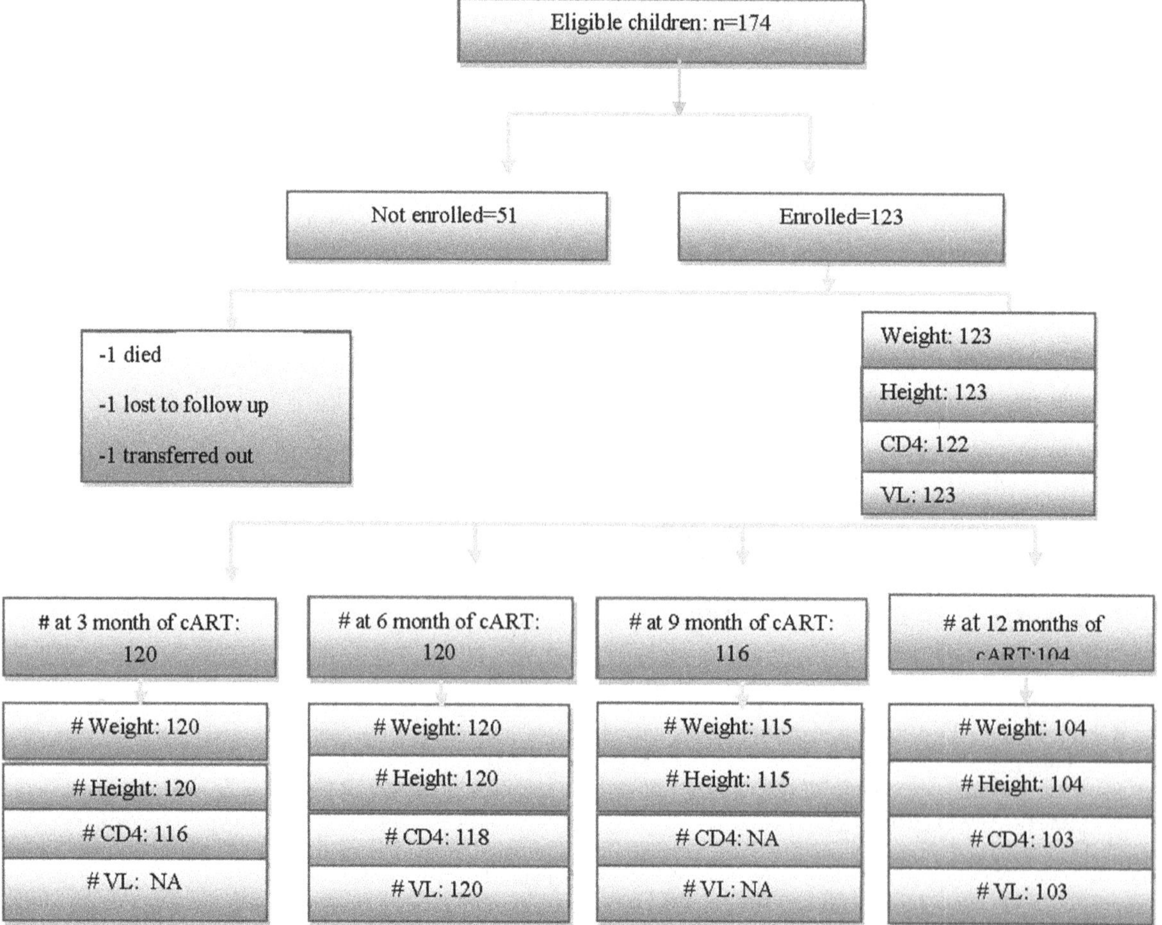

Figure 1. Flowchart summarizing the number of children at each stage of the study.

Table 1. Baseline characteristics at cART initiation (n = 123).

	<5 years (n = 49)	≥5 years (n = 74)	N
DEMOGRAPHIC AND SOCIAL			
Median (IQR) age, years	2.5(1.8–3.5)	11.0(9.0–13.4)	**123**
Female n (%)	28(57)	39(53)	**123**
Perinatal infection n (%)	49(100)	74(100)	**123**
Children exposed to PMTCT, n (%)	15(33)	10(15)	**110**
Parent status n (%)*			**123**
Both parents alive	28(57)	34(46)	
Only mother alive	7(14)	12(16)	
Only father alive	4(8)	6(8)	
Both parents died	10(20)	22(30)	
Guardians/caregivers n (%)			**123**
Both parents	19(39)	20(27)	
Mother only	15(31)	25(34)	
Father only	2(4)	3(4)	
Other family member	11(23)	23(31)	
Other	2(4)	3(4)	
Caregiver's educational status n (%)**			**123**
No education/few years primary school	17(34.7)	28(37.85)	
At least primary school completed	32(65.3)	46(62.2)	
Distance from healthcare center n (%)***			**123**
Living in Kigali	39(79.6)	16(21.6)	
Living outside of Kigali	10(20.4)	58(78.4)	
Tested and Diagnosed n (%)			**123**
PMTCT services	15	10	
Family member died/sick	15	25	
Symptoms	19	39	
CLINICAL			
Weight-for-age z-score			**123**
Mean (SD)	−2.04(1.6)	−1.49(1.1)	
z-score ≤−2 n (%)	26(53)	25(34)	
Height-for-age z-score			**123**
Mean (SD)	−2.5(1.4)	−1.7(0.9)	
z-score ≤−2 n (%)	34(69)	29(39)	
WHO stage, n (%)			**122**
Stage 1 & II	5(10.2)	18(24.7)	
Stage III & IV	44(89.8)	55(75.3)	
Tuberculosis at cART, n (%)	11(22)	19(26)	123
LABORATORY			
Immunological status at baseline			**119**
Median (IQR) CD4 values	20(13–28)	337/mm3(236–484)	
Children with CD4<15% or <350/mm3, n (%)	13(28)	41 (57)	
Virological status at baseline			**123**
Median (IQR) HIV-1 RNA copies/mL	283,000(59,800–1,100,000)	90,600(12,800–268,000)	
Biochemistry & Hematology at baseline			**122**
Median (IQR) ALT, UI/l	20(15–32)	19(15–25)	
Median (IQR) AST, UI/l	40(34–50)	34(29–40)	
Median (IQR) Hemoglobin, g/dL	11(10.2–11.6)	12(11.7–12.8)	
INITIAL cART REGIMEN n (%)			**123**
AZT/3TC/NVP	38(77.5)	46(62.2)	
ABC/3TC/NVP	1(2	2(2.7)	

Table 1. Cont.

	<5 years (n = 49)	≥5 years (n = 74)	N
D4T/3TC/NVP	2(4)	11(15.0)	
AZT/3TC/EFV	4(8)	12(16.2)	
D4T/3TC/EFV	2(4)	2(2.7)	
ABC/3TC/LPV/r	2(4)	1(1.4)	
Treatment switch	9(18.4)	12(16.2)	

*Orphan status was defined as having at least one biological parent vs. none.
**Caregiver's educational level was categorized as non-educated/few years of primary school vs. completed at least primary school.
***Distance to the clinic was defined as living in Kigali vs. outside of Kigali.

50.0) IU/mL and rose to 22.0 (15.0, 30.0) and 54.1 (29.9, 91.9) IU/mL at 12 months, respectively. The median (range) hemoglobin at cART initiation was 11.6 (11.3, 12.0) g/dL and increased to 12.3 (12.1, 12.5) at 12 months of cART.

Both age groups, above and below 5 years at cART initiation, had a significant increase in HAZ z-scores on therapy, but improvement was better in children above 5 years of age (GEE OR: 3.7 (95% CI: 1.8, 7.6)). Children who were not underweight when initiating cART were more likely to experience a significant HAZ and reduction of stunting overtime (GEE OR: 4.1 (95% CI: 1.9, 8.6)) as compared to those who were underweight (data not presented). WAZ increase was observed in both children with good and poor adherence, but the increase was slightly better in children with good adherence than children with poor adherence (GEE OR: 1.2 (95% CI: 0.9, 1.7)). Children who initiated treatment with CD4 ≥350 cells/µ/L or CD4 ≥15% had better improvement in WAZ scores compared to children who initiated treatment with CD4 below these cut offs (GEE OR: 1.9 (95% CI: 0.9, 3.8)). Children who achieved viral suppression compared to children with virological failure had significant WAZ (GEE OR:

Table 2. Changes of WAZ, HAZ, Hemoglobin, CD4 values and HIV RNA overtime.

	Baseline (n = 123)	3 Months (n = 119)	6 Months (n = 119)	12 Months (n = 104)	P-values
Nutritional status					
WAZ (mean, 95%CI*)	−1.73(−1.95,−1.50)	−1.38(−1.59,−1.17)	−1.28(−1.47,−1.08)	−1.17(−1.38,−0.96)	**<0.001**
Underweight (WAZ<−2) (n, %)	52(42)	36 (30)	31(26)	21(20)	**<0.001**
HAZ (mean, 95%CI*)	−2.01(−2.23,−1.80)	−1.93(−2.15,−1.71)	−1.82(−2.04,−1.60)	−1.75(−1.98,−1,51)	**<0.001**
Stunting (HAZ<−2) (n, %)	63(51)	57(47)	53(44)	43(41)	**0.001**
Hemoglobin (mean, 95 CI*), g/dL	11.6(11.3-12.0)	12.1(11.8-12.4)	12.2(12.0-12.4)	12.3(12.1-12.5)	**<0.001**
Immunological status					
Children ≥5 years, n = 74					
CD4 T-cells (median, IQR)	337(236–484)	500(345–675)	567(365–765)	620(375–880)	**<0.001**
CD4 T-cells <500, n (%),	57(79)	34(49)	29(40)	22(34)	**<0.001**
Children <5 years, n = 49					
CD4 T-cell % (median, IQR)	20(13–28)	29(22–36)	33(26–39)	36(28–41)	**<0.001**
CD4T-cell <25%, n (%),	30(65)	17(38)	11(24)	5(13)	**<0.001**
Virological status (HIV-RNA)					
<40 (copies/mL), n (%)	0(0)	Not determined	52(43)	79(76)	**<0.001**
>1000 copies/mL, n (%)	123(100)		46(38)	17(16)	**<0.001**

P values bold: Changes over time for all variables were statistically significant at p<0.05 using a univariate Generalized estimating equation model for categorical, normal and no normal distributed outcomes.

2.3 (95% CI: 1.6, 3.3)) and HAZ increases over time (GEE OR: 1.3 (95% CI: 1.1, 1.5)). A small percentage of children did not show any improvement in WAZ (4%) and HAZ (9%) after 12 months of cART. Out of 5 children who did not have increased WAZ, three had virological and immunological failure, and 4 had poor adherence. Out of 12 who did not have increased HAZ, 9 had virological failure, 7 had immunological failure, and 7 had poor adherence.

Immunological and virological responses

A significant increase in CD4 T- cells was observed in both children younger than 5 years of age as well as in those over 5 years of age. The median CD4 T-cell percent for younger children increased from 20% to 36% and the median CD4 T-cell count for children above 5 years increased from 337 to 620cells/mm^3 by 12 months follow-up; the proportion of children who achieved immunological success was 87% for children under 5 years and 66% for children 5 years of age and above. In bivariable models, independent predictors of immunological success included age and CD4 T-cell baseline value, with children below 5 years and those having a CD4 T-cell baseline value above 350/mm^3 showing a more robust increase in median CD4 T-cells (GEE OR: 1.9 (95% CI: 1.1, 4.1) and 7.0 (4.3, 11.6), respectively). PMTCT exposure, WHO stage at baseline, poor adherence, and socio-economic characteristics were not statistically associated with CD4 T-cell recovery in the first 12 months of cART.

The mean changes in HIV RNA plasma concentration over time are presented in Table 2. After 12 months of cART, 24% had detectable HIV RNA (>40 copies/mL), including 16% with virologic failure (>1000 copies/mL). In bivariable analyses, independent predictors of virological failure were being less than 5 years old at baseline (GEE OR: 2.6 (95% CI: 1.3, 5.2)), exposure to PMTCT (GEE OR: 3.4 (95% CI: (1.5, 7.8)), poor adherence during the first six months of treatment (GEE OR: 2.5 (95% CI: 1.3, 5.0)) and initiating cART with viral load ≥50.000 copies/mL (GEE OR: 4.6 (95% CI: 2.3, 156.2)). Other medical and social characteristics were not significantly associated with HIV RNA change over time (Table 3).

Adverse effects of treatment and treatment switches

There were 158 cumulative adverse effects reported in 52 (42%) children during the period of 12 months. The highest number was reported at month two of treatment in 40 (33%) of the children. The majority (47 out of 52) of children reported the same adverse effect at 2 or more time points; 41 children had mild and transient adverse effects which recovered without stopping treatment, 11/ 123 (9%) children experienced persistent side effects and/or worsening over time and underwent cART regimen changes as a result. The incidence of side-effects was higher within the first 6 months of cART initiation than thereafter (Figure 2a, 2b). The most common side effects were nausea and vomiting (14.8%), nevirapine-associated skin rash and hypersensitivity (13.2%), any grade of anemia (7%), diarrhea (6%), and dizziness and fatigue (5%) (Table 4). Eighty six percent of mild/moderate side effects improved without additional therapy.

During the follow-up period of 18 months, 21 (17%) children switched their initial cART regimen. Reasons for switching included persistent side effects (n = 11), virological failure (n = 3), tuberculosis treatment (replacement of nevirapine by efavirenz, n = 2), replacement of stavudine following a change of the Rwandan cART guidelines (n = 3), and replacement due to stock-out issues (n = 2). The children who developed nevirapine-associated skin-related side effects and/or significant liver enzyme elevations stopped treatment and their symptoms abated after treatment cessation; they resumed treatment with an efavirenz-based regimen. In three children with significant anemia, zidovudine was replaced by abacavir or tenofovir, hemoglobin improved to ≥10 g/dl within 6 months after treatment change. Two adolescents on a stavudine-based regimen developed signs of lipoatrophy (n = 1) and lipohypertrophy (n = 1) during the second year of treatment, and switched from stavudine to tenofovir. Eighteen out of the 21 treatment modifications were from one drug to another within the first line; 3 children switched from the first line NNRTI based regimen to a second line with lopinavir/ ritonavir because of virologic failure.

Adherence assessment

Adherence as estimated by self-report was high, with a median >95% at all-time points. In only 77 (11%) out of 710 scheduled visits at least one missed dose was reported by self-report. Incorrect dosage of any drug or change of time of taking medication was reported in 44 (6%) of all scheduled visits. Poor adherence on self-report was highly predictive of poor adherence on pill count (data not shown); however, good adherence by self-report was often not confirmed by pill count data. Pill count data showed that pills or scheduled visits were missed at 269 (38%) of visits. The proportion of children who were poor adherent according to pill count and recorded missed visits (adherence <95%) decreased over time, from 38% at month 3 to 20% by 12 months.

In bivariable analysis, after 6 months of cART 48% of children with good adherence had an undetectable viral load while only 34% of children with poor adherence had an undetectable viral load. The proportion of children with an undetectable viral load increased to 80% in the adherent group and to 57% in the less adherent group after 12 months of cART.

In bivariable analysis, lower caregiver educational status (GEE OR: 1.2 (95% CI: (1.1, 9.8)) and being an orphan ((GEE OR: 1.6 (95% CI): (1.2, 8.3)) were associated with lower adherence. None of the other factors, including gender, age, regimen or distance to the clinic were found to be statistically associated with adherence over time.

Discussion

The majority of children in this study showed good clinical and immunologic recovery, good adherence to cART and retention in care, as well as improved height and weight after 12 months of cART. Although the study showed overall treatment success after 12 months, HIV viral load was not fully suppressed in nearly a quarter of children, and immunologic recovery was less successful in children 5 years or older and those with more advanced HIV disease at cART initiation. Approximately one in 10 children developed severe side effects resulting in temporary cART cessation and regimen switches.

At baseline, slightly more than half of children were stunted and 40% were underweight. These proportions were higher than those reported by various recent national surveys in children regardless of HIV status, in which 27–44% of children were stunted, and up to 12% of children were underweight, depending on the area of the survey [22,23]. The lowest proportion of underweight children (6%) was found in Kigali district [22]. However, in our study, the number of children stunted and underweight after 12 months of cART was close to these survey figures. Furthermore, the overall

Table 3. Number of children with virological failure* over time.

	Month 6	Month 12	p-values**	Odds Ratio(95%%CI)
Parent status				
Both died	12(38)	6(21)	0.872	0.9(0.4–2.0)
At least one lives	34(39)	11(15)		
Caregiver's educational status				
Completed at least Primary school	17(37)	9(19)	0.678	0.6(0.3–3.1)
Non educated	30(39)	16(20)		
Distance from healthcare center				
Living in Kigali	22(40)	9(17)	0.567	0.8(0.5–2.7)
Outside of Kigali	28(41)	13(19)		
Age group				
Age ≥5 years at cART initiation	21(29)	7(11)	**0.006**	**2.6(1.3–5.2)**
Age <5 years at cART initiation	25(52)	10(25)		
Immunological status at baseline				
CD4≥15% or 350/mm3	21(34)	6(12)	0.282	1.5(0.7–2.9)
CD4<15% or <350/mm3	23(43)	10(20)		
WHO stage at baseline				
Baseline WHO I&II	8(35)	0	0.171	1.7(0.8–3.9)
Baseline WHO III&IV	37(39)	16(19)		
95% Adherence				
Adherent	26(32)	12(15)	**0.009**	**2.5(1.3–5.0)**
Non-adherent	20(53)	5(24)		
PMTCT exposure				
No-exposure	26(31)	9(12)	**0.003**	**3.4(1.5–7.9)**
Exposure	14(58)	6(38)		
Regimen switch up to 6 or 9 months				
No treatment change	40(37)	12(14)	0.337	1.6(0.6–4.3)
Treatment change	6(54)	7(49)		

*Virological failure defined as VL≥1000 copies/mL for one measurement;
**between group comparisons.
P values bold: significant difference at p<0.05.

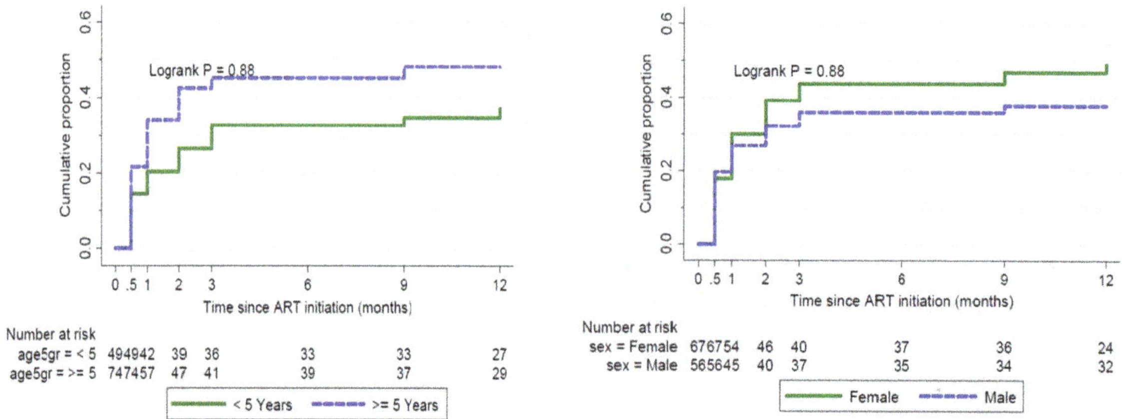

Figure 2. Cumulative of proportion of children with any side effect by sex (left) and age group (right) from baseline to 12 months of Treatment.

Table 4. Clinical and laboratory side effects.

	Day 15	Month 1	Month 2	Month 3	Month 6	Month 9	Month 12
Clinical side effects, n (%)							
Skin, mucosa and nails							
Hypersensitivity/Skin rash	16(13)	31(26)	26(21)	18(15)	6(5)	5(4)	2(2)
Nail pigmentation	-	-	-	2(2)	7(6)	9(8)	9(9)
Gastro-intestinal							
Nausea and vomiting, n (%)	21(17)	30(25)	34(28)	18(15)	4(3)	2(2)	1(1)
Diarrhea, n(%)	12(10)	13(11)	15(13)	11(9)	-	-	-
Abdominal pain, n (%)	4(3)	1(1)	2(2)	1(1)	-	-	-
Neurological							
Dizziness, n(%)	3(2)	6(5)	6(5)	6(5)	2(2)	2(2)	1(1)
Insomnia, n(%)	-	-	-	2(2)	2(2)	2(2)	1(1)
Laboratory							
Anemia (Hb<10 g/dl)	NA	NA	19(16)	6(5)	4(3)	2(2)	2(2)
Liver functions elevated (ALT), n (%)	7(6)	13(10)	8(7)	8(7)	3(3)	2(2)	-
Other*, n (%)	4(3)	2(2)	5(4)	3(2)	1(1)	-	-

*other included fatigue, anxiety and nightmares.

increase in weight among all children, and increase of height by baseline nutrition status and age are comparable to increases reported in other studies from similar resource constrained settings [9,24,25,26,27,28,29]. These findings reflect the efficacy of cART and offer reassuring evidence of its safety and tolerability in Rwandan children in which regular clinical monitoring is routine. Children who did not show any improvement in WAZ and HAZ after 12 months of treatment also showed poor ART adherence, poor immunologic recovery and virological failure.

In our study, children above 5 years of age were more likely to have impaired immunological recovery after 12 months of cART; conversely those under five were more likely to experience virologic failure. The robust immunologic recovery that we observed in young children may be partially explained by the superior ability of young infants to repopulate T lymphocytes [30,31], or by the hypothesis that later initiation of cART allows for more architectural damage to lymphatic tissues, which in turn hampers immune reconstitution [4,32]. The relationship between young age and virological failure has been documented in other studies in sub-Saharan Africa [13,33]. It is also consistent with earlier observations that infants and young children often present with high viral load and that it takes longer to fully suppress viral replication [34,35,36,37,38]. Prospective studies with longer follow-up periods should be conducted to determine whether the association between age at cART initiation and suboptimal virologic suppression is maintained after a longer period on cART. Not surprisingly, age and immune status at cART initiation were the factors most strongly associated with immunological success [9,39]. This observation emphasizes the fact that efforts should be made to diagnose and treat HIV infected children as early as possible.

The proportion of children with a detectable viral load and virological failure after 12 months of cART in this study is a serious finding that needs urgent attention. Poor adherence to cART and nevirapine exposure during PMTCT were associated with cART failure in our study as has been shown in other studies [40,41]. Previous studies confirmed that one in two infants exposed to single dose nevirapine prophylaxis develop nevirapine resistance, which in turn may expose children to more resistant viral strains and compromise therapy with NNRTI-containing regimens [42,43,44,45,46,47]. The finding that non-adherence measured by pill count was a strong predictor of virologic response reiterates the importance of adherence to cART and adherence monitoring through other means than self-report, in which patients are more likely to report high adherence [48]. Although it is obvious that adherence is paramount for achieving and maintaining viral suppression, and prevention of drug-resistance [49,50], it seems that the specific challenges regarding adherence in pediatric populations have not yet been sufficiently tackled. Issues such as drug administration in young children, adolescent behavior, socio-economic status and the dependency on the caregiver [51,52] may all play a role and are often difficult to solve. Additionally, the pharmacokinetic properties of ARVs in young children are not well known; underdosing or increased metabolism may lead to suboptimal plasma drug levels and thereby influence virologic outcomes. In an earlier study conducted in Rwanda, we observed that 14% of children using efavirenz were not adequately dosed [53], and other studies have shown similar results for other drug combinations [54,55].

The incidence of mild and moderate side effects in this study, mainly associated with nevirapine use, were similar to the findings from Uganda by Tukei [56], but were higher than what was reported by Lapphra in Thai children [57] and by Oumar in Malian children [58]. Most of the severe symptoms reported were reversed after discontinuation of the suspected drug and treatment changes to potentially less toxic medication as has been reported previously by Shubber et al [59]. The number of children with severe and/or persistent side effects leading to drug substitution was higher in our study compared to the studies mentioned previously [56,57,58]. Side effects and treatment switches may impact on treatment adherence, and potentially undermine the success of cART [60,61]. The side effects and regimen changes may have contributed to the relatively high percentage of children with treatment failure that we have seen in our study. More than half of the children without viral suppression had persistent side effects and/or regimen switches. Careful monitoring of the safety of cART remains needed, especially during the first months of cART, and we strongly support the national ART guidelines recommending PI-based regimens for all children <3 years of age [15].

This study has a number of limitations. Due to funding constraints, the sample size was relatively small; results for the present study on 123 children may not be generalizable to the larger population of children in Rwanda, given that data were only collected from children in one center in Kigali. Moreover, data for this study were collected a few years ago, current practice, validity and implication of some recommendations may be affected. However, the study presents more comprehensive information on cART outcomes in children than is available from national Rwandan HIV programs. The study highlights an important point that treatment failures are common in Rwandan children and emphasizes the importance of close virological monitoring. Another limitation is that the duration of follow-up was shorter than originally planned. This means that we were unable to assess the long term impact of cART on growth, immune and virologic responses, and long term toxicity. Studies with a longer duration of follow up are needed to inform national programs. Furthermore, we could not attribute the incidence of anemia solely to use of zidovudine as coexisting nutritional deficiencies and other chronic diseases may also have played a role [56,62,63]. Finally, we could not assess cART drug resistance in this particular study, but an earlier study in Rwanda showed that >90% of children with a viral load ≥1000 copies/mL after 12 months of cART were reported to have at least one NRTI or NNRTI's major mutations [10].

In conclusion, the importance of timely initiation of cART before profound immunodeficiency occurs in children should not be underestimated, as has been reported previously [9,11,12,13,14]. The Ministry of Health in Rwanda has recognized this and has adjusted its guidelines accordingly. Initiation of cART is now recommended for all children under 5 regardless of clinical condition and CD4 status, and for all children and adults older than 5 years with CD4 T-cells $<500/mm^3$. However, several challenges related to side effects, and achieving long-term adherence and virologic suppression remain. To be truly successful, pediatric HIV programs must aim to find HIV infected children before disease progression occurs, initiate cART timely, and monitor treatment success and side effects closely. Furthermore, the main causes of virologic failure should be further investigated, so that strategies for early recognition of children at high risk and appropriate interventions can be developed [64,65].

Acknowledgments

The authors would like to thank all the patients and families from Treatment and Research for AIDS Center participating in this study and the team of the INTERACT Project and the Rwandan Ministry of Health. Laboratory technicians from the National Reference Laboratory, Rwanda are kindly acknowledged for the analysis of laboratory tests that were performed for the purpose of this study.

Author Contributions

Conceived and designed the experiments: PRM NM JMAL JvdW AA PR SPMG. Performed the experiments: PRM KRB NM DT. Analyzed the data: PRM KRB BAK. Contributed reagents/materials/analysis tools: PRM KRB NM JMAL JvdW BAK DT PR SPMG. Wrote the paper: PRM KRB NM JMAL JvdW AA BAK DT PR SPMG.

References

1. HHS Panel on Antiretroviral Therapy and Medical Management of HIV-Infected Children (2012) Guidelines for the Use of Antiretroviral Agents in Pediatric HIV Infection. Available: http://aidsinfonihgov/contentfiles/lvguidelines/pediatricguidelinespdf Accessed September 2013
2. Mofenson LM, Brady MT, Danner SP, Dominguez KL, Hazra R, et al. (2009) Guidelines for the Prevention and Treatment of Opportunistic Infections among HIV-exposed and HIV-infected children: recommendations from CDC, the National Institutes of Health, the HIV Medicine Association of the Infectious Diseases Society of America, the Pediatric Infectious Diseases Society, and the American Academy of Pediatrics. MMWR Recomm Rep 58: 1–166.
3. Penazzato M, Crowley S, Mofenson L, Franceschetto G, Nannyonga MM, et al. (2012) Programmatic impact of the evolution of WHO pediatric antiretroviral treatment guidelines for resource-limited countries (Tukula Fenna Project, Uganda). J Acquir Immune Defic Syndr 61: 522–525.
4. Puthanakit T, Kerr S, Ananworanich J, Bunupuradah T, Boonrak P, et al. (2009) Pattern and predictors of immunologic recovery in human immunodeficiency virus-infected children receiving non-nucleoside reverse transcriptase inhibitor-based highly active antiretroviral therapy. Pediatr Infect Dis J 28: 488–492.
5. Sutcliffe CG, van Dijk JH, Munsanje B, Hamangaba F, Siniwymaanzi P, et al. (2011) Risk factors for pre-treatment mortality among HIV-infected children in rural Zambia: a cohort study. PLoS One 6: e29294.
6. Yotebieng M, Van Rie A, Moultrie H, Meyers T (2010) Six-month gain in weight, height, and CD4 predict subsequent antiretroviral treatment responses in HIV-infected South African children. AIDS 24: 139–146.
7. Clavel F, Hance AJ (2004) HIV drug resistance. N Engl J Med 350: 1023–1035.
8. Musiime V, Kaudha E, Kayiwa J, Mirembe G, Odera M, et al. (2013) Antiretroviral drug resistance profiles and response to second-line therapy among HIV type 1-infected Ugandan children. AIDS Res Hum Retroviruses 29: 449–455.
9. Musoke PM, Mudiope P, Barlow-Mosha LN, Ajuna P, Bagenda D, et al. (2010) Growth, immune and viral responses in HIV infected African children receiving highly active antiretroviral therapy: a prospective cohort study. BMC Pediatr 10: 56.
10. Mutwa PR, Boer KR, Rusine J, Muganga N, Tuyishimire D, et al. (2014) Long-term effectiveness of combination antiretroviral therapy and prevalence of HIV drug resistance in HIV-1-infected children and adolescents in Rwanda. Pediatr Infect Dis J 33: 63–69.
11. Sutcliffe CG, van Dijk JH, Munsanje B, Hamangaba F, Sinywimaanzi P, et al. (2011) Weight and height z-scores improve after initiating ART among HIV-infected children in rural Zambia: a cohort study. BMC Infect Dis 11: 54.
12. Ndumbi P, Falutz J, Pant Pai N, Tsoukas CM (2014) Delay in cART Initiation Results in Persistent Immune Dysregulation and Poor Recovery of T-Cell Phenotype Despite a Decade of Successful HIV Suppression. PLoS One 9: e94018.
13. Okomo U, Togun T, Oko F, Peterson K, Townend J, et al. (2012) Treatment outcomes among HIV-1 and HIV-2 infected children initiating antiretroviral therapy in a concentrated low prevalence setting in West Africa. BMC Pediatr 12: 95.
14. Mossdorf E, Stoeckle M, Mwaigomole EG, Chiweka E, Kibatala PL, et al. (2011) Improved antiretroviral treatment outcome in a rural African setting is associated with cART initiation at higher CD4 cell counts and better general health condition. BMC Infect Dis 11: 98.
15. Rwdanda Ministry of Health (2012) National Guidelines for Comprehensive Care of People Living with HIV in Rwanda.
16. Rwdanda Ministry of Health (2012) National Annual Report on HIV&AIDS July 2011–June 2012. Available: http://wwwrbcgovrw/spipphp?article503 Accessed August 2013.
17. Rwdanda Ministry of Health (2007) Guide de Prise en Charge des Personnes Infectées par le VIH au Rwanda. Available: http://wwwaidstar-onecom/focus_areas/treatment/resources. Accessed July 2013.
18. World Health Organization (2006) Antiretroviral Therapy of HIV infection in Infants and Children: Towards universal access Recommendations for a public health approach. Available: http://wwwhoint/hiv/pub/guidelines/art/en/ Accessed August 2013
19. Rwdanda Ministry of Health (2009) Guidelines for the provision of comprehensive care to persons infected by HIV in Rwanda.
20. (2004) Division of AIDS Table for Grading the Severity of adult and Pediatric Adverse Events Available: http://rsctech-rescom/safetyandpharmacovigilance/gradingtablesaspx Accessed November 2013 Version 1.0.
21. Phan V, Thai S, Choun K, Lynen L, van Griensven J (2012) Incidence of treatment-limiting toxicity with stavudine-based antiretroviral therapy in Cambodia: a retrospective cohort study. PLoS One 7: e30647.
22. National Institute of Statistics of Rwanda/Ministry of Finance and Economic Planning Kigali R (2010) Rwanda Demographic and Health Survey. Available: http://wwwstatisticsgovrw/survey/demographic-and-health-survey-dhs Accessed September 2013.
23. National Institute of Statistics of Rwanda/Ministry of Finance and Economic Planning R (2012) Comprehensive Food Security and Vulnerability Analysis and Nutrition Survey Available: http://wwwstatisticsgovrw/publications/comprehensive-food-security-and-vulnerability-analysis-and-nutrition-survey-cfsva-2012 Accessed November 2013
24. Bolton-Moore C, Mubiana-Mbewe M, Cantrell RA, Chintu N, Stringer EM, et al. (2007) Clinical outcomes and CD4 cell response in children receiving antiretroviral therapy at primary health care facilities in Zambia. JAMA 298: 1888–1899.
25. Davies MA, Keiser O, Technau K, Eley B, Rabie H, et al. (2009) Outcomes of the South African National Antiretroviral Treatment Programme for children: the IeDEA Southern Africa collaboration. S Afr Med J 99: 730–737.
26. Essajee SM, Kim M, Gonzalez C, Rigaud M, Kaul A, et al. (1999) Immunologic and virologic responses to HAART in severely immunocompromised HIV-1-infected children. AIDS 13: 2523–2532.
27. Kamya MR, Mayanja-Kizza H, Kambugu A, Bakeera-Kitaka S, Semitala F, et al. (2007) Predictors of long-term viral failure among ugandan children and adults treated with antiretroviral therapy. J Acquir Immune Defic Syndr 46: 187–193.
28. Sutcliffe CG, Moss WJ (2010) Do children infected with HIV receiving HAART need to be revaccinated? Lancet Infect Dis 10: 630–642.
29. Wamalwa DC, Farquhar C, Obimbo EM, Selig S, Mbori-Ngacha DA, et al. (2007) Early response to highly active antiretroviral therapy in HIV-1-infected Kenyan children. J Acquir Immune Defic Syndr 45: 311–317.
30. Franco JM, Leon-Leal JA, Leal M, Cano-Rodriguez A, Pineda JA, et al. (2000) CD4+ and CD8+ T lymphocyte regeneration after anti-retroviral therapy in HIV-1-infected children and adult patients. Clin Exp Immunol 119: 493–498.
31. Soh CH, Oleske JM, Brady MT, Spector SA, Borkowsky W, et al. (2003) Long-term effects of protease-inhibitor-based combination therapy on CD4 T-cell recovery in HIV-1-infected children and adolescents. Lancet 362: 2045–2051.
32. Walker AS, Doerholt K, Sharland M, Gibb DM, Collaborative HIVPSSC (2004) Response to highly active antiretroviral therapy varies with age: the UK and Ireland Collaborative HIV Paediatric Study. AIDS 18: 1915–1924.
33. Wittkop L, Ngo-Giang_huong N, Team E-C-EP (2013) Prevalence and impact of transmitted drug resistance (TDR) on response to ART in children. Abstract Presented at 7th Conference on HIV Pathogenesis, treatment and Prevention.
34. van Rossum AM, Geelen SP, Hartwig NG, Wolfs TF, Weemaes CM, et al. (2002) Results of 2 years of treatment with protease-inhibitor–containing antiretroviral therapy in dutch children infected with human immunodeficiency virus type 1. Clin Infect Dis 34: 1008–1016.
35. Starr SE, Fletcher CV, Spector SA, Yong FH, Fenton T, et al. (1999) Combination therapy with efavirenz, nelfinavir, and nucleoside reverse-transcriptase inhibitors in children infected with human immunodeficiency virus type 1. Pediatric AIDS Clinical Trials Group 382 Team. N Engl J Med 341: 1874–1881.
36. Nachman SA, Stanley K, Yogev R, Pelton S, Wiznia A, et al. (2000) Nucleoside analogs plus ritonavir in stable antiretroviral therapy-experienced HIV-infected children: a randomized controlled trial. Pediatric AIDS Clinical Trials Group 338 Study Team. JAMA 283: 492–498.
37. Pelton SI, Johnson D, Chadwick E, Baldwin Z, Yogev R (1999) A one year experience: T cell responses and viral replication in children with advanced human immunodeficiency virus type 1 disease treated with combination therapy including ritonavir. Pediatr Infect Dis J 18: 650–652.
38. Palumbo PE, Kwok S, Waters S, Wesley Y, Lewis D, et al. (1995) Viral measurement by polymerase chain reaction-based assays in human immunodeficiency virus-infected infants. J Pediatr 126: 592–595.
39. Lewis J, Walker AS, Castro H, De Rossi A, Gibb DM, et al. (2012) Age and CD4 count at initiation of antiretroviral therapy in HIV-infected children: effects on long-term T-cell reconstitution. J Infect Dis 205: 548–556.
40. Teasdale CA, Abrams EJ, Coovadia A, Strehlau R, Martens L, et al. (2013) Adherence and viral suppression among infants and young children initiating protease inhibitor-based antiretroviral therapy. Pediatr Infect Dis J 32: 489–494.
41. Nachega JB, Hislop M, Nguyen H, Dowdy DW, Chaisson RE, et al. (2009) Antiretroviral therapy adherence, virologic and immunologic outcomes in

adolescents compared with adults in southern Africa. J Acquir Immune Defic Syndr 51: 65–71.
42. Persaud D, Bedri A, Ziemniak C, Moorthy A, Gudetta B, et al. (2011) Slower clearance of nevirapine resistant virus in infants failing extended nevirapine prophylaxis for prevention of mother-to-child HIV transmission. AIDS Res Hum Retroviruses 27: 823–829.
43. Palumbo P, Lindsey JC, Hughes MD, Cotton MF, Bobat R, et al. (2010) Antiretroviral treatment for children with peripartum nevirapine exposure. N Engl J Med 363: 1510–1520.
44. Mphatswe W, Blanckenberg N, Tudor-Williams G, Prendergast A, Thobakgale C, et al. (2007) High frequency of rapid immunological progression in African infants infected in the era of perinatal HIV prophylaxis. AIDS 21: 1253–1261.
45. Lockman S, Shapiro RL, Smeaton LM, Wester C, Thior I, et al. (2007) Response to antiretroviral therapy after a single, peripartum dose of nevirapine. N Engl J Med 356: 135–147.
46. Coovadia A, Abrams EJ, Stehlau R, Meyers T, Martens L, et al. (2010) Reuse of nevirapine in exposed HIV-infected children after protease inhibitor-based viral suppression: a randomized controlled trial. JAMA 304: 1082–1090.
47. Arrive E, Newell ML, Ekouevi DK, Chaix ML, Thiebaut R, et al. (2007) Prevalence of resistance to nevirapine in mothers and children after single-dose exposure to prevent vertical transmission of HIV-1: a meta-analysis. Int J Epidemiol 36: 1009–1021.
48. Vyankandondera J, Mitchell K, Asiimwe-Kateera B, Boer K, Mutwa P, et al. (2013) Antiretroviral therapy drug adherence in Rwanda: perspectives from patients and healthcare workers using a mixed-methods approach. AIDS Care 25: 1504–1512.
49. Mofenson LM, Cotton MF (2013) The challenges of success: adolescents with perinatal HIV infection. J Int AIDS Soc 16: 18650.
50. Mghamba FW, Minzi OM, Massawe A, Sasi P (2013) Adherence to antiretroviral therapy among HIV infected children measured by caretaker report, medication return, and drug level in Dar Es Salaam, Tanzania. BMC Pediatr 13: 95.
51. Vreeman RC, Wiehe SE, Ayaya SO, Musick BS, Nyandiko WM (2008) Association of antiretroviral and clinic adherence with orphan status among HIV-infected children in Western Kenya. J Acquir Immune Defic Syndr 49: 163–170.
52. Azmeraw D, Wasie B (2012) Factors associated with adherence to highly active antiretroviral therapy among children in two referral hospitals, northwest Ethiopia. Ethiop Med J 50: 115–124.
53. Mutwa PR, Fillekes Q, Malgaz M, Tuyishimire D, Kraats R, et al. (2012) Mid-dosing interval efavirenz plasma concentrations in HIV-1-infected children in Rwanda: treatment efficacy, tolerability, adherence, and the influence of CYP2B6 polymorphisms. J Acquir Immune Defic Syndr 60: 400–404.
54. Menson EN, Walker AS, Sharland M, Wells C, Tudor-Williams G, et al. (2006) Underdosing of antiretrovirals in UK and Irish children with HIV as an example of problems in prescribing medicines to children, 1997–2005: cohort study. BMJ 332: 1183–1187.
55. King JR, Kimberlin DW, Aldrovandi GM, Acosta EP (2002) Antiretroviral pharmacokinetics in the paediatric population: a review. Clin Pharmacokinet 41: 1115–1133.
56. Tukei VJ, Asiimwe A, Maganda A, Atugonza R, Sebuliba I, et al. (2012) Safety and tolerability of antiretroviral therapy among HIV-infected children and adolescents in Uganda. J Acquir Immune Defic Syndr 59: 274–280.
57. Lapphra K, Vanprapar N, Chearskul S, Phongsamart W, Chearskul P, et al. (2008) Efficacy and tolerability of nevirapine- versus efavirenz-containing regimens in HIV-infected Thai children. Int J Infect Dis 12: e33–38.
58. Oumar AA, Diallo K, Dembele JP, Samake L, Sidibe I, et al. (2012) Adverse drug reactions to antiretroviral therapy: prospective study in children in sikasso (mali). J Pediatr Pharmacol Ther 17: 382–388.
59. Shubber Z, Calmy A, Andrieux-Meyer I, Vitoria M, Renaud-Thery F, et al. (2013) Adverse events associated with nevirapine and efavirenz-based first-line antiretroviral therapy: a systematic review and meta-analysis. AIDS 27: 1403–1412.
60. Moh R, Danel C, Messou E, Ouassa T, Gabillard D, et al. (2007) Incidence and determinants of mortality and morbidity following early antiretroviral therapy initiation in HIV-infected adults in West Africa. AIDS 21: 2483–2491.
61. Padua CA, Cesar CC, Bonolo PF, Acurcio FA, Guimaraes MD (2006) High incidence of adverse reactions to initial antiretroviral therapy in Brazil. Braz J Med Biol Res 39: 495–505.
62. Pryce C, Pierre RB, Steel-Duncan J, Evans-Gilbert T, Palmer P, et al. (2008) Safety of antiretroviral drug therapy in Jamaican children with HIV/AIDS. West Indian Med J 57: 238–245.
63. Shah I (2006) Adverse effects of antiretroviral therapy in HIV-1 infected children. J Trop Pediatr 52: 244–248.
64. Scanlon ML, Vreeman RC (2013) Current strategies for improving access and adherence to antiretroviral therapies in resource-limited settings. HIV AIDS (Auckl) 5: 1–17.
65. Gusdal AK, Obua C, Andualem T, Wahlstrom R, Chalker J, et al. (2011) Peer counselors' role in supporting patients' adherence to ART in Ethiopia and Uganda. AIDS Care 23: 657–662.

Serotype Distribution and Antibiotic Susceptibility of *Streptococcus pneumoniae* Strains Carried by Children Infected with Human Immunodeficiency Virus

Dodi Safari[1]*, Nia Kurniati[2], Lia Waslia[3], Miftahuddin Majid Khoeri[1], Tiara Putri[4], Debby Bogaert[5], Krzysztof Trzciński[5]

1 Eijkman Institute for Molecular Biology, Jakarta, Indonesia, **2** Department of Child Health, Dr. Cipto Mangunkusumo Hospital/Faculty of Medicine Universitas Indonesia, Jakarta, Indonesia, **3** Eijkman Oxford Clinical Research Unit, Jakarta, Indonesia, **4** Faculty of Biology, Gajah Mada University, Yogyakarta, Indonesia, **5** Department of Pediatric Immunology and Infectious Diseases, Wilhelmina's Children Hospital, University Medical Center Utrecht, Utrecht, the Netherlands

Abstract

Background: We studied the serotype distribution and antibiotic susceptibility of *Streptococcus pneumoniae* isolates carried by children infected with HIV in Jakarta, Indonesia.

Methods: Nasopharyngeal swabs were collected from 90 HIV infected children aged 4 to 144 months. *S. pneumoniae* was identified by conventional and molecular methods. Serotyping was performed with sequential multiplex PCR and antibiotic susceptibility with the disk diffusion method.

Results: We identified *S. pneumoniae* carriage in 41 children (46%). Serotype 19F was most common among 42 cultured strains (19%) followed by 19A and 6A/B (10% each), and 23F (7%). Most isolates were susceptible to chloramphenicol (86%), followed by clindamycin (79%), erythromycin (76%), tetracycline (43%), and sulphamethoxazole/trimethoprim (41%). Resistance to penicillin was most common with only 33% of strains being susceptible. Strains of serotypes targeted by the 13-valent pneumococcal conjugate polysaccharide vaccine (PCV13) were more likely to be multidrug resistant (13 of 25 or 52%) compared to non-PCV13 serotype isolates (3 of 17 or 18%; Fisher exact test $p = 0.05$).

Conclusion: Our study provides insight into the epidemiology of pneumococcal carriage in young HIV patients in Indonesia. These findings may facilitate potential preventive strategies that target invasive pneumococcal disease in Indonesia.

Editor: Adam J. Ratner, Columbia University, United States of America

Funding: This study was supported by a small grant from International Society of Infectious Disease (ISID). The funders had no role in study design, data collection and analysis, decision to publish, or preparation of the manuscript.

Competing Interests: DB has received consulting fees from Pfizer. KT has received consulting fees from Pfizer and grant support for studies onpneumococcal carriage from Pfizer.

* Email: safari@eijkman.go.id

Introduction

Streptococcus pneumoniae is a leading cause of bacterial pneumonia, meningitis, and sepsis worldwide. An estimated 1.6 million people die from invasive pneumococcal disease (IPD) each year, one million of whom are children [1]. Incidence of IPD varies substantially by age, genetic background, socioeconomic status, immune status, and geographical location [2]. Capsular polysaccharide is considered to be the ultimate virulence factor of *S. pneumoniae* as un-encapsulated strains are virtually absent among *S. pneumoniae* causing IPD [3,4]. Over 90 *S. pneumoniae* serotypes have been identified based on the capsule chemical structure and immunogenicity [5] and capsular oligosaccharides are used as vaccine antigens in pneumococcal vaccines.

Current pneumococcal conjugate vaccines cover only a selected set of serotypes, e.g. PCV7 (7 serotypes), PCV10 (10 serotypes) and PCV13 (13 serotypes). The introduction of the PCV7 vaccine targeting the serotypes 4, 6B, 9V, 14, 18C, 19F, and 23F significantly reduced the burden of pneumococcal disease in many populations [6]. Despite high efficacy against disease caused by the vaccine serotypes (VTs), the net effect of vaccination is often reduced due to serotype replacement [6,7]. In a number of geographical locations including the USA, Germany, The Netherlands, England and Wales [8–11], serotype 19A was reported to be the most commonly emerging non-vaccine serotype (NVT) following PCV7 introduction. Colonization of the upper respiratory tract is the obligatory first step in the pathogenesis of pneumococcal disease, and therefore considered the most important risk factor for IPD [12]. It also provides the basis for horizontal spread of pneumococci in the community, making it an important target for preventive measures [13,14].

Currently, epidemiological data on *S. pneumoniae* carriage and invasive disease is limited for the Indonesian population. In 2001, Soewignjo *et al.* reported that the prevalence of *S. pneumoniae* carriage was 48% in healthy children in Lombok Island, Indonesia [15]. Recently, Farida *et al.* reported that in Semarang, Indonesia, prevalence of *S. pneumoniae* in 2010 was 43% and 11% in children aged 6–60 months and adults aged 45–75 years, respectively [17]. One of the risk factors for IPD is infection with human immunodefficiency virus (HIV) [16]. So far, no data are available on *S. pneumoniae* carriage in high-risk populations in Indonesia. Currently, pneumococcal vaccination is not part of the expanded program on immunization (EPI) for infants in Indonesia. Both the PCV13 (targeting all PCV7 serotypes plus serotypes 1, 3, 5, 6A, 7F and 19A) and the 23-valent pneumococcal polysaccharide vaccine (PPV23) are available at a commercial price. The use of pneumococcal vaccines is not monitored in any systemic way in Indonesia.

In this present study, we investigate the carriage of *S. pneumoniae* in children infected with HIV in Jakarta, Indonesia. We expect our results to guide the modification of existing, and the implementation of potentially new preventive strategies targeting pneumococcal disease in the country.

Methods

Study population

A cross-sectional study on *S. pneumoniae* nasopharyngeal colonization was performed from January to July 2012 among children infected with human immunodeficiency virus (HIV) during their routine clinic visits at the Cipto Mangunkusumo Hospital, Jakarta – Indonesia. The study has been reviewed and approved by the ethical committee of Faculty of Medicine, Universitas Indonesia, Jakarta, Indonesia. The children's parents signed informed consent forms and provided clinical and demographic information, such as age, sex, family size and in which region they were living. Detailed medical information on the CD4 lymphocyte count within the past 3 months and the use of antibiotics was recorded during the study. Parents were also asked whether any person living with a child is smoking. No other environmental exposure factors were recorded. According to the study's protocol children with symptoms of a respiratory tract infection and children who were immunized with one or more doses of any pneumococcal vaccine were excluded from the study.

Sample collection

Nasopharyngeal (NP) swabs were collected using a flexible nasopharyngeal flocked swab (Copan, Italy no 503SC01) as recommended by WHO [14,18]. Swabs were placed into 1.0 ml of skim milk tryptone glucose glycerol (STGG) transport medium, shipped on wet ice directly to the Eijkman Institute, Jakarta. Upon arrival at the lab, 20 µl of each STGG sample was plated onto a 5% sheep blood agar supplemented with 5 mg/L gentamicin (SB-Gent), and incubated at 35°C for 24 h with 5% CO_2. In the case of alpha-hemolytic colonies growth on the SB-Gent plate, a single colony was re-cultured and tested by Gram-staining, and also tested for susceptibility to optochin [13]. Gram-positive, optochin-sensitive isolates were stored in STGG at −80°C for further analysis.

DNA extraction

Bacterial DNA was extracted as described previously [19]. Briefly, pneumococcal isolates were retrieved from storage by subculture on the SB-Gent. The bacterial cells suspension was heated at 100°C for 10 minutes and instantly frozen at −20°C for 10 minutes. Lysates were centrifuged at 1000×g for 10 minutes, after which the supernatant was collected and stored at −20°C until further use.

Molecular detection of pneumococcal surface antigen A gene

The polymerase chain reaction (PCR) targeting the pneumococcal surface antigen A gene (*psa*A) was performed as described by Morrison et al. [20]. In short, the reaction mixture contained GoTaq Green Master Mix (Promega), forward (5′-CTTTCTGC-AATCATTCTTG-3′) and reverse (3′-GCCTTCTTTACCTT-GTTCTGC-5′) primers at 10 µM concentration, and 1.0 µl of DNA template. The presence of 838 bp amplicon was detected by electrophoresis of 5 µl of PCR product on 1% agarose gels stained with ethidium bromide, and visualized in UV light.

Serotyping

Serotype determination was performed by a sequential multiplex PCR (smPCR), as published by Pai *et al.* [19]. Briefly, seven smPCRs were performed, each in a 25 µl reaction mixture of GoTaq Green Master Mix (Promega) and up to five pairs of primers specific for a particular serotype or serotypes cluster and an internal positive control targeting 160 bp fragment of capsule transcriptional regulator gene *wzg* (*cps*A) universally present in *cps* operons of almost all serotypes and using 1.0 µl of cell lysate extract as DNA template. The primers set used in the study allowed for identification of 40 serotypes, including all serotypes targeted by PCV13 and were published by the CDC (USA) [21].

Antibiotic susceptibility testing

Antibiotic susceptibility tests were carried out for all of the pneumococcus isolates using the disk diffusion method according to CLSI standard [22], and antimicrobial disks (Oxoid) with chloramphenicol, clindamycin, erythromycin, sulfamethoxazole/trimethoprim, and tetracycline. Susceptibility to penicillin was tested with the oxacillin disk [22]. Strains expressing lack of susceptibility to three or more antimicrobial agents of different classes were considered multidrug resistant (MDR) in the study.

Statistical methods

Statistical analyses were conducted using GraphPad Prism V5.0 (GraphPad Software, San Diego, CA, USA).

Results

Streptococcus pneumoniae isolates were cultured from 41 of 90 (46%) nasopharyngeal samples collected in the study from children infected with HIV in Jakarta, Indonesia. All strains were susceptible to optochin and positive for the *psa*A gene by PCR. The patient characteristics are described in Table 1. There were no differences in carriage rates within gender, family size, use of antibiotics, or tobacco smoking in the household. Although, *S. pneumoniae* carriage rates were higher in children with a CD4 lymphocyte count less than 25% (59%), compared to children with a CD4 count >25% (37%) the difference did not reach statistical significance (Fisher exact test $p = 0.086$) (Table 1). There was no correlation between child age and CD4 count (Pearson; $r = 0.09$, $p = 0.46$) neither of the differences in carriage rates between age groups in the study were significant. There were no exclusions from the study based on a child's previous immunization with any pneumococcal vaccine.

Altogether, we cultured 42 *S. pneumoniae* strains from 41 samples, with a single sample from one child positive simultaneously for strains of serotype 3 and 9V. The most commonly observed was serotype 19F (8 of 42 cultured pneumococcal strains; 19%) followed by 9A and 6A/B (4 carriers each; 10%), 23F (3

Table 1. Patient characteristics related to pneumococcal carriage.

Characteristics		N	N (%) of children carrying *S. pneumoniae*
HIV-infected children		90	41 (46)
Age (month)			
	0–24	9	3 (33)
	25–60	33	15 (46)
	61–144	48	23 (48)
Sex			
	Male	44	18 (49)
	Female	46	23 (51)
Exposure to cigarette			
	Yes	41	18 (44)
	No	49	23 (47)
No of family member			
	[1–3]	34	17 (50)
	[4–6]	28	11 (39)
	[>7]	12	6 (50)
	no data	16	7 (44)
Current antibiotics use			
	Yes	20	9 (45)
	No	70	32 (46)
CD4 lymphocyte count[a]			
	<25%	34	20 (59)
	≥ 25%	30	11 (37)
	no data	26	10 (39)

[a]CD4 lymphocyte count measured within 3 months prior to nasopharyngeal sampling.

carriers; 7%), 9V, 35B, 11A (two carriers each; 5%) and serotypes 18C, 3, 12F, 15B/C and 35F (single carrier each; 2%) (Table 2). We found that eleven isolates (26%) were untypeable using the SM-PCR method, with six of those 11 (14% of all) also being PCR-negative for the *cpsA* gene. In this study, strains that could be covered by the pneumococcal conjugate vaccine varied between 45% to 60% for PCV7 and PCV13 vaccines, respectively.

The majority of strains were susceptible to chloramphenicol (86%), clindamycin (79%), erythromycin (76%), sulphamethoxazole/trimethoprim (41%) and tetracycline (43%) (Table 3). Meanwhile, only 33% of strains were susceptible to penicillin (Table 3). Use of the oxacillin disc to screen isolates for lack of susceptibility to penicillin could be considered as a limitation in our study as it does not allow to distinguish low level from high level resistance with low level resistant strains often retaining sensitivity to a range of beta-lactams, including aminopenicllins [22]. Compared to strains of other serotypes, isolates of PCV13 serotypes detected in the study (3, 6A/B, 7F, 9V, 14, 18C, 19A, 19F, and 23F) were less susceptible to any of the six antimicrobial agents tested, although the difference was significant only for penicillin (Table 3). In this study, we found 16 of isolates expressed a lack of susceptibility to three or more antimicrobial agents of different classes thus considered multi-drug resistant (MDR) (Table 4). With 13 (52%) of 25 strains of PCV13 serotypes versus three (18%) of 17 non-PCV13 serotype strains classified as MDR in our study, the multidrug resistance was more common, however the difference did not reach statistical significance (Fisher exact test $p = 0.0504$) among isolates of serotypes targeted by the vaccine.

Discussion

Since limited data was available on the epidemiology of *S. pneumoniae* carriage in the Indonesian population, especially in high-risk children, we studied *S. pneumoniae* carriage in children infected with HIV. Our findings of 46% of *S. pneumoniae* carriage in HIV-positive children (aged 4 to 144 months) in Jakarta are in line with a previously published report on carriage in healthy children in Lombok Island and Semarang, Indonesia, where 48% of children (aged 0–25 months) and 43% of children (aged 6–60 months) carried pneumococci [15,17]. *S. pneumoniae* carriage in children with this acquired immunodeficiency varies in different geographical locations. In comparison to other studies in which nasopharyngeal carriage of *S. pneumoniae* was detected in HIV-infected children using the WHO-recommended culture method, the prevalence of pneumococcal carriage in Jakarta was lower compared to 66% recorded in Tanzania (children aged 12–168 months) and 77% reported in Kenya (3–59 months) [23,24], but higher than in Romania (children aged 39–106 months), Brazil (0–228 months), and USA with the reported carriage rates of 30%, 29%, and 20%, respectively [25–27]. There is relatively little known about possible impact of the HIV infection on pneumococcal carriage. Abdullahi *et al.* [24] reported higher carriage prevalence in Kenya among HIV-positive versus HIV-negative children whereas infection with HIV has no effect on pneumococcal carriage reported in adults in South Africa by Shiri *et al.* [28]. Although we observed a trend towards higher *S. pneumoniae* carriage rates in children with lower CD4 lymphocyte count, both Mwenya, *et al.* [29] and Anthony *et al.* [23] reported lack of any

Table 2. Serotype distribution and vaccine coverage among 42 *S. pneumoniae* carriage isolates of HIV-infected children in Jakarta.

Serotype		N (%) of isolates
19F		8 (19)
19A		4 (10)
6A/B		4 (10)
23F		3 (7)
11A		2 (5)
9V		2 (5)
sg18		2 (5)
12F		1 (2)
15B/C		1 (2)
3		1 (2)
35B		1 (2)
35F		1 (2)
7F		1 (2)
untypeable		
	cps-positive	5 (12)
	cps-negative	6 (14)
PCV-7 coverage		19 (45)
PCV-13-coverage		25 (60)

association between CD4 levels and pneumococcal carriage in HIV-infected children.

Pneumococcal conjugate vaccines are reported to provide substantial protection against IPD and clinical pneumonia when given to HIV-infected infants [30]. Despite PCV7 vaccine being available in Indonesia since 2008 and PCV13 since 2011, their use is limited as it is evident from lack of any exclusion from the study based on child previous immunization against pneumococcal disease but also from a relatively high prevalence of vaccine serotypes in carriage. We observed that serotype 19F isolates were the most common in carriage in this study. Meanwhile in 2001, Soewignjo *et al.* reported that in healthy children from Lombok, Indonesia, the most common were strains of serogroup 6 (25%) followed by serogroup 23 (21%) and serogroup 19 (6%) [15]. Farida *et al.* reported that in healthy children from Semarang, Indonesia, the most common were strains of serotype 6A/B (19%) followed by serotype 15B/C and 11A (10%), 23F(9%), and 19F(8%) [17]. In our study, serogroup 19 isolates (serotypes 19F and 19A together) accounted for over a quarter (12 out of 42 or 29%) of all the pneumococcal strains cultured from HIV-infected children. Interestingly, eleven isolates were classified as untypeable in the study, with six strains of PCR-negative for the *cpsA* gene. It either indicates over-representation of untypeable strains when carriage is detected by conventional culture [31], reflects significant circulation of strains expressing capsular types not targeted by SM-PCR, or indicates low sensitivity of the protocol used to determine the serotype of pneumococcal strains.

We identified susceptibility to sulfamethoxazole/trimethoprim in 41%, and to penicillin in 33% carriage isolates in this study, whereas susceptibility to sulfamethoxazole/trimethoprim and penicillin was still common (91% and 100% respectively) in the study conducted in 1997 in Lombok [15]. Meanwhile in Semarang, Indonesia in 2010, 24% of *S. pneumoniae* strains were penicillin non-susceptible, and 45% were resistant to sulfamethoxazole/trimethoprim [17].

Table 3. Antimicrobial susceptibility of *Streptococcus pneumoniae* strains carried by children infected with HIV.

Antimicrobial Agent	Number (%) of susceptible isolates			*p*-Value (Fisher exact test)
	All (n = 42)	**PCV13 serotype strains[a] (n = 25)**	**non-PCV13 serotype strains (n = 17)**	
Chloramphenicol	36 (86)	20 (80)	16 (94)	0.3739
Clindamycin	33 (79)	18 (72)	15 (88)	0.2708
Erythromycin	32 (76)	16 (64)	16 (94)	0.0312
Sulphamethoxazole/ trimethoprim	17 (41)	7 (28)	10 (59)	0.0605
Penicillin[b]	14 (33)	5 (20)	9 (53)	0.0448
Tetracycline	18 (43)	8 (32)	10 (59)	0.1169

[a]Strains of serotypes targeted by thirteen-valent conjugated polysaccharide pneumococcal vaccine: 1, 3, 4, 5, 6A, 6B, 7F, 9V, 14, 18C, 19A, 19F, 23F.
[b]Susceptibility to penicillin was determined with oxacillin disk [22].

Table 4. Serotype of multi-drug resistant *S. pneumoniae* strains.

Isolate	Serotype	Antimicrobial susceptibility profile [22]					
		Chloramphenicol	**Clindamycin**	**Erythromycin**	**Sulphamethoxazole/trimethoprim**	**Penicillin[a]**	**Tetracycline**
ISID-77	19F	S	R	R	R	R	R
ISID-107	19F	S	S	R	R	R	R
ISID-1	19F	S	R	R	R	R	R
ISID-16	19F	S	R	R	R	R	R
ISID-31	19F	S	S	R	R	R	R
ISID-12	19F	S	R	R	R	R	R
ISID-8	19A	S	S	S	R	R	R
ISID-6	19A	S	S	S	R	R	R
ISID-24	19A	S	S	S	R	R	R
ISID-110	6A/B	S	R	R	R	R	R
ISID-11	6A/B	S	R	R	R	R	R
ISID-36	12 F	R	S	S	R	S	R
ISID-47	11A	S	R	R	R	S	R
ISID-104	23F	R	R	R	R	R	R
ISID-75-R	9V	R	S	S	R	R	R
ISID-111	untypeable	S	R	S	R	S	R

S – susceptible; R – non-suceptible.
[a]Susceptibility to penicillin was determined with oxacillin disk [22].

We also found that serotype 19F isolates along isolates of serogroup 6A/B were more frequently resistant to antimicrobial drugs tested in the study compared to strains of other serotypes. This is in agreement with ANSORP (Asian Network for Surveillance of Resistant Pathogens) data reporting a 59% multidrug resistance among *S. pneumoniae* invasive isolates collected in the region, with 19F being the major multidrug resistant serotype (24% of all MDR strains from IPD) [32]. Furthermore, recent Malaysian data showed that serotype 19F was correlated with increased resistance against penicillin [33].

We observed strains of serotypes targeted by PCV13 to be more frequently resistant to antipneumococcal drugs tested in the study compared to non-PCV13 strains. Immunization with PCVs would target not only serotypes common in carriage in the studied population, but also strains of serotypes less susceptible to anti-pneumococcal drugs. In geographical locations with high rates of antibiotics resistance among *S. pneumoniae* strains, introduction of PCVs lowered not only incidence of IPD, but also lowered (at least temporarily) rates of resistance to particular antimicrobial agents in strains circulating in carriage and causing pneumococcal diseases [34–36]. Similar effects could be expected in our study population. In conclusion, our study gives insight into the population of *S. pneumoniae* strains circulating in carriage in patients who are at high risk for IPD due to age and comorbidity. We expect our results to be helpful in shaping preventive strategies targeting IPD in Indonesia both on a national and local level.

Acknowledgments

We are grateful to the children and parents for participating in the study, and the staff of the Department of Child Health, Dr. Cipto Mangunkusumo Hospital, Jakarta. We also thank Dr. Decy Subekti, Siti Mudaliana, and Stephany Tumewu for technical assistance and discussion.

Author Contributions

Conceived and designed the experiments: DS NK DB KT. Performed the experiments: DS NK LW MMK TP. Analyzed the data: DS NK DB KT. Contributed reagents/materials/analysis tools: NK LW MMK TP. Wrote the paper: DS KT.

References

1. O'Brien KL, Wolfson LJ, Watt JP, Henkle E, Deloria-Knoll M, et al. (2009) Burden of disease caused by *Streptococcus pneumoniae* in children younger than 5 years: global estimates. Lancet 374: 893–902. doi:10.1016/S0140-6736(09)61204-6.
2. Van der Poll T, Opal SM (2009) Pathogenesis, treatment, and prevention of pneumococcal pneumonia. Lancet 374: 1543–1556. doi:10.1016/S0140-6736(09)61114-4.
3. Browall S, Norman M, Tångrot J, Galanis I, Sjöström K, et al. (2014) Intraclonal variations among *Streptococcus pneumoniae* isolates influence the likelihood of invasive disease in children. J Infect Dis 209: 377–388. doi:10.1093/infdis/jit481.
4. Jansen AGSC, Rodenburg GD, van der Ende A, van Alphen L, Veenhoven RH, et al. (2009) Invasive pneumococcal disease among adults: associations among serotypes, disease characteristics, and outcome. Clin Infect Dis 49: e23–e29. doi:10.1086/600045.
5. Oliver MB, van der Linden MPG, Küntzel SA, Saad JS, Nahm MH (2013) Discovery of *Streptococcus pneumoniae* serotype 6 variants with glycosyltransferases synthesizing two differing repeating units. J Biol Chem 288: 25976–25985. doi:10.1074/jbc.M113.480152.
6. Weinberger DM, Malley R, Lipsitch M (2011) Serotype replacement in disease after pneumococcal vaccination. Lancet 378: 1962–1973. doi:10.1016/S0140-6736(10)62225-8.
7. Feikin DR, Kagucia EW, Loo JD, Link-Gelles R, Puhan MA, et al. (2013) Serotype-specific changes in invasive pneumococcal disease after pneumococcal conjugate vaccine introduction: a pooled analysis of multiple surveillance sites. PLoS Med 10: e1001517. doi:10.1371/journal.pmed.1001517.
8. Van der Linden M, Reinert RR, Kern WV, Imöhl M (2013) Epidemiology of serotype 19A isolates from invasive pneumococcal disease in German children. BMC Infect Dis 13: 70. doi:10.1186/1471-2334-13-70.
9. Spijkerman J, van Gils EJM, Veenhoven RH, Hak E, Yzerman EPF, et al. (2011) Carriage of *Streptococcus pneumoniae* 3 years after start of vaccination program, the Netherlands. Emerg Infect Dis 17: 584–591. doi:10.3201/eid1704.101115.
10. Miller E, Andrews NJ, Waight PA, Slack MP, George RC (2011) Herd immunity and serotype replacement 4 years after seven-valent pneumococcal conjugate vaccination in England and Wales: an observational cohort study. Lancet Infect Dis 11: 760–768. doi:10.1016/S1473-3099(11)70090-1.
11. Kaplan SL, Barson WJ, Lin PL, Stovall SH, Bradley JS, et al. (2010) Serotype 19A Is the most common serotype causing invasive pneumococcal infections in children. Pediatrics 125: 429–436. doi:10.1542/peds.2008-1702.
12. Bogaert D, De Groot R, Hermans PWM (2004) *Streptococcus pneumoniae* colonisation: the key to pneumococcal disease. Lancet Infect Dis 4: 144–154. doi:10.1016/S1473-3099(04)00938-7.
13. Auranen K, Rinta-Kokko H, Goldblatt D, Nohynek H, O'Brien KL, et al. (2013) Colonisation endpoints in *Streptococcus pneumoniae* vaccine trials. Vaccine 32: 153–158. doi:10.1016/j.vaccine.2013.08.061.
14. Satzke C, Turner P, Virolainen-Julkunen A, Adrian PV, Antonio M, et al. (2013) Standard method for detecting upper respiratory carriage of *Streptococcus pneumoniae*: Updated recommendations from the World Health Organization Pneumococcal Carriage Working Group. Vaccine 32: 165–179. doi:10.1016/j.vaccine.2013.08.062.
15. Soewignjo S, Gessner BD, Sutanto A, Steinhoff M, Prijanto M, et al. (2001) *Streptococcus pneumoniae* nasopharyngeal carriage prevalence, serotype distribution, and resistance patterns among children on Lombok Island, Indonesia. Clin Infect Dis 32: 1039–1043. doi:10.1086/319605.
16. Gilks CF, Ojoo SA, Ojoo JC, Brindle RJ, Paul J, et al. (1996) Invasive pneumococcal disease in a cohort of predominantly HIV-1 infected female sex-workers in Nairobi, Kenya. Lancet 347: 718–723.
17. Farida H, Severin JA, Gasem MH, Keuter M, Wahyono H, et al. (2014) Nasopharyngeal carriage of *Streptococcus pneumonia* in pneumonia-prone age groups in Semarang, Java Island, Indonesia. PLoS ONE 9: e87431. doi:10.1371/journal.pone.0087431.
18. O'Brien KL, Nohynek H, World Health Organization Pneumococcal Vaccine Trials Carriage Working Group (2003) Report from a WHO Working Group: standard method for detecting upper respiratory carriage of *Streptococcus pneumoniae*. Pediatr Infect Dis J 22: e1–e11. doi:10.1097/01.inf.0000049347.42983.77.
19. Pai R, Gertz RE, Beall B (2006) Sequential multiplex PCR approach for determining capsular serotypes of *Streptococcus pneumoniae* isolates. J Clin Microbiol 44: 124–131. doi:10.1128/JCM.44.1.124-131.2006.
20. Morrison KE, Lake D, Crook J, Carlone GM, Ades E, et al. (2000) Confirmation of psaA in all 90 serotypes of *Streptococcus pneumoniae* by PCR and potential of this assay for identification and diagnosis. J Clin Microbiol 38: 434–437.
21. CDC website. Available: http://www.cdc.gov/ncidod/biotech/files/pcr-oligonucleotide-primers.pdf. Accessed 2014 September 17.
22. Clinical and Laboratory Standards Institute (2007) Performance Standards for Antimicrobial Susceptibility Testing: Seventeenth Informational Supplement. Wayne, PA: CLSI.
23. Anthony L, Meehan A, Amos B, Mtove G, Mjema J, et al. (2012) Nasopharyngeal carriage of *Streptococcus pneumoniae*: prevalence and risk factors in HIV-positive children in Tanzania. Int J Infect Dis 16: e753–e757. doi:10.1016/j.ijid.2012.05.1037.
24. Abdullahi O, Karani A, Tigoi CC, Mugo D, Kungu S, et al. (2012) The prevalence and risk factors for pneumococcal colonization of the nasopharynx among children in Kilifi District, Kenya. PloS One 7: e30787. doi:10.1371/journal.pone.0030787.
25. Polack FP, Flayhart DC, Zahurak ML, Dick JD, Willoughby RE (2000) Colonization by *Streptococcus penumoniae* in human immunodeficiency virus-infected children. Pediatr Infect Dis J 19: 608–612.
26. Cardoso VC, Cervi MC, Cintra OAL, Salathiel ASM, Gomes ACLF (2006) Nasopharyngeal colonization with *Streptococcus pneumoniae* in children infected with human immunodeficiency virus. J Pediatr (Rio J) 82: 51–57. doi:10.2223/JPED.1437.
27. Leibovitz E, Dragomir C, Sfartz S, Porat N, Yagupsky P, et al. (1999) Nasopharyngeal carriage of multidrug-resistant *Streptococcus pneumoniae* in institutionalized HIV-infected and HIV-negative children in northeastern Romania. Int J Infect Dis 3: 211–215.
28. Shiri T, Auranen K, Nunes MC, Adrian PV, van Niekerk N, et al. (2013) Dynamics of pneumococcal transmission in vaccine-naive children and their HIV-infected or HIV-uninfected mothers during the first 2 years of life. Am J Epidemiol 178: 1629–1637. doi:10.1093/aje/kwt200.
29. Mwenya DM, Charalambous BM, Phillips PPJ, Mwansa JCL, Batt SL, et al. (2010) Impact of cotrimoxazole on carriage and antibiotic resistance of *Streptococcus pneumoniae* and *Haemophilus influenzae* in HIV-infected children in Zambia. Antimicrob Agents Chemother 54: 3756–3762. doi:10.1128/AAC.01409-09.

30. Bliss SJ, O'Brien KL, Janoff EN, Cotton MF, Musoke P, et al. (2008) The evidence for using conjugate vaccines to protect HIV-infected children against pneumococcal disease. Lancet Infect Dis 8: 67–80. doi:10.1016/S1473-3099(07)70242-6.
31. Valente C, de Lencastre H, Sá-Leão R (2013) Selection of distinctive colony morphologies for detection of multiple carriage of *Streptococcus pneumoniae*. Pediatr Infect Dis J 32: 703–704. doi:10.1097/INF.0b013e31828692be.
32. Kim SH, Song J-H, Chung DR, Thamlikitkul V, Yang Y, et al. (2012) Changing trends in antimicrobial resistance and serotypes of *Streptococcus pneumoniae* isolates in Asian countries: an Asian Network for Surveillance of Resistant Pathogens (ANSORP) study. Antimicrob Agents Chemother 56: 1418–1426. doi:10.1128/AAC.05658-11.
33. Le C-F, Palanisamy NK, Mohd Yusof MY, Sekaran SD (2011) Capsular serotype and antibiotic resistance of *Streptococcus pneumoniae* isolates in Malaysia. PloS One 6: e19547. doi:10.1371/journal.pone.0019547.
34. Kyaw MH, Lynfield R, Schaffner W, Craig AS, Hadler J, et al. (2006) Effect of introduction of the pneumococcal conjugate vaccine on drug-resistant *Streptococcus pneumoniae*. N Engl J Med 354: 1455–1463. doi:10.1056/NEJMoa051642.
35. Dagan R (2009) Impact of pneumococcal conjugate vaccine on infections caused by antibiotic-resistant *Streptococcus pneumoniae*. Clin Microbiol Infect 15 Suppl 3: 16–20. doi:10.1111/j.1469-0691.2009.02726.x.
36. Link-Gelles R, Thomas A, Lynfield R, Petit S, Schaffner W, et al. (2013) Geographic and temporal trends in antimicrobial nonsusceptibility in *Streptococcus pneumoniae* in the post-vaccine era in the United States. J Infect Dis 208: 1266–1273. doi:10.1093/infdis/jit315.

Why Children with Severe Bacterial Infection Die: A Population–Based Study of Determinants and Consequences of Suboptimal Care with a Special Emphasis on Methodological Issues

Elise Launay[1,2*], Christèle Gras-Le Guen[1,3], Alain Martinot[4], Rémy Assathiany[5], Elise Martin[1], Thomas Blanchais[1], Catherine Deneux-Tharaux[2], Jean-Christophe Rozé[6], Martin Chalumeau[2,7]

1 CHU Nantes, Hôpital de la Mère et de l'Enfant, Clinique médicale pédiatrique, Faculté de médecine de Nantes, Nantes, France, **2** Inserm U1153, Obstetrical, Perinatal and Pediatric Epidemiology Research Team, Research Center for Epidemiology and Biostatistics Sorbonne Paris Cité (CRESS), Paris Descartes University, Paris, France, **3** CHU Nantes, Hôpital de la Mère et de l'Enfant, Urgences pédiatriques, Faculté de médecine de Nantes, Nantes, France, **4** CHU de Lille, Hôpital R. Salengro, Unité d'urgences pédiatriques et de maladies infectieuses, Université de Lille-Nord de France, Lille, France, **5** Association pour le Recherche et l'Enseignement en Pédiatrie Générale (AREPEGE); Association Française de Pédiatrie Ambulatoire (AFPA), Cabinet de Pédiatrie, Issy-les-Moulineaux, France, **6** CHU Nantes, Hôpital de la Mère et de l'Enfant, Réanimation pédiatrique et néonatale, Faculté de médecine de Nantes, Nantes, France, **7** Hôpital Necker Enfants Malades, AP-HP, Service de pédiatrie générale, Paris Descartes University, Paris, France

Abstract

Introduction: Suboptimal care is frequent in the management of severe bacterial infection. We aimed to evaluate the consequences of suboptimal care in the early management of severe bacterial infection in children and study the determinants.

Methods: A previously reported population-based confidential enquiry included all children (3 months- 16 years) who died of severe bacterial infection in a French area during a 7-year period. Here, we compared the optimality of the management of these cases to that of pediatric patients who survived a severe bacterial infection during the same period for 6 types of care: seeking medical care by parents, evaluation of sepsis signs and detection of severe disease by a physician, timing and dosage of antibiotic therapy, and timing and dosage of saline bolus. Two independent experts blinded to outcome and final diagnosis evaluated the optimality of these care types. The effect of suboptimal care on survival was analyzed by a logistic regression adjusted on confounding factors identified by a causal diagram. Determinants of suboptimal care were analyzed by multivariate multilevel logistic regression.

Results: Suboptimal care was significantly more frequent during early management of the 21 children who died as compared with the 93 survivors: 24% vs 13% ($p = 0.003$). The most frequent suboptimal care types were delay to seek medical care (20%), under-evaluation of severity by the physician (20%) and delayed antibiotic therapy (24%). Young age (under 1 year) was independently associated with higher risk of suboptimal care, whereas being under the care of a paediatric emergency specialist or a mobile medical unit as compared with a general practitioner was associated with reduced risk.

Conclusions: Suboptimal care in the early management of severe bacterial infection had a global independent negative effect on survival. Suboptimal care may be avoided by better training of primary care physicians in the specifics of pediatric medicine.

Editor: Susanna Esposito, Fondazione IRCCS Ca' Granda Ospedale Maggiore Policlinico, Università degli Studi di Milano, Italy

Funding: The authors received no specific funding for this work. Inserm Unit 1153 received a grant from the Bettencourt Foundation (Coups d'élan pour la recherche française) in support of its research activities. The funders had no role in study design, data collection and analysis, decision to publish, or preparation of the manuscript.

Competing Interests: The authors have declared that no competing interests exist.

* Email: elise.launay@chu-nantes.fr

These authors contributed equally to this work.

Introduction

Bacterial infection remains a major cause of childhood mortality in industrialised countries. [1] In 2009, Harndern et al. reviewed pediatric deaths in 5 regions of the United Kingdom and found that among the 15% of deaths related to infection, failure to recognise and manage severe bacterial infection (SBI) was the most common avoidable primary care factor. [2] In 2010, we published a population-based study evaluating optimality of care for 21 children who died due to SBI: the initial medical management was suboptimal in 76% of cases, with a delay in seeking medical care in 33%. [3] These alarming frequencies in suboptimal initial care in pediatric patients with SBI do not allow for drawing conclusions on the relationship between suboptimal care and outcomes because both studies focused on patients who died.

The consequences of suboptimal care in pediatric patients with SBI have been examined in 4 studies. [4,5,6,7] All found clinically meaningful and statistically significant associations between suboptimal care and morbidity and mortality. [4,5,6,7] However, the results were limited by methodological concerns such as selection bias related to hospital-based recruitment, [6] classification bias related to arbitrary definition of diagnosis delay as consultation more than once before hospitalisation, [5] non-independent evaluation of the optimality of care, [7] non-justified use of continuous variables in multivariable models, [4,5,7] and/or selection of non-appropriate variables for adjustment (without using a causal diagram that could help deal with co-variables that could be confounders or intermediate variables). [8,9] No study examined the determinants of this suboptimal care to inform corrective actions for parents and healthcare workers.

The aim of the present study was to evaluate the determinants and consequences of suboptimal care in the initial management of SBI in children, using appropriate methodological approaches, to evaluate the relevance of future targeted corrective actions for parents and healthcare workers.

Methods

General methodology

The present study is an extension of a previously published population-based confidential enquiry into the quality of initial care in children age from 3 months to 16 years who died of SBI from January 2000 to March 2006 in a geographic zone of France comprising two adjoining administrative districts. [3] The definition of SBI (bacterial infection leading to admission to the pediatric intensive care unit [PICU]), the strategy of identification of cases, and the assessment of exhaustiveness were described in detail in the previous publication. Pediatric care in this area was provided by one university hospital center (in Nantes), four general hospitals, pediatricians in private practice, general practitioners (GPs), and two call centers for medical emergencies that could send emergency mobile medical teams (including physicians specialized in emergency medicine) to the patient's home. For the present study, we defined a control group of pediatric patients who survived a SBI during the same period and in the same geographic region. The organization of care called for all children older than 3 months and requiring hospitalization for SBI to be transferred to the PICU of the Nantes university hospital. Thus, controls were all pediatric patients hospitalised for SBI in the PICU of the hospital during the study period. Controls were identified by discharge codes and the microbiology laboratory electronic files as described previously. [3] The initial research was approved by Institutional Review Committee (Comité de Protection des Personnes Ile de France III) and this extension was approved by the ethics committee of the Nantes university hospital (Groupe Nantais d'Ethique dans le Domaine de la Santé), which approved a waiver of the need for consent. The results were reported according to the STROBE checklist for reporting observational studies. [10]

Data were collected as previously described from the complete patient medical file: a pre-established template reconstructed the timed and dated medical observations with blinding to final diagnosis or outcome. [3] Children whose files were too incomplete to trace the clinical history with sufficient precision were identified and excluded.

Optimality of care evaluation

Two experts (an experienced pediatrician in private practice and a pediatric intensive care specialist who supervises a pediatric emergency department), blinded to final diagnosis and outcome, independently determined the suboptimal character of the initial management as described previously. [3] These two experts were not involved in the management of any included children. Experts had to justify their final conclusion by giving details on the optimality (optimal or not optimal) of each care in terms of specific criteria selected from national and international clinical practice guidelines applicable during the study period: [11,12,13] the timing of administration of antibiotics for meningococcemia (immediate in case of extensive purpura) and the modality of administration of hemodynamic support in septic shock (bolus up to 40 mL/kg in the first hour). As in the study by Nadel *et al.*, [6] which evaluated suboptimal care for meningococcal disease, we defined delay in seeking medical care by parents as the absence of immediate consultation in cases of fever with a purpuric rash or accompanied by other signs of severity: cyanosis, moaning, convulsions, confusion, impairment of higher functions, intense headaches, intense muscle or articular pain, marked asthenia, persistent vomiting, or cold hands or feet. We also arbitrarily considered the failure to seek medical care when a high fever lasted more than 48 hr as a delay in seeking medical care. For each child, we were then able to evaluate the optimality of 6 different key types of care: 1) seeking medical care by parents; 2) evaluation of sepsis signs and detection of severe disease by a physician, 3) timing of antibiotic therapy, 4) dosage of antibiotic therapy, 5) timing of saline bolus, and 6) dosage of saline bolus.

Analyses

We described the children studied, their demographic characteristics, and their final diagnoses, especially bacteriologic. We analyzed signs of severe disease: signs of sepsis (tachycardia, bradycardia, and tachypnea), [14] presence of tonus disorders, impaired vigilance, respiratory distress, moaning, or other signs of potential SBI, such as meningism or extensive purpura. We described the sequence of care of children (first medical contact and number of consultations before hospitalization).

We assessed the degree of agreement between the two experts for each type of care by calculating the κappa coefficient interpreted with the Landis and Koch scale. [15] In cases of disagreement, the optimal nature of the care was determined by a third expert. We analyzed the 6 categories of suboptimal care by outcome and physicians' qualification. We also analyzed risk factors for death (relation between suboptimal care and death) and determinants of suboptimal medical care (excluding seeking medical care).

We analyzed the crude and adjusted association between number of suboptimal care and death. The number of suboptimal care was the sum of the 6 above-mentioned types for each child and thus ranged from 0 to 6. To identify confounding variables,

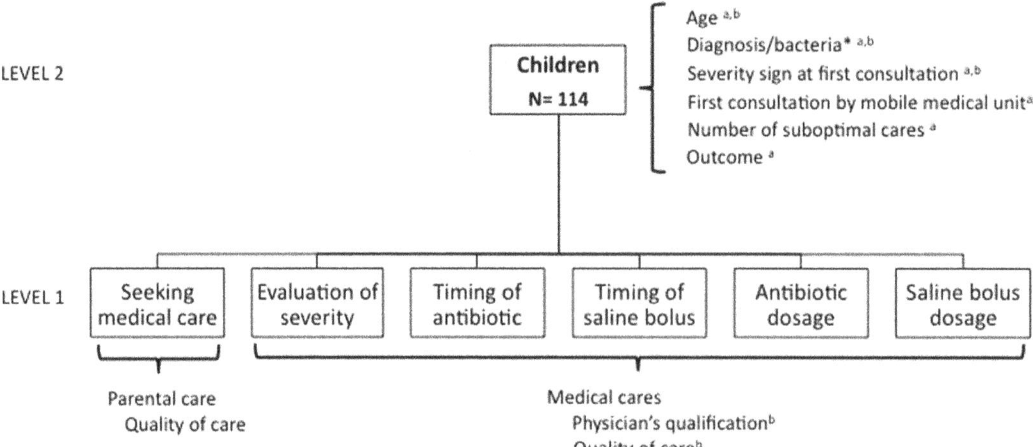

Figure 1. Structure of data. a = co-variables used in the study of the consequences of suboptimal care. b = co-variables used in the study of the determinants of medical sub-optimal care.

we built a theorical causal diagram between optimality of care and outcome (dead/alive at discharge from hospital) based on the published pathophysiological concepts of severe sepsis (Figure S1) and adapted from this a "realistic" causal diagram between optimality of initial care (before admission to a PICU) and outcome considering the available data and using DAGitty software (Figure S2). [16,17] Clinical phenotype was defined by diagnosis (meningitis versus other diagnosis) and two other variables reflecting the measurable intrinsic severity of the disease: presence of severity sign at the first consultation and first consultation by a mobile medical unit (this unit is reserved for patients with the most severe condition in France). Covariables tested on univariate analysis were age of children, diagnosis, sign of severe disease at the first consultation, and first consultation by a mobile medical unit (Figure 1). Relevant variables according to the causal diagram were included in multivariate analyses.

To evaluate the determinants of the quality of initial medical care, we considered each of the 5 medical care types by children. We used a hierarchical regression model that took into account the hierarchical structure of the data (i.e., non-independence of the variables for the 5 care types), and allowed us to include characteristics of care at the care level (level 1; i.e., quality of each care [optimal/suboptimal] and qualification of physician giving the care) and characteristics of the children at the level of the child (level 2; i.e., age of children, diagnosis, and presence of signs of severe disease at first consultation [Figure 1]). We included variables considered associated with suboptimal care (Figure S2). First, we estimated a random intercept model without any variable ("empty" model) to obtain the baseline children-level variance and to test the effect of children. Then, we included care and children characteristics and estimated the association of these variables and quality of care. We calculated the proportion of the model's variance explained by level 1 and level 2 variables defined as (variance of the model with level 1 variables − variance of the empty model)/variance of empty model and (variance of the model with level 1 and level 2 variables − variance of the empty model)/variance of empty model, respectively. Quantitative variables were tested for linearity and transformed into polynomials of the smallest degree when deviation was observed. Analyses involved use of Stata 11 (StataCorp, College Station, TX, USA).

Results

Patients and care pathway

In total, 119 patients were eligible; five (4%) were excluded because of incomplete charts, for 114 patients analysed (Figure S3). Overall, 21 children died (18%, 95% confidence interval [95% CI] 11–25) before PICU admission (n = 1) or PICU discharge (n = 20), and 93 survived. The clinical characteristics of the 21 children who died were described elsewhere. [3] The median age of the 114 included children was 2.4 years [interquartile range 0.7–6.7 years], the sex ratio was 1.3 (M/F) and one half had known serious medical conditions at the time of diagnosis (Table 1). More than a half of the children (63%) presented signs of severe disease at the first medical contact. Meningitis was the most frequent diagnosis (57%), followed by purpura fulminans (35%). Meningococcus was found in 47% of cases. The first medical contact was a GP in 66% of cases, an emergency physician in 25%, and a mobile medical unit in 9%; 60% of children were hospitalized after this first medical contact. Children whose first medical contact was the mobile medical unit were more likely to have severity signs at this first medical contact (100% versus 60%, $p = 0.01$).

Optimality of care

Agreement between experts was "moderate" for evaluation of the optimality of the delay to seek medical care and for saline bolus dosage, with a κ coefficient of 0.40 ± 0.06 and 0.46 ± 0.09, respectively ($p < 0.001$). Agreement with the optimality of the 4 other medical care types (severity evaluation, antibiotic therapy timing and dosage, and saline bolus timing) was "substantial" or "almost perfect," with κ 0.78 ± 0.09; 0.78 ± 0.09; 0.67 ± 0.09 and 0.88 ± 0.09, respectively ($p < 0.001$). Overall, 52% of children received at least one care type evaluated as suboptimal, and 25% received two or more suboptimal care types (Table 1). Among the 684 individual care types delivered, 104 (15%, 95% CI 12–18%) were suboptimal. Parental delay in seeking medical care and physician underestimation of severity and delayed antibiotic administration accounted for 70% of this suboptimal care (22%, 22% and 26%, respectively). The frequency of suboptimal care in the initial management did not significantly decrease over the years (19% to 15% from 2000 to 2005; p for trend$>$0.8) nor did the frequency of each type of care ($p > 0.2$).

Table 1. Patient characteristics and care pathways before admission to a pediatric intensive care unit, quality of care and their association with outcome by dead and alive children and univariate and multivariate analysis.

	Total n = 114 (%)	Dead n = 21 (%)	Alive n = 93 (%)	Univariate analysis			Multivariate analysis[§]		
				OR	95% CI	p	aOR	95% CI	p
PATIENTS									
Age, yr									
Median[a] [IQR]	2.4 [0.7–6.7]	2.0 [0.9–2.8]	2.9 [0.7–7.1]	0.85	0.73–1.0	0.057	0.82	0.68–0.99	0.04
<1 yr	32 (28)	7 (33)	25 (27)						
1 to 2 yr	21 (18)	4 (19)	17 (18)			0.01			
2 to 5 yr	27 (24)	9 (43)	18 (19)						
≥5 yr	34 (30)	1 (5)	33 (36)						
Sex ratio M/F	1.28	1.33	1.27			0.92			
Underlying medical conditions, n (%)	39 (52)	7 (33)	32 (34)			0.93			
Severity signs at first medical contact[b], n (%)	72 (63)	16 (76)	56 (60)			0.17			
Final diagnosis, n (%)									
Purpura fulminans and others[c]	49 (43)	14 (67)	35 (38)	1	-	-	1	-	-
Meningitis	65 (57)	7 (33)	58 (62)	0.30	0.11–0.85	0.02	0.31	0.10–0.98	0.047
Bacteria involved, n (%)									
Streptococcus pneumoniae	31 (27)	3 (14)	28 (30)						
Neisseria meningitidis	54 (47)	12 (57)	42 (45)						
Other[d]	11 (10)	4 (19)	7 (8)			0.17			
No documentation	18 (16)	2 (10)	16 (17)						
with purpura fulminans	10 (55)	1 (50)	9 (56)						
CARE PATHWAYS									
First medical contact									
GP or emergency physician, n (%)	104 (91)	15 (71)	89 (96)	1	-	-	1	-	-
Mobile medical unit	10 (9)	6 (29)	4 (4)	8.9	2.05–38.6	<0.001	8.72	1.76–43.28	0.008
No of medical contacts, n (%)									
1	68 (60)	15 (71)	53 (57)						
2	37 (32)	6 (29)	31 (33)			0.43			
>2	9 (8)	0	9 (10)						
QUALITY OF CARES									
No. of suboptimal care, by children									
Median [IQR][a]	1 [0–1]	1 [0–2]	0 [0–1]	1.55	1.06–2.26	0.025	1.65	1.07–2.54	0.022
0	55 (48)	7 (33)	48 (52)						
1	31 (27)	5 (24)	26 (28)						
2	17 (15)	5 (24)	12 (13)						

Table 1. Cont.

	Total n = 114 (%)	Dead n = 21 (%)	Alive n = 93 (%)	Univariate analysis			Multivariate analysis[§]		
				OR	95% CI	p	aOR	95% CI	p
3	5 (4)	1 (5)	4 (4)						
4	6 (5)	3 (14)	3 (3)						
No suboptimal care/no care, % [95% CI]	15 [12–18]	24 [16–32]	13 [10–16]			0.003			
Care types									
Parental care, n (%)									
Seeking medical care									
Suboptimal	23 (20)	6 (29)	17 (18)	1.79	0.60–5.34	0.29			
Optimal	91 (80)	15 (71)	76 (82)	1	-	-			
Medical care, n (%)									
Evaluation of severity									
Suboptimal	23 (20)	7 (33)	16 (17)	2.40	0.82–7.03	0.10			
Optimal	91 (80)	14 (67)	77 (83)	1	-	-			
Antibiotic therapy timing									
Suboptimal	27 (24)	5 (24)	22 (24)	1	0.33–3.08	0.98			
Optimal	87 (76)	16 (76)	71 (76)	1	-	-			
Saline bolus timing									
Suboptimal	14 (12)	5 (24)	9 (10)	2.92	0.84–10.1	0.08			
Optimal	100 (88)	16 (76)	84 (90)	1	-	-			
Saline bolus dosage									
Suboptimal	12 (11)	7 (33)	5 (5)	**8.80**	2.23–34.7	0.002			
Optimal	102 (89)	14 (67)	88 (95)	1	-	-			
Antibiotic therapy dosage									
Suboptimal	5 (4)	0 (0)	5 (5)	0.67	0.01–6.03	0.29			
Optimal	109 (96)	21 (100)	88 (95)	1	-	-			

aOR, adjusted odds ratio; 95% CI, 95% confidence interval; IQR, interquartile range.

[§]Logistic regression model.

[a]Age and no. of suboptimal care were treated as continuous variables (no deviation to linearity).

[b]Severity signs were hemodynamic failure, purpura, conscientiousness impairment, respiratory distress, meningism, behavioural changes or hypotonia.

[c]Others were 2 pneumonia with pleural effusion and a septic shock following pyelonephritis in a child with malformative uropathy in the deceased group, and 2 septic shock on bacterial cellulitis and a bacterial tracheitis in the survivor group.

[d]Others were, for survivors, *Haemophilus influenzae* (n = 3), Group B *Streptococcus* (n = 1), *Staphylococcus aureus* (n = 1), and for deceased children, *E.coli* (n = 1), Group A *Streptococcus* (n = 1), *Salmonella spp (n = 1)* and *Mycoplama pneumoniae* (n = 1).

Table 2. Risk factors for medical suboptimal care.

	Optimal n = 489 (%)	Suboptimal n = 81 (%)	Univariate analysis			Multivariate analysis *,**		
			OR	95% CI	p	aOR	95% CI	p
Age								
<1 yr	125 (26)	35 (43)	1			1		
1–2	95 (19)	10 (12)	0.38	0.18–0.81	0.009	0.32	0.11–0.98	0.046
2–5 yr	119 (24)	16 (20)	0.48	0.25–0.92	0.02	0.37	0.14–0.98	0.045
≥5 yr	150 (31)	20 (25)	0.48	0.26–0.87	0.01	0.24	0.09–0.64	0.004
Physician qualification, n (%)								
General practitioner	55 (11)	27 (33)	1			1		
Adult emergency	16 (3)	7 (9)	0.90	0.33–2.44	0.82	0.63	0.15–2.62	0.53
Pediatric emergency	322 (66)	37 (46)	0.23	0.13–0.42	<0.001	0.16	0.08–0.35	<0.001
Mobile medical unit	83 (17)	6 (7)	0.15	0.05–0.40	<0.001	0.09	0.03–0.31	<0.001
Pediatric ward	13 (3)	4 (5)	0.63	0.18–2.13	0.45	0.65	0.11–3.67	0.63
Severity signs at first consultation, n (%)								
No	182 (87)	28 (13)	1			1		
Yes	307 (85)	53(15)	1.12	0.68–1.84	0.6	1.3	0.59–2.90	0.51
Final diagnosis, n (%)								
Other	210 (86)	35 (14)	1			1		
Meningitis	279 (86)	46 (14)	0.99	0.62–1.59	0.9	0.73	0.34–1.59	0.43

*Multivariate analysis involved a hierarchical logistic regression model with random intercept and effects.
**Significant associations remained when age was transformed into polynomials (X = 10/[age − 2.5]), aOR for age 1.04, 95% CI 1.01–1.07, p = 0.003.

Factors associated with outcome

As compared with children who died, survivors were more frequently older than 5 years ($p<0.05$; Table 1) and diagnosed as having meningitis (62% vs 33%). The two groups did not differ in other demographic, clinical or bacteriologic characteristics or total number of medical contacts before admission to the ICU ($p>0.1$, Table 1). For children who died, the first medical contact was frequently a mobile medical unit (vs GP office or hospital emergency department): 29% vs 4% ($p<0.001$). The proportion of suboptimal care among all care types during the initial management was higher for children who died than survived: 24% vs 13% (95% CI of the risk difference: 9–13%). On univariate analysis, insufficient saline bolus was significantly associated with death (OR = 8.8; 95% CI: 2.23–34.7), under-evaluation of severity and delay to administer saline bolus was associated but not significantly with death (OR = 2.74; 95% CI: 0.82–7.03 and 2.92; 95% CI: 0.84–10.1 respectively) (Table 1).

After adjustment for confounders, each suboptimal care (continuous variable, no deviance to linearity) increased the odds of death by 65% (adjusted odds ratio [aOR] 1.65, 95% CI 1.08–2.54, p = 0.02) (Table 1). Each year of age (continuous variable, no deviation to linearity) decreased the odds of death (aOR 0.82, 95% CI 0.68–0.99, p = 0.04), as did having meningitis as compared with other diagnoses (aOR 0.31, 95% CI 0.10–0.98, p = 0.047). A first medical contact by the mobile medical unit was associated with an adverse outcome (aOR 8.72, 95% CI 1.76–43.28, p = 0.008) (Table 1).

Determinants of optimality of medical care

Among the 570 cares received by children during their initial management (Table 2), the repartition of suboptimal care differed by physician qualification. The proportion of suboptimal care was 33% for those provided by a GP, 30% for those in adult emergency settings, 24% for those in pediatric wards, 10% for those in pediatric emergency care and 7% for those in the mobile medical unit ($p<0.001$). The proportion of under-evaluation of severity was 30% for a GP, 9% for pediatric emergency care and 0% for the mobile medical unit (p = 0.001). The proportion of delayed antibiotic therapy was 50% for a GP, 20% for pediatric emergency care and 0% for the mobile medical unit (p = 0.02). The other types of care (antibiotic therapy dosage and timing and dosage of saline bolus) did not differ by physician qualification.

On univariate analysis, younger children (<1 year) were at increased risk of suboptimal care (see Table 2), and odds of suboptimal care were lower with pediatric emergency or mobile medical unit care than GP care (OR 0.23, 95% CI 0.13–0.42; and OR 0.15, 95% CI 0.05–0.40, respectively) (Table 2). We found no association between final diagnosis or presence of severity sign at first medical contact and quality of care. The optimality of care varied significantly between children (i.e., children effect, empty model, $p<0.001$). After adjustment in a multilevel multivariate model, the association between optimality of care and age of children (dichotomised in 4 classes or transformed in polynomials) and physician qualification remained stable (Table 2). The variance of the empty model was 1.56, that of the model with a level 1 variable (physician qualification) was 1.54 and that of the full model (level 1 and 2 variables) was 1.21. Level 1 variables explained 2% of the variance, whereas level 1 and 2 variables explained 21% of the variance.

Discussion

We found a strong association of suboptimal medical care and death for children with an SBI: each suboptimal care increased the odds of death by 65%. Some types of care, particularly the dosage of saline bolus, were associated more with death than others. The gold standard to demonstrate causality in medical research is a controlled double blind randomised trial, but such studies are obviously not ethical in the case of SBI. Observational study analysis of causal association requires being aware of the risk of bias. [18] Here, we studied the determinants and consequences of suboptimal care in the early management of SBI in pediatric patients using an adequate approach to deal with the structure and type of data, including multilevel analysis and fractional polynomials [19,20,21] while minimizing the selection bias for children who died by using a population recruitment pattern with exhaustivity checking. As recommended by methodological standards, [22] suboptimality of care was evaluated by two independent experts who were blinded to the final diagnosis and outcome, with an overall high level of agreement between experts.

The strength of the significant association between suboptimal care and death remained nearly unchanged after adjustment for potential confounders: age of children, final diagnosis and initial severity of disease (represented as having a first medical contact by a mobile medical unit). However, some variables were inaccurately measured and/or some explanatory variables were lacking in the model. Indeed, we show a gap between the number of variables in the theoretical causal diagram and the one used (Figure S1 and Figure S2). For example, we could have explained more accurately the risk of death by considering genetic susceptibility to infection or bacterial virulence. [23,24] We were also limited in the evaluation of initial severity of the infection because of the retrospective design of the study. First medical contact by a mobile medical unit is an objective and reliable evaluation of clinical severity because in France, the mobile medical unit aims to care for children with the most severe disease who could not be transported to the hospital before receiving emergency care. Nevertheless, the presence of a severity sign at the first medical examination is a more arguable reflection of intrinsic severity because of the retrospective design of the study. For example, data on vital signs at the first medical contact, which are a key point to evaluate clinical severity in children in the context of SBI, [25] were sometimes missing, which led to inaccurate evaluation of severity of the disease for statistical analysis and also difficulty for the expert to accurately assess the optimality of the severity evaluation. Experts evaluated only misinterpretation of vital signs when they were mentioned. Here, we demonstrated the significant and independent global effect of suboptimal care on outcome, but we cannot affirm that suboptimal care in the early management was directly responsible for death because suboptimal care in the PICU was not assessed. Moreover, we analyzed only six types of care for each management and not all types. We could not examine the time effect and the total number of care. The total number of care could be the result of intrinsic severity (severely ill children requiring more care and sometimes showing a fulminant evolution) or the result of previous suboptimal care (inadequate care could lead to worsened disease, which then requires more care). The time effect could have been considered in a marginal structural model (Figure S1), but such a model requires timely detailed information that cannot be obtained with a retrospective study. [26]

We did not include children with SBI who survived but were not hospitalized in a PICU. It could be argued that we over-evaluated the frequency of suboptimal care because children with SBI admitted to a PICU may have received more suboptimal care, which caused clinical worsening and then admission to a PICU as compared with children who received adequate care and would not have required admission to a PICU. Thus, this selection bias could have led to an under-evaluation of the association of suboptimal care and death because these children not hospitalized in a PICU and having received potentially more optimal care would most probably have survived.

The generalization of our results may be limited because the bacterial epidemiology may have changed since the study period. In France, conjugate vaccines against *Haemophilus influenzae, Neisseria meningitidis C and Streptococcus pneumoniae* with 7 and 13 valences were routinely recommended for all children by health authorities in 1992, 2009, 2002 and 2009, respectively. Invasive infection due to *H. influenzae* had almost disappeared during the study period. Reported cases of invasive pneumococcal infection decreased after vaccination introduction for only children younger than 2 years old. Incidences were 29 per 100 000 in 2001, 25 per 100 000 in 2004 and 18 per 100 000 in 2012 (meningitis and bacteremia). No significant changes were observed for older children. [27] Vaccine against meningococcus C had a too low coverage in the pediatric population to evidence a decrease in invasive infection due to *N. meningitidis* C since study period. [28] Thus, since the study period, the pattern of SBI may have changed for invasive pneumococcal infection in children less than 2 years old.

We did not observe a significant decrease in suboptimality of care across the years even though French recommendations concerning immediate administration of antibiotic therapy with purpura fuminans were largely diffused in 2000 and the Surviving Sepsis campaign began in 2003. [29,30] This finding highlights that simple diffusion of written recommendations are not enough to quickly modify practices of a large healthcare professional public. [31]

The analysis of suboptimal care determinants allowed us to identify potential targets for corrective actions. Young age (<1 year) was independently associated with increased risk of suboptimal care, whereas being under the care of a paediatric emergency specialist or a mobile medical unit physician was associated with reduced risk. Similar conclusions were reached by Dhamar *et al.* in a retrospective review of the quality of care received by 304 children with serious illnesses receiving treatment in 5 emergency departments in California between 2000 and 2003: after adjustment for confounding factors with a hierarchical model, younger children were at increased risk of receiving suboptimal care, and quality of care was better when provided by pediatric emergency physicians as compared with a GP. [32] Young age of children also appeared to be a barrier to optimal management of critical illness in community hospitals according to a qualitative study. [33] Corrective actions should then target the GP, in training and established, and focus on clinical evaluation of the youngest children.

Seeking medical care was considered delayed in 20% of our cases and accounted for 22% of the suboptimal care. We could not study the determinants of this delay, but French parents were previously found to poorly recognise purpuric rash. [34] Nevertheless, methods to recognize purpuric rash are warranted for not missing severe bacterial infections. [35] Parents worrying about their child's health has also been identified as a good marker of severe infection, although this sign is often missing, even with severe infection. [36] The better understanding of why parents are worried or not could be helpful to optimize early detection of sepsis.

Conclusions

Thanks to an adequate strategy for data analysis, we showed a significant association of suboptimal care for children with SBI and death. We identified determinants that could be acted on to optimize early management of SBI in children and then hopefully reduce the incidence of death. Physicians who are in charge of febrile children should pay particular attention to children younger than 1 year and systematically evaluate vital signs (pulse, respiratory rate, consciousness, capillary refill) that allow for early recognition of severe sepsis. Physicians and parents could be warned via widely distributed flyers or even television, as has been efficient in United Kindom by the meningitis research foundation. [37] Physicians who rarely experience vital emergency situations could also benefit from a simulated training program. [38]

Supporting Information

Figure S1 Theoretical causal diagrams between optimality of care and death reflecting time-dependance of exposure and confounding factors. a: summarized diagram with C representing confounding factors; E, exposition (optimality of care); F, risk factors for exposition (determinants of optimality); and Y, outcome (survival status). b: more complete diagram with H representing host factors (age, genetic and non-genetic susceptibility to infection); B, bacterial factors (type of infection, bacterial specie/serotype, virulence, inoculum); O, optimality of care; S, clinical severity; P, physician characteristics (qualification, clinical experience etc.); Pa, parent characteristics (educational/ socioeconomic status, facility of access to health care systems etc.). Indices represent different time points (from 0 to k) (Inspired by Robins et al, Epidemiology, September 2000, Vol. 11 No. 5).

Figure S2 "Realistic" causal diagram between optimality of care before admission to a pediatric intensive care unit (PICU) and death. This diagram was established with DAGitty considering available variables. [16] The green circle with triangle inside represents exposure; blue circle with stick inside, outcome; green circles, exposure ancestors; pink circles, confounding factors; pink vectors, biasing pathway; green vectors, causal pathways; grey vectors, ancestor pathway. Clinical phenotype was represented by final diagnosis, severity signs at the first medical contact and first medical contact by a medical mobile unit.

Figure S3 Study flowchart.

Acknowledgments

This article is dedicated to the memory of Ms Albertine Aouba, MD, CépiDc-Inserm, Centre d'épidémiologie sur les causes médicales de décès, Le Vésinet, France.

Author Contributions

Conceived and designed the experiments: EL CGL CDT JCR MC. Performed the experiments: AM RA. Analyzed the data: EL CGL EM TB MC. Contributed reagents/materials/analysis tools: EL CGL MC. Contributed to the writing of the manuscript: EL MC. Critical revision of the manuscript for important intellectual concept: CGL AM RA CDT JCR.

References

1. Hartman ME, Linde-Zwirble WT, Angus DC, Watson RS (2013) Trends in the epidemiology of pediatric severe sepsis. Pediatr Crit Care Med 14: 686–693.
2. Harndern A, Mayon-White R, Mant D, Kelly D, Pearson G (2009) Child deaths: confidential enquiry into the role and quality of UK primary care. Br J Gen Pract 59: 819–824.
3. Launay E, Gras-Le Guen C, Martinot A, Assathiany R, Blanchais T, et al. (2010) Suboptimal care in the initial management of children who died from severe bacterial infection: a population-based confidential inquiry. Pediatr Crit Care Med 11: 469–474.
4. Han YY, Carcillo JA, Dragotta MA, Bills DM, Watson RS, et al. (2003) Early reversal of pediatric-neonatal septic shock by community physicians is associated with improved outcome. Pediatrics 112: 793–799.
5. McIntyre PB, Macintyre CR, Gilmour R, Wang H (2005) A population based study of the impact of corticosteroid therapy and delayed diagnosis on the outcome of childhood pneumococcal meningitis. Arch Dis Child 90: 391–396.
6. Nadel S, Britto J, Booy R, Maconochie I, Habibi P, et al. (1998) Avoidable deficiencies in the delivery of health care to children with meningococcal disease. J Accid Emerg Med 15: 298–303.
7. Ninis N, Phillips C, Bailey L, Pollock JI, Nadel S, et al. (2005) The role of healthcare delivery in the outcome of meningococcal disease in children: case-control study of fatal and non-fatal cases. BMJ 330: 1475.
8. Hernan MA, Cole SR (2009) Invited Commentary: Causal diagrams and measurement bias. Am J Epidemiol 170: 959–962; discussion 963–954.
9. Ahrens KA, Schisterman EF (2013) A time and place for causal inference methods in perinatal and paediatric epidemiology. Paediatr Perinat Epidemiol 27: 258–262.
10. von Elm E, Altman DG, Egger M, Pocock SJ, Gotzsche PC, et al. (2008) The Strengthening the Reporting of Observational Studies in Epidemiology (STROBE) statement: guidelines for reporting observational studies. J Clin Epidemiol 61: 344–349.
11. Conseil supérieur d'hygiène publique Opinion from the French High Committee on Public Health, Mars 10, 2000. Available: http://www.sante.gouv.fr/htm/dossiers/cshpf/a_mt_100300_meningite_01.htm. Accessed 2007 Dec 22.
12. Health Protection Agency (2006) Guidance for public health management of meningococcal disease in the UK. Health Protection Agency Meningococcus Forum.
13. Société de Réanimation de Langue Française Use of catecholamines during septic shock (adults and children). XV consensus conference of the French Society of Intensive cares 1996. Available: http://www.sfar.org/article/33/utilisation-des-catecholamines-au-cours-du-choc-septique-adultes-enfants-cc-1996. Accessed 2014 Jan 8.
14. Goldstein B, Giroir B, Randolph A (2005) International pediatric sepsis consensus conference: definitions for sepsis and organ dysfunction in pediatrics. Pediatr Crit Care Med 6: 2–8.
15. Landis JR, Koch GG (1977) The measurement of observer agreement for categorical data. Biometrics 33: 159–174.
16. Textor J, Hardt J, Knuppel S (2011) DAGitty: a graphical tool for analyzing causal diagrams. Epidemiology 22: 745.
17. Angus DC, van der Poll T (2013) Severe sepsis and Septic Shock. N Engl J Med 369: 840–851.
18. Launay E, Morfouace M, Deneux-Tharaux C, Gras le-Guen C, Ravaud P, et al. (2013) Quality of reporting of studies evaluating time to diagnosis: a systematic review in paediatrics. Arch Dis Child doi:101136.
19. Altman DG, Royston P (2006) The cost of dichotomising continuous variable. BMJ 332: 1080.
20. Ambler G, Royston P (2001) Fractional polynomial model selection procedures: investigation of type i error rate. J Statist Comput Simul 69: 89–108.
21. Snijders T, Bosker R (1999) Multilevel analysis: An introduction to basic and advanced multilevel modeling: London: Sage Publications Ltd.
22. Bouvier-Colle MH (2002) Confidential enquiries and medical expert committees: a method for evaluating healthcare. The case of Obstetrics. Rev Epidemiol Sante Publique 50: 203–217.
23. Casanova JL, Abel L (2007) Human genetics of infectious diseases: a unified theory. EMBO J 26: 915–922.
24. Peterson JW (1996) Bacterial Pathogenesis. In: Baron S, editor. Medical Microbiology 4th edition. 2011/03/18 ed.
25. Thompson M, Mayon-White R, Harnden A, Perera R, McLeod D, et al. (2008) Using vital signs to assess children with acute infections: a survey of current practice. Br J Gen Pract 58: 236–241.
26. Robins JM, Hernan MA, Brumback B (2000) Marginal Structural Models and Causal Inference in Epidemiology. Epidemiology 11: 550–560.
27. Varon E, Janoir C, Gutmann L (2012) Centre national de référence du pneumocoque. Rapport d'activités 2013. Available: http://www.cnr-pneumo.fr/docs/rapports/CNRP2013.pdf. Accessed 2014 July 22.
28. Stahl J, Cohen R, Denis F, Gaudelus J, Lery T, et al. (2013) Vaccination against meningococcus C. Vaccinal coverage in the French target population. Med Mal Infect 43: 75–80.
29. Ministère des affaires sociales et de la santé Aide mémoire sur les infections invasives à méningocoque. Available: http://www.sante.gouv.fr/IMG/pdf/Annexe_-_Fiche_aide_memoire_sur_les_infections_invasives_a_meningocoques.pdf. Accessed 2014 Jan 8.
30. Slade E, Tamber PS, Vincent JL (2003) The Surviving Sepsis Campaign: raising awareness to reduce mortality. Crit Care 7: 1–2.
31. Giguere A, Legare F, Grimshaw J, Turcotte S, Fiander M, et al. (2012) Printed educational materials: effects on professional practice and healthcare outcomes. Cochrane Database Syst Rev 10: CD004398.
32. Dharmar M, Marcin JP, Romano PS, Andrada ER, Overly F, et al. (2008) Quality of care of children in the emergency department: association with hospital setting and physician training. J Pediatr 153: 783–789.
33. Gilleland J, McGugan J, Brooks S, Dobbins M, Ploeg J (2013) Caring for critically ill children in the community: a needs assessment. BMJ Qual Saf.
34. Aurel M, Dubos F, Motte B, Pruvost I, Leclerc F, et al. (2011) Recognising haemorrhagic rash in children with fever: a survey of parents' knowledge. Arch Dis Child 96: 697–698.
35. Mant D, Van den Bruel A (2011) Should we promote the tumbler test? Arch Dis Child 96: 613–614.
36. Van den Bruel A, Haj-Hassan T, Thompson M, Buntinx F, Mant D (2010) Diagnostic value of clinical features at presentation to identify serious infection in children in developed countries: a systematic review. Lancet 375: 834–845.
37. Meningitis Research Fondation Meningitis research fondation's website. Available: http://www.meningitis.org. Accessed 2014 July 22.
38. Katznelson J, Mills W, Forsythe C, Shaikh S, Tolleson-Rinehart S (2014) Project CAPE: a high-fidelity, in situ simulation program to increase critical access hospital emergency department provider comfort with seriously ill pediatric patients. Pediatr Emerg Care 30: 397–402.

21

Estimating the Timing of Mother-to-Child Transmission of the Human Immunodeficiency Virus Type 1 Using a Viral Molecular Evolution Model

Antoine Chaillon[1,2*], Tanawan Samleerat[1,3], Faustine Zoveda[4], Sébastien Ballesteros[4], Alain Moreau[1], Nicole Ngo-Giang-Huong[5,6], Gonzague Jourdain[5,6], Sara Gianella[2], Marc Lallemant[5,6], Frantz Depaulis[4], Francis Barin[1]

1 Université François-Rabelais, Institut National de la Santé et de la Recherche Médicale - Unité 966 et Laboratoire de Virologie, Centre Hopsitalier Universitaire Bretonneau, Tours, France, **2** University of California San Diego, Department of Pathology, San Diego, California, United States of America, **3** Faculty of Associated Medical Sciences, Chiang Mai University, Chiang Mai, Thailand, **4** Laboratoire Ecologie et Evolution, Centre National de la Recherche Scientifique - Unité Mixte de Recherche 7625-Ecole Normale Supérieure, Paris, France, **5** Institut de Recherche pour le Développement, Chiang Mai, Thailand, **6** Harvard School of Public Health, Department of Immunology and Infectious Diseases, Boston, Massachusetts, United States of America

Abstract

Background: Mother-to-child transmission (MTCT) is responsible for most pediatric HIV-1 infections worldwide. It can occur during pregnancy, labor, or breastfeeding. Numerous studies have used coalescent and molecular clock methods to understand the epidemic history of HIV-1, but the timing of vertical transmission has not been studied using these methods. Taking advantage of the constant accumulation of HIV genetic variation over time and using longitudinally sampled viral sequences, we used a coalescent approach to investigate the timing of MTCT.

Materials and Methods: Six-hundred and twenty-two clonal *env* sequences from the RNA and DNA viral population were longitudinally sampled from nine HIV-1 infected mother-and-child pairs [range: 277–1034 days]. For each transmission pair, timing of MTCT was determined using a coalescent-based model within a Bayesian statistical framework. Results were compared with available estimates of MTCT timing obtained with the classic biomedical approach based on serial HIV DNA detection by PCR assays.

Results: Four children were infected during pregnancy, whereas the remaining five children were infected at time of delivery. For eight out of nine pairs, results were consistent with the transmission periods assessed by standard PCR-based assay. The discordance in the remaining case was likely confused by co-infection, with simultaneous introduction of multiple maternal viral variants at the time of delivery.

Conclusions: The study provided the opportunity to validate the Bayesian coalescent approach that determines the timing of MTCT of HIV-1. It illustrates the power of population genetics approaches to reliably estimate the timing of transmission events and deepens our knowledge about the dynamics of viral evolution in HIV-infected children, accounting for the complexity of multiple transmission events.

Editor: Jean-Pierre Vartanian, Institut Pasteur, France

Funding: This work was supported by funds from the Agence Nationale de Recherches sur le Sida et les Hépatites (ANRS, Paris, France), the Institut de Recherche pour le Développement (IRD, Paris, France), the National Institutes of Health (5 R01 HD 33326), and the Agence Nationale de Recherche (ANR biodiversité). T Samleerat was supported by a doctoral fellowship from the French Ministry of Foreign Affairs and the Thai Ministry of Higher Education. The funders had no role in study design, data collection and analysis, decision to publish, or preparation of the manuscript.

Competing Interests: The authors have declared that no competing interests exist.

* E-mail: achaillon@ucsd.edu

Introduction

The prevention of mother-to-child transmission (MTCT) of the human immunodeficiency virus (HIV) is one of the main global health issues and is one of the World Health Organization's key priorities. HIV-1 still infects about two million children worldwide, with 330,000 new infections reported in children in 2011 (Report on the Global AIDS Epidemic 2012, Geneva, World Health Organization). Without preventive intervention, probability of MTCT is 15–30% in high-income countries and up to 25–40% in sub-Saharan Africa, mainly due to differences in infant feeding practices [1]. In non-breastfeeding populations, and in the absence of chemoprophylaxis and targeted obstetrical prevention measures, transmission occurs *in utero* in approximately one third of the cases (mostly late in the third trimester of pregnancy) and *intrapartum* in the remaining two thirds [1,2].

Application of various phylogenetic approaches to HIV-1 has led to reconstruction of HIV-1 evolutionary history within and between hosts with good precision [3]. At the epidemiological level, history and origin of the HIV-1 epidemic have been successfully explored through molecular phylogeny [4–6], and these approaches also provided insights into clusters of HIV-1 transmission [7–9]. Moreover, application of these molecular evolutionary processes at the intra-host scale were implemented to investigate HIV-1 compartmentalization dynamics, disease progression, and adaptive response to drug therapy [10–14]. If traditional phylogenetic analyses establish evolutionary relatedness, recent developments that incorporate sample date information have permitted new approaches [15]. Specifically, the introduction of molecular clock in phylogenetic inference allowed more precise investigations into the evolutionary processes in order to infer molecular phylodynamics of HIV-1 [16]. Additionally, longitudinally obtained sequences from patients have been more recently used to investigate transmission direction and to estimate date of infection [17–21].

Aside from the descriptions of rare early *in utero* transmission events [22], the timing of transmission has been mostly estimated using partially indirect dynamic models [2]. Such probabilistic approaches exclusively rely on the virus detection at successive sampling time points after delivery [23]. Molecular variability constitutes valuable additional information, and viral sequences sampled at different time points can be used to investigate the rate and population dynamics of intra-host HIV-1 evolution [6,24–30]. We hypothesized that this approach could provide a good approximation of the timing of MTCT by estimating the time of most recent common ancestor (TMRCA) of viruses in the child. In this study, we used a coalescent approach within a Bayesian statistical framework to investigate the timing of MTCT. Using time series of cellular HIV-1 DNA and plasma HIV-1 RNA *env* sequences from nine mother-child pairs, we compared these quantitative results with the classic biomedical definition based on serial PCR that more qualitatively discriminates between transmission periods (i.e. *in utero vs. intrapartum*).

Materials and Methods

Ethics Statement

The initial protocol and its amendments were approved by the ethics committees of the Thai Ministry of Public Health, Chiang Mai University, and the Harvard School of Public Health. All study sites complied with regulations of the Department of Health and Human Services for the protection of research subjects. Women were enrolled at 28 weeks' gestation if they provided written informed consent.

Biological material

Nine mother-infant pairs, enrolled in the Perinatal HIV Prevention Trial-1 (PHPT-1) in Thailand were studied [31].The infants were not breastfed. HIV-1 infection status was determined by PCR-based HIV-1 proviral DNA detection, using DNA extracted from peripheral blood collected longitudinally within 48 hours of birth, at six weeks, four months, and six months of age. We considered the infant to have been infected *in utero* if the first test (using blood collected within 48 hours of birth) was positive and *intrapartum* if the first test result was negative but the following test results were positive [23]. HIV-1 *env* gene sequences were obtained from the mothers at delivery and from sequential samples collected at different times in their babies starting from the first positive PCR result up to several months or several years after birth (table 1). Extraction, amplification, cloning, and sequencing of *env* genes were done as previously described [32]. Briefly, genomic DNA was extracted from peripheral blood and viral RNA was extracted from plasma samples. A 1.2 kb fragment covering almost the entire HIV-1 *env* gp120 gene (from upstream V1 to downstream V5) was amplified by nested polymerase chain reaction (PCR) or PCR following reverse transcription (RT-PCR) using subtype-specific primers [32]. For each sample, several independent PCRs were pooled before cloning and sequencing in order to be representative of the viral diversity. All sequences were deposited in GenBank under accession numbers HM121341 to HM121962. A preliminary phylogenetic analysis using reference sequences from all the major HIV-1 clades showed that all individuals were infected by CRF01_AE strains, the predominant lineage in Thailand.

Data analyses

Sequences were aligned with the MAFFT v7.13 software [33] in both multiple and pairwise alignments, using an HIV-B and a consensus of HIV-1 CRF01_AE sequence as reference sequences. The resulting alignments were visually inspected with JALVIEW v2.0 [34]. The partition of genetic variation (diversity) was investigated through a molecular analysis of variance (AMOVA; [35]) implemented in ARLEQUIN v3.0 [36] to assess which fraction of genetic variation was accounted by various factors: mother-and-child pairs, sampling times, and DNA vs. RNA, (table 2). For the whole dataset of nine mother-and-child pair, a maximum likelihood (ML) tree was constructed using PHYML v2.4 [37] with a GTR+Gamma mutational model as assessed by the mutational model selection procedure implemented in HYPHY v2.2 [38,39]. Branch support was evaluated with 1000 bootstrap replicates (Figure 1).

Finally, to assess the impact of putative recombination on our phylogenetic analyses, we applied the method of Genetic Algorithm implemented in GARD [40] looking for potential topological tree incongruence (i.e. the impact of recombination on tree reconstruction) and tested for significance using Kishino Hasegawa (KH) topological incongruence analysis [41].

Coalescent Bayesian Markov Chain Monte Carlo (MCMC) estimates of the transmission timing

We used the BEAST package v1.7 [42] to estimate MTCT timing with a combination of probability models of gene trees and Bayesian statistical framework. Analysis were conducted under the best-fitting set of molecular, coalescent and demographic models (i.e. GTR+Gamma and an extended Bayesian skyline plot), as indicated by a Bayes Factor >20 (Table S1) [43,44]. For each mother infant pair, three chains were run assuming an uncorrelated lognormal relaxed molecular clock that allows the rate of evolution to vary across the tree [15]. Three independent chains were run for each pair with similar prior but different initial states, checking that such replicates reached similar results in order to assess convergence. Mixing and convergence (i.e. effective sample size greater than 200 for all parameters) were assessed in Tracer v1.5. All chains reached stationarity before 50,000,000 steps (except for pair 0779, which analysis had to be rerun with 100,000,000 steps for convergence). The Logcombiner v1.7.5 tool was then used to combine the chains. The first 10% of the chains were discarded (*burn in* period). Subsequently, the chain was regularly sampled to get an average estimate of parameter values and associated uncertainty [95% highest posterior density (HPD)]. Maximum clade credibility tree was selected with the software TREEANNOTATOR v1.7.4, after a 10% burn in. Trees were visualized in FIGTREE v.1.3.1.

Table 1. Pairs sampling informations.

Pair ID (IU/ IP*)	Mother (M)/ Infant (I)	Time points (days after delivery)/DNA (D) or RNA (R)/number of clones								Total sequences
		1	2	3	4	5	6	7	8	
0779 (IP)	M	0/D/15								84
	I		124/R/7	224/D/10	278/D/10 278/R/10	376/R/9	852/D/4	936/R/10	1034/R/9	
0858 (IU)	M	0/D/12								92
	I	0/R/14	128/D/10 128/R/4	183/D/10	370/D/10	482/D/7 482/R/9	575/D/10	860/D/6		
0939 (IP)	M	0/D/6								55
	I		44/R/6	126/D/10	187/D/11	231/D/11	861/D/11			
1005 (IU)	M	0/D/23 0/R/9								101
	I	0/D/10	47/R/17	122/D/10	185/D/10	355/R/11	543/D/11			
1021 (IP)	M	0/D/6								56
	I		68/R/6	124/R/10	429/R/9	551/D/5	611/R/10	820/R/10		
1110 (IU)	M	0/D/8								29
	I	0/R/10	475/D/11							
1224 (IU)	M	0/D/15								65
	I	0/R/11	122/D/11 122/R/8	185/D/10	277/D/10					
1333 (IP)	M	0/D/11								66
	I		87/D/11 87/R/11	115/D/9	185/D/8 185/R/10	350/D/6				
1391 (IP)	M	0/D/11								74
	I		47/R/10	128/D/9 128/R/10	184/D/9	459/R/10	526/D/8	755/D/7		

IU: *in utero* transmission - IP: *intrapartum* transmission.

Results

MTCT timing according to reference diagnostic procedures

The timing of MTCT was estimated using qualitative PCR assays for HIV-1 DNA detection in sequential samples collected from the infants. According to these data, four infants were infected during pregnancy (pairs 0858, 1005, 1110, 1224; *in utero* transmission), whereas five infants were infected at delivery or perinataly (pairs 0779, 0939, 1021, 1333, 1391; *intrapartum* transmission) (table 1).

Sequences analysis

A mean of 6 sequential samples per infant was included in the study (*range* = 2–8) with a mean follow-up period of 664 days (range: 277–1034 days; table 1). A total of 622 *env* sequences were analyzed, with a mean number of 12 clones per time-point (n = 4–32) and a mean of 69 clones for each mother-infant pair (range: 29–101). Among them, 61.4% were issued from cellular DNA, and 38.6% were issued from plasma viral RNA (382 and 240 sequences, respectively; Table 1).

Population structure was explored through an analysis of the molecular variance (AMOVA). The genetic variability between viral sequences (diversity) was explained by order of importance by: (*i*) mother-child pair, (*ii*) mother *vs* infant within each pair, (*iii*) the temporal stratification of the data, and (*iv*) the DNA or RNA origin of the sequences (Table 2). For instance, the percentage of molecular variance attributed to the nature of the sequences' origin (i.e. either cellular DNA or plasma viral RNA) was 3.9%, compared to 10.1% and 79.0% for the temporal stratification of the data and the nature of the pair, respectively. This finding suggests that the origin of the sequences (i.e. cellular DNA or plasma viral RNA) had moderate influence on the results.

Since recombination could strongly influence the population structure of sequences dataset, sequences were screened for recombination before phylogenetic analysis using GARD [45]. Though we found evidenced of single recombination events for most of the pairs, topological incongruence analysis using the KH test was not significant, indicating the signal for recombination was likely due to substitution rate variation, rather than differing phylogenetic history [41].

Phylogenetic analysis

As expected, the phylogeny of the entire data set (Figure 1) showed well supported (monophyletic) subtrees for each mother-infant pair, since each child viral sequence was directly and uniquely derived from the corresponding mother. Each mother-infant tree can therefore be considered separately (Figure 2). Two topological patterns corresponding to two different types of transmission events could be distinguished: eight of nine pairs supported a single viral transmission event with child sequences constituting a well-differentiated (monophyletic) subtree (Figure 2: pairs 0779, 1021, 1333, 1391 0858, 1005 and 1110) and were supported by high posterior probabilities (Figure 2). In these cases,

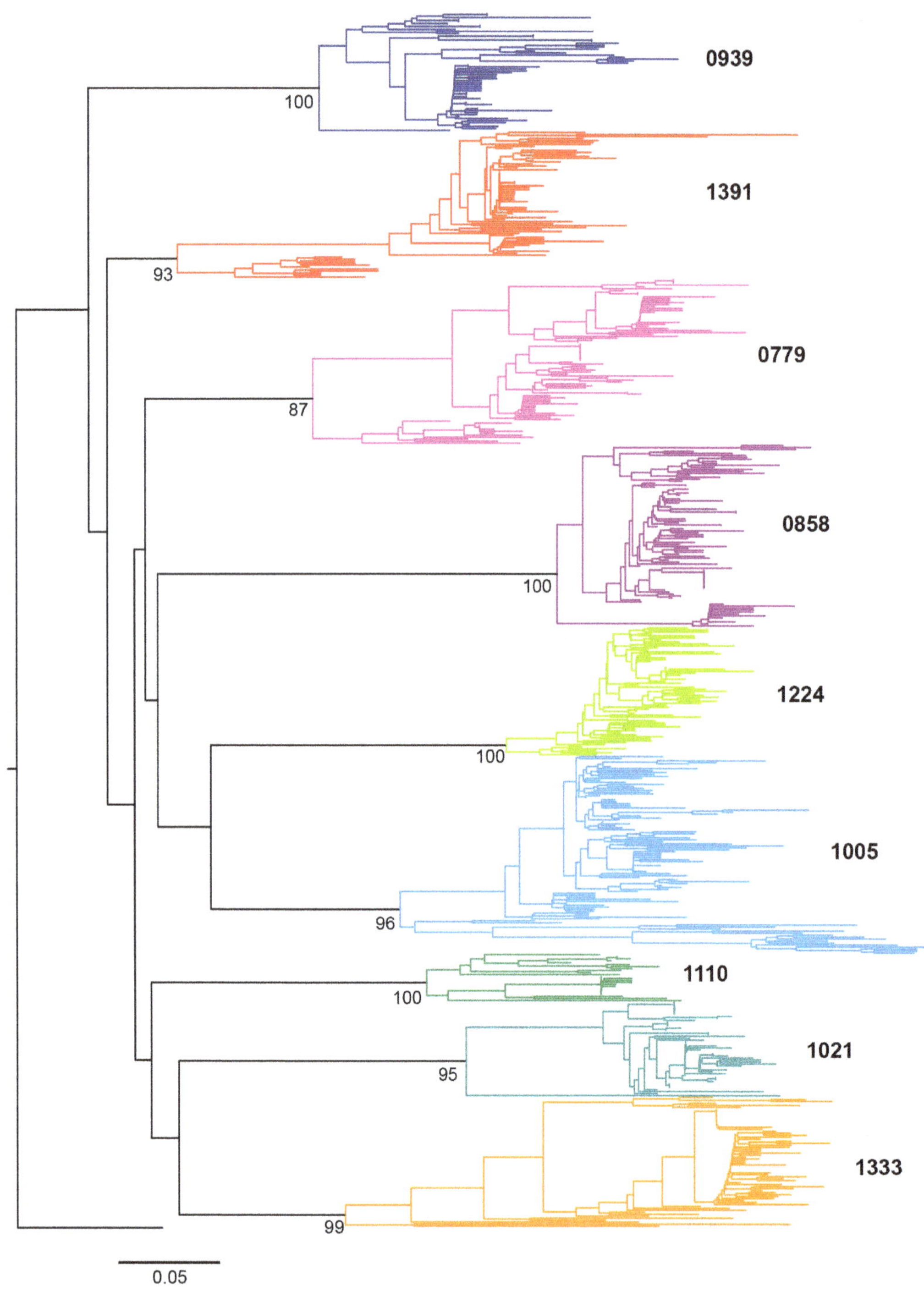

Figure 1. Rooted phylogenetic tree of the entire dataset (mothers and children of the nine pairs), reconstructed specifying a GTR+Gamma model. Each color represents a different pair. The external group (black) belongs to the CRF01_AE subtype. The scale corresponds to 5% of divergence between sequences. The bootstrap values are indicated.

a unique viral ancestor was likely transmitted from the mother to child. In contrast, viral lineages in the infants were intermixed with the mother lineages for pairs 0939, and 1224 (Figure 2). Such polyphyly of the child subtrees can be a consequence of (*i*) a poor phylogenetic resolution or (ii) transmission of several maternal variants. According to this second hypothesis, the TMRCA estimate would trace back to some point during the course of the maternal viral evolution. This kind of pattern would then provide support for multiple transmission variants that may have occurred during a single event (co-infection), or as several successive events (super-infections). Biological data obtained from the reference diagnostic PCR-based procedure may help to distinguish between these possibilities. Infection of infant 0939, which occurred perinatally, might be related to a single transmission event. Indeed, transmission of multiple variants during this time-limited period is more likely to have occurred

Table 2. Effect of different factors (mother-infant pair, duration of follow up and DNA/RNA origin of the viral sequences) on molecular variance analyzed by AMOVA.

Data	Molecular variance due to M/I pair relative to duration of follow-up			Molecular variance due to M/I pair relative to origin of sequences (times pooled)	
	DNA	RNA	DNA & RNA		
Pairs	81.25%*	77.24%*	79.23%*	**Pairs**	79.02%*
Time within each pair	6.47%*	14.93%*	10.06%*	**DNA/RNA within each pair**	3.87%*
Residual	12.28%*	7.83%*	10.71%*	**Residual**	17.12%*

*p<0.001.
AMOVA: analysis of the molecular variance.

during a single event (co-infection) rather than successive events (superinfections).

In contrast, infection of infant 1224, which occurred *in utero*, might have resulted from either a co-infection by several variants during a simple event or super-infections due to several sequential events (Figure 3).

Coalescent Bayesian Markov Chain Monte Carlo (MCMC) estimate of transmission timing

For the nine pairs, the posterior distribution of the child viral population TMRCA was inferred. The resulting estimate of the TMRCA closely corresponded to the transmission timing according to standard assays (Figure 3). The genealogical inferences were consistent with the biological diagnosis based on timing of HIV-1 proviral detection for eight of nine pairs. The 95% HPD of possible infant root age overlapped birth when viral transmission occurred *intrapartum* according to the reference biological diagnosis (Figure 3: four bottom grey boxes) and excluded it when transmission occurred *in utero* (Figure 3: four top open boxes). Variance of TMRCA largely varied among the pairs. Though the inferred TMRCA results were consistent for five pairs (0779, 1021, 1333, 1391 and 1005; HPD range extending to roughly two months), others showed a greater variance. This variance extended to almost five months for pairs 0858 and 1224. Pair 1110 showed an extremely large range extending close to birth but was documented with only 29 sequences, including 62% of sequences issued from cellular DNA. Of note, pair 0939 range excluded birth and was discordant with the biomedical diagnostic assay. However, the corresponding phylogenetic tree suggested infection with multiple viral variants (Figure 2). The 95% HPD largely preceded birth, extending even before pregnancy, thereby reinforcing the probable infection by several maternal variants.

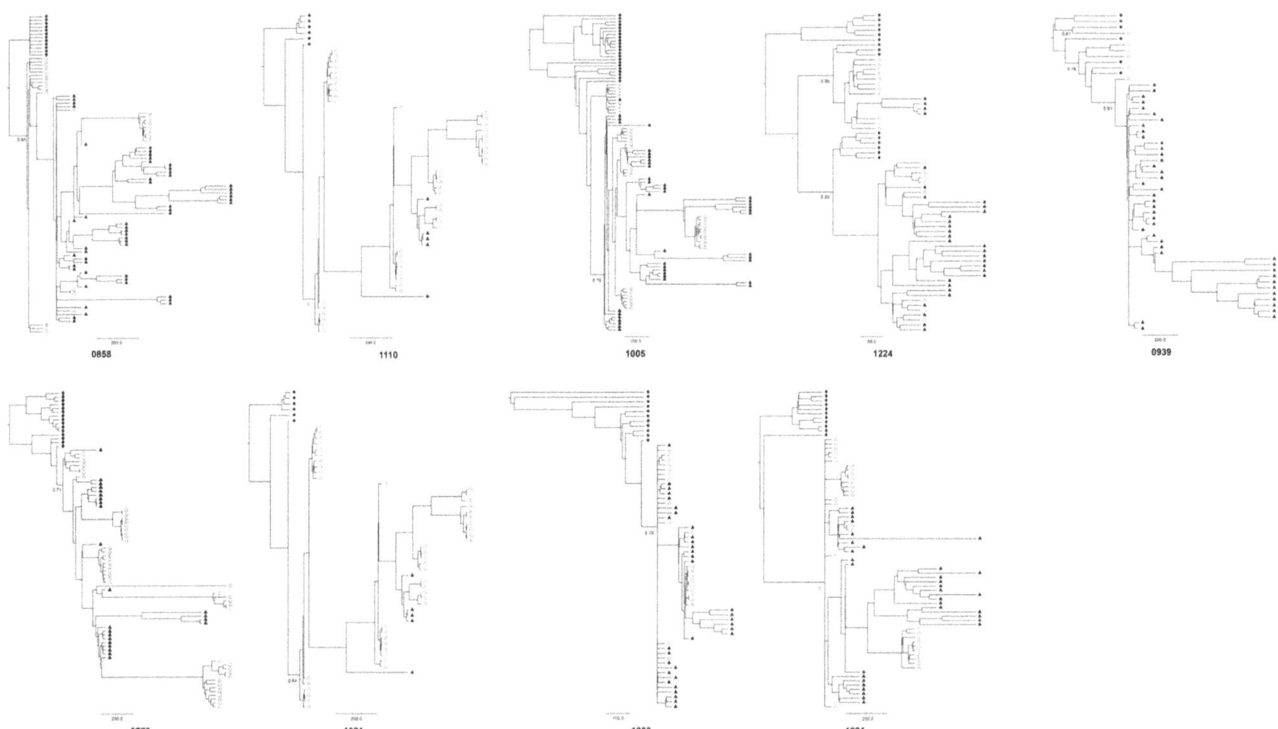

Figure 2. Bayesian MCMC phylogenetic trees. Maternal and child sequences are represented by diamonds and triangles respectively. Filled and unfilled symbols refer to DNA and RNA samples respectively. Time scale expressed in days is indicated below each tree. Posterior probabilities of the main lineages are indicated at the root.

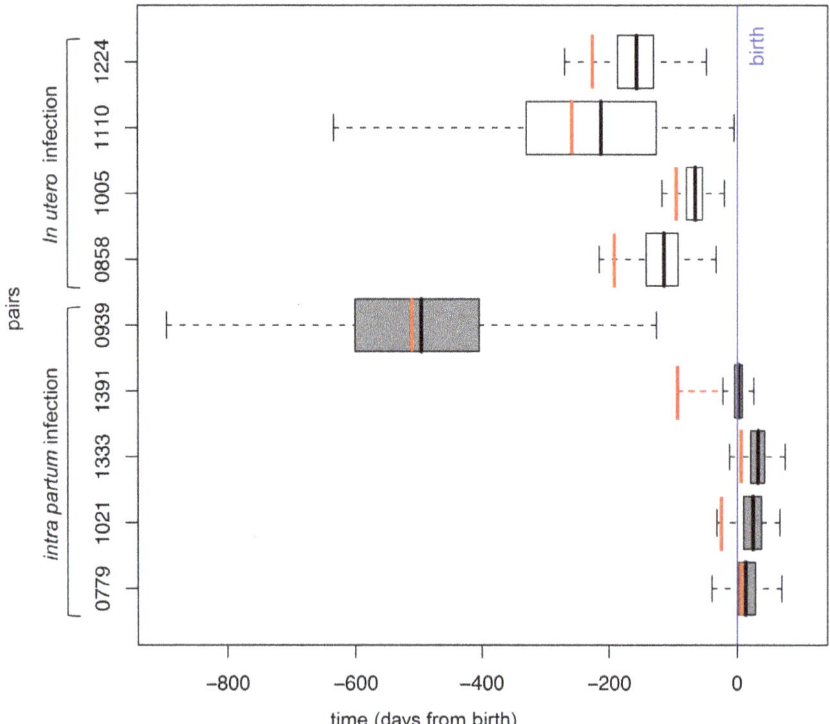

Figure 3. Boxplots of the TMRCA posterior distributions. Dashed lines represent the 95% High Posterior Density (HPD). First (25%) and third (75%) quartiles (limits of the rectangle) and median (thick line) are also indicated. According to the biomedical reference diagnostic method, the four top infants with white boxplots were infected *in utero*, whereas the five bottom infants with grey boxplots were infected *intra partum*. Vertical red lines indicate the maximum estimates of TMRCA.

The MRCA of the viral variants should then trace back to the mother's viral population and may even precede pregnancy. If the timing assumed by the biomedical diagnosis was correct, it is possible that several maternal variants were transmitted at birth in child 0939.

Considering the "children-only" dataset, parameter estimates were still consistent with those obtained with the entire dataset. Inferred TMRCA were mutually highly consistent for 7 of the 9 pairs and in a lesser extent for pairs 1224, 1333 who were also distinct by the shortest duration of follow-up (respectively 277 and 350 days) (Figure 4). This finding was expected considering that the child TMRCA could be estimated regardless of the maternal sequence data (Figure 4).

Discussion

HIV-1 pediatric infection is a challenging health issue worldwide, and a primary goal of HIV-1 prevention programs is to limit acquisition of HIV-1 during mother-to-child transmission [1]. Although it has been shown that MTCT of HIV-1 can occur both during pregnancy and at delivery [2], the exact timing of MTCT remains difficult to determine precisely with biomedical methods based on serial PCR and indirect probabilistic approaches [23]. To our knowledge, time-measured Bayesian MCMC analyses of longitudinally sampled sequences have never been used to investigate this question. The well-documented sample of longitudinally collected sequences from nine HIV-1 infected mother-infant pairs included in this study represents a unique opportunity to investigate MTCT timing and to validate Bayesian inference.

The maternal and infant viral populations within each pair were significantly differentiated, thus reflecting a drastic bottleneck associated with transmission [32,46–56]. This bottleneck and the subsequent molecular evolution within the infected child provided the basis for our proposed approach. Tree topologies suggested different types of transmission: six pairs showed well-supported monophyletic subtrees claiming for a single transmission event of a single viral variant. In contrast, the data suggested transmission of several variants, as indicated by several separate branches, for the three remaining pairs.

Transmission time estimates using a time-scaled Bayesian phylogenetic approach were shown to be reliable. Despite the short time scales involved (from 277 to 1034 days depending of the mother-infant pair), they were qualitatively highly consistent with the reference diagnostic procedures based on timing of HIV-1 proviral DNA detection. In eight of nine cases, our inferences of the timing of transmission corroborated the PCR results, including four *in utero* and four *intrapartum* infected infants. These results validate the time-scaled Bayesian approach to date MTCT of HIV-1. The single discordant case concerned a pair for which TMRCA was not consistent with the biomedical diagnosis that argued for *intrapartum* transmission. Transmission of multiple maternal variants was strongly suggested by the phylogenetic analysis of this mother-infant pair. The introduction of several variants in a single transmission event or closely related events could lead to large uncertainty in the estimated timing of transmission, leading the ancestry among viral lineages to trace further back in time in the mother's population. However, it remains difficult to distinguish between this hypothesis supported by the PCR results and a possible misclassification by the standard diagnostic assay.

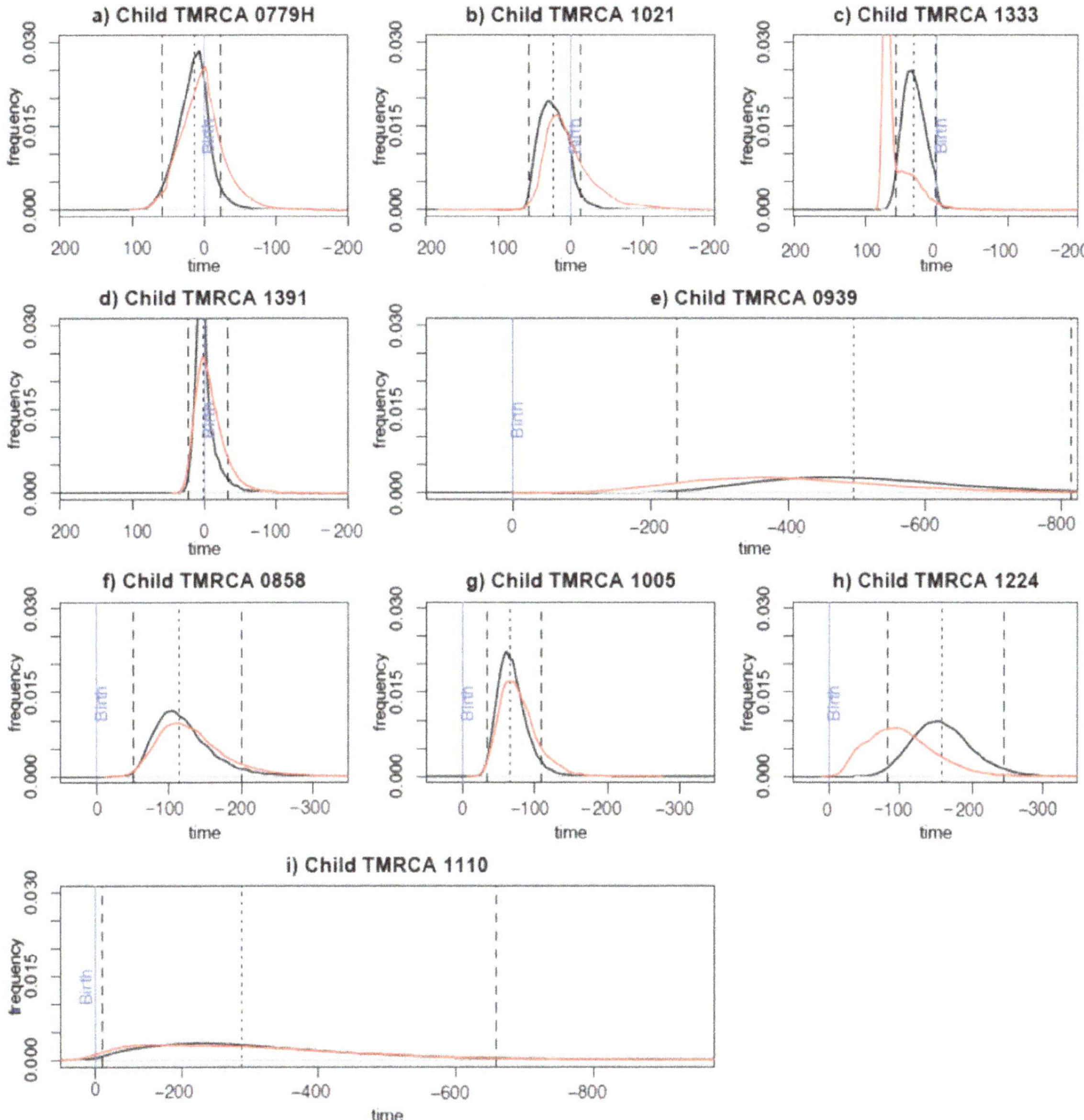

Figure 4. Comparative TMRCA posterior distributions. Red curves correspond to posterior distribution of children-only data. Black curves refer to posterior distribution of pair (mother and child) data. Dashed lines represent the 95% confidence interval. Median (hashed line) is indicated. The blue vertical line indicates birth and times on the x axis are expressed in days since birth. Y axis: TMRCA density; X axis: time in days. a to e: infants infected *intrapartum*. f to i: infants infected *in utero*.

The observed TMRCA variance largely varied among the pairs and could be partially linked to the time of transmission; the more recent the transmission, the more precise the estimate. Hence, TMRCA estimates were consistent (corresponding to a greater coefficient of variance) for five pairs, particularly for the *intrapartum* infected children. Interestingly, a wide confidence interval was observed for two infants (pair 1110, and pair 1224 albeit at a lesser extent), considered to have been infected *in utero* according to the PCR results. This uncertainty might be explained by both the transmission of several variants for the two cases and a low number of available sequences for pair 1110.

We must consider that the transmission of several variants might be attributed either to introduction of several maternal variants in a single transmission event (co-infection) or to several successive introductions of maternal variants (super-infection) that could occur during pregnancy (*in utero*) or during pregnancy and then at delivery (*in utero* and *intrapartum*). Discrimination between these two possibilities remains a challenging objective. Unlike phylogenetic methods that follow a lineage backwards to coalescence, probabilistic models were implemented to detect if transmission occurred because of one or several variants [57]. To our knowledge, superinfection during pregnancy has never been modeled through time. A model introducing migration and divergence processes between the viral populations of the mother and its child might distinguish co-infection from superinfection.

This study was limited by the inclusion of sequences issued from both cellular DNA and plasma viral RNA, which may reflect different tempos of HIV-1 evolution. However, our AMOVA analysis suggested that the origin of the sequences (i.e. cellular DNA or plasma viral RNA) did not play a major role on the observed molecular variance. Additionally, the use of a relaxed clock model partially accommodates for the potential different evolution rate of sequences present in cellular DNA and plasma viral RNA. The reappearance of archived viral population must be considered [58,59]. For example, the phylogenetic tree of pair 1391 showed that proviral DNA sequences sampled at time $t = 755$ days in the child were extremely close to RNA sequences present earlier in his plasma, at 47 and 184 days after birth. This finding suggests the possibility of continuous re-emergence of variants from putative viral reservoirs in children. If DNA reservoirs contribute to the RNA pool recurrently, it appears relevant to consider both DNA and RNA sequences to avoid features of HIV-1 evolution. The potential bias introduced by the maternal sequences must be considered also. They were issued from cellular DNA since RNA sequences were not available for most mothers as a consequence of the low plasma viral load at delivery in response to antiretroviral prophylaxis during pregnancy [31]. However, the inferred TMRCA using RNA-derived sequence only were still consistent with the full analysis when considering the seven mother-infant pairs for which the number of sequences issued from plasma RNA was sufficient. Sampling times lead to a local rescaling of rates of substitutions through the local clock model and branching. Even if it constraints the relative nodes positions along the trees, the time estimate of the child's root provided confidence in the TMRCA inference and was confirmed by the congruence with the biomedical assays. Another limitation may be linked to the technical strategy used. Indeed, the sequences were not obtained using the single genome amplification technology that is considered as a gold standard since it avoid recombination events during the PCR from bulk DNA and it limits the non proportional representation of target sequences due to template resampling [60–62]. However, and as discussed above, the concordance between the molecular evolution approach and the reference biomedical diagnosis suggest that this limitation did not have a drastic effect.

Conclusions

This study has benefited from the temporal anchoring of HIV-1 sequences to infer transmission timing and evolutionary rates in mother-infant pairs. Thanks to the validation based on the determination of the transmission period through the reference diagnostic procedure, our study offered a unique opportunity to validate the Bayesian coalescent framework on documented cases. It confirms that time series of viral sequences can provide powerful insights to draw inference about transmission timing. Such theoretical approaches could also provide insight into multiple infections processes (i.e. coinfection or superinfection) not readily detectable with the current diagnostic assays.

Acknowledgments

The authors would like to acknowledge Dr Joel O.Wertheim for his critical comments during the preparation of this paper.

Author Contributions

Conceived and designed the experiments: AC FZ SB FD. Performed the experiments: AC TS AM. Analyzed the data: AC FZ SB FD. Contributed reagents/materials/analysis tools: AC NNGH GJ ML. Wrote the paper: AC SG FD FB.

References

1. Prendergast A, Tudor-Williams G, Jeena P, Burchett S, Goulder P (2007) International perspectives, progress, and future challenges of paediatric HIV infection. Lancet 370: 68–80. doi:10.1016/S0140-6736(07)61051-4.
2. Rouzioux C, Costagliola D, Burgard M, Blanche S, Mayaux MJ, et al. (1995) Estimated timing of mother-to-child human immunodeficiency virus type 1 (HIV-1) transmission by use of a Markov model. The HIV Infection in Newborns French Collaborative Study Group. Am J Epidemiol 142: 1330–1337.
3. Rambaut A, Posada D, Crandall KA, Holmes EC (2004) The causes and consequences of HIV evolution. Nat Rev Genet 5: 52–61. doi:10.1038/nrg1246 nrg1246 [pii].
4. Holmes EC, Nee S, Rambaut A, Garnett GP, Harvey PH (1995) Revealing the history of infectious disease epidemics through phylogenetic trees. Philos Trans R Soc Lond B Biol Sci 349: 33–40. doi:10.1098/rstb.1995.0088.
5. Junqueira DM, de Medeiros RM, Matte MCC, Araújo LAL, Chies JAB, et al. (2011) Reviewing the history of HIV-1: spread of subtype B in the Americas. PloS One 6: e27489. doi:10.1371/journal.pone.0027489.
6. Worobey M, Gemmel M, Teuwen DE, Haselkorn T, Kunstman K, et al. (2008) Direct evidence of extensive diversity of HIV-1 in Kinshasa by 1960. Nature 455: 661–664. doi:10.1038/nature07390.
7. Edwards CTT, Holmes EC, Wilson DJ, Viscidi RP, Abrams EJ, et al. (2006) Population genetic estimation of the loss of genetic diversity during horizontal transmission of HIV-1. BMC Evol Biol 6: 28. doi:10.1186/1471-2148-6-28.
8. Hué S, Pillay D, Clewley JP, Pybus OG (2005) Genetic analysis reveals the complex structure of HIV-1 transmission within defined risk groups. Proc Natl Acad Sci U S A 102: 4425–4429. doi:10.1073/pnas.0407534102.
9. Lemey P, Rambaut A, Pybus OG (2006) HIV evolutionary dynamics within and among hosts. AIDS Rev 8: 125–140.
10. Castro-Nallar E, Pérez-Losada M, Burton GF, Crandall KA (2012) The evolution of HIV: inferences using phylogenetics. Mol Phylogenet Evol 62: 777–792. doi:10.1016/j.ympev.2011.11.019.
11. Nickle DC, Jensen MA, Shriner D, Brodie SJ, Frenkel LM, et al. (2003) Evolutionary Indicators of Human Immunodeficiency Virus Type 1 Reservoirs and Compartments. J Virol 77: 5540–5546. doi:10.1128/JVI.77.9.5540-5546.2003.
12. Rachinger A, Stolte IG, van de Ven TD, Burger JA, Prins M, et al. (2010) Absence of HIV-1 superinfection 1 year after infection between 1985 and 1997 coincides with a reduction in sexual risk behavior in the seroincident Amsterdam cohort of homosexual men. Clin Infect Dis Off Publ Infect Dis Soc Am 50: 1309–1315. doi:10.1086/651687.
13. Shankarappa R, Margolick JB, Gange SJ, Rodrigo AG, Upchurch D, et al. (1999) Consistent viral evolutionary changes associated with the progression of human immunodeficiency virus type 1 infection. J Virol 73: 10489–10502.
14. Zhu T, Wang N, Carr A, Nam DS, Moor-Jankowski R, et al. (1996) Genetic characterization of human immunodeficiency virus type 1 in blood and genital secretions: evidence for viral compartmentalization and selection during sexual transmission. J Virol 70: 3098–3107.
15. Drummond AJ, Ho SYW, Phillips MJ, Rambaut A (2006) Relaxed phylogenetics and dating with confidence. PLoS Biol 4: e88. doi:10.1371/journal.pbio.0040088.
16. Lewis F, Hughes GJ, Rambaut A, Pozniak A, Leigh Brown AJ (2008) Episodic sexual transmission of HIV revealed by molecular phylodynamics. PLoS Med 5: e50. doi:10.1371/journal.pmed.0050050.
17. Bernard EJ, Azad Y, Vandamme AM, Weait M, Geretti AM (2007) HIV forensics: pitfalls and acceptable standards in the use of phylogenetic analysis as evidence in criminal investigations of HIV transmission. HIV Med 8: 382–387. doi:10.1111/j.1468-1293.2007.00486.x.
18. Poon AFY, McGovern RA, Mo T, Knapp DJHF, Brenner B, et al. (2011) Dates of HIV infection can be estimated for seroprevalent patients by coalescent analysis of serial next-generation sequencing data. AIDS Lond Engl 25: 2019–2026. doi:10.1097/QAD.0b013e32834b643c.
19. English S, Katzourakis A, Bonsall D, Flanagan P, Duda A, et al. (2011) Phylogenetic analysis consistent with a clinical history of sexual transmission of HIV-1 from a single donor reveals transmission of highly distinct variants. Retrovirology 8: 54. doi:10.1186/1742-4690-8-54.
20. Kaye M, Chibo D, Birch C (2009) Comparison of Bayesian and maximum-likelihood phylogenetic approaches in two legal cases involving accusations of transmission of HIV. AIDS Res Hum Retroviruses 25: 741–748. doi:10.1089/aid.2008.0306.

21. Rachinger A, Groeneveld PHP, van Assen S, Lemey P, Schuitemaker H (2011) Time-measured phylogenies of gag, pol and env sequence data reveal the direction and time interval of HIV-1 transmission. AIDS Lond Engl 25: 1035–1039. doi:10.1097/QAD.0b013e3283467020.
22. Brossard Y, Aubin JT, Mandelbrot L, Bignozzi C, Brand D, et al. (1995) Frequency of early in utero HIV-1 infection: a blind DNA polymerase chain reaction study on 100 fetal thymuses. AIDS Lond Engl 9: 359–366.
23. Bryson YJ, Luzuriaga K, Sullivan JL, Wara DW (1992) Proposed definitions for in utero versus intrapartum transmission of HIV-1. N Engl J Med 327: 1246–1247. doi:10.1056/NEJM199210223271718.
24. Gilbert MTP, Rambaut A, Wlasiuk G, Spira TJ, Pitchenik AE, et al. (2007) The emergence of HIV/AIDS in the Americas and beyond. Proc Natl Acad Sci U S A 104: 18566–18570. doi:10.1073/pnas.0705329104.
25. Hughes GJ, Fearnhill E, Dunn D, Lycett SJ, Rambaut A, et al. (2009) Molecular phylodynamics of the heterosexual HIV epidemic in the United Kingdom. PLoS Pathog 5: e1000590. doi:10.1371/journal.ppat.1000590.
26. Pybus OG, Rambaut A, Harvey PH (2000) An integrated framework for the inference of viral population history from reconstructed genealogies. Genetics 155: 1429–1437.
27. Drummond A, Pybus OG, Rambaut A (2003) Inference of viral evolutionary rates from molecular sequences. Adv Parasitol 54: 331–358.
28. Hudson RR (1983) Properties of a neutral allele model with intragenic recombination. Theor Popul Biol 23: 183–201.
29. Grenfell BT, Pybus OG, Gog JR, Wood JLN, Daly JM, et al. (2004) Unifying the epidemiological and evolutionary dynamics of pathogens. Science 303: 327–332. doi:10.1126/science.1090727.
30. Rosenberg NA, Nordborg M (2002) Genealogical trees, coalescent theory and the analysis of genetic polymorphisms. Nat Rev Genet 3: 380–390. doi:10.1038/nrg795.
31. Lallemant M, Jourdain G, Le Coeur S, Kim S, Koetsawang S, et al. (2000) A trial of shortened zidovudine regimens to prevent mother-to-child transmission of human immunodeficiency virus type 1. Perinatal HIV Prevention Trial (Thailand) Investigators. N Engl J Med 343: 982–991.
32. Samleerat T, Braibant M, Jourdain G, Moreau A, Ngo-Giang-Huong N, et al. (2008) Characteristics of HIV type 1 (HIV-1) glycoprotein 120 env sequences in mother-infant pairs infected with HIV-1 subtype CRF01_AE. J Infect Dis 198: 868–876. doi:10.1086/591251.
33. Katoh K, Asimenos G, Toh H (2009) Multiple alignment of DNA sequences with MAFFT. Methods Mol Biol Clifton NJ 537: 39–64. doi:10.1007/978-1-59745-251-9_3.
34. Waterhouse AM, Procter JB, Martin DMA, Clamp M, Barton GJ (2009) Jalview Version 2–a multiple sequence alignment editor and analysis workbench. Bioinforma Oxf Engl 25: 1189–1191. doi:10.1093/bioinformatics/btp033.
35. Excoffier L, Smouse PE, Quattro JM (1992) Analysis of molecular variance inferred from metric distances among DNA haplotypes: application to human mitochondrial DNA restriction data. Genetics 131: 479–491.
36. Excoffier L, Laval G, Schneider S (2005) Arlequin (version 3.0): an integrated software package for population genetics data analysis. Evol Bioinforma Online 1: 47–50.
37. Guindon S, Gascuel O (2003) A simple, fast, and accurate algorithm to estimate large phylogenies by maximum likelihood. Syst Biol 52: 696–704.
38. Delport W, Poon AFY, Frost SDW, Kosakovsky Pond SL (2010) Datamonkey 2010: a suite of phylogenetic analysis tools for evolutionary biology. Bioinforma Oxf Engl 26: 2455–2457. doi:10.1093/bioinformatics/btq429.
39. Pond SLK, Frost SDW, Muse SV (2005) HyPhy: hypothesis testing using phylogenies. Bioinforma Oxf Engl 21: 676–679. doi:10.1093/bioinformatics/bti079.
40. Kosakovsky Pond SL, Posada D, Gravenor MB, Woelk CH, Frost SDW (2006) Automated phylogenetic detection of recombination using a genetic algorithm. Mol Biol Evol 23: 1891–1901. doi:10.1093/molbev/msl051.
41. Kishino H, Hasegawa M (1989) Evaluation of the maximum likelihood estimate of the evolutionary tree topologies from DNA sequence data, and the branching order in hominoidea. J Mol Evol 29: 170–179.
42. Drummond AJ, Suchard MA, Xie D, Rambaut A (2012) Bayesian Phylogenetics with BEAUti and the BEAST 1.7. Mol Biol Evol 29: 1969–1973. doi:10.1093/molbev/mss075.
43. Heled J, Drummond AJ (2008) Bayesian inference of population size history from multiple loci. BMC Evol Biol 8: 289. doi:10.1186/1471-2148-8-289.
44. Kass RE, Raftery AE (1995) Bayes Factors. J Am Stat Assoc 90: 773–795. doi:10.1080/01621459.1995.10476572.
45. Kosakovsky Pond SL, Posada D, Gravenor MB, Woelk CH, Frost SDW (2006) GARD: a genetic algorithm for recombination detection. Bioinforma Oxf Engl 22: 3096–3098. doi:10.1093/bioinformatics/btl474.
46. Ahmad N, Baroudy BM, Baker RC, Chappey C (1995) Genetic analysis of human immunodeficiency virus type 1 envelope V3 region isolates from mothers and infants after perinatal transmission. J Virol 69: 1001–1012.
47. Briant L, Wade CM, Puel J, Brown AJ, Guyader M (1995) Analysis of envelope sequence variants suggests multiple mechanisms of mother-to-child transmission of human immunodeficiency virus type 1. J Virol 69: 3778–3788.
48. Dickover RE, Garratty EM, Plaeger S, Bryson YJ (2001) Perinatal transmission of major, minor, and multiple maternal human immunodeficiency virus type 1 variants in utero and intrapartum. J Virol 75: 2194–2203. doi:10.1128/JVI.75.5.2194-2203.2001.
49. Kishko M, Somasundaran M, Brewster F, Sullivan JL, Clapham PR, et al. (2011) Genotypic and functional properties of early infant HIV-1 envelopes. Retrovirology 8: 67. doi:10.1186/1742-4690-8-67.
50. Kwiek JJ, Russell ES, Dang KK, Burch CL, Mwapasa V, et al. (2008) The molecular epidemiology of HIV-1 envelope diversity during HIV-1 subtype C vertical transmission in Malawian mother-infant pairs. AIDS Lond Engl 22: 863–871. doi:10.1097/QAD.0b013e3282f51ea0.
51. Pasquier C, Cayrou C, Blancher A, Tourne-Petheil C, Berrebi A, et al. (1998) Molecular evidence for mother-to-child transmission of multiple variants by analysis of RNA and DNA sequences of human immunodeficiency virus type 1. J Virol 72: 8493–8501.
52. Renjifo B, Chung M, Gilbert P, Mwakagile D, Msamanga G, et al. (2003) In-utero transmission of quasispecies among human immunodeficiency virus type 1 genotypes. Virology 307: 278–282.
53. Russell ES, Kwiek JJ, Keys J, Barton K, Mwapasa V, et al. (2011) The genetic bottleneck in vertical transmission of subtype C HIV-1 is not driven by selection of especially neutralization-resistant virus from the maternal viral population. J Virol 85: 8253–8262. doi:10.1128/JVI.00197-11.
54. Scarlatti G, Leitner T, Halapi E, Wahlberg J, Jansson M, et al. (1993) Analysis of the HIV-1 envelope V3-loop sequences from ten mother-child pairs. Ann N Y Acad Sci 693: 277–280.
55. Wolinsky SM, Wike CM, Korber BT, Hutto C, Parks WP, et al. (1992) Selective transmission of human immunodeficiency virus type-1 variants from mothers to infants. Science 255: 1134–1137.
56. Zhang H, Tully DC, Hoffmann FG, He J, Kankasa C, et al. (2010) Restricted genetic diversity of HIV-1 subtype C envelope glycoprotein from perinatally infected Zambian infants. PloS One 5: e9294. doi:10.1371/journal.pone.0009294.
57. Lee HY, Giorgi EE, Keele BF, Gaschen B, Athreya GS, et al. (2009) Modeling sequence evolution in acute HIV-1 infection. J Theor Biol 261: 341–360. doi:10.1016/j.jtbi.2009.07.038.
58. Shen L, Siliciano RF (2008) Viral reservoirs, residual viremia, and the potential of highly active antiretroviral therapy to eradicate HIV infection. J Allergy Clin Immunol 122: 22–28. doi:10.1016/j.jaci.2008.05.033.
59. Zhang J, Nielsen R, Yang Z (2005) Evaluation of an improved branch-site likelihood method for detecting positive selection at the molecular level. Mol Biol Evol 22: 2472–2479. doi:10.1093/molbev/msi237.
60. Lahr DJG, Katz LA (2009) Reducing the impact of PCR-mediated recombination in molecular evolution and environmental studies using a new-generation high-fidelity DNA polymerase. BioTechniques 47: 857–866. doi:10.2144/000113219.
61. Eckert KA, Kunkel TA (1991) DNA polymerase fidelity and the polymerase chain reaction. PCR Methods Appl 1: 17–24.
62. Horton RM (1995) PCR-mediated recombination and mutagenesis. SOEing together tailor-made genes. Mol Biotechnol 3: 93–99. doi:10.1007/BF02789105.

22

HIV in Children in a General Population Sample in East Zimbabwe: Prevalence, Causes and Effects

Erica L. Pufall[1]*, Constance Nyamukapa[1,2], Jeffrey W. Eaton[1], Reggie Mutsindiri[2], Godwin Chawira[2], Shungu Munyati[2], Laura Robertson[1], Simon Gregson[1]

1 Department of Infectious Disease Epidemiology, Imperial College London, St. Mary's Campus, Norfolk Place, London, United Kingdom, **2** Biomedical Research and Training Institute, Avondale, Harare, Zimbabwe

Abstract

Background: There are an estimated half-million children living with HIV in sub-Saharan Africa. The predominant source of infection is presumed to be perinatal mother-to-child transmission, but general population data about paediatric HIV are sparse. We characterise the epidemiology of HIV in children in sub-Saharan Africa by describing the prevalence, possible source of infection, and effects of paediatric HIV in a southern African population.

Methods: From 2009 to 2011, we conducted a household-based survey of 3389 children (aged 2–14 years) in Manicaland, eastern Zimbabwe (response rate: 73.5%). Data about socio-demographic correlates of HIV, risk factors for infection, and effects on child health were analysed using multi-variable logistic regression. To assess the plausibility of mother-to-child transmission, child HIV infection was linked to maternal survival and HIV status using data from a 12-year adult HIV cohort.

Results: HIV prevalence was (2.2%, 95% CI: 1.6–2.8%) and did not differ significantly by sex, socio-economic status, location, religion, or child age. Infected children were more likely to be underweight (19.6% versus 10.0%, p = 0.03) or stunted (39.1% versus 30.6%, p = 0.04) but did not report poorer physical or psychological ill-health. Where maternal data were available, reported mothers of 61/62 HIV-positive children were deceased or HIV-positive. Risk factors for other sources of infection were not associated with child HIV infection, including blood transfusion, vaccinations, caring for a sick relative, and sexual abuse. The observed flat age-pattern of HIV prevalence was consistent with UNAIDS estimates which assumes perinatal mother-to-child transmission, although modelled prevalence was higher than observed prevalence. Only 19/73 HIV-positive children (26.0%) were diagnosed, but, of these, 17 were on antiretroviral therapy.

Conclusions: Childhood HIV infection likely arises predominantly from mother-to-child transmission and is associated with poorer physical development. Overall antiretroviral therapy uptake was low, with the primary barrier to treatment appearing to be lack of diagnosis.

Editor: Delmiro Fernandez-Reyes, Brighton and Sussex Medical School, United Kingdom

Funding: ELP received a Doctoral Foreign Study Award from the Canadian Institutes for Health Research (http://www.cihr-irsc.gc.ca/e/193.html). JWE thanks the Bill and Melinda Gates foundation for funding support via a grant to the HIV Modelling Consortium (http://www.gatesfoundation.org/). The Manicaland HIV/STD Prevention Project is supported by a grant from the Wellcome Trust (grant 050517/z/97abc, http://www.wellcome.ac.uk/). The funders had no role in study design, data collection and analysis, decision to publish, or preparation of the manuscript.

Competing Interests: The authors have declared that no competing interests exist.

* Email: e.pufall11@imperial.ac.uk

Introduction

In 2012, it was estimated that over 85% of children who became infected with HIV were living in sub-Saharan Africa (SSA) [1]. However, general population data about epidemiology and health effects of paediatric HIV in SSA are sparse. The most common data about HIV prevalence in SSA, Demographic and Health Surveys (DHS) and community-based cohort studies, have typically only included persons over age 15 years. As a result, estimates for HIV in children are generally extrapolated from data about pregnant women using mathematical models [2]. In Zimbabwe, UNAIDS estimated that 2.8% (95% CI: 1.6–3.7%) of children 0–14 were HIV-positive in 2012 [2,3]. Direct empirical data about the epidemiology, sources and impacts of HIV in children will improve confidence in estimates and ensure that health and social care systems are able to meet the needs of infected children.

Most infected children are believed to have acquired HIV perinatally from their HIV-positive mothers. Untreated HIV infection in infants is typically characterised by rapid disease progression and death at a median of two years of age or less, with survival depending at what stage (*e.g.* perinatally, breastfeeding) the infant becomes vertically infected [4,5], but it is estimated that perhaps up to a third of vertically infected children survive into adolescence [6–8] and clinical reports have provided evidence of non-sexually acquired infections in adolescents [9–12]. However, debate continues as to whether or not these children are actually long-term survivors of mother-to-child transmission (MTCT) or have acquired HIV horizontally. Other studies have reported instances of horizontal HIV transmission in children [13–15]; however, these studies used non-representative samples or were conducted in highly localised areas.

In this study, we aim to: (i) describe patterns of HIV infection in a representative general population sample of children aged 2–14 years in a large-scale generalised HIV epidemic in rural areas of eastern Zimbabwe; (ii) investigate possible sources of horizontal HIV transmission in childhood; (iii) assess whether the observed age-pattern of HIV-positive children is consistent with that expected from survival of children infected from MTCT (given recent trends in adult prevalence and prevention of mother-to-child transmission (PMTCT) program scale-up); (iv) assess the impact of HIV on children's mental and physical health and nutritional status; and (v) investigate the levels and determinants of antiretroviral treatment (ART) coverage in children.

Methods

Study Population and Data Collection

The Manicaland HIV/STD Prevention Project is a population-based, open cohort study in eastern Zimbabwe [16–18]. Each round of the survey involves a census of all households in the 12 study sites (4 subsistence farming areas; 4 large-scale commercial estates; 2 small towns; and 2 roadside settlements), followed by interviews with individual household members and collection of dried blood spot samples for HIV testing.

In the most recent round (2009–2011) of the Manicaland survey, all children (aged 2–14 years) in a randomly selected 1/3 of households were invited to participate in an investigation of HIV prevalence amongst children. Children were interviewed about their welfare, health, and healthcare using a structured questionnaire. Children under seven answered with assistance from their primary caregiver. Questions on HIV testing and knowledge of HIV status were addressed to the child's primary caregiver in the presence of the child if he or she was over the age of seven. Additionally, the questionnaire was administered by a nurse who had HIV Testing and Counselling certificates, which include training in how to respond if a child becomes distressed. More sensitive questions were asked only of older children and were answered without their caregiver being present: children aged 7–14 years were asked questions on sexual abuse and on psychological health. If a child reported abuse then the interviewer notified the supervising nurse who would subsequently investigate in the company of a social worker. The information from the supervisor and social worker was then fed back to the Child Protection committee in the study area. All maternal data (religion and HIV status) were collected in the general (adult) survey and linked to child data based on children reporting who their biological mother was, and confirmed through fertility histories and the household roster. In cases where a link could not be made, or if the child was a maternal orphan, maternal data was coded as missing. Dried blood spot samples were collected and tested for HIV in an offsite laboratory using the COMBAIDS-RS HIV 1+2 Immunodot Assay (Span Diagnostics, India); for cases in which the child tested HIV-positive but had an uninfected mother, the HIV test results were confirmed using Vironostika HIV Uni-form II Plus O (Biomérieux, France) ELISA tests. Data used in the manuscript are provided in the supporting information file Dataset S1.

Ethics Statement

Ethical approval for the Manicaland HIV/STD Prevention Project was obtained from the Research Council of Zimbabwe (Number 02187), the Biomedical Research and Training Institute Zimbabwe's institutional review board (Number AP6/97), and the Imperial College London Research Ethics Committee (Number ICREC 9_3_13). Written informed consent was obtained prior to survey participation from each child's primary caregiver. In addition, children aged 7–14 years provided verbal or written assent, respectively. Participants and guardians were informed that, at any point, they could refuse to answer a question or decline to continue the interview.

Data Analysis

In this analysis of children aged 2–14 years old, we tested for associations of HIV infection with socio-demographic characteristics (sex, age-group, household socio-economic status (SES), community type, and mother's religion) using logistic regression. Socio-economic status was measured using a summed asset-based wealth index developed for the study population in Manicaland [19]. The mother's self-reported religious affiliation was classified into "Christian", "Traditional", "Spiritual", "Other", or "none", as in previous analyses of Manicaland data [20].

To test the hypothesis that HIV infection in children occurs primarily through MTCT, where available, we examined maternal survival/infection status (deceased, alive and HIV-negative, alive and HIV-positive, alive with unknown HIV status) by child HIV status to establish the plausibility of vertical HIV transmission. The odds ratios of being a maternal orphan and of being a maternal orphan or having an HIV-positive mother amongst infected and uninfected children were evaluated using a one-sided Fisher's exact test. We tested for associations between HIV infection and risk factors for horizontal HIV transmission, which included blood transfusion, vaccination, non-vaccination medical injections, breastfed by a non-biological mother, cared for a sick relative, and sexual abuse.

To assess whether the observed age-pattern of HIV prevalence in children is consistent with that which would be expected in Zimbabwe if infections were due to mother-to-child transmission, we compared the age-specific HIV prevalence data to national estimates of child HIV prevalence reported by UNAIDS [1]. These estimates are derived using the Spectrum model [21–23], which assumes MTCT is the source of paediatric HIV and reflects the declining trends in HIV prevalence recorded in pregnant women, rates of mother-to-child transmission, patterns of paediatric survival by time of infection, national data on PMTCT and anti-retroviral therapy (ART) scale-up, and effectiveness of PMTCT regimens [4]. The Spectrum file that we used in this analysis can be downloaded from http://apps.unaids.org/spectrum/.

The impact of HIV on measures of physical and mental health was evaluated using linear (continuous outcomes) or logistic (binary outcomes) regression, adjusting for age. Z-scores for height- and weight-for-age and weight-for-height were calculated using WHO child growth standards [24,25]. Z-scores below -2 were considered to indicate stunting (low height-for-age), being underweight (low weight-for-age) and wasting (low weight-for-height). Comparisons were made for stunting and being underweight for all children, while wasting was only compared in children aged 2–5 years, as these were the ages for which reference data were available [24]. Psychological wellbeing scores were calculated in children aged 7–14 years using principal components analysis of psychological distress measures as described by

Nyamukapa *et al.*, 2010 [26]. All analyses were conducted in Stata version 12.1 (StataCorp LP, USA).

Results

Demographic Profile of Infected Children

Four thousand six hundred and eleven children aged 2–14 years were enumerated and selected for inclusion in the study, of which 3389 (73.5%) completed the survey and gave a dried blood spot for HIV testing. Children who did not complete the survey did not have significantly different age or gender distributions and their household of residence did not have significantly different mean SESs than those who completed the questionnaire (all $p>0.05$). Reasons given for non-response included: away from home for work (7.4%), away from home for school (7.0%), another reason for being away from home (67.1%), whereabouts unknown (1.1%), refused (12.3%), and other (5.0%). Seventy-three (2.2%, 95% CI: 1.7–2.6%) were HIV-positive. Prevalence was 1.6% (11/688), 2.5% (33/1296), and 1.8% (25/1405) among children aged 2–4 years, 5–9 years, and 10–14 years, respectively. Demographic characteristics of children aged 2–14 years by HIV status are presented in Table 1. HIV prevalence did not differ significantly ($p<0.05$) by sex, age-group, or any other demographic characteristics (household SES, community type, and maternal religion).

Sources of HIV Infection

All but one HIV-positive child were either maternal orphans or had an HIV-positive surviving mother, consistent with the primary source of childhood infection being MTCT (Table 2). HIV-positive children were significantly more likely to be a maternal orphan (OR: 6.56, 95% CI: 4.03–10.66) and/or have an HIV-positive mother (OR: 76.03, 95% CI: 18.54–311.79)) than HIV-negative children. The one child who was HIV-positive but for whom the woman identified as his biological mother was HIV-negative (Table 2) was a three year-old male reported to be living with both biological parents. He did not report any of the risk factors for non-sexual horizontal transmission (blood transfusions, non-medical injections, breastfeeding by a non-biological mother, caring for a sick relative, or child abuse). Overall, 26.9% (902/3360) of participants who answered the survey questions reported any of the selected risk factors for horizontal HIV transmission (Table 3), excluding vaccination-related injections, of which 99.7% (3364/3374) of children reported having had. Item non-response ranged from 0.1% (ever cared for a sick relative) to 27.1% (ever had a blood transfusion) and did not differ between HIV-negative and HIV-positive children (all $p>0.05$). HIV-positive children were significantly more likely to report non-vaccination injections than HIV-negative children (41.1% vs. 26.2%, $p=0.01$). Otherwise, no significant differences in reporting of risk factors (blood transfusions, breastfeeding by a non-biological mother, caring for a sick relative, child abuse or sexual activity) were found between HIV-positive and uninfected children.

Comparison of Observed Age-Specific HIV Prevalence with National Estimates from the Spectrum Model

HIV prevalence in children aged 2–14 observed in Manicaland was lower than the national estimates for Zimbabwe as a whole in 2010 from the Spectrum model (3.6%). However, the age-pattern of HIV prevalence amongst children observed in the data was consistent with the model estimates (Figure 1). This suggests that the age-patterns of HIV in Manicaland are in line with what would be expected if MTCT were the main source of child

Table 1. Association between demographic characteristics and HIV infection in children.

Category	Sub-category	HIV+	N in Sub-category	OR (95% CI)[†]	*p*-value[‡]
Gender	Male	2.34%	1712	Referent	0.21
	Female	1.73%	1677	0.75 (0.46–1.21)	
Age Group	2–4	1.60%	688	Referent	0.27
	5–9	2.54%	1296	1.61 (0.81–3.20)	
	10–14	1.78%	1405	1.11 (0.55–2.28)	
Household SES	Poorest quintile	1.75%	688	Referent	0.33
	Second quintile	2.38%	632	1.37 (0.64–2.95)	
	Middle quintile	0.70%	143	0.40 (0.05–3.07)	
	Fourth quintile	2.70%	1063	1.58 (0.80–3.13)	
	Least poor quintile	1.85%	863	1.06 (0.50–2.26)	
Community type	Subsistence farming	2.44%	1391	Referent	0.38
	Roadside trading	1.93%	671	0.79 (0.41–1.50)	
	Agricultural estate	1.36%	811	0.54 (0.27–1.08)	
	Commercial centre	2.13%	516	0.87 (0.44–1.73)	
Mother's religion[a]	Christian	1.44%	967	Referent	0.95
	Traditional	0%	13	N/A	
	Spiritual	1.53%	849	1.02 (0.48–2.19)	
	Other	1.69%	301	1.15 (0.41–3.21)	
	None	0%	67	N/A	

[†]Unadjusted odds ratio.
[‡]Fisher's exact test for difference of proportions.
[a]Total respondents (N = 2206) is lower than other categories due to maternal orphans (n = 348), unlinked records (n = 722) and question non-response (n = 113).

Table 2. Maternal mortality and HIV status in children.

	Child HIV status	
Maternal status	**HIV- (N = 3316)**	**HIV+ (N = 73)**
Mother deceased	318 (9.59%)	30 (41.09%)
Mother alive, HIV+	390 (11.76%)	31 (42.47%)
Mother alive, HIV-	1765 (53.23%)	1 (1.37%)
Mother alive, unknown HIV status	843 (25.42%)	11 (15.07%)

infections, accounting for the declining trend in adult HIV prevalence and the scale-up of PMTCT programmes in Zimbabwe.

HIV Status and Child Health

HIV-positive children were significantly more likely to be underweight (low weight-for-age) (AOR: 2.20; 95% CI: 1.08–4.47) and stunted (AOR: 1.69; 95% CI: 1.02–2.81) than HIV-negative children, but were not more likely to be wasted (low weight-for-height) (AOR: 0.43; 95% CI: 0.05–3.34) or to report a recent illness (AOR: 1.31; 95% CI: 0.64–2.66) (Table 4). HIV status was also not associated with psychological wellbeing (Coefficient: −0.06; 95% CI: −0.21 – +0.09) (Table 4).

Of the 73 HIV-positive children, 26.0% (19/73) reported that they knew their HIV status. Of the HIV-negative children, 114/3309 (3.5%) had had an HIV test, significantly less than reported testing prevalence in HIV-positive children ($p<0.001$). Children of mothers who reported that they knew they were HIV-positive were 5.17 times (95% CI: 2.27–11.76) more likely to have had an HIV test and know the result than children of mothers who self-reported as HIV-negative. Knowledge of HIV status was not associated with psychological wellbeing score for HIV-positive children (change in psychological wellbeing score: +0.01; 95% CI: −0.131 – +0.33). All but two of the children (17/19) who were aware of their HIV-positive status reported taking drugs that stop HIV from causing AIDS (*i.e.* were on anti-retroviral therapy (ART)). Despite high ART coverage when HIV status is known, overall, less than a quarter (23.3%, 17/73) of the HIV-positive children was receiving ART.

Discussion

This study describes the prevalence and consequences of HIV in children living in a rural area of southern Africa. In eastern Zimbabwe, from 2009–2011, 2.2% (95% CI: 1.7–2.6%) of children aged 2–14 years tested positive for HIV, at a time when HIV prevalence was 11% and 17%, respectively, amongst male and female adults (15–54 years) in the same population. This estimate, from a representative general-population sample, is lower than those from a sample of children in 2005 in Chimanimani district in southern Manicaland, where HIV prevalence was 3.2% (41/1290) in children aged 2–14 years [27]. Such a reduction between 2005 and 2010 is expected based on the decline in adult HIV prevalence and the increase in PMTCT coverage since 2005. A study conducted with 4,386 primary school children in Harare in 2010 found an HIV prevalence of 2.7% (95% CI: 2.2–3.1%) in children aged 6–13 years [28], which is close to the prevalence of 2.2% found in our study for a slightly different age-group in a different region. As was the case in the Chimanimani study [27] and in studies in similar age-groups elsewhere in SSA [29–31], including a large national population survey in South Africa conducted in 2008 [32], we

Table 3. Association between HIV status and potential horizontal risk factors for HIV.

Horizontal risk factors	**Exposure**	**N**	**HIV+%**	**AOR (95% CI)** †	***p*-value**‡
Ever had a blood transfusion	No	3,355	2.15%	Referent	0.14
	Yes	7	14.3%	6.51 (0.80–53.34)	
Lifetime number of non-vaccination injections	0	2491	1.73%	Referent	0.004
	>0	873	3.44%	2.19 (1.23–3.89)	
Received tuberculosis, polio, measles, and/or diphtheria vaccination	No	10	0%	Referent	0.81
	Yes	3364	2.11%	N/A	
Breastfed by non-biological mother	No	3359	2.14%	Referent	0.71
	Yes	16	0%	N/A	
Cared for a sick relative (ages 6–14)	No	2403	2.29%	Referent	0.45
	Yes	35	0%	N/A	
Ever been sexually abused (ages 7–14)	No	2180	2.25%	Referent	N/A
	Yes	4	0%	N/A	

†Adjusted odds ratio; adjusted for age, gender, SES, and site type.
‡Fisher's exact test for difference of proportions.
NB: Different Ns are due to different question non-response rates.

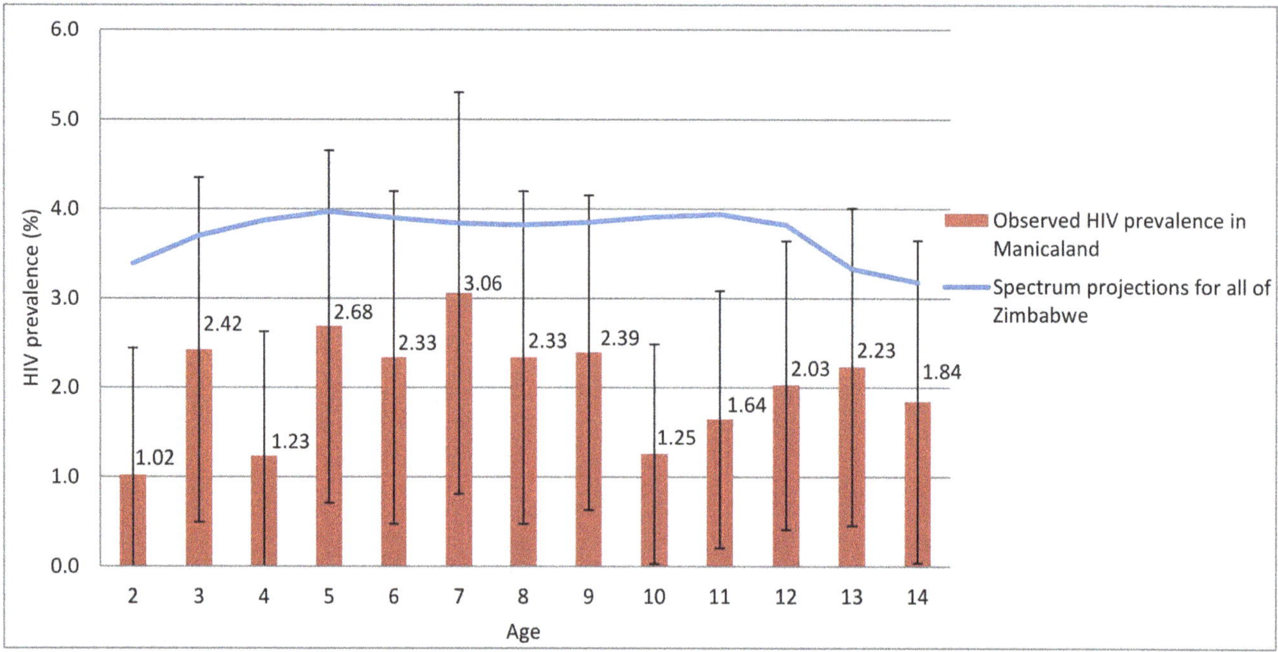

Figure 1. Comparison of observed HIV prevalence by age in Manicaland, with 95% confidence intervals, to the Zimbabwe national HIV estimates from UNAIDS and the Zimbabwe Ministry of Health and Child Welfare.

found no significant differences in HIV prevalence with respect to sex or age.

Our finding of a relatively even pattern of HIV prevalence by age is consistent with official national estimates derived from the Spectrum model. Survival data for children infected with HIV through MTCT suggest high mortality [7] and, in a stable epidemic with little horizontal transmission and no PMTCT intervention, HIV prevalence will decline as children age into adolescence. However, the decline in HIV prevalence in pregnant women since the late 1990s (from 25.7% in 2002 to 16.1% 2009 [33]) and the scale-up of PMTCT services from the mid-2000s explain reduced prevalence in younger children to the levels observed in the current study. The pattern of HIV prevalence we saw with age is also consistent with that reported by Eaton et al. in 15–17 year-olds in the same population at different time points (2009–2011 here and 2006–2008 in Eaton et al.) [12]. That is, it supports the hypothesis that MTCT is the main source of HIV infection in children and adolescents in this population.

Our data further confirm the belief that MTCT is the primary mode of HIV transmission in children in eastern Zimbabwe [12]. Mothers of HIV-infected children were significantly more likely than mothers of uninfected children to be deceased or HIV-positive. One child, for whom we could not identify a plausible source of infection, did not report any vertical, sexual, or other horizontal risk factors for transmission. Exposure to potential modes of transmission may have been under-reported and data were not collected on all possible sources of infection, such as scarification and hospital and dental visits, which have previously

Table 4. Effects of HIV status on physical and mental health outcomes in children and adolescents.

Health outcome	HIV status	N	%	AOR (95% CI)[†]	*p-value*
Ill in last two weeks	HIV−	3320	11.55%	Referent	0.11
	HIV+	69	19.61%	1.31 (0.64–2.66)	
Low height-for-age	HIV−	3222	30.60%	Referent	0.04
	HIV+	69	39.13%	1.69 (1.02–2.81)	
Low weight-for-age	HIV−	2225	9.97%	Referent	0.03
	HIV+	51	19.61%	2.20 (1.08–4.47)	
Low weight-for-height[‡]	HIV−	833	11.64%	Referent	0.42
	HIV+	16	6.25%	0.43 (0.05–3.34)	
Psychological wellbeing score[a]	HIV−	2385	0.01	Referent	0.45
	HIV+	55	−0.05	−0.06 (−0.21–+0.09)	

[†]Adjusted odds ratio; adjusted for age, gender, SES, and community type.
[‡]Children 2-5 only.
[a]Mean and change in score between HIV− and HIV+; ages 6-14 only.

been identified as sources of HIV in children [13–15]. Sexual abuse has also been identified as a potential mode of HIV acquisition in select cases in children [34–39], however, due to ethical reasons, little research has been conducted into the proportion of children infected with HIV through sexual abuse, even though sexual abuse has been reported to be common in South Africa [40,41]. While we cannot be certain about the accuracy of reporting about the child's biological mother, without biological tests, for which this study did not have consent, the identification of the biological mother was consistent with information reported on the household roster and the child was named on the mother's fertility history.

The need to understand HIV infection in children is particularly important given that HIV is increasingly becoming a cause of hospitalisation amongst adolescents in SSA [11] and this trend is likely to continue as more HIV-positive children age into adolescence. We found that HIV-positive children were significantly more likely to report non-vaccination medical injections than HIV-negative individuals, most likely because HIV-positive children are more likely to seek healthcare for managing their infection or to treat HIV-associated illnesses [11]. Thus, this association should therefore not be misconstrued as evidence for medical injections as a source of horizontal transmission, particularly as 27 of the 30 (90%) of the HIV-positive children who reported having had medical injections also reported being a maternal orphan or having a mother who was HIV-positive. Stunting and wasting in HIV-positive children, as well as being underweight, have been reported previously in SSA [11,42,43]. We found HIV-positive children to be significantly more likely to be underweight and stunted, indicative of the long-term harm of HIV infection on health and nutritional status. Perhaps unsurprisingly, we did not find a significant relationship with wasting, which measures recent severe weight loss, often associated with acute starvation and severe disease.

There are few data from SSA on the psychological manifestations of HIV infection in children, although studies from developed countries report significantly higher incidence of psychiatric admissions for HIV-positive children than HIV-negative children, with knowledge of HIV status increasing the risk of admission [44]. A previous study in Zimbabwe found that 56% of HIV-positive adolescents reported psychosocial problems, but that these problems were not common in younger children [45]. These data, however, were collected from children and adolescents visiting facilities offering HIV care services, and many respondents were already presenting with AIDS-related illnesses. Because the results were from a clinical study and were not compared to an HIV-negative population, it is not possible to conclude that there was a significant increase in psychosocial distress based on HIV status. Although we found no significant association between HIV status and psychological wellbeing, the lack of data from SSA in this area and the findings of Ferrand *et al.* (2010) [45] suggest that this is an important topic for future investigation.

Only a quarter of HIV-positive children in our study were aware of their HIV status. Across southern and eastern Africa, ART coverage among children is a major problem and high priority for many governments as it continues to lag behind adult coverage (33% versus 65% in the 22 priority countries, of which 21 are in Africa) [46]. So long as they remain undiagnosed, and therefore untreated, HIV-positive children are at higher risk for AIDS-related illnesses and early mortality. In the longer term, knowledge of HIV status is important to mitigate the risk of passing the infection on to sexual partners. Despite the low coverage of HIV testing, we found that if children or their guardians were aware of the child's HIV-positive status there was a 90% chance that the child would be on ART. This suggests that, despite the fear, potential stigma and associated costs, a positive diagnosis does result in the initiation of treatment. One way to help increase treatment amongst children might be to increase HIV-testing of women, as we found that when a mother knew herself to be HIV-positive, her child was significantly more likely to have had an HIV test themselves – suggesting that getting more mothers diagnosed through PMTCT programs will improve child testing. Other possible ways to increase infant diagnosis of HIV in this population are the new point-of-care tests currently being developed. New tests include a rapid p24 antigen test and a nucleic-acid amplification test, both of which can be performed in under half an hour [47]. Currently, many infants go undiagnosed due to the long turnaround times or poor infrastructure associated with dried blood spot sample testing [48]. Early infant HIV diagnosis is important, as the high ART coverage when children are aware of their status implies that lack of knowledge of HIV status is a contributing factor to the low coverage of ART in children that has been noted in Zimbabwe (39.5% according to the 2011 national estimates [49]) and more broadly in most of sub-Saharan Africa.

Conclusion

These findings provide evidence that MTCT is the principal source of HIV infection in children in southern Africa and that current initiatives to increase the availability and effectiveness of PMTCT should result in reductions in HIV prevalence in children over time. Effort should be made to encourage HIV testing in children because, despite low overall ART coverage, children who are aware of their HIV status were highly likely to be on treatment.

Acknowledgments

We thank Janet Dzangare and Elizabeth Gonese (Zimbabwe Ministry of Health and Child Welfare) and Mary Mahy (UNAIDS) for assistance with the Zimbabwe Spectrum file. We thank John Stover for advice regarding HIV prevalence estimates from the Spectrum software. We are grateful to all participants in the Manicaland HIV/STD Prevention Project.

Author Contributions

Conceived and designed the experiments: ELP CN JWE SM LR SG. Analyzed the data: ELP JWE. Wrote the paper: ELP CN JWE RM LR SG SM GC. Organised the data collection: CN RM GC SG.

References

1. UNAIDS (2013) Global report: UNAIDS report on the global AIDS epidemic 2013.
2. Zimbabwe National Statistics Agency (ZIMSTAT), ICF International. (2012) Zimbabwe demographic and health survey 2010–11.
3. UNAIDS (2012) Global AIDS response progress report 2012: Follow-up to the 2011 political declaration on HIV/AIDS: Intensifying our efforts to eliminate HIV/AIDS: Zimbabwe country report.
4. Rollins N, Mahy M, Becquet R, Kuhn L, Creek T, et al. (2012) Estimates of peripartum and postnatal mother-to-child transmission probabilities of HIV for

use in spectrum and other population-based models. Sex Transm Infect (Suppl 2): i44–i51.

5. Becquet R, Marston M, Dabis F, Moulton LH, Gray G, et al. (2012) Children who acquire HIV infection perinatally are at higher risk of early death than those acquiring infection through breastmilk: A meta-analysis. PLOS One 7(2): e28510.
6. Newell ML, Coovadia H, Cortina-Borja M, Rollins N, Gaillard P, et al. (2004) Mortality of infected and uninfected infants born to HIV-infected mothers in Africa: A pooled analysis. Lancet 364(9441): 1236–1243.
7. Ferrand RA, Corbett EL, Wood R, Hargrove J, Ndhlovu CE, et al. (2009) AIDS among older children and adolescents in southern Africa: Projecting the time course and magnitude of the epidemic. AIDS 23(15): 2039–2046.
8. Marston M, Zaba B, Salomon JA, Brahmbhatt H, Bagenda D (2005) Estimating the net effect of HIV on child mortality in African populations affected by generalized HIV epidemics. J Acquir Immune Defic Syndr 38(2): 219–227.
9. Ferrand RA, Luethy R, Bwakura F, Mujuru H, Miller RF, et al. (2007) HIV infection presenting in older children and adolescents: A case series from Harare, Zimbabwe. Clin Infect Dis 44(6): 874–878.
10. Ferrand RA, Munaiwa L, Matsekete J, Bandason T, Nathoo K, et al. (2010) Undiagnosed HIV infection among adolescents seeking primary health care in Zimbabwe. Clin Infect Dis 51(7): 844–851.
11. Ferrand RA, Bandason T, Musvaire P, Larke N, Nathoo K, et al. (2010) Causes of acute hospitalization in adolescence: Burden and spectrum of HIV-related morbidity in a country with an early-onset and severe HIV epidemic: A prospective survey. PLoS Med 7(2): e1000178.
12. Eaton J, Garnett GP, Takavarasha F, Mason P, Robertson L, et al. (2013) Increasing adolescent HIV prevalence in eastern zimbabwe - evidence of long-term survivors of mother-to-child transmission? PLoS One 8(8): e70447.
13. Okinyi M, Brewer DD, Potterat JJ (2009) Horizontally-acquired HIV infection in kenyan and swazi children. Int J STD AIDS 20(12): 852–857.
14. Gomo E, Chibatamoto PP, Chandiwana SK, Sabeta CT (1997) Risk factors for HIV infection in a rural cohort in Zimbabwe: A pilot study. Cent Afr J Med 43(12): 350–354.
15. Shisana O, Connolly C, Rehle TM, Mehtar S, Dana P (2008) HIV risk exposure among South African children in public health facilities. AIDS Care 20(7): 755–763.
16. Gregson S, Garnett GP, Nyamukapa CA, Hallett TB, Lewis JJ, et al. (2006) HIV decline associated with behaviour change in eastern Zimbabwe. Science 311(5761): 664–666.
17. Lopman B, Nyamukapa CA, Mushati P, Wambe M, Mupambireyi Z, et al. (2008) HIV incidence after 3 years follow-up in a cohort recruited between 1998 and 2000 in Manicaland, Zimbabwe: Contributions of proximate and underlying determinants to transmission. Int J Epidemiol 37(1): 88–105.
18. Gregson S, Nyamukapa C, Garnett GP, Mason PR, Zhuwau T, et al. (2002) Sexual mixing patterns and sex-differentials in teenage exposure to HIV infection in rural Zimbabwe. Lancet 359: 1896–1903.
19. Lopman B, Lewis JJ, Nyamukapa CA, Mushati P, Chandiwana SK, et al. (2007) HIV incidence and poverty in Manicaland, Zimbabwe. AIDS 21(Supplement 7): S57–S66.
20. Manzou R, Schumacher C, Gregson S (2014) Temporal dynamics of religion as a determinant of HIV infection in East Zimbabwe: A serial cross-sectional analysis. PLoS One 9(1): e86060.
21. Stover J (2009) AIM: A computer program for making HIV/AIDS projections and examining the demographic and social impacts of AIDS.
22. Stover J, Kirmeyer S (2009) DemProj: A computer program for making population projections.
23. Stover J, Brown T, Marston M (2012) Updates to the spectrum/estimation and projection package (EPP) model to estimate HIV trends for adults and children. Sex Transm Infect (Suppl 2): i11–i16.
24. WHO Multicentre Growth Reference Study Group (2006) WHO child growth standards: Length/height-for-age, weight-for-age, weight-for-length, weight-for-height and body mass index-for-age: Methods and development: 312.
25. de Onis M, Onyango AW, Borghi E, Siyam A, Nishida C, et al. (2007) Development of a WHO growth reference for school-aged children and adolescents. Bull World Health Organ 85(9): 660–667.
26. Nyamukapa CA, Gregson S, Wambe M, Mushore P, Lopman B, et al. (2010) Causes and consequences of psychological distress among orphans in eastern Zimbabwe. AIDS Care 22(8): 988–996.
27. Gomo E, Rusakaniko S, Mashange W, Mutsvangwa J, Chandiwana B, et al. (2006) Household survey of HIV-prevalence and behaviour in Chimanimani district, Zimbabwe, 2005.
28. Bandason T, Langhaug LF, Makamba M, Laver S, Hatzold K, et al. (2013) Burden of HIV among primary school children and feasibility of primary school-linked HIV testing in Harare, Zimbabwe: A mixed methods study. AIDS Care 25(12): 1520–1526.
29. [Anonymous] (2005) South African national HIV prevalence, HIV incidence, behaviour and communication survey, 2005.
30. Tsheko GN, Odirile LW, Segwabe M, Bainame K (2005) A census of orphans and vulnerable children in two villages in Botswana.
31. Munyati S, Rusakaniko S, Mupambireyi PF, Mahati ST, Chibatamoto PP, et al. (2006) A census of orphans and vulnerable children in two zimbabwean districts.
32. Shisana O, Rehle T, Simbayi LC, Zuma K, Jooste S, et al. (2009) South african national HIV prevalence, incidence, behaviour and communication survey 2008: A turning tide among teenagers?
33. Zimbabwe Ministry of Health and Child Welfare (2010) Antenatal clinic HIV surveillance report 2009.
34. Bechtel K (2010) Sexual abuse and sexually transmitted infections in children and adolescents. Curr Opin Pediatr 22(1): 94–99.
35. Girardet RG, Lahoti S, Howard LA, Fajman NN, Sawyer MK, et al. (2009) Epidemiology of sexually transmitted infections in suspected child victims of sexual assault. Pediatrics 124(1): 79–86.
36. Gellert GA, Durfee MJ, Berkowitz CD, Higgins KV, Tubiolo VC (1993) Situational and sociodemographic characteristics of children infected with human immunodeficiency virus from pediatric sexual abuse. Pediatrics 91(1): 39–44.
37. Hammerschlag MR (1998) Sexually transmitted diseases in sexually abused children: Medical and legal implications. Sex Transm Infect 74(3): 167.
38. Lindegren ML, Hanson IC, Hammett TA, Beil J, Fleming PL, et al. (1998) Sexual abuse of children: Intersection with the HIV epidemic. Pediatrics 102(4): E461–E4610.
39. Schaaf HS (2004) Human immunodeficiency virus infection and child sexual abuse. S Afr Med J 94(9): 782–785.
40. Jewkes R, Levin J, Mbananga N, Bradshaw D (2002) Rape of girls in South Africa. Lancet 359(9303): 319–320.
41. Meel BL (2003) A study on the prevalence of HIV-seropositivity among rape survivals in Transkei, South Africa. J Clin Forensic Med 10(2): 65–70.
42. Nalwoga A, Maher D, Todd J, Karabarinde A, Biraro S, et al. (2012) Nutritional status of children living in a community with high HIV prevalence in rural Uganda: A cross-sectional population-based survey. Trop Med Int Health 15(4): 414–422.
43. Chiabi A, Lebela J, Kobela M, Mbuagbaw L, Obama MT, et al. (2012) The frequency and magnitude of growth failure in a group of HIV-infected children in Cameroon. Pan Afr Med J 11: 15.
44. Gaughan DM, Hughes MD, Oleske JM, Malee K, Gore CA, et al. (2004) Psychiatric hospitalizations among children and youths with human immunodeficiency virus infection. Pediatrics 113(6): e544–e551.
45. Ferrand RA, Lowe S, Whande B, Munaiwa L, Langhaug L, et al. (2010) Survey of children accessing HIV services in a high prevalence setting: Time for adolescents to count? Bull World Health Organ 88(6): 428–434.
46. WHO UNICEF, UNAIDS (2013) Global update on HIV treatment 2013: Results, impact and opportunities.
47. Haleyur Giri Setty MK, Hewlett IK (2014) Point of care technologies for HIV. AIDS Res Treat 2014(497046).
48. Mori Y, Kitao M, Tomita N, Notomi T (2004) Real-time turbidimetry of LAMP reaction for quantifying template DNA. J Biochem Biophys Methods 59(2): 145–157.
49. Zimbabwe Ministry of Health and Child Welfare (2012) Zimbabwe national HIV and AIDS estimates 2011 (draft).

Induction with Lopinavir-Based Treatment Followed by Switch to Nevirapine-Based Regimen versus Non-Nucleoside Reverse Transcriptase Inhibitors-Based Treatment for First Line Antiretroviral Therapy in HIV Infected Children Three Years and Older

Gerardo Alvarez-Uria*, Raghavakalyan Pakam, Praveen Kumar Naik, Manoranjan Midde

Department of Infectious Diseases, Rural Development Trust Hospital, Bathalapalli, AP, India

Abstract

Background: The World Health Organization recommends non-nucleoside reverse transcriptase inhibitors (NNRTIs)-based antiretroviral therapy (ART) for children three years and older. In younger children, starting ART with lopinavir boosted with ritonavir (LPVr) results in lower risk of virological failure, but data in children three years and older are scarce, and long-term ART with LPVr is problematic in resource-poor settings.

Methodology: Retrospective cohort of children three years and older who started triple ART including LPVr or a NNRTI between 2007 and 2013 in a rural setting in India. Children who started LPVr were switched to nevirapine-based ART after virological suppression. We analysed two outcomes, virological suppression (HIV-RNA <400 copies/ml) within one year of ART using logistic regression, and time to virological failure (HIV-RNA >1000 copies/ml) after virological suppression using Cox proportional hazard regression. A sensitivity analysis was performed using inverse probability of treatment weighting (IPTW) based of propensity score methods.

Findings: Of 325 children having a viral load during the first year of ART, 74/83 (89.2%) in the LPVr group achieved virological suppression *versus* 185/242 (76.5%) in the NNRTI group. In a multivariable analysis, the use of LPVr-based ART was associated with higher probability of virological suppression (adjusted odds ratio 3.19, 95% confidence interval [CI] 1.11–9.13). After IPTW, the estimated risk difference was 12.2% (95% CI, 2.9–21.5). In a multivariable analysis including 292 children who had virological suppression and available viral loads after one year of ART, children switched from LPVr to nevirapine did not have significant higher risk of virological failure (adjusted hazard ratio 1.18, 95% CI 0.36–3.81).

Conclusions: In a cohort of HIV infected children three years and older in a resource-limited setting, an LPVr induction-nevirapine maintenance strategy resulted in more initial virological suppression and similar incidence of virological failure after initial virological suppression than NNRTI-based regimens.

Editor: Nicolas Sluis-Cremer, University of Pittsburgh, United States of America

Funding: The authors have no support or funding to report.

Competing Interests: The authors have declared that no competing interests exist.

* Email: gerardouria@gmail.com

Introduction

Due to higher viral loads, pharmacokinetic variability and suboptimal adherence because of complex regimens and frequent dosing adjustments, suppression of viral replication after initiation of antiretroviral therapy (ART) is more difficult to achieve in children than in adults [1]. Compared with non-nucleoside reverse transcriptase inhibitors (NNRTIs), protease inhibitors (PIs) have a higher genetic barrier [2]. Studies performed in adults in resource-limited settings show that boosted PI-based regimens result in less NRTI resistances [3,4]. In children <3 years, randomized control trials have demonstrated that the use of lopinavir boosted with ritonavir (LPVr) based regimens has lower risk of virological failure than ART containing nevirapine (NVP) [5,6]. In children >3 years, observational studies in resource-limited setting suggest that the use of PI-based ART is also associated with lower risk of virological failure, but data are scarce [7,8].

Once virological suppression is achieved, the risk of virological failure of ART with NNRTIs is considerably reduced [5,9]. In children taking PI-based regimens, switching to a NNRTI-based regimen after virological suppression can result in multiple benefits, such as alignment with adult ART, lower cost, better metabolic profile, simplification of ART with fixed-dose combinations, and preserving PIs for second line treatment [10]. In this study, we compared the virological response of children who received NNRTI-based ART with those treated with LPVr-based ART followed by switch to NVP-based treatment in an HIV cohort study in India.

Methods

This study was approved by the Ethical Committee of the Rural Development Trust (RDT) Hospital. Written informed consent was given by caretakers for their information to be stored in the study database and used for research.

Setting

The study was performed in Anantapur, a district situated in the South border of Andhra Pradesh, India. Anantapur has a population of approximately four million people, and 72% of them live in rural areas [11]. RDT is a non-governmental organization that provides medical care to HIV infected people free of charge, including medicines, consultations, and hospital admission charges. In our setting, the HIV epidemic is largely driven by heterosexual transmission and it is characterized by poor socio-economic conditions and high levels of illiteracy [12]. Although the vast majority of children acquire HIV perinatally, 8% of female children acquire HIV through sexual contacts and 90% of them are diagnosed after aged 18 months. Near half of children have lost one or both of their parents [12].

Study design and definitions of variables of interest

The Vicente Ferrer HIV Cohort Study (VFHCS) is an open cohort study of all HIV infected patients who have attended Bathalapalli RDT Hospital. The baseline characteristics of the cohort have been described in detail elsewhere [12,13]. The cohort is fairly representative of the HIV population in the district, as it covers approximately 70% of all HIV infected people registered in the district [14]. For this study, we selected HIV infected children aged 3 to 16 years who started first-line ART from January 1st 2007 to December 31st 2013 from the VFHCS database. The selection of patients from the database was executed on June 14th 2014 (end of the follow-up period).

ART was started by clinical criteria (clinical stage 3 or 4 of the World Health Organization [WHO]) or by immunological criteria (CD4 count <750 cells/µl or <20% in children aged 36–59 months, and CD4 count <350 cells/µl in children aged >59 months) according to the Indian National Guidelines [15]. Children started ART with two NRTIs and a NNRTI (NVP or efavirenz) or LPVr. Children who started LPVr were switched to a NVP-based regimen after achieving virological suppression. To facilitate dose calculations, we used weight band-based dosing of paediatric LPVr tablets (100 mg/25 mg) to achieve an approximate dose of 300 mg/m^2/dose (10–20 kg, 2-0-2; 20–30 kg, 3-0-3; >30 kg, 4-0-4) [16,17]. Paediatric LPVr tablets were substituted by larger adult tablets (200 mg/50 mg) if the child was able to swallow them (in these cases, the dosing in the 20–30 kg band was 2-0-1 adult tablets). Caretakers and children were instructed not to break LPVr tablets. We did not use liquid formulation of LPVr due to its poorer palatability, and cold-chain requirements. Other anti-retroviral drugs were given as per WHO and National guidelines [18].

Viral load was performed every six months after ART initiation. High viral load at baseline was defined as having >100,000 copies/ml of HIV-RNA [19]. Initial virological suppression was defined as having <400 copies/ml of HIV-RNA during the first year of ART. Following the WHO definition, virological failure was defined as having >1,000 copies/ml of HIV-RNA after six months of ART in two consecutive viral load determinations [20]. However, children having a single viral load >1,000 copies/ml only in the last viral load determination were considered to have virological failure.

Designation of the community of patients was performed by self-identification. Scheduled caste community is marginalised in the traditional Hindu caste hierarchy and, therefore, suffers social and economical exclusion and disadvantage [21]. Scheduled tribe community is generally geographically isolated with limited economical and social contact with the rest of the population [21]. Scheduled castes and scheduled tribes are considered socially disadvantaged communities and are supported by positive discrimination schemes operated by the Government of India [22].

Clinical staging was performed following WHO guidelines for HIV disease in children [20].

In HIV infected children <5 years, the CD4 lymphocyte percentage has generally been preferred for monitoring the immune status because of the variability of the CD4 cell count during the first years of life [18]. However, an analysis of the HIV Paediatric Prognostic Markers Collaborative Study (HPPMCS) demonstrated that the CD4 percentage provides little or no additional prognostic value compared with the CD4 cell count in children [23]. Therefore, the immune status of children was calculated using the 12-month risk of AIDS used by the HPPMCS, which uses the CD4 cell count and the age of children to calculate the level of immunodeficiency (i.e., high 12-month risk of AIDS indicates low CD4 cell counts for the age and *vice versa*) [24]. Because of the small number of older children included in the HPPMCS, children older than 12 years were considered to be 12 years old to calculate the 12-month AIDS risk [25].

Statistical analysis

To compare the effectiveness of NNRTI-based ART (NNRTI group) *versus* LPVr-based ART followed by switch to NVP-based ART after achieving virological suppression (LPVr induction-NVP maintenance group), we performed two analyses. For the first analysis, we studied the proportion of children who achieved virological suppression (HIV-RNA <400 copies/ml) during the first year of ART. Secondly, we performed a time-to-event analysis from ART initiation to virological failure among those children who achieved virological suppression and had available viral loads after one year of ART.

Continuous variables were compared using the rank sum test and categorical variables were compared using the χ^2 test. Univariate and multivariable analysis of factors associated with initial virological suppression were performed using logistic regression. Univariate and multivariable analysis of factors associated with time to virological failure after initial virological suppression were performed using Cox proportional hazard regression. To include all children in the multivariable models, missing values were imputed using multiple imputations by chained equation assuming missing at random [26].

In a sensitivity analysis to minimize the effect of confounding and obtain an unbiased estimate of the treatment effect, differences in baseline characteristics of the two groups were balanced using propensity score methods to estimate the average treatment effect. To include non-linear effects and interactions, propensity scores were estimated via boosted models using the "twang" package in the R statistical computing environment (R

Table 1. Characteristics of 325 HIV infected children initiating antiretroviral therapy in Anantapur, India.

	NNRTI group n = 242	LPVr group n = 83	P-value
Categorical variables	**N (%)**	**N (%)**	**χ^2**
Gender			0.346
Male	134 (55.4)	41 (49.4)	
Female	108 (44.6)	42 (50.6)	
Disadvantaged community			0.738
No	188 (77.7)	63 (75.9)	
Yes	54 (22.3)	20 (24.1)	
Living with parents			0.064
No	72 (29.8)	16 (19.3)	
Yes	170 (70.2)	67 (80.7)	
WHO clinical stage			0.012
1–2	152 (62.8)	39 (47)	
3–4	90 (37.2)	44 (53)	
Baseline viral load			0.973
<100,000 copies/ml	20 (45.5)	9 (45)	
>100,000 copies/ml	24 (54.5)	11 (55)	
Missing values (N)	198	63	
NRTIs			<0.001
d4T+3TC	148 (61.2)	29 (34.9)	
AZT+3TC	86 (35.5)	52 (62.7)	
ABC+3TC	8 (3.3)	2 (2.4)	
Liquid formulations			<0.001
No	181 (74.8)	79 (95.2)	
Yes	61 (25.2)	4 (4.8)	
Continuous variables	**Median (IQR)**	**Median (IQR)**	**Rank sum**
Age	7.8 (5.2–10.9)	8.9 (6.1–10.7)	0.173
12-month AIDS risk	3.7 (3.2–5.5)	3.6 (3.2–4.9)	0.481
Missing values (N)	4	0	

3TC, lamivudine; ABC, abacavir; AZT, zidovudine; IQR, interquartile range; LPVr, lopinavir boosted with ritonavir; NNRTI, non-nucleoside reverse transcriptase inhibitor; NRTI, nucleoside reverse transcriptase inhibitor.

Foundation for Statistical Computing, Vienna, Austria) [27]. To select the optimal interation of generalized boosted models, we set to minimize the means of the absolute standardized difference [28]. The propensity scores were used to estimate the inverse probability of treatment weights (IPTW) [28]. As two variables had missing values, multiple imputations were performed to obtain twenty complete datasets. IPTW were computed for each dataset and then, we calculated the average of the IPTWs [29]. These sampling weights were used to compare the initial virological suppression and the time to virological failure of the two groups using robust variance to account for the weighted nature of the sample [30].

Except for the estimation of propensity scores, the statistical analysis was performed using Stata Statistical Software (Stata Corporation. Release 12.1, College Station, Texas, USA).

Results

During the study period, 466 children started ART. 55 children were excluded because they died or were lost to follow up before having a viral load determination (10 in the LPVr induction-NVP maintenance group and 45 in the NNRTI group). Although previous exposure to NVP was not an exclusion criterion, none of the caretakers of children included in the study referred previous exposure to NVP.

Eighty-six children who had viral load determinations after one year of ART but not during the first year were not included in the first analysis. Therefore, 325 were included in the analysis of virological suppression during the first year of ART, 83 in the LPVr induction-NVP maintenance group and 242 in the NNRTI group (205 were on NVP and 37 were on efavirenz). In the LPVr induction-NVP maintenance group, the median duration of LPVr before switch to NVP was 213 days (interquartile range 180–250). Differences between the two groups are presented in **Table 1**. The proportion of children in WHO clinical stage 3 or 4 was higher in the LPVr induction-NVP maintenance group. Children in the NNRTI group used more commonly liquid formulation and stavudine in their ART regimens.

74/83 (89.2%) of children in the LPVr induction-NVP maintenance group achieved virological suppression during the first year of ART *versus* 185/242 (76.4%) in the NNRTI group (p = 0.013; unadjusted odds ratio [OR] 2.53, 95% confidence

Table 2. Factors associated with virological suppression (HIV-RNA <400 copies/ml) during the first year of antiretroviral therapy.

	OR (95% CI)	aOR (95% CI)[†]
Female gender	1.41 (0.81–2.45)	2.06* (1.08–3.91)
Age (years)	0.98 (0.91–1.06)	0.91 (0.81–1.02)
Disadvantaged community	0.67 (0.36–1.23)	0.44 (0.14–1.40)
Living with parents	1.34 (0.74–2.41)	1.16 (0.47–2.83)
WHO clinical stage 3–4	1.40 (0.80–2.46)	1.54 (0.75–3.17)
Baseline VL>100,0000 c/ml	0.39 (0.1–1.59)	0.24 (0.02–2.49)
NRTIs		
d4T+3TC	1 (reference)	1 (reference)
AZT+3TC	0.70 (0.41–1.21)	0.53 (0.27–1.03)
ABC+3TC	1.99 (0.24–16.24)	1.66 (0.17–16.08)
Use of liquid formulations	0.44* (0.24–0.81)	0.47 (0.21–1.05)
12-month AIDS risk (%)	1.00 (0.96–1.03)	1.01 (0.96–1.06)
LPVr vs. NNRTI	2.53* (1.19–5.38)	3.19* (1.11–9.13)

3TC, lamivudine; aOR, adjusted odds ratio; ABC, abacavir; AZT, zidovudine; CI, confidence interval; LPVr, lopinavir boosted with ritonavir; NNRTI, non-nucleoside reverse transcriptase inhibitor; NRTI, nucleoside reverse transcriptase inhibitor; VL, viral load.
*P-value<0.05;
[†]To include all patients in the multivariable model, missing values of baseline viral load and 12-month AIDS risk were imputed using chained equations (64 children had complete data available).

interval [CI] 1.19–5.38). Univariate and multivariable analysis of factors associated with initial virological suppression are presented in **Table 2**. In the univariate analysis, the use of liquid formulations in the ART regimen was associated with lower probability of virological suppression. In the multivariable analysis with multiple imputation of missing values of the baseline viral load and the 12-month AIDS risk, female gender was associated with virological suppression (adjusted odds ratio [aOR] 2.06, 95% CI 1.08–3.91). The use of LPVr *versus* NNRTI was associated with higher probability of virological suppression (aOR 3.19, 95% CI 1.11–9.13). In sensitivity analyses, removing high baseline viral load from the model and imputing only missing values of 12-month AIDS risk (aOR 2.42, 95% CI 1.08–5.42) or using only complete cases (aOR 2.49, 95% CI 1.11–5.58) showed similar results. In the IPTW model, the use of LPVr was also associated with higher probability of virological suppression (OR 2.41, 95% CI 1.1–5.4), and the estimated risk difference was 12.2% (95% CI, 2.9–21.5).

In the second analysis of time to virological failure, we included 292 children who achieved virological suppression and had viral load determination after one year of ART, 66 in the LPVr induction-NVP maintenance group and 226 in the NNRTI group (197 were on NVP and 29 were on efavirenz). Differences between the two groups were similar to the ones found in the analysis of initial virological suppression (**Table 3**). The Kaplan-Meier estimates of the incidence of virological failure showed no significant differences between the two groups (**Figure 1**). Univariate and multivariable analysis of factors associated with initial virological failure are presented in **Table 4**. In the multivariable analysis with multiple imputation of missing values of the baseline viral load and the 12-month AIDS risk, we did not find statistically significant differences in time to virological failure between the LPVr induction-NVP maintenance group and the NNRTI group (adjusted hazard ratio [aHR] 1.18, 95% CI 0.36–3.81). In sensitivity analyses, removing high baseline viral load from the model and imputing only missing values of 12-month AIDS risk (aHR 1.00, 95% CI 0.35–2.91) or using only complete cases (aHR 0.98, 95% CI 0.34–2.83) showed similar results. In the IPTW model, we also did not find statistically significant differences in time to virological failure between the LPVr induction-NVP maintenance group and the NNRTI group (HR 1.48, 95% CI 0.54–4.01; p-value = 0.443).

Among 71 children in the NNRTI group and 12 in the LPVr induction-NVP maintenance group who had virological failure, genotypic resistance testing was available in 44 children of the NNRTI group and in three of the LPVr induction-NVP maintenance group (**Table 5**). The median time to virological failure was 395 days (interquartile range [IQR] 279–731) in the NNRTI group and 245.5 days (IQR, 211.5–556) in the LPVr induction-NVP maintenance group. While in the LPVr induction-NVP maintenance group only one child had two-class resistance (NNRTI and NRTI), 36 (82%) children in the NNRTI group had two-class resistance.

Discussion

In this cohort study using routine clinical data of children three years and older from a resource-limited setting, the use of LPVr-based ART was associated with an increased probability of initial virological suppression and a subsequent switch from LPVr to NVP was not associated with a higher risk of virological failure compared with children starting NNRTI-based ART. The results of this study are in contrast with the 2013 guidelines of the WHO, which recommend NNRTI-based regimens for first line ART in children three years and older [20]. If our findings are confirmed in other settings, the results of this study could have important public health implications to help reduce virological failures among children starting ART in developing countries.

The higher proportion of children achieving initial virological suppression with LPVr induction therapy is in accordance with an international multisite clinical trial in children younger than three years [31]. In this clinical trial, children in the NVP group had higher risk of virological failure, and those who experienced

Table 3. Characteristics of 292 HIV infected children who achieved virological suppression (HIV-RNA <400 copies/ml) after antiretroviral therapy initiation in Anantapur, India.

	NNRTI group	NVP switch group	P-value
	n = 226	n = 66	
Categorical variables	N (%)	N (%)	χ^2
Gender			0.316
Male	122 (54)	31 (47)	
Female	104 (46)	35 (53)	
Disadvantaged community			0.717
No	176 (77.9)	50 (75.8)	
Yes	50 (22.1)	16 (24.2)	
Living with parents			0.036
No	75 (33.2)	13 (19.7)	
Yes	151 (66.8)	53 (80.3)	
WHO clinical stage			0.003
1–2	151 (66.8)	31 (47)	
3–4	75 (33.2)	35 (53)	
Baseline viral load			0.456
<100,000 copies/ml	22 (57.9)	8 (47.1)	
>100,000 copies/ml	16 (42.1)	9 (52.9)	
Missing values (N)	188	49	
NRTIs			<0.001
d4T+3TC	154 (68.1)	22 (33.3)	
AZT+3TC	71 (31.4)	43 (65.2)	
ABC+3TC	1 (0.4)	1 (1.5)	
Liquid formulations			0.017
No	185 (81.9)	62 (93.9)	
Yes	41 (18.1)	4 (6.1)	
Continuous variables	**Median (IQR)**	**Median (IQR)**	**Rank sum**
Age	7.9 (5.5–10.4)	8.3 (6.1–10.4)	0.595
12-month AIDS risk	3.8 (3.2–5.5)	3.6 (3.3–4.9)	0.453
Missing values (N)	8	0	

3TC, lamivudine; ABC, abacavir; AZT, zidovudine; IQR, interquartile range; NNRTI, non-nucleoside reverse transcriptase inhibitor; NRTI, nucleoside reverse transcriptase inhibitor, NVP, nevirapine.

virological failure had more drug resistances [31]. In our study, we observed fewer resistances in the LPVr induction-NVP maintenance group too, but the number of children with available drug resistance testing was small. While protease inhibitors have a relatively high barrier to the development of resistance, there are several single-gene mutations that lead to NNRTI resistance. NNRTI resistance occurs early after starting ART, when viral load and viral replication are high and, therefore, the chances of development of NNRTI mutations are also higher [32]. Once the viral load is low, the risk of developing NNRTI mutations is considerably reduced.

After virological suppression, the incidence of virological failure was similar in both groups, indicating that children switched from LPVr to NVP-based regimens did not have higher risk of virological failure than those children who started ART with NNRTI-based regimens and achieved virological suppression. However, in our study none of the children was exposed to NVP for prevention of vertical transmission, so switching from LPVr to NVP in previously exposed children may require more intense virological monitoring [33].

Viral load monitoring is not readily available in developing countries, so the implementation of this induction-maintenance strategy might be problematic where viral load is not available. However, the 2013 WHO guidelines, which recommend using viral load monitoring in HIV patients on ART, and the commercialization of new low-cost and simple viral load technologies might lead National HIV programmes in low- and middle-countries to scale-up viral load monitoring in the near future [20,34]. On the other hand, the majority of children in our study received six to nine months of LPVr-based ART before switch to NVP-based regimens, resulting in lower rates of virological failure and resistance. In setting where viral load is not available, induction therapy with LPVr-based ART during six or nine months followed by switch to NVP-based ART instead of ART initiation with NNRTI-based regimens could be beneficial, but new studies are needed to confirm this hypothesis.

Table 4. Factors associated with virological failure (HIV-RNA >1000 copies/ml) in children who achieved initial virological suppression.

	HR (95% CI)	aHR (95% CI)[†]
Female gender	1.00 (0.52–1.93)	1.19 (0.52–2.73)
Age (years)	1.10 (0.99–1.22)	1.07 (0.94–1.23)
Disadvantaged community	0.30* (0.09–0.97)	0.32 (0.09–1.12)
Living with parents	0.88 (0.44–1.76)	1.03 (0.44–2.42)
WHO clinical stage 3–4	1.36 (0.70–2.63)	1.77 (0.69–4.57)
Baseline VL>100,0000 c/ml	0.24 (0.01–5.74)	0.12 (0.00–7.88)
AZT+3TC vs. others	0.85 (0.42–1.73)	0.70 (0.30–1.68)
Use of liquid formulations	0.52 (0.18–1.48)	0.61 (0.19–1.90)
12-month AIDS risk (%)	1.02 (0.97–1.07)	1.06 (0.97–1.16)
NVP switch vs. NNRTI	0.96 (0.36–2.53)	1.18 (0.36–3.81)

3TC, lamivudine; aHR, adjusted hazard ratio; AZT, zidovudine; CI, confidence interval; NNRTI, non-nucleoside reverse transcriptase inhibitor; NRTI, nucleoside reverse transcriptase inhibitor; NVP, nevirapine; VL, viral load.
*P-value<0.05;
[†]To include all patients in the multivariable model, missing values of baseline viral load and 12-month AIDS risk were imputed using chained equations (55 children had complete data available).

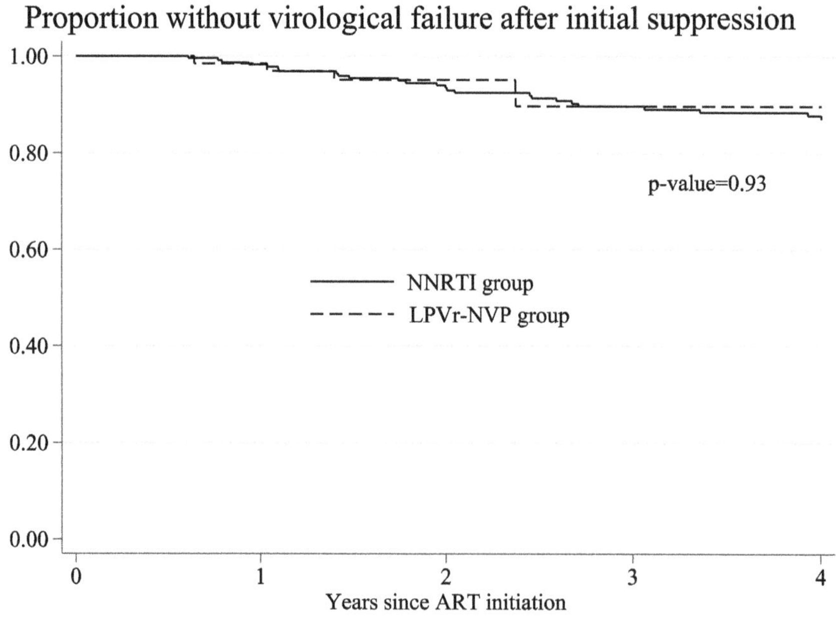

Figure 1. Proportion of children without virological failure after initial virological suppression over time. LPVr-NVP, ritonavir boosted lopinavir-based regimen followed by switch to nevirapine-based regimen; NNRTI, non-nucleoside reverse transcriptase inhibitor-based regimen.

Table 5. Drug resistance in children with virological failure.

ARV Resistances	NNRTI group (count)	LPVr-NVP group (count)
No resistance	0	1
NNRTI	8	0
3TC	0	1
NNRTI+3TC	18	1
NNRTI+3TC+other NRTIs	18	0

3TC, lamivudine (mutation M184V); ARV, antiretroviral; LPVr-NVP, ritonavir boosted lopinavir-based regimen followed by switch to nevirapine-based regimen; NNRTI, non-nucleoside reverse transcriptase inhibitor; NRTI, nucleoside reverse transcriptase inhibitor;

The study has some limitations. Our results reflect the "real life" of HIV infected children in a resource-limited setting. However, unlike clinical trials, observational studies can be biased due to unknown confounders. The selection of treatment was not randomized, so factors not included in the multivariable analyses might have influenced the outcomes of study. In addition, we did not have complete data for all cases; particularly many children had missing values of baseline HIV viral load. Nevertheless, we performed extensive sensitivity analyses, which showed similar results with different statistical methods. Our findings need to be confirmed by observational studies performed in other settings or, ideally, by a randomized clinical trial.

Conclusions

In a large cohort of HIV infected children three years and older from a resource-limited setting and without previous exposure to NVP, starting ART with LPVr-based regimens was associated with higher probability of virological suppression than starting with NNRTI-based regimens. Once virological suppression was achieved, children switched from LPVr to NVP-based treatment did not have a higher risk of virological failure than children who started NNRTI-based ART and achieved virological suppression. If these results are confirmed in other settings, this LPVr induction- NVP maintenance strategy could help reduce virological failures among HIV infected children three years and older starting ART.

Author Contributions

Conceived and designed the experiments: GAU. Analyzed the data: GAU. Contributed reagents/materials/analysis tools: GAU RP MM PKN. Contributed to the writing of the manuscript: GAU RP MM PKN.

References

1. Kamya MR, Mayanja-Kizza H, Kambugu A, Bakeera-Kitaka S, Semitala F, et al. (2007) Predictors of long-term viral failure among ugandan children and adults treated with antiretroviral therapy. J Acquir Immune Defic Syndr 46: 187–193. doi:10.1097/QAI.0b013e31814278c0.
2. Sigaloff KCE, Calis JCJ, Geelen SP, van Vugt M, de Wit TFR (2011) HIV-1-resistance-associated mutations after failure of first-line antiretroviral treatment among children in resource-poor regions: a systematic review. Lancet Infect Dis 11: 769–779. doi:10.1016/S1473-3099(11)70141-4.
3. Dlamini JN, Hu Z, Ledwaba J, Morris L, Maldarelli FM, et al. (2011) Genotypic resistance at viral rebound among patients who received lopinavir/ritonavir-based or efavirenz-based first antiretroviral therapy in South Africa. J Acquir Immune Defic Syndr 58: 304–308. doi:10.1097/QAI.0b013e3182278c29.
4. Lockman S, Hughes M, Sawe F, Zheng Y, McIntyre J, et al. (2012) Nevirapine-versus lopinavir/ritonavir-based initial therapy for HIV-1 infection among women in Africa: a randomized trial. PLoS Med 9: e1001236. doi:10.1371/journal.pmed.1001236.
5. Violari A, Lindsey JC, Hughes MD, Mujuru HA, Barlow-Mosha L, et al. (2012) Nevirapine versus ritonavir-boosted lopinavir for HIV-infected children. N Engl J Med 366: 2380–2389. doi:10.1056/NEJMoa1113249.
6. Palumbo P, Lindsey JC, Hughes MD, Cotton MF, Bobat R, et al. (2010) Antiretroviral treatment for children with peripartum nevirapine exposure. N Engl J Med 363: 1510–1520. doi:10.1056/NEJMoa1000931.
7. Jaspan HB, Berrisford AE, Boulle AM (2008) Two-year outcomes of children on non-nucleoside reverse transcriptase inhibitor and protease inhibitor regimens in a South African pediatric antiretroviral program. Pediatr Infect Dis J 27: 993–998. doi:10.1097/INF.0b013e31817acf7b.
8. Estripeaut D, Mosser J, Doherty M, Acosta W, Shah H, et al. (2013) Mortality and long-term virologic outcomes in children and infants treated with lopinavir/ritonavir. Pediatr Infect Dis J 32: e466–472. doi:10.1097/INF.0b013e3182a09276.
9. Alvarez-Uria G, Naik PK, Pakam R, Midde M (2012) Early HIV viral load determination after initiating first-line antiretroviral therapy for indentifying patients with high risk of developing virological failure: data from a cohort study in a resource-limited setting. Trop Med Int Health 17: 1152–1155. Available: http://www.ncbi.nlm.nih.gov/pubmed/22487689. Accessed 2012 Sep 7.
10. Arpadi S, Shiau S, Strehlau R, Martens L, Patel F, et al. (2013) Metabolic abnormalities and body composition of HIV-infected children on Lopinavir or Nevirapine-based antiretroviral therapy. Arch Dis Child 98: 258–264. doi:10.1136/archdischild-2012-302633.
11. Office of The Registrar General & Census Commissioner, India (2011) Census of India.
12. Alvarez-Uria G, Midde M, Pakam R, Naik PK (2012) Gender differences, routes of transmission, socio-demographic characteristics and prevalence of HIV related infections of adults and children in an HIV cohort from a rural district of India. Infect Dis Rep 4: e19. doi:10.4081/idr.2012.e19.
13. Alvarez-Uria G, Midde M, Pakam R, Kannan S, Bachu L, et al. (2012) Factors Associated with Late Presentation of HIV and Estimation of Antiretroviral Treatment Need according to CD4 Lymphocyte Count in a Resource-Limited Setting: Data from an HIV Cohort Study in India. Interdiscip Perspect Infect Dis 2012: 293795. doi:10.1155/2012/293795.
14. Alvarez-Uria G, Midde M, Pakam R, Bachu L, Naik PK (2012) Effect of Formula Feeding and Breastfeeding on Child Growth, Infant Mortality, and HIV Transmission in Children Born to HIV-Infected Pregnant Women Who Received Triple Antiretroviral Therapy in a Resource-Limited Setting: Data from an HIV Cohort Study in India. ISRN Pediatr 2012: 763591. doi:10.5402/2012/763591.
15. National AIDS Control Organisation (2006) Guidelines for HIV Care and Treatment in Infants and Children. Available: http://www.nacoonline.org/NACO/About_NACO/Policy__Guidelines/Policies__Guidelines1/. Accessed 2013 Jul 31.
16. Sáez-Llorens X, Violari A, Deetz CO, Rode RA, Gomez P, et al. (2003) Forty-eight-week evaluation of lopinavir/ritonavir, a new protease inhibitor, in human immunodeficiency virus-infected children. Pediatr Infect Dis J 22: 216–224. doi:10.1097/01.inf.0000055061.97567.34.
17. Ramos J (2009) Boosted protease inhibitors as a therapeutic option in the treatment of HIV-infected children. HIV Med 10: 536–547. doi:10.1111/j.1468-1293.2009.00728.x.
18. World Health Organization (2010) Antiretroviral therapy for HIV infection in infants and children: Towards universal access. Available: http://www.who.int/hiv/pub/paediatric/infants2010/en/index.html. Accessed 2011 Feb 10.
19. PENTA Steering Committee, Welch S, Sharland M, Lyall EGH, Tudor-Williams G, et al. (2009) PENTA 2009 guidelines for the use of antiretroviral therapy in paediatric HIV-1 infection. HIV Med 10: 591–613. doi:10.1111/j.1468-1293.2009.00759.x.
20. World Health Organization (2013) Consolidated guidelines on the use of antiretroviral drugs for treating and preventing HIV infection. Available: http://www.who.int/hiv/pub/guidelines/arv2013/en/index.html. Accessed 2013 Jul 20.
21. Gang IN, Sen K, Yun MS (2002) Caste, Ethnicity, and Poverty in Rural India. IZA.
22. Alvarez-Uria G, Midde M, Naik PK (2012) Socio-demographic risk factors associated with HIV infection in patients seeking medical advice in a rural hospital of India. J Public health Res 1: e14. doi:10.4081/jphr.2012.e14.
23. HIV Paediatric Prognostic Markers Collaborative Study, Boyd K, Dunn DT, Castro H, Gibb DM, et al. (2010) Discordance between CD4 cell count and CD4 cell percentage: implications for when to start antiretroviral therapy in HIV-1 infected children. AIDS 24: 1213–1217. doi:10.1097/QAD.0b013e3283389f41.
24. HIV Paediatric Prognostic Markers Collaborative Study (2006) Predictive value of absolute CD4 cell count for disease progression in untreated HIV-1-infected children. AIDS 20: 1289–1294. doi:10.1097/01.aids.0000232237.20792.68.
25. www.hppmcs.org (n.d.). Available: http://www.hppmcs.org/. Accessed 2013 Aug 11.
26. Royston P (2009) Multiple imputation of missing values: Further update of ice, with an emphasis on categorical variables. Stata Journal 9: 466–477.
27. Ridgeway G, McCaffrey D, Morral A, Burgette L, Griffin BA (2013) Toolkit for Weighting and Analysis of Nonequivalent Groups: A tutorial for the twang package. R vignette RAND.
28. McCaffrey DF, Griffin BA, Almirall D, Slaughter ME, Ramchand R, et al. (2013) A tutorial on propensity score estimation for multiple treatments using generalized boosted models. Stat Med 32: 3388–3414. doi:10.1002/sim.5753.
29. Hill J (2004) Reducing bias in treatment effect estimation in observational studies suffering from missing data. Available: http://academiccommons.columbia.edu/catalog/ac:129151. Accessed 2 July 2014.
30. Austin PC (2013) A tutorial on the use of propensity score methods with survival or time-to-event outcomes: reporting measures of effect similar to those used in randomized experiments. Stat Med. doi:10.1002/sim.5984.
31. Violari A, Lindsey JC, Hughes MD, Mujuru HA, Barlow-Mosha L, et al. (2012) Nevirapine versus ritonavir-boosted lopinavir for HIV-infected children. N Engl J Med 366: 2380–2389. doi:10.1056/NEJMoa1113249.
32. PENPACT-1 (PENTA 9/PACTG 390) Study Team, Babiker A, Castro nee Green H, Compagnucci A, Fiscus S, et al. (2011) First-line antiretroviral therapy with a protease inhibitor versus non-nucleoside reverse transcriptase inhibitor

and switch at higher versus low viral load in HIV-infected children: an open-label, randomised phase 2/3 trial. Lancet Infect Dis 11: 273–283. doi:10.1016/S1473-3099(10)70313-3.

33. Kuhn L, Coovadia A, Strehlau R, Martens L, Hu C-C, et al. (2012) Switching children previously exposed to nevirapine to nevirapine-based treatment after initial suppression with a protease-inhibitor-based regimen: long-term follow-up of a randomised, open-label trial. Lancet Infect Dis 12: 521–530. doi:10.1016/S1473-3099(12)70051-8.

34. UNITAID (n.d.) HIV/AIDS Diagnostics Technology Landscape 4th Edition. Available: http://www.unitaid.eu/images/marketdynamics/publications/UNITAID-HIV_Diagnostic_Landscape-4th_edition.pdf.

Rhinovirus-16 Induced Release of IP-10 and IL-8 Is Augmented by Th2 Cytokines in a Pediatric Bronchial Epithelial Cell Model

Julie A. Cakebread[1*¤], **Hans Michael Haitchi**[1], **Yunhe Xu**[1], **Stephen T. Holgate**[1,2], **Graham Roberts**[1,2], **Donna E. Davies**[1,2]

1 Academic Unit of Clinical and Experimental Sciences, University of Southampton Faculty of Medicine, University Hospital Southampton, Southampton, United Kingdom, 2 NIHR Respiratory Biomedical Research Unit, University Hospital Southampton, Southampton, United Kingdom

Abstract

Background: In response to viral infection, bronchial epithelial cells increase inflammatory cytokine release to activate the immune response and curtail viral replication. In atopic asthma, enhanced expression of Th2 cytokines is observed and we postulated that Th2 cytokines may augment the effects of rhinovirus-induced inflammation.

Methods: Primary bronchial epithelial cell cultures from pediatric subjects were treated with Th2 cytokines for 24 h before infection with RV16. Release of IL-8, IP-10 and GM-CSF was measured by ELISA. Infection was quantified using RTqPCR and $TCID_{50}$. Phosphatidyl inositol 3-kinase (PI3K) and P38 mitogen activated protein kinase (MAPK) inhibitors and dexamethasone were used to investigate differences in signaling pathways.

Results: The presence of Th2 cytokines did not affect RV replication or viral titre, yet there was a synergistic increase in IP-10 release from virally infected cells in the presence of Th2 cytokines. Release of IL-8 and GM-CSF was also augmented. IP-10 release was blocked by a PI3K inhibitor and IL-8 by dexamethasone.

Conclusion: Th2 cytokines increase release of inflammatory cytokines in the presence of rhinovirus infection. This increase is independent of effects of virus replication. Inhibition of the PI3K pathway inhibits IP-10 expression.

Editor: Stephania Ann Cormier, University ofTennessee Health Science Center, United States of America

Funding: This work was funded by Asthma UK, (http://www.asthma.org.uk/) a Medical Research Council (UK) grant (G0501506)(http://www.mrc.ac.uk/index.htm) and the Asthma, Allergy & Inflammation Research Charity (http://www.aaircharity.org/). The funders had no role in study design, data collection and analysis, decision to publish or preparation of the manuscript.

Competing Interests: STH and DED are founders and shareholders of Synairgen, a University spin-out company that is developing inhaled interferon beta for treatment of virus-induced exacerbations of asthma and COPD. STH and DED are also consultants to Synairgen. The other authors have no conflicts to declare.

* E-mail: Julie.Cakebread@agresearch.co.nz

¤ Current address: Ruakura Research Centre, Hamilton, New Zealand

Introduction

Asthma is a complex respiratory disease characterized by variable airflow obstruction, bronchial hyper-responsiveness and airway inflammation. In atopic asthma, the Th2 type cytokines interleukin (IL)-13 and IL-4 [1] are key players in allergic responses, playing a pivotal role in inflammatory and remodelling aspects of asthma pathogenesis [2,3]. Th2 cytokines can impair immune responses to viral infections. It has been shown that adults with a 'less atopic phenotype' have a greater ability to clear human rhinovirus (RV) compared to atopic adults [4,5].

Although atopic asthma is the more dominant form of asthma during school years and into young adulthood [6–8], exacerbation of asthma has been strongly linked to respiratory infection alone, with 44% to 80% of childhood asthma exacerbations being triggered by RV infection [9]. RV is the most common pathogen associated with asthma exacerbations in children [10]. Furthermore, a combination of sensitization, high exposure to one or more allergens, *and* viral detection significantly increases the risk of hospitalization for asthma [11,12].

The mechanisms behind the association of atopy and virus co-morbidity are as yet, unclear. Some studies have provided evidence that Th2 cytokines and viral pathogen associated molecular patterns (PAMPs) trigger release of the Th2 polarizing cytokine thymic stromal lymphopoietin [13], whilst other studies have shown that the epithelial effects of Th2-associated cytokines, such as IL13 and IL4, are dominant over the effects of the Th1-associated cytokines such as interferon-gamma [14]. Like allergen and RV, IL-13 and IL-4 have been shown to enhance expression of ICAM-1 [14,15], the cellular receptor for major group RVs. Th2 cytokines have the potential to facilitate entry of major group RV into airway cells of atopic subjects and to favour migration and activation of immune effector cells into the airway. This study uses epithelial monolayer cultures from a non asthmatic pediatric population to investigate whether the presence of Th2 cytokines modulates virus-induced inflammation; we also examine the ability of signaling pathway inhibitors to suppress these responses.

Methods

Ethics statement

Ethical approval was given by the Southampton and South West Hampshire Research Ethics Committee (07/Q1704/21). Parents of participants provided written informed consent. Procedures, including consent, was approved by the ethics committee.

Primary Cell culture

Bronchial brushings were obtained by fibreoptic bronchoscopy from pediatric subjects, not diagnosed with asthma, following current guidelines [16]. Subjects were recruited when attending hospital for clinically indicated bronchoscopy or other planned surgical procedure under a general anaesthetic. The subject group comprised 8 males (mean age 7.3 years; range 2–15 years), and 7 females (mean age 8.4 years; range 1–15 years). Details of patient phenotypes are in table 1. Brushings were processed for primary bronchial epithelial cell (pBEC) culture in Bronchial Epithelial Growth Medium (BEGM) (Lonza, Wokingham, United Kingdom,) as previously described [17]. Pediatric pBECs (ppBECs) were plated onto collagen coated (30 µg/ml PureCol, Inamed Biomaterials, Fremont, USA) 12-well plates (Nunc, Fisher Scientific, Loughborough, United Kingdom), at passage 2. For experiments minimal medium, BEBM, was used.

Virus culture

RV16 (a gift from Professor Sebastian L. Johnston, Imperial College, London) was amplified as previously described [18]. Virus strain was confirmed by qPCR (Primer Design, Southampton, UK) and infectivity determined with HeLa titration assay and 50% tissue culture infective dose ($TCID_{50}$)/ml.: Ultra violet treated virus controls (UV) were obtained by irradiating live virus stocks (1200 mJ/cm2 on ice for 50 min). Inactivation of virus was confirmed by $TCID_{50}$.

Infection of cells with RV

pBECs were infected with RV16 (Dose: 1×10^{6} $TCID_{50}$ units/10^{6} cells) for 1 hour at room temperature. Cells were washed to remove residual viral particles and the cultures replenished with BEBM. Different multiplicities of infection (MOIs) were not tested due to limitations in sample availability. Based on previous experience we chose a moderate dose of virus for infection. RV16 was chosen since it has minimal cytotoxic effects, as seen in figure S1.

Cytokine treatments

Cultures were pretreated with 10 ng/ml [19] of IL-13, IL-4 or both, for 24 h prior to infection. Cytokines were replenished with BEBM after washing, post-infection.

Controls of UV irradiated RV16, medium alone and Th2 only controls were included in all experiments.

Inhibitor treatments

Inhibitors were added to cultures 30 minutes before infection with RV16 and were refreshed after infection. Inhibitors of PI3K (LY294002, Calbiochem, Merck Millipore, UK) and p38 (SB03580, Sigma-Aldrich, Dorset, UK) were used at 10 µM, and dexamethasone (Sigma-Aldrich, Dorset, UK) at 1 µM. Vehicle control (DMSO) was used in all experiments.

Extraction of total RNA and mRNA quantification

Cells were harvested into TRIzol reagent (Invitrogen,UK) and total RNA was isolated using standard protocols. RNA (1 µg) was reverse-transcribed using Precision reverse transcription kit (Primer Design, Southampton, UK) according to the manufacturer's instructions. cDNA was amplified by PCR using Perfect Probe or Double Dye assays (Primer Design, Southampton, UK). Expression levels of cytokines were calculated relative to

Table 1. Summary of clinical and physiological characteristics of subjects studied.

Subject	Age (yrs)	Gender	Indication/operation
1	1	F	Bronchoscopy - recurrent chest symptoms & intermittent stridor
2	11	M	Bronchoscopy - recurrent severe croup
3	3	M	Bronchoscopy - recurrent croup and stridor
4	5	M	Bronchsocopy- recurrent cough, prematurity, tracheomalacia
5	3	M	Bronchoscopy - tracheomalacia
6	1	F	Bronchoscopy - recurrent chronic cough
7	2	M	Bronchoscopy - tracheomalacia
8	6	M	Adenoidectomy and tonsillectomy, gromit insertion
9	14	M	Surgery for nasal septum deviation
10	10	F	Dental procedure
11	12	F	Dental procedure
12	15	F	Dental procedure
13	7	F	Dental procedure
14	13	F	Dental procedure
15	15	M	Dental procedure

Subjects were recruited when attending hospital for clinically indicated bronchoscopy or other planned surgical procedure under a general anaesthetic. Bronchial brushings were obtained by fibreoptic bronchoscopy from pediatric subjects not diagnosed with asthma following current guidelines [16]. Mean age (years) 7.9 (range 1–15), M = 8 F = 7.

housekeeping genes GAPDH and UBC using the ΔΔCT method. Viral RNA was quantified using a reference standard (Primer Design, Southampton, UK).

Cytokine analysis

Protein secretion of IL-8, Interferon gamma-induced protein (IP-10), and Granulocyte macrophage colony-stimulating factor (GM-CSF) into cell-conditioned media was measured by ELISA (R&D, Abingdon, United Kingdom), following the manufacturer's instructions.

Statistical analysis

Normality of distribution was assessed using the Shapiro Wilk test (Sigmaplot) and parametric (ANOVA) or non parametric (Friedman repeated measures ANOVA on Ranks) tests undertaken for within group comparisons, as appropriate to detect any overall changes with different treatments. Where significant differences were identified, pairwise tests (paired T-test (T-test) or Wilcoxon signed rank test (Wilcoxon) respectively were used to investigate between-treatment differences. To assess to possibility of synergistic effects, the sum of cytokine release of single treatments (Th2 and virus) and cytokine release observed in combined treatment was compared using the same methodological approaches. $P<0.05$ was considered statistically significant. Whiskers on boxplots represent 5th-95th centile.

Results

Th2 cytokines enhance RV16-induced IP-10 release

Upregulation of IL-8 expression by IL-13 (10 ng/ml) and IL-4 (10 ng/ml) treatment was confirmed by ELISA. Initial experiments showed cultures treated with IL-4, IL-13 or both cytokines released significantly higher amounts of IL-8 than no treatment (NT) controls ($p<0.001$, Figure 1A, $n=9$) but there was no difference between treatments. This demonstrates that the cells, originating from subjects without asthma, are responsive to Th2 cytokines. The combination of IL-13 and IL-4 induced expression of IL-8 (Figure 1B, $p<0.05$, $n=15$) but not IP-10.

We next assessed the effect of Th2 cytokines on RV16-induced inflammatory responses. pBECs were treated with Th2 cytokines, or not, for 24 hours before infecting with RV16 (1×10^6 $TCID_{50}$ units/10^6 cells (MOI 1). Both IL-8 ($p<0.01$) and IP-10 $p<0.01$) release were significantly stimulated by RV16 infection alone (Figure 2A and 2B respectively). No induction of IL-8 or IP-10 was observed with UV irradiated virus (UV), suggesting cytokine induction to be a result of viral replication. The secretion of IL-8 and IP-10 protein was augmented in cultures pretreated with Th2 cytokines (Figure 2A: IL-8, $p<0.05$, 2B: IP-10, $p<0.01$). The increase in virus-induced IP-10 expression was synergistic in the presence of Th2 cytokines compared to the sum of the values of single challenges ($p<0.01$), whilst the increase in IL-8 was additive. We also investigated GM-CSF because of its involvement with dendritic cell recruitment and maturation, linking innate and adaptive immune responses. We saw no significant increase in protein release in response to Th2 cytokines alone but up-regulation of GM-CSF ($p<0.05$) was observed in response to virus infection. The presence of RV16 and Th2 cytokines resulted in an additive effect on GM-CSF release ($p<0.01$) compared to virus alone (Figure 2C).

Viral replication is not moderated by Th2 cytokines

We hypothesised that the presence of Th2 cytokines favoured viral replication, causing the observed increase in IL-8, IP-10 and GM-CSF release. However, we did not see any differences in viral

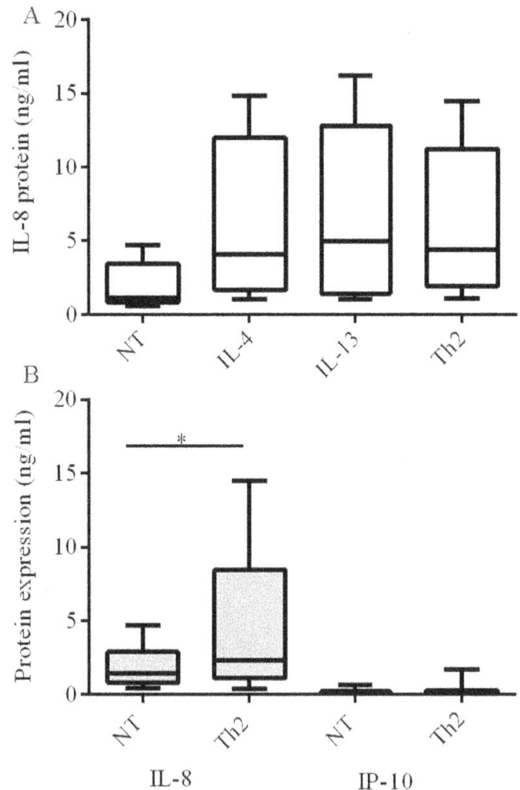

Figure 1. Induction of IL-8 but not IP-10 in response to Th2 stimulation. ppBECs were treated for 24 hours with IL-13 (10 ng/ml) and IL-4 (10 ng/ml) for 24 hours. Protein secretion in cell supernatant was measured by ELISA (R&D). Statistical analysis 1A $n=9$ ANOVA $P<0.05$. 1B $n=15$, Wilcoxon, $p<0.05$. NT-no treatment.

copy number when cells were infected in the absence or presence of the Th2 cytokines (Figure 3) (RV16 copy number (median (range) = 2.0×10^4 (2.2×10^2–1.4×10^5) *versus* 1.4×10^4 (3.0×10^2–1.4×10^5) $n=15$, respectively). Viral titre (virus released into the supernatant) was measured using $TCID_{50}$ and again we could detect no difference between cells pretreated in the absence or presence of Th2 cytokines (RV16 titre (median (range)) = 2.8×10^5 (2.8×10^4–1.5×10^6) *versus* 5×10^5 (1.5×10^4–8.9×10^6) $n=15$, respectively). Absence of replicating virus in the UV controls was confirmed using the same methods.

Major group RVs such as RV16 are reported to have less cytotoxicity than minor group virus [20] and in keeping with this we did not see cytopathic effects in our cultures at 24 hours (Figure S1). We measured Lactate Dehydrogenase (LDH), an enzyme found in the cytosol of cells and released into supernatant upon cell damage or lysis. We did not detect a difference in LDH levels between cells infected with virus in the presence of Th2 cytokine compared to virus alone (data not shown).

We also examined expression of ICAM-1, the cellular receptor for RV16. There was no detectable change in expression following 24hr Th2-cytokine treatment. (Figure S2). Together these data are consistent with the view that the observed increases in cytokine expression in the presence of Th2 cytokines is not a consequence of increased entry of virus, or increased viral replication.

Inhibition of inflammatory pathways

The combined effects of Th2 cytokines and RV16 infection produced different effects depending on the response being

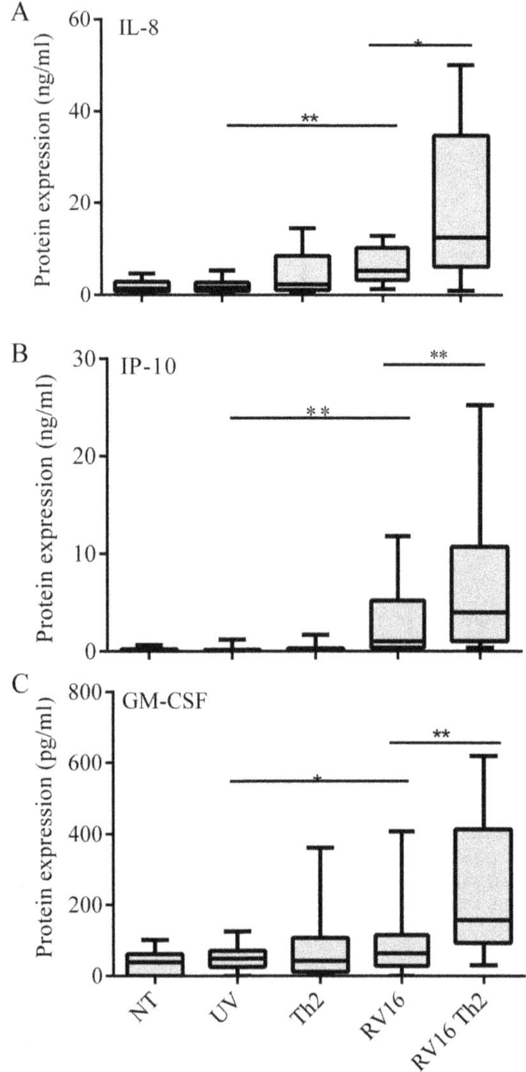

Figure 2. Synergistic increase in virus-induced IP-10 release in the presence of Th2 cytokines. ppBECs were pretreated with IL-13 + IL-4 or not for 24 hours prior to infection with RV16 at 1×10^6 $TCID_{50}$ units/10^6 cells (n = 15). Protein secretion in cell culture supernatants was measured after 24 h using ELISA (R&D). Statistical analysis used ANOVA for within group comparison, followed by 2A) IL-8, T-test, 2B) IP-10, Wilcoxon and 2C) GM-CSF, Wilcoxon.*P<0.05 **P<0.01. NT-no treatment.

measured. IP-10 release was synergistic while IL-8 and GM-CSF release were additive. One explanation could be that these cytokines are stimulated by distinct signaling pathways. We therefore repeated our experiments using inhibitors of PI3K (LY294002) [21] and p38 MAPK (SB203580) pathways [22] and also Dexamethasone [23]. LY294002 is being considered for development as a cancer drug [24] and has potential in respiratory disease. SB203580 was chosen since activation of p38 MAP kinases occurs early in RV infection so participates in signalling cascades controlling cellular responses to cytokines and stress [25]. Dexamethasone was chosen since it is used as an anti inflammatory treatment for asthma and has been shown to inhibit IL-8 in previous studies [26,27].

A significant change in virus-induced IL-8 and IP-10 protein expression was observed in the presence of inhibitors, with or without Th2 cytokines (ANOVA: IL-8 p = 0.001, IP-10 p = 0.04). Dexamethasone significantly inhibited RV16-induced IL-8 release both in the absence (p = 0.008) or presence (p = 0.03) of Th2 cytokines (Figure 4A). The potent inhibitory effect of dexamethasone on IL-8 release is in keeping with our previous observations [28]. The PI3K inhibitor had only a modest inhibitory effect on IL-8 release but significantly reduced RV16-induced IP-10 expression in the absence (p = 0.016) or presence (p = 0.017) of Th2 cytokines (Figure 4B). Dexamethasone was much less effective at inhibiting RV16-induced IP-10 than the PI3K inhibitor, and the effect was reduced further in the presence of Th2 cytokines. We saw no significant inhibitory effects on IL-8 or IP-10 with the p38 MAPK inhibitor.

RV16-induced GM-CSF expression was almost completely suppressed by dexamethasone both in the absence (p<0.05) or presence (p<0.01) of Th2 cytokines (Figure 4C). Virus replication and release were not altered by the presence of inhibitors in the cultures (Figure S3). This suggests that the inhibitors were acting on signal transduction pathways linked to cytokine expression and was not a result of suppression of virus replication.

We show that RV-induced IP-10 release is synergistically enhanced in the presence of Th2 cytokines, and that this effect can be blocked by inhibition of the PI3K pathway.

Discussion

In this study, we used primary epithelial cells from a non-asthmatic pediatric population and experimentally promoted a Th2 environment using exogenous Th2 cytokines. We show that, in undifferentiated pediatric bronchial epithelial cell cultures, Th2 cytokines do not increase entry or replication of virus but do augment the release of inflammatory mediators following RV infection.

The complexity of interactions between environment, host and pathogen make it difficult to assess the contribution of individual components of asthma or atopy but several attempts have been made to tease apart these interactions [29–31]. For simplicity we chose to use non-differentiated cultures to mimic the basal cells of the pseudostratifed bronchial epithelium [32] with a combination of both cytokines to more closely model *in vivo* conditions [14,33,34]. It is known that these cells are exposed in asthmatic bronchial epithelium due to epithelial damage and/or fragility [35]. When we designed the study we did not collect data on atopy since this would incur additional skin and blood tests which we felt would be unreasonable in such a young cohort. We recognize that this is a limitation of the study. Further, to our knowledge there are no data comparing responses of very young children with older teenagers. The wide age range used in this study was unavoidable given the difficulty in recruiting pediatric subjects and we cannot exclude age effects on the responses of the cells.

Our aim was to investigate whether Th2 cytokines, IL-13 and IL-4, modulate the effects of RV infection in bronchial epithelial monolayers. We confirmed previously reported RV-induced up-regulation of inflammatory cytokines IL-8 and IP-10 observed in a cell line [36] and in pBECs taken from adult subjects (Figure 2) [28]. In the study by Wark *et al* rhinovirus induced IP-10 and IL-8 expression of pBECs from adult subjects with allergic asthma was not significantly different to nonatopic healthy controls [28] and this may also be true of pediatric cultures. To our knowledge a similar comparison in a pediatric population has not been performed and unfortunately samples were not readily available for comparison in this study [19,37].

Using ppBECs from non asthmatic subjects we demonstrate that infection in the presence of Th2 cytokines stimulated a

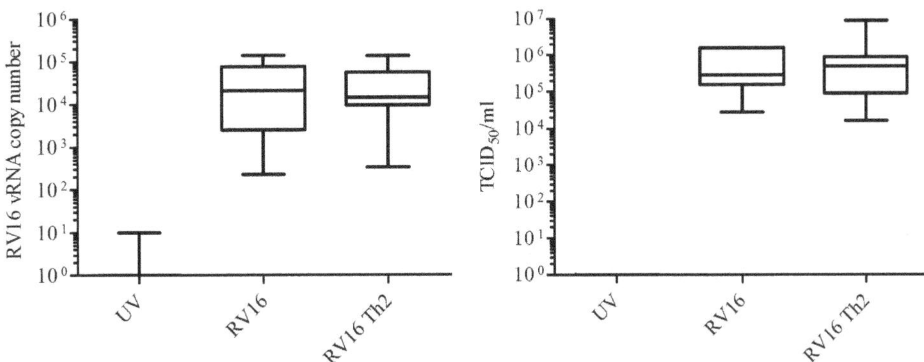

Figure 3. Replication of RV was not modified in the presence of Th2 cytokines. ppBECs were pretreated with IL-13 + IL-4 or not for 24 hours prior to infection with RV16 at 1×10^6 $TCID_{50}$ units/10^6 cells. Viral RNA was quantified and expressed as copy number relative to known standards (n = 15). Viral release into the supernatant was measured using $TCID_{50}$ assay (n = 15).

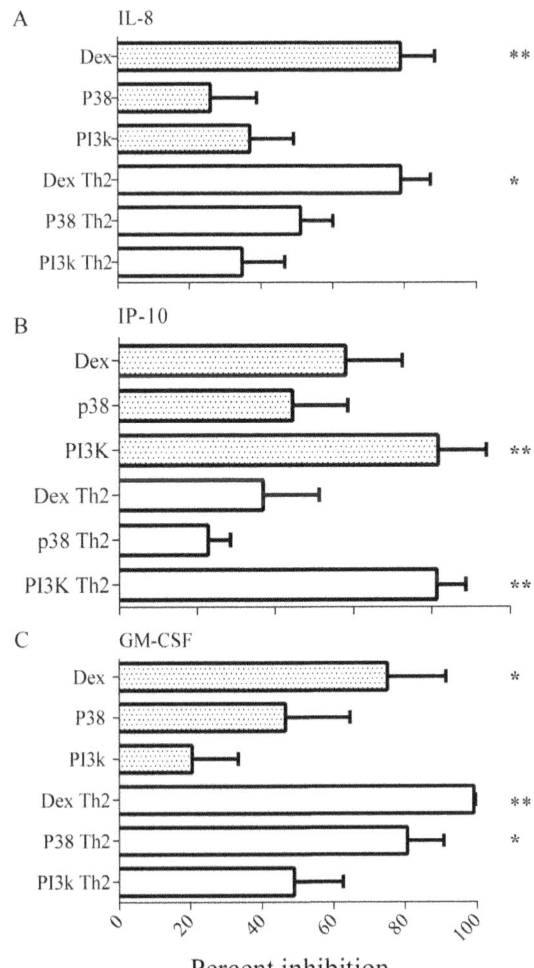

Figure 4. Inhibition of inflammatory pathways suppress virus- induced cytokines. ppBECs were pretreated with IL-13 + IL-4 (clear bars) or not (shaded bars) for 24 hours prior to infection with RV16 (n = 8). Inhibitors were added 30 minutes prior to infection. Protein secretion in cell supernatant was measured using ELISA (R&D). Statistical analysis used ANOVA (*$p<0.05$) followed by 4A) IL-8, Wilcoxon (absence) or T-test (presence) of Th2 cytokines, 4B IP-10 Wilcoxon (absence) or T-test (presence) of Th2 cytokines and 4C) GM-CSF, T-test. Data were normalized relative to no treatment and cytokine only controls. Total inhibition is shown as 100% and no inhibition as $<1\%$.

significant increase in IL-8, IP-10 and GM-CSF release. This appeared to be unrelated to a direct effect of the Th2 cytokines on viral replication, since no significant increase in viral RNA expression or viral titre was observed. Most importantly, the effect of RV infection and Th2 cytokines on IP-10 release was synergistic and this effect could be inhibited by blocking the activity of PI3K. Further investigations are important to ascertain the basis of this enhancement, but this is beyond the scope of the present study.

It has been reported that expression of ICAM-1, the cellular receptor for major group RVs such as RV16 is up-regulated by IL-4 and IL-13 following 24 hour incubation [14,34]. Such an increase in ICAM-1 would be expected to make the cells more vulnerable to RV16 infection, with increased binding and entry of virus into the cells leading to enhanced viral replication. We saw variability in the level of ICAM-1 expression in cultures taken from a small subset of 6 children (ages 1–15) used in the study but we did not see any significant up-regulation of ICAM-1 expression following 24 hr stimulation with Th2 cytokines. Whilst these results differ from some previous publications, this may be explained by the different models used [14,34].

We did not observe differences in cytopathic effects or LDH release in our cultures at 24 hours (Figure S1) suggesting that the increases in IL-8, IP-10 and GM-CSF were not caused by increased cell death or enhanced viral replication. This supports the findings of Wood *et al* who performed a study in an asthmatic population presenting to hospital with acute asthma exacerbation. They reported that expression of IP-10 is maintained when non-replicating virus is present (ie. viral persistence) and concluded that cellular inflammation caused by viral infection rather than viral replication itself was responsible for the clinical manifestations of a viral induced exacerbation of asthma [38].

We have previously reported that IP-10 expression is much less sensitive to suppression by dexamethasone and that IP-10 levels in serum remain elevated in subjects admitted to the emergency room with a virus-induced asthma exacerbation [28]. We found that dexamethasone was a poor inhibitor of IP-10 release from RV16 infected pBECs but confirmed potent inhibition of IL-8 release, in keeping with other studies [26,27].

We show that IP-10 release can be blocked by inhibition of PI3K. IP-10 expression is known to be corticosteroid refractory, and our finding that inhibition of PI3K in pBECs potently suppresses IP-10 expression may have therapeutic implications, having the potential to attenuate IP-10 and bring inflammation under control where dexamethasone has no effect. PI3Ks play important roles in tumorigenesis, so there is considerable interest in development of PI3K inhibitors as cancer potential therapeutic agents [39]. LY294002 acts as a competitive ATP binder [40] and has significant *in vivo* antitumor efficacy [24]. Recent studies elucidating the crystal structure of LY294002 provides a basis for development of its therapeutic potential [41].

In conclusion we show that Th2 cytokines, IL-13 and IL-4, synergistically enhance release of RV-induced IP-10, independent of replicating virus. This release can be inhibited by blocking the PI3K pathway.

Supporting Information

Figure S1 Phenotypes of cell cultures under the different conditions. pBECs were pretreated with IL-13 + IL-4 or SFM for 24 hours prior to infection with RV16 at 1×10^6 $TCID_{50}$ units/10^6 cells (n = 15). After 1 hr, infection medium was removed and the cells washed with PBS. Starvation medium was replaced +/− cytokines. No differences were seen between the different treatments. Pictures are representative of all the cultures.

Figure S2 ICAM-1 receptor expression was not altered following 24hr stimulus with Th2 cytokines. pPBECs were treated for 24 hours with IL-13 10 ng/ml, IL-4 10 ng/ml or both. ICAM-1 expression was assessed using flow cytometry. Data are plotted as ICAM-1 expression relative to isotype control, or as percent positive cells n = 6. No treatment controls were included for comparison.

Figure S3 Replication of virus was not moderated by inhibitors. pBECs were pretreated with IL-13 + IL-4 or SFM for 24 hours prior to infection with RV16 at 1×10^6 $TCID_{50}$ units/10^6 cells (n = 8). Inhibitors were added 30 minutes before infection. After 1 hr, infection medium was removed and the cells washed with PBS. Starvation medium was replaced +/− cytokines and/or inhibitors. Viral release into cell culture supernatants was measured using $TCID_{50}$ assay. Expression of viral RNA was quantified using RT-qPCR and expressed as copy number relative to known standards.

Acknowledgments

We are grateful to our clinicians for their assistance with this study, to the Wellcome Trust Clinical Research Facility, at Southampton University Hospital Trust for supporting the study and to all the participants and their families.

Author Contributions

Conceived and designed the experiments: JAC DED GR HMH STH. Performed the experiments: JAC YX. Analyzed the data: JAC DED GR. Contributed reagents/materials/analysis tools: JAC DED HMH YX GR. Wrote the paper: JAC DED.

References

1. Kim HY, DeKruyff RH, Umetsu DT (2010) The many paths to asthma: phenotype shaped by innate and adaptive immunity. Nat Immunol 11: 577–584. ni.1892 [pii];10.1038/ni.1892 [doi].
2. Brightling CE, Symon FA, Birring SS, Bradding P, Pavord ID, et al. (2002) TH2 cytokine expression in bronchoalveolar lavage fluid T lymphocytes and bronchial submucosa is a feature of asthma and eosinophilic bronchitis. J Allergy Clin Immunol 110: 899–905. S0091674902014732 [pii].
3. Robinson DS (2000) Th-2 cytokines in allergic disease. Br Med Bull 56: 956–968.
4. Gern JE, Vrtis R, Grindle KA, Swenson C, Busse WW (2000) Relationship of upper and lower airway cytokines to outcome of experimental rhinovirus infection. Am J Respir Crit Care Med 162: 2226–2231.
5. Parry DE, Busse WW, Sukow KA, Dick CR, Swenson C, et al. (2000) Rhinovirus-induced PBMC responses and outcome of experimental infection in allergic subjects. J Allergy Clin Immunol 105: 692–698. S0091-6749(00)36224-8 [pii];10.1067/mai.2000.104785 [doi].
6. Hollams EM, Deverell M, Serralha M, Suriyaarachchi D, Parsons F, et al. (2009) Elucidation of asthma phenotypes in atopic teenagers through parallel immunophenotypic and clinical profiling. J Allergy Clin Immunol 124: 463–470. S0091-6749(09)00952-X [pii];10.1016/j.jaci.2009.06.019 [doi].
7. Sly PD, Boner AL, Bjorksten B, Bush A, Custovic A, et al. (2008) Early identification of atopy in the prediction of persistent asthma in children. Lancet 372: 1100–1106. S0140-6736(08)61451-8 [pii];10.1016/S0140-6736(08)61451-8 [doi].
8. Stern DA, Morgan WJ, Halonen M, Wright AL, Martinez FD (2008) Wheezing and bronchial hyper-responsiveness in early childhood as predictors of newly diagnosed asthma in early adulthood: a longitudinal birth-cohort study. Lancet 372: 1058–1064. S0140-6736(08)61447-6 [pii];10.1016/S0140-6736(08)61447-6 [doi].
9. Jackson DJ, Johnston SL (2010) The role of viruses in acute exacerbations of asthma. J Allergy Clin Immunol 125: 1178–1187. S0091-6749(10)00689-5 [pii];10.1016/j.jaci.2010.04.021 [doi].

10. Johnston SL, Pattemore PK, Sanderson G, Smith S, Lampe F, et al. (1995) Community study of role of viral infections in exacerbations of asthma in 9-11 year old children. BMJ 310: 1225–1229.
11. Green RM, Custovic A, Sanderson G, Hunter J, Johnston SL, et al. (2002) Synergism between allergens and viruses and risk of hospital admission with asthma: case-control study. BMJ 324: 763.
12. Subrata LS, Bizzintino J, Mamessier E, Bosco A, McKenna KL, et al. (2009) Interactions between innate antiviral and atopic immunoinflammatory pathways precipitate and sustain asthma exacerbations in children. J Immunol 183: 2793–2800. jimmunol.0900695 [pii];10.4049/jimmunol.0900695 [doi].
13. Bulek K, Swaidani S, Aronica M, Li X (2010) Epithelium: the interplay between innate and Th2 immunity. Immunol Cell Biol 88: 257–268. icb2009113 [pii];10.1038/icb.2009.113 [doi].
14. Bianco A, Sethi SK, Allen JT, Knight RA, Spiteri MA (1998) Th2 cytokines exert a dominant influence on epithelial cell expression of the major group human rhinovirus receptor, ICAM-1. Eur Respir J 12: 619–626.
15. Papi A (1997) Epithelial ICAM-1 regulation and its role in allergy. Clin Exp Allergy 27: 721–724.
16. Hurd SZ (1991) Workshop summary and guidelines: investigative use of bronchoscopy, lavage, and bronchial biopsies in asthma and other airway diseases. J Allergy Clin Immunol 88: 808–814.
17. Bucchieri F, Puddicombe SM, Lordan JL, Richter A, Buchanan D, et al. (2002) Asthmatic bronchial epithelium is more susceptible to oxidant-induced apoptosis. Am J Respir Cell Mol Biol 27(2): 179–185.
18. Papi A, Johnston SL (1999) Rhinovirus infection induces expression of its own receptor intercellular adhesion molecule 1 (ICAM-1) via increased NF-kappaB-mediated transcription. J Biol Chem 274: 9707–9720.
19. Andrews AL, Nasir T, Bucchieri F, Holloway JW, Holgate ST, et al. (2006) IL-13 receptor alpha 2: a regulator of IL-13 and IL-4 signal transduction in primary human fibroblasts. J Allergy Clin Immunol 118: 858–865.
20. Bossios A, Psarras S, Gourgiotis D, Skevaki CL, Constantopoulos AG, et al. (2005) Rhinovirus infection induces cytotoxicity and delays wound healing in bronchial epithelial cells. Respir Res 6: 114.
21. Vlahos CJ, Matter WF, Hui KY, Brown RF (1994) A specific inhibitor of phosphatidylinositol 3-kinase, 2-(4-morpholinyl)-8-phenyl-4H-1-benzopyran-4-one (LY294002). J Biol Chem 269: 5241–5248.
22. Kumar S, Jiang MS, Adams JL, Lee JC (1999) Pyridinylimidazole compound SB 203580 inhibits the activity but not the activation of p38 mitogen-activated protein kinase. Biochem Biophys Res Commun 263: 825–831. 10.1006/bbrc.1999.1454 [doi];S0006-291X(99)91454-7 [pii].
23. Chang MM, Juarez M, Hyde DM, Wu R (2001) Mechanism of dexamethasone-mediated interleukin-8 gene suppression in cultured airway epithelial cells. Am J Physiol Lung Cell Mol Physiol 280: L107–L115.
24. Hu L, Zaloudek C, Mills GB, Gray J, Jaffe RB (2000) In vivo and in vitro ovarian carcinoma growth inhibition by a phosphatidylinositol 3-kinase inhibitor (LY294002). Clin Cancer Res 6: 880–886.
25. Griego SD, Weston CB, Adams JL, Tal-Singer R, Dillon SB (2000) Role of p38 mitogen-activated protein kinase in rhinovirus-induced cytokine production by bronchial epithelial cells. J Immunol 165: 5211–5220.
26. Edwards MR, Johnson MW, Johnston SL (2006) Combination therapy: Synergistic suppression of virus-induced chemokines in airway epithelial cells. Am J Respir Cell Mol Biol 34: 616–624. 2005-0385OC [pii];10.1165/rcmb.2005-0385OC [doi].
27. Skevaki CL, Christodoulou I, Spyridaki IS, Tiniakou I, Georgiou V, et al. (2009) Budesonide and formoterol inhibit inflammatory mediator production by bronchial epithelial cells infected with rhinovirus. Clin Exp Allergy 39: 1700–1710. CEA3307 [pii];10.1111/j.1365-2222.2009.03307.x [doi].
28. Wark PA, Bucchieri F, Johnston SL, Gibson PG, Hamilton L, et al. (2007) IFN-gamma-induced protein 10 is a novel biomarker of rhinovirus-induced asthma exacerbations. J Allergy Clin Immunol 120: 586–593. S0091-6749(07)01025-1 [pii];10.1016/j.jaci.2007.04.046 [doi].
29. Korpi-Steiner NL, Valkenaar SM, Bates ME, Evans MD, Gern JE, et al. (2010) Human monocytic cells direct the robust release of CXCL10 by bronchial epithelial cells during rhinovirus infection. Clin Exp Allergy 40: 1203–1213. CEA3546 [pii];10.1111/j.1365-2222.2010.03546.x [doi].
30. Lachowicz-Scroggins ME, Boushey HA, Finkbeiner WE, Widdicombe JH (2010) Interleukin-13-induced mucous metaplasia increases susceptibility of human airway epithelium to rhinovirus infection. Am J Respir Cell Mol Biol 43: 652–661. 2009-0244OC [pii];10.1165/rcmb.2009-0244OC [doi].
31. Xatzipsalti M, Psarros F, Konstantinou G, Gaga M, Gourgiotis D, et al. (2008) Modulation of the epithelial inflammatory response to rhinovirus in an atopic environment. Clin Exp Allergy 38: 466–472. CEA2906 [pii];10.1111/j.1365-2222.2007.02906.x [doi].
32. Jakiela B, Brockman-Schneider R, Amineva S, Lee WM, Gern JE (2008) Basal cells of differentiated bronchial epithelium are more susceptible to rhinovirus infection. Am J Respir Cell Mol Biol 38: 517–523.
33. Grunig G, Warnock M, Wakil AE, Venkayya R, Brombacher F, et al. (1998) Requirement for IL-13 independently of IL-4 in experimental asthma. Science 282: 2261–2263.
34. Striz I, Mio T, Adachi Y, Heires P, Robbins RA, et al. (1999) IL-4 induces ICAM-1 expression in human bronchial epithelial cells and potentiates TNF-alpha. Am J Physiol 277: L58–L64.
35. Puddicombe SM, Polosa R, Richter A, Krishna MT, Howarth PH, et al. (2000) Involvement of the epidermal growth factor receptor in epithelial repair in asthma. FASEB J 14: 1362–1374.
36. Subauste MC, Jacoby DB, Richards SM, Proud D (1995) Infection of a human respiratory epithelial cell line with rhinovirus. Induction of cytokine release and modulation of susceptibility to infection by cytokine exposure. J Clin Invest 96: 549–557. 10.1172/JCI118067 [doi].
37. Lordan JL, Bucchieri F, Richter A, Konstantinidis A, Holloway JW, et al. (2002) Cooperative effects of Th2 cytokines and allergen on normal and asthmatic bronchial epithelial cells. J Immunol 169: 407–414.
38. Wood LG, Powell H, Grissell TV, Davies B, Shafren DR, et al. (2011) Persistence of rhinovirus RNA and IP-10 gene expression after acute asthma. Respirology 16: 291–299. 10.1111/j.1440-1843.2010.01897.x [doi].
39. Liu P, Cheng H, Roberts TM, Zhao JJ (2009) Targeting the phosphoinositide 3-kinase pathway in cancer. Nat Rev Drug Discov 8: 627–644. nrd2926 [pii];10.1038/nrd2926 [doi].
40. Marone R, Cmiljanovic V, Giese B, Wymann MP (2008) Targeting phosphoinositide 3-kinase: moving towards therapy. Biochim Biophys Acta 1784: 159–185. S1570-9639(07)00260-9 [pii];10.1016/j.bbapap.2007.10.003 [doi].
41. Walker EH, Pacold ME, Perisic O, Stephens L, Hawkins PT, et al. (2000) Structural determinants of phosphoinositide 3-kinase inhibition by wortmannin, LY294002, quercetin, myricetin, and staurosporine. Mol Cell 6: 909–919. S1097-2765(05)00089-4 [pii].

Risk Factors Associated with Death in In-Hospital Pediatric Convulsive Status Epilepticus

Tobias Loddenkemper[1,☯], Tanvir U. Syed[2,☯], Sriram Ramgopal[1*], Deepak Gulati[2], Sikawat Thanaviratananich[2], Sanjeev V. Kothare[1], Amer Alshekhlee[3], Mohamad Z. Koubeissi[2,4]

1 Department of Neurology, Children's Hospital Boston and Harvard Medical School, Boston, Massachusetts, United States of America, **2** Department of Neurology, Case Western Reserve University and University Hospitals, Cleveland, Ohio, United States of America, **3** Department of Neurology, St Louis University, St. Louis, Missouri, United States of America, **4** Department of Neurology, George Washington University, Washington, D.C., United States of America

Abstract

Objective: To evaluate in-patient mortality and predictors of death associated with convulsive status epilepticus (SE) in a large, multi-center, pediatric cohort.

Patients and Methods: We identified our cohort from the KID Inpatient Database for the years 1997, 2000, 2003 and 2006. We queried the database for convulsive SE, associated diagnoses, and for inpatient death. Univariate logistic testing was used to screen for potential risk factors. These risk factors were then entered into a stepwise backwards conditional multivariable logistic regression procedure. *P*-values less than 0.05 were taken as significant.

Results: We identified 12,365 (5,541 female) patients with convulsive SE aged 0–20 years (mean age 6.2 years, standard deviation 5.5 years, median 5 years) among 14,965,571 pediatric inpatients (0.08%). Of these, 117 died while in the hospital (0.9%). The most frequent additional admission ICD-9 code diagnoses in addition to SE were cerebral palsy, pneumonia, and respiratory failure. Independent risk factors for death in patients with SE, assessed by multivariate calculation, included near drowning (Odds ratio [OR] 43.2; Confidence Interval [CI] 4.4–426.8), hemorrhagic shock (OR 17.83; CI 6.5–49.1), sepsis (OR 10.14; CI 4.0–25.6), massive aspiration (OR 9.1; CI 1.8–47), mechanical ventilation >96 hours (OR9; 5.6–14.6), transfusion (OR 8.25; CI 4.3–15.8), structural brain lesion (OR7.0; CI 3.1–16), hypoglycemia (OR5.8; CI 1.75–19.2), sepsis with liver failure (OR 14.4; CI 5–41.9), and admission in December (OR3.4; CI 1.6–4.1). African American ethnicity (OR 0.4; CI 0.2–0.8) was associated with a decreased risk of death in SE.

Conclusion: Pediatric convulsive SE occurs in up to 0.08% of pediatric inpatient admissions with a mortality of up to 1%. There appear to be several risk factors that can predict mortality. These may warrant additional monitoring and aggressive management.

Editor: Joshua L. Bonkowsky, University of Utah School of Medicine, United States of America

Funding: TL serves on the Laboratory Accreditation Board for Long Term (Epilepsy and ICU) Monitoring (ABRET), serves as an Associate Editor for Seizure, serves on the American Board of Clinical Neurophysiology, and on the Council of the American Clinical Neurophysiology Society, performs Video EEG longterm monitoring, EEGs, and other electrophysiological studies at Children's Hospital Boston and bills for these procedures (20%), receives support from National Institutes of Health (NIH)/National Institute of Neurological Disorders and Stroke (NINDS) 1R21NS076859-01 (2011-2013), is supported by a Career Development Fellowship Award from Harvard Medical School and Children's Hospital Boston, by the Program for Quality and Safety at Children's Hospital Boston, from the Payer Provider Quality Initiative, the Translational Research Project at Children's Hospital Boston, receives funding from the Epilepsy Foundation of America (EF-213583 & EF-213882), and from the Center for Integration of Medicine & Innovative Technology (CIMIT/DoD), and received investigator initiated research support from Eisai and Lundbeck. Drs. TS, SR, DG, and ST have nothing to disclose. Dr. SK performs Video EEG longterm monitoring, EEGs, and other electrophysiological studies at Children's Hospital Boston and bills for these procedures, is interim medical director of the Center for Pediatric Sleep Disorders at Children's Hospital Boston, and has received research support from National Institute of Health (1 RC1 HL099749-01 (R21) (2009-12), and RFA-HL-09-001 (2010-14) and the Harvard Catalyst (2010-11). He also serves on the editorial board of the journal Pediatric Neurology. Dr. AA has nothing to disclose. Dr. MK has no conflict of interest related to the current work, has received grant support from the Coulter Foundation, and is on the Speakers' Bureaus of UCB and Pfizer. The funders had no role in study design, data collection and analysis, decision to publish, or preparation of the manuscript.

Competing Interests: TL serves on the Laboratory Accreditation Board for Long Term (Epilepsy and ICU) Monitoring (ABRET), performs Video EEG longterm monitoring, EEGs, and other electrophysiological studies at Children's Hospital Boston and bills for these procedures (20%). He has received investigator initiated research support from Eisai Inc. Dr. SK performs Video EEG longterm monitoring, EEGs, and other electrophysiological studies at Children's Hospital Boston and bills for these procedures. He also serves on the editorial board of the Journal of Pediatric Neurology. Dr. MK is on the Speakers' Bureaus of UCB and Pfizer. There are no patents, products in development or marketed products to declare.

* E-mail: Sriram.ramgopal@childrens.harvard.edu

☯ These authors contributed equally to this work.

Introduction

Status epilepticus (SE) is characterized by prolonged seizures or by multiple seizures without full restoration of consciousness between events [1]. The condition is associated with significant morbidity and mortality. SE is thought to have a fatality rate of approximately 2% [2,3]. Complications of SE are also significant and include refractory epilepsy, neurologic deficits and repeated episodes of SE [4].

While a number of studies have identified associations for poor outcomes in SE [5,6], the use of publically available hospital databases with large sample sizes may allow for better determination of morbidity and mortality risk factors for patients with this condition. In this study, we investigate potential risk factors leading to death in children presenting with generalized convulsive SE.

Patients and Methods

Study Population

This study utilized patient data acquired from the Kids' Inpatient Database (KID). The KID dataset has been set up through the Healthcare Cost and Utilization Project (HCUP) and is the only all-payer inpatient care database for children in the United States. Data from both insured and uninsured pediatric patients, defined as individuals less than 20 years of age, are collected. Data collected from KID include demographic information, including patient age, gender, race, median income and ZIP code, primary and secondary diagnoses, procedures, payment information, and patient length of stay. KID also collects information on factors including hospital size, teaching status, type of hospital and hospital location. We used data from the years 1997, 2000, 2003 and 2006. The 1997 database includes data from 2,521 hospitals in 22 states, the 2000 database includes data from 2,784 hospitals in 27 states, the 2003 database includes data from 3,438 hospitals in 36 states, and the 2006 database includes data from 3,739 hospitals in 38 states. Twenty percent of normal newborn births and 80% of the inpatient admissions from each institution are included in the dataset as a systematic random sample [7].

Standard Protocol Approvals

Prior to data analysis, the Institutional Review Boards of Case Western Reserve University and University Hospitals, Cleveland, OH, and Boston Children's Hospital, Boston, MA, granted exempt status to this study. Informed consent was not required. This study was done in accordance with the HCUP user agreement.

Data Acquisition

We queried KID for cases with a diagnostic code of generalized convulsive status epilepticus via usage of the International Statistical Classification of Diseases and Related Health Problems, 9th revision (ICD-9) code 345.3. This code corresponds to "grand mal status". No other ICD-9 codes were used. Data pertaining to month of admission, admission source (from the emergency room, at birth, from outside the hospital and from outside the facility), sex, elective admission or not, age, length of stay, ethnicity, income level (assessed as median income per ZIP code), hospital type (general hospital, children's hospital, or general hospital with a children's unit), hospital bed size, hospital location (rural versus urban and geographic region), and teaching status of hospital were collected. We also used ICD-9 codes to collect data pertaining to patient comorbidities, interventions and complications (table 1). Outcomes pertaining to mortality, which were listed separately in the KID dataset, were collected for each patient.

Statistical Analysis

Univariate logistic testing was used to screen for significant risk factors of death. Risk factors with an associated p-value less than 0.20 were entered into a stepwise backwards conditional multivariable logistic regression procedure. The multivariable model only retained risk factors with an associated p-value less than 0.05. Two-way interaction terms were entered one at a time into the resulting multivariable model and were retained if the associated p-value was less than 0.05. Model validity was assessed using the Hosmer and Lemeshow goodness-of-fit test with p-value greater than 0.05 indicating adequate model fit of data. All statistical analyses were performed in Stata 11.0 (Statacorp, College Station, TX).

Results

Description of Patient Population and Mortality Rate

A total of 14,965,571 patients were included based on the KID datasets from 1997, 2000, 2003 and 2006. Of these, 12,365 patients (0.083%) were diagnosed with convulsive SE, including 5,541 (44.8%) girls. Five patients (<0.0001%) were excluded from the study due to insufficient data for the tested variables. Mean patient age was 6.2±5.5 years (range <1–20 years, median 5 years). One-hundred-and-seventeen patients (0.95%) with convulsive SE died during their inpatient admission. Additional demographic data are provided in table 2.

Risk Factor Analysis

Logistic testing was done to identify potential risk factors for death in convulsive status epilepticus, and those risk factors associated with a p-value of 0.20 were entered into a multivariate model. Factors with a p-value of less than 0.05 were taken as significant following model verification. Univariate and multivariate calculations are provided in tables 1, 3 and 4.

Risk Factors Based on Demographic Data

African American children were at a significantly lower risk of mortality following an episode of convulsive SE ($p = 0.009$). Patients in other racial groups did not have an associated increase or decrease in mortality. No association was found between patient age and mortality risk. Household income, calculated as the average income in a ZIP code region, was also not a significant risk factor for death.

Risk Factors Based on Hospital Admission

Using univariate analysis, cases referred from outside hospitals were associated with a higher rate of mortality, as were Children's Hospitals, Teaching Hospitals, and General Hospitals with a Children's Unit. These findings were not significant in multivariate analysis. Patient length of stay, weekend versus weekday admission, hospital size and geographic region of hospital were not associated with an increased risk of mortality. None of these factors emerged as significant in multivariate analysis.

Risk Factors Based on Comorbidities

A number of patient comorbidities corresponded to a greater mortality risk in convulsive SE. Sepsis ($p<0.001$), hypoglycemia ($p = 0.004$), near-drowning episode ($p = 0.001$), hemorrhagic shock ($p<0.001$), structural brain lesions ($p<0.001$), massive aspiration ($p = 0.008$), and postoperative sepsis with liver failure ($p<0.001$)

Table 1. Univariate calculations of complications and comorbidities from the KID database.

Predictor	ICD-9 Code	Total N	Predictor N	OR	Lower 95%	Upper 95%	P
Metabolic							
Hyponatremia	276.1	12360	238	3.31	1.52	7.18	0.002
Hypoxia	799.0, 770.8, 768, 348.1, 768.5, 768.6, 768.9	12360	293	12.35	8.01	19.04	<.001
Drug overdose	966	12360	12	-	-	-	
Hepatic encephalopathy	572.2	12360	<10	-	-	-	-
Metabolic derangements	277, 348.31	12360	105	4.26	1.54	11.76	0.005
Severe malnutrition	260, 261, 262, 263	12360	60	3.65	0.88	15.14	0.074
Toxic	349.82, 323.7, 983, 984, 985, 988, 989	12360	19	-	-	-	-
Hypoglycemia	250.8, 251.0, 251.1, 251.2, 300.19, 775.6	12360	67	8.77	3.46	22.23	<.001
Drug withdrawal	292.0, 779.5	12360	<10	-	-	-	-
Infectious							
Sepsis	038, 771.8, 995.91 995.92, 771.81	12360	44	33.56	16.17	69.66	<.001
Cerebral malaria	084.9	12365	<10	-	-	-	-
Disseminated tuberculosis	018	-	-	-	-	-	-
Acute viral encephalitis	049.9, 062, 064, 139.0, 323.0, 323.01	12360	34	10.37	3.12	34.40	<0.001
Central nervous system infections	V12.42	12365	<10	-	-	-	-
Meningoencephalitis	323.0, 323.4	12360	<10	-	-	-	-
Bacterial meningitis	320, 320.7, 320.8, 320.81, 320.82, 320.9	12360	<10	-	-	-	-
Infectious encephalopathy	136.9, 323.5, 323.9, 348.3	12360	394	2.57	1.29	5.10	<.007
Severe malaria	084, 084.9, 084.4, 084.5, 084.6, 084.7, 084.8	12330	-	-	-	-	-
Pneumonia	480, 480.8, 480.9, 481, 482, 482.8, 483, 485, 011.6	12360	51	6.69	2.05	21.78	0.002
Meningitis	013.0, 036.0, 320, 047.8, 047.9, 320.1, 321, 320.8, 322	12360	44	-	-	-	-
Bacteremia	790.7, 771.83	12360	58	-	-	-	-
Viral encephalitis	062, 063, 064, 139.0, 323.0, 049.9	12360	34	10.37	3.12	34.39	<.001
RSV infection	079.6	12360	42	2.57	0.35	18.81	0.354
Postoperative sepsis and liver failure	998.59	12360	26	59.93	26.14	137.42	<.001
Septic shock	785.52, 785.59	12360	46	57.93	30.35	110.59	<.001
Hemodynamic							
Congenital heart disease	746.9	12360	<10	-	-	-	-
Hypotension	458, 458.0, 458.1, 458.2, 458.29, 458.8, 458.9	12360	146	15.96	9.28	27.47	<.001
Intractable hypertension	401, 403, 403.0, 405, 405.0	12360	104	5.48	2.19	13.71	<.001
Cardiac failure	428.9	12360	<10	-	-	-	-
Hemorrhagic shock	785.59, 958.4	12360	29	50.93	22.67	114.39	<.001
Post cardiac arrest	997.1	12360	<10	-	-	-	-
Neurologic							
Cerebral palsy	333.71, 343, 343.0, 343.1, 343.2, 343.3, 343.8, 343.9	12360	2132	0.64	0.37	1.12	0.118
Subdural Hematoma	432.1, 767.0	12360	21	11.19	2.58	48.59	<0.001
Cerebrovascular accident	434.01, 434.11, 434.91	12360	36	37.07	17.32	82.07	<.007
Brain trauma	850, 767.0, 850.9 854, 310.2	12360	14	-	-	-	-
Acute cerebrovascular disease	436, 437, 437.1, 437.8, 437.9 438, 438.8, 438.9	12360	46	2.34	0.32	17.10	0.403

Table 1. Cont.

Predictor	ICD-9 Code	Total N	Predictor N	OR	Lower 95%	Upper 95%	*P*
Brain death	348.8	12360	119	9.19	4.54	18.61	<.001
Brainstem tumor	191.7, 225.9	12360	<10	-	-	-	-
Structural brain lesion	348.8	12360	119	9.19	4.54	18.61	<.001
Intracranial hemorrhage	800.3, 800.8	12360	<10	-	-	-	-
Brainstem herniation	348.4	12360	33	24.46	9.90	60.40	<.001
Epilepsy	345	12360	376	0.84	0.26	2.65	0.763
Generalized Convulsive Epilepsy	345.1	12360	38	-	-	-	-
Generalized Non-Convulsive Epilepsy	345.0	12360	19	-	-	-	-
Infantile spasms	345.6	12360	<10	-	-	-	-
Hydrocephalus	331	12360	832	0.62	0.25	1.51	0.291
Obstructive hydrocephalus	331.4	12360	472	0.89	0.33	2.42	0.821
Communicating hydrocephalus	331.3	12360	16	-	-	-	-
Idiopathic hydrocephalus	331.5	12360	<10	-	-	-	-
Congenital hydrocephalus	742.3	12360	349	0.30	0.04	2.12	0.224
CNS Malformation in fetus	655.0	12360	<10	-	-	-	-
Tuberous sclerosis	759.5	12360	124	0.85	0.12	6.13	0.871
Rasmussen encephalitis	323.81	12360	<10	-	-	-	-
	Other						
Non compliance	V15.81	12360	<10	-	-	-	-
Near drowning	994.1	12360	<10	26.38	2.93	237.80	0.004
Congenital malformations	V13.6, V13.69	12360	<10	-	-	-	-
Massive aspiration	507, 770.1, 770.18, E879.4	12360	711	2.25	1.28	3.96	0.005
Esophageal tear	530.89	12360	<10	-	-	-	-
Fever	780.6	12360	612	1.04	0.45	2.37	0.929
Interventions							
Transfusion	99.01–99.09	12360	110	36.48	22.21	59.93	<0.001
Ventriculoperitoneal shunt	2.31–2.39	12360	23	4.79	0.64	35.82	0.127
Intubation	96.04	12360	19	-	-	-	-
Mechanical ventilation	96.71	12360	3351	12.64	7.87	20.30	<0.001
Mechanical ventilation 96 hours	96.72	12360	426	22.74	15.53	33.30	<0.001

ICD-9 – International Classification of Disease, 9th edition, RSV – respiratory syncytial virus.

were associated with increased mortality. Though risk factors such as hypertension, subdural hemorrhage, viral encephalitis, and infectious encephalopathy were significant risk factors in univariate analysis, they did not emerge as significant factors following multivariate calculations. Other comorbidities, including a previous diagnosis of epilepsy, antiepileptic medication withdrawal, fever, esophageal tears, post-cardiac arrest status, brainstem tumors, infantile spasms, other encephalitis, and hydrocephalus were not associated with increased mortality.

Risk Factors Based on Procedures

The need for blood transfusion was associated with greater risk of death ($p<0.001$). While intubation was not a risk factor for death, mechanical ventilation for more than 96 hours was associated with a higher mortality ($p<0.001$). Ventriculoperitoneal shunt placement was not associated with higher mortality.

Discussion

Summary

This retrospective study utilized the KID dataset to identify a number of risk factors for poor outcome in pediatric patients diagnosed with convulsive status epilepticus. Higher risk was associated with end-of-year hospital admissions, various patient-related comorbidities, blood transfusion and prolonged mechanical ventilation. African American ethnicity was associated with a lower risk of mortality. A review of the literature is presented in table 5.

Mortality rate

The mortality rates of convulsive SE in previous studies vary. Some studies report a less than 2% mortality [2,3] whereas other studies provide figures over 30% [8]. The mortality rate of convulsive SE in our study was approximately 1%. This finding corresponds to mortality rates from previous research. A state-wide study based in California utilized a dataset including over

Table 2. Patient Population.

Total patient population	**14,965,571**	
Cases of Convulsive SE (%)	12,365 (0.083%)	
Number of Females with SE	5,541 (44.8%)	
Mean Age (SD; range)	6.2 (5.5; 0–20)	
Deaths in SE Cases	117 patients	
Case Fatality Rate	0.95%	
Patient Demographics	***patients***	***percent***
Caucasian	4,697	49.11%
African American	1,943	20.35%
Hispanic	2,044	21.37%
Asian or Pacific Islander	275	2.88%
Native American	71	0.74%
Other	531	5.55%

SE – Status epilepticus; SD – standard deviation.

19,000 adults and children admitted for SE and found an in-hospital mortality rate of 1.9% [3]. A prospective study evaluating intractable epilepsy in 613 children found a death rate of 1.6% over 4 years [9]. Another prospective study found a mortality rate of 2% in 47 pediatric patients with SE [10]. Studies with higher mortality rates may have analyzed high-risk subgroups, such as SE patients with pediatric intensive care unit (ICU) admissions [8] or cases of refractory SE only [11]. Because prolonged seizures are thought to be a risk factor for complications and death, studies that maintained criteria of a minimum seizure length of 30 or more minutes may have subsequently reported higher fatality rates [12,13]. Investigators who studied mortality over months to years of follow-up reported higher fatality rates [12]. Most studies of SE do not specifically investigate pediatric patients. Because the mortality of SE may rise with age [5,14], the inclusion of adult patients can result in a higher case-fatality rate. However, the age-specific incidence of epilepsy is highest in infancy and early childhood and decreases progressively as children grow up [15].

Demographic data

Race. Children of African American ethnicity were found to have lower mortality rates in convulsive SE compared to children of other ethnic groups. In a retrospective study analyzing risk factors for mortality in status epilepticus in Richmond, Virginia, African American ethnicity was found to correlate with decreased mortality risk in univariate, though not multivariate, analysis [14]. While they may have decreased risk of mortality compared to other racial groups, African American children have also been noted to present in SE disproportionately more frequently [3,16]. Because decreased mortality in status persisted in spite of consideration of socioeconomic factors, a heritable resistance to seizure-related mortality in this population cannot be ruled out.

Sex. The importance of gender in the risk assessment of SE is debated. While some studies have identified that males are more likely to present in status [17], other studies have found the opposite [18]. Mortality outcomes in status epilepticus between males and females are similarly conflicting [3,5,6]. While our study found that more males presented in SE than females, we did not find sex to be a significant risk factor in predicting mortality outcomes.

Age. Some studies have found an association between SE mortality and children of younger ages [19], whereas others have noted that older patients have a higher risk of death during SE [5,14]. SE is also noted to occur more frequently in younger patients [5]. Age was not found to be a significant independent risk factor for death in our study.

Hospital Data

Time of Year. We tested each month individually as a predictor of mortality and subsequently tested statistically significant months in the multivariable mortality model to account for potential seasonal variations in disease severity, as may occur with infectious or epidemic disease processes. Hospital admissions for convulsive SE during the month of December were associated with an increased risk of mortality. More research will be needed to verify these data and to identify possible causes. Seasonal variations in infections such as bacterial meningitis [20] and viral encephalitis [21] and other respiratory tract infections may have played a role in this annual variation.

Teaching and Children's Hospitals. The univariate analysis identified a significant association between deaths and admission into Teaching Hospitals, Children's Hospitals and General Hospitals with a Children's unit. In addition, referrals from outside hospitals are also associated with significant mortality. None of these factors emerged as significant in the multivariate analysis. We believe that some these findings may be related to referral bias, as more severe cases of SE are likely to be referred to Children's Hospitals and teaching institutions.

Comorbidities

Symptomatic epilepsy. Structural brain lesions, as demonstrated by imaging or autopsy findings, emerged as a risk factor for death in our study. This finding is in concordance with results from previous studies suggesting higher mortality in convulsive SE patients with structural lesions, such as brain tumors [6], cerebral dysgenesis [12,22]_ENREF_13, neurodegenerative disease [6], cerebral palsy [12] or other brain malformations [19]. Mortality may be higher in patients with acute symptomatic SE and neurological injury [23].

Pulmonary complications. Aspiration was a common comorbid condition associated with death in pediatric patients

Table 3. Univariate calculations of hospital and demographic data from the KID database.

Predictor	Total N	Predictor N	OR	Lower 95%	Upper 95%	*P*
January Admission	12360	957	1.00			
February Admission	12360	983	1.95	0.67	5.74	0.22
March Admission	12360	992	2.13	0.74	6.16	0.16
April Admission	12360	878	1.97	0.66	5.90	0.23
May Admission	12360	963	1.59	0.52	4.89	0.42
June Admission	12360	934	1.85	0.62	5.54	0.27
July Admission	12360	935	1.44	0.45	4.54	0.54
August Admission	12360	899	2.14	0.73	6.28	0.17
September Admission	12360	883	1.08	0.31	3.75	0.90
October Admission	12360	999	1.73	0.58	5.18	0.33
November Admission	12360	963	0.99	0.29	3.44	0.99
December Admission	12360	1042	4.11	1.55	10.89	0.01
Admission Source	121999					
Emergency room		7674	1.00	-	-	-
Birth		2197	1.53	0.94	2.48	0.084
Outside Hospital		2042	2.07	1.32	3.23	0.001
Outside Facility		286	2.46	0.98	6.21	0.055
Weekend Admission	12146	3389	1.36	0.93	2.00	0.114
Female	12360	5537	1.17	0.81	1.69	0.392
Elective Admission	11333	738	1.34	0.67	2.66	0.48
Age in years (if more than 1 year old)	12319	-	1.03	0.99	1.06	0.108
Age in Days (if less than 1 year old)	801	-	1.00	0.99	1.00	0.327
Length of Stay	12360	-	1.03	1.02	1.04	<0.001
Race	12360					
White		4697	1.00			
Black		1943	0.49	0.24	1.01	0.053
Hispanic		2044	0.78	0.43	1.41	0.412
Other		3676	1.43	0.95	2.15	0.088
Urban/Rural by ZIP Code	7506					
Large		4306	1.00			
Small		2187	1.27	0.76	2.10	0.361
Metropolitan		638	1.21	0.54	2.73	0.639
Non-core		375	1.18	0.42	3.32	0.754
Income per ZIP Code	12006					
1st quartile		3076	1.00			
2nd quartile		3133	1.11	0.64	1.92	0.722
3rd quartile		2776	1.53	0.90	2.59	0.115
4th quartile		3012	1.28	0.74	2.19	0.376
Hospital Type	11693					
General		4897	1.00			
General with children's unit		4125	1.60	1.01	2.54	0.045
Children's		2671	2.14	1.32	3.44	0.002
Hospital Bed Size	11936					
Small		1696	1.00			
Medium		3430	1.20	0.64	2.25	0.563
Large		6810	1.16	0.65	2.07	0.62
Urban Hospital	11936	11265	3.33	0.82	13.51	0.092
Hospital Region	12360					
Northeast		2528	1.00			

Table 3. Cont.

Predictor	Total N	Predictor N	OR	Lower 95%	Upper 95%	P
Midwest		2488	1.39	0.77	2.53	0.273
South		4125	1.13	0.65	1.98	0.669
West		3219	1.54	0.88	2.68	0.13
Teaching Hospital	11936	9156	2.16	1.23	3.79	0.007

with convulsive SE. The risk of aspiration was specifically found to be an independent risk factor for mortality in our study. Pneumonia was identified as a cause of death in a prior retrospective pediatric study [22], a pediatric prospective study [24], and in a pediatric drug trial for management of status epilepticus [25]. In our population it is unclear how many cases of pneumonia were causes or consequences of SE.

Sepsis and hemodynamic compromise. Sepsis emerged as an important risk factor for death in our pediatric population. Sepsis may occur as a consequence of pneumonia or from other infective foci. A retrospective study on pediatric ICU patients identified sepsis to be a major cause of death in children with prolonged (>45 minute) episodes of SE [8]. Another study on emergency management procedures in children presenting with SE also identified sepsis as a risk factor for death [26].

Infections may also be an important cause of SE, particularly in cases that were presumably induced by febrile illness or pneumonia [27]. Our study also identified postoperative sepsis with liver failure to be significant enough to constitute an independent risk factor, and this finding is also backed by a previous pediatric case series [28] and by another series on refractory pediatric SE [4]. Hemorrhagic shock was identified as a risk factor for death. In a trial comparing the use of phenytoin and midazolam in school-age children, hemorrhagic shock was noted as a cause of death [25].

Metabolic complications. Hypoglycemia emerged as an independent risk factor for death in pediatric convulsive SE. Hypoglycemia increased the risk of neurological sequelae in a prospective study in children [29]. Hypoglycemia may also be a cause of SE [10,16]. Metabolic complications were associated with an increased risk of mortality using univariate analysis. Previous work has noted similar findings [25] and has more specifically associated deaths to hyponatremia [26]. Liver dysfunction, as mentioned above, is another potential source of metabolic dysfunction.

Near drowning. Convulsive SE related to near-drowning episodes constituted an independent risk factor for mortality in our series and other studies [30]. Near-drowning episodes may occur as a consequence of seizures [31]. Conversely, SE may also occur as a result of cerebral anoxia following such an event [32].

Intracranial infections. The importance of brain infections in leading to SE or resulting in mortality has been noted in previous studies. A prospective pediatric study identified meningitis and encephalitis as causes of SE. Meningitis was also an

Table 4. Significant risk factors for death in pediatric patients with convulsive status epilepticus following multivariate analysis.

Predictor	Odds Ratio	P Value	Lower 95%	Upper 95%
African American Race	0.36	0.009	0.17	0.78
December Admission	3.38	<0.001	2.01	5.67
Admission Source				
Emergency Room	1.00	-	-	-
Birth	1.34	0.279	0.79	2.29
Outside Hospital	1.58	0.073	0.96	2.60
Outside Facility	2.05	0.159	0.75	5.56
Comorbidities				
Sepsis	10.14	<0.001	4.02	25.57
Hypoglycemia	5.79	0.004	1.75	19.16
Near Drowning	43.17	0.001	4.37	426.82
Hemorrhagic Shock	17.83	0.001	6.47	49.12
Structural Brain Lesion	7.01	<0.001	3.07	15.98
Massive Aspiration	9.11	0.008	1.77	47.01
Postoperative Sepsis with Liver Failure	14.44	<0.001	4.98	41.86
Procedures				
Transfusion	8.25	<0.001	4.32	15.78
Mechanical Ventilation >72 hours	9.03	<0.001	5.59	14.60

Table 5. Selected historical studies of status epilepticus with salient findings.

Author, Year and Study Design	Follow up	Mortality rate	Predictors/Risk Factors
Aicardi et al, 1970 [12] *Retrospective*	Discharge Unclear	4.2% (10/239) 11% (27/239)	Prolonged SE, cerebral disease
Chevrie et al, 1978 [19] *Prospective*	<4 year f/u	21/334 in 1st year	Symptomatic seizures, age <6 months
Dunn et al, 1988 [13] *Prospective*	Discharge	8.24% (8/97)	Severe pre-existing brain damage, meningitis and encephalopathy
Maytal et al, 1989 [41] *Retrospective with prospective follow-up*	13.2 months	7.2% (7/97)	Prolonged SE
DeLorenzo et al, 1992 [14] *Retrospective and prospective*	7 years	2.3% of children 25% in adults	Tumor, hematological disease, anoxia, metabolic and congenital malformations
Scholtes et al, 1996 [42] *Retrospective*	Discharge	11.5% (13/112)	Anoxia, presence of >1 complication, insufficient therapy, prolonged duration (>8 hrs)
Logroscino et al, 1997 [6] *Retrospective*	19 years	21% (38/184)	<1 year age, acute illness
Barnard et al, 1999 [22] *Retrospective*	Discharge 53 months	9.6% (5/52) 15.4% (8/52)	Brain tumors, metabolic disorder, multi-organ failure
Mah et al, 1999 [10] *Retrospective*	5 years	2% SE group 1.5% in NSE group	Drug overdose, sepsis, disseminated tuberculosis, congenital heart disease
Waterhouse et al, 1999 [34] *Prospective*	-	17.8% (5.2 in pediatric and 24%)	CNS infection, hypoxia, drug withdrawal, continuous SE
Berg et al, 2001 [9] *Prospective*	4 years	1.6% (10/613)	Neurodegenerative conditions, coexisting medical conditions
Callenbach et al, 2001 [24] *Retrospective*	4 years	1.9% (9/472)	Respiratory insufficiency, RSV infection, aspiration, brain herniation
Kim et al, 2001 [43] *Case series*	4 years	43.5% (10/23)	Acute symptomatic etiology, especially anoxia
Sahin et al, 2001 [4] Retrospective	8 years	31.8% (7/22)	Remote symptomatic and progressive encephalopathy
Tabarki et al, 2001 [44] *Retrospective*	7 years	15.8% (22/139)	Acute symptomatic seizure, progressive encephalopathy
Logroscino G et al 2002 [39] *Retrospective*	Unclear	43%	Prolonged SE (>24 hr), acute symptomatic etiology, myoclonic SE
Ogutu et al, 2002 [45] *Pharmacokinetics and clinical effects measurements*	Discharge	13.1% (5/38)	Intracranial hypertension, intractable convulsions
Sillanpää et al, 2002 [2] *Prospective*	Long follow up	16% (24/150)	Remote symptomatic cause, young patient (<6 yrs), partial seizures, history of febrile seizure
Singhi et al, 2002 [46] *Prospective*	Discharge	25% (10/40)	Early intubation and ventilation, meningoencephalitis, acute hyponatremia, hepatic encephalopathy
Wu et al, 2002 [3] *Retrospective*	Discharge	1.9% (55/2885)	Female sex, older age (>75)
KarasallhoGlu et al, 2003 [47] *Retrospective*	1 month	7.2% (6/83)	Polypharmacy, discontinuation of AEDs, neuromotor retardation, generalized background abnormality on EEG
Berg et al, 2004 [30] *Prospective*	Unclear	2.1% (13/613)	Neurodegenerative disorder ± epileptic encephalopathy, prolonged SE
Chin et al, 2004 [26] *Retrospective*	Discharge	5.1% (5/98)	Younger age, intubation, CNS infection, hyponatremia, hypoxia, sepsis, subdural hematoma
Asadi-Pooya et al, 2005 [48] *Retrospective*	Discharge	10.4% (14/135)	Prolonged febrile seizure, CNS infection, metabolic/AED withdrawal, symptomatic epilepsy, prolonged stay
Brevoord et al, 2005 [25] *Retrospective*	Discharge	5.7% (7/205)	Near drowning episode, pneumococcal meningitis, cardiac failure, brainstem tumor, hemorrhagic shock, metabolic defect
Gulati et al, 2005 [8] *Retrospective*	Discharge	30% (9/30)	Prolonged SE (>45 min), septic shock

Table 5. Cont.

Author, Year and Study Design	Follow up	Mortality rate	Predictors/Risk Factors
Kang et al, 2005 [23] *Retrospective*	Unclear	3%	Higher mortality in acute symptomatic SE versus remote symptomatic SE
Maegaki et al, 2005 [49] *Retrospective*	Discharge	3.8% (9/241)	Prolonged SE (>2 hr), moderate-severe asthma
Ozdemir et al, 2005 [11] *Retrospective*	Discharge	19% (5/27)	Acute symptomatic SE, progressive encephalopathy, underlying disease
Ahmad et al, 2006 [50] *Randomized controlled trial*	Discharge	17.5% (N = 160)	Progressive infection, cerebral malaria, febrile convulsions, acute bacterial meningitis, metabolic derangements
Chen et al, 2006 [51] *Population based study*	Discharge	3.1% (7/226)	Febrile illness, acute bacterial meningitis, progressive neurological disorders, intermittent SE.
Morrison et al, 2006 [33] *Retrospective*	Discharge	18% (3/17)	Subdural hematoma, birth asphyxia, post-cardiac arrest
Hayashi et al, 2007 [52] *Retrospective*	Discharge	2.1% (10/479)	Encephalitis, cerebrovascular disease
Muchochi et al, 2007 [53] *Non-randomized controlled*	Discharge	11.54% (3/26)	Pre-existing cerebral malaria, convulsions
Mpimbaza et al, 2008 [54] *Randomized controlled trial*	Discharge	6% (20/330)	Malaria, severe malnutrition, immunosuppression, pneumonia
Sadarangani et al, 2008 [29] *Retrospective*	Discharge	Confirmed convulsive SE: 19% (11/58) Probable convulsive SE: 11% (13/120)	Acute bacterial meningitis, age <1 year, hypoglycemia, focal onset seizures
Siddiqui et al, 2008 [55] *Retrospective*	Discharge	12% (15/125)	Acute intracranial infections, age <5 years, prolonged SE (5.93±5.76 hours)
Lin et al, 2009 [56] *Retrospective*	Stay in ICU Unclear	8.51% (12/141) 9.2% (13/141)	Febrile illness
Mei Li et al, 2009 [36] *Retrospective*	1 month	15.8% (32/203)	Mechanical ventilation, complications, SE duration after admission, hyponatremia, recurrent SE
Molinero et al, 2009 [27] *Prospective*	Discharge	13% (6/47)	Infectious cause, cerebrovascular accident, long seizure duration

AED – antiepileptic drug; SE – status epilepticus; CNS – central nervous system; ICU – intensive care unit; RSV – respiratory syncytial virus.

important risk factor for death [13]. Similar findings have been noted in prospective [29] and retrospective [26] pediatric studies. Human immunodeficiency virus-associated encephalitis was identified as a cause of SE in one previous pediatric study [4]. In our present data sample, we found intracranial infections, such as viral encephalitis and infectious encephalopathy, to be associated with mortality. These factors did not emerge as independent risk factors for death in multivariate analysis in this series.

Other comorbidities. Brain herniation was associated with an increased risk of death. Transtentorial herniation was identified as a long-term cause of death in a prior retrospective pediatric study [24]. Similarly, subdural hematoma, noted as a cause of death in a previous pediatric case series [33], was associated with mortality in our study. However, these factors were not found to be a significant risk factor for death in multivariate analysis. Unlike prior studies [34], patients with status following drug withdrawal did not have a higher mortality rate in this dataset.

Procedures

Blood Transfusion. We identified blood transfusion as a factor for fatalities. This additional risk is probably not a result of the transfusion in itself but is likely a marker for the poor clinical condition of certain patients who subsequently require greater intervention. While this finding was not corroborated by prior research, studies investigating patients with related markers of disease severity, such as those investigating ICU patients, have similarly high death rates [8,25].

Mechanical Ventilation. The need for ventilatory support in convulsive SE may arise from poor respiratory drive resulting from seizure complications or in the context of pharmacological coma induction. The risk of death in mechanical ventilation may be related to the risk of aspiration and impaired mucociliary clearance, leading to pneumonia [35]. Additionally, mechanical ventilation is also associated with complications such as pneumothorax and ventilator-associated lung injury. We confirmed mechanical ventilation as an independent risk factor for death in SE. Mechanical ventilation was associated with death in a prospective study that included adolescents and children [36]. Similar findings were noted in a randomized control trial comparing antiepileptic medications in the treatment of SE [37].

Risk factors assessment in SE. We investigated diagnostic entities due to their known association with high risk of mortality. The KID mentions all diagnoses encountered during a hospital admission irrespective of the cause-effect relationship between SE and associated diagnoses. Entities such as near drowning, hemorrhagic shock, structural brain lesion, and hypoglycemia (likely causes of SE), as well as sepsis, prolonged mechanical ventilation, and transfusion (likely resulting from SE or its treatment) increased mortality in children with convulsive SE. Awareness of these risks may thus promote more improved targeted management towards correcting these conditions.

Challenges. The findings of this study need to be interpreted in the setting of data acquisition and subsequent analysis. Misclassification of seizures and comorbidities in the ICD-9 coding system is a potential source of error, as it is with all large databases studies. Multiple criteria exist to diagnose SE. While the Working Group of SE of the Epilepsy Foundation of America defines SE as a seizure of at least 30 minutes duration or multiple seizures without full recovery of consciousness in between [1], other investigators advocate a cutoff time as short as five minutes [38]. Individual physicians may not use the same operational definitions, leading to variations in case reporting. The KID dataset lacks information on the timing of procedures, such as blood transfusion and intubation, which may also be important variables in determining the risk of death in SE. Patients who suffer from SE are noted to have an increased risk of dying that extends to weeks, and possibly years, after discharge [39]. This information is unavailable in the KID dataset. Because there are no unique patient identifiers in the KID dataset, it was not possible to account for multiple episodes of SE in the same patient. While neonates were included in this study, there is a lack of consensus on the definition of SE in these patients. This study was unable to investigate certain variables, such as seizure duration, and some etiologies, such as cerebrovascular accidents and malaria, which have been identified as important risk factors in other studies due to few numbers of these cases.

Conclusion

Convulsive SE is a rare but serious condition and results in approximately 0.1% of all pediatric inpatient hospital admissions. It is fatal in approximately 1% of cases. The rarity of this condition makes it a difficult subject to study. The use of large nationwide databases, such as the KID dataset permits identification of factors associated with increased mortality.

The findings from this study suggest new directions for research. Research should be done to determine which interventions may lead to improved outcomes. More data are needed to ascertain risk factors for long-term mortality in pediatric SE. Parallel research using large groups of adults should be done to establish risk factors for poor outcomes in this group. This may also help to identify risk factors that overlap between pediatric and adult populations. Prospective multicenter studies evaluating children presenting in SE may assist in better determination of risk factors for death and identify those interventions which best promote patient survival.

Our results may also carry implications for improvement of patient care. It is likely that in-hospital mortality of SE is largely a function of the underlying cause of the SE, while other factors may also have an impact on outcome. Some of these risk factors may be ameliorated with specific therapy. Mild induced hypothermia, for example, may be beneficial in patients with near-drowning episodes [40]. Early identification and treatment of some of these aggravating factors may not only prevent immediate mortality, but it may also reduce long-term complications and limit neurological dysfunction. Beyond these implications, the development of treatment paradigms may also help reduce variability in care and outcomes and thereby decrease hospital costs. This research may lead the development of warning algorithms which may in turn promote early interventions that reduce ICU admissions, other medical complications, and even death. Identification of risk factors is thus an important first step towards providing improved care when caring for pediatric patients with SE.

Acknowledgments

The authors would like to acknowledge the Healthcare Cost and Utilization and Project (HCUP) for provision of the KID Inpatient Database for this study.

Author Contributions

Conceived and designed the experiments: TL TS SR DG ST SK AA MK. Performed the experiments: TS DG ST AA. Analyzed the data: TS DG ST AA. Wrote the paper: SR TL MK TS.

References

1. Working Group on Status Epilepticus (1993) Treatment of convulsive status epilepticus. Recommendations of the Epilepsy Foundation of America's Working Group on Status Epilepticus. JAMA 270: 854–859.
2. Sillanpaa M, Shinnar S (2002) Status epilepticus in a population-based cohort with childhood-onset epilepsy in Finland. Ann Neurol 52: 303–310.
3. Wu YW, Shek DW, Garcia PA, Zhao S, Johnston SC (2002) Incidence and mortality of generalized convulsive status epilepticus in California. Neurology 58: 1070–1076.
4. Sahin M, Menache CC, Holmes GL, Riviello JJ (2001) Outcome of severe refractory status epilepticus in children. Epilepsia 42: 1461–1467.
5. Koubeissi M, Alshekhlee A (2007) In-hospital mortality of generalized convulsive status epilepticus: a large US sample. Neurology 69: 886–893.
6. Logroscino G, Hesdorffer DC, Cascino G, Annegers JF, Hauser WA (1997) Short-term mortality after a first episode of status epilepticus. Epilepsia 38: 1344–1349.
7. Agency for Healthcare Research and Quality (2011) Overview of the Kids' Inpatient Database (KID). Available: http://www.hcup-us.ahrq.gov/kidoverview.jsp. Accessed 2011 Dec 20.
8. Gulati S, Kalra V, Sridhar MR (2005) Status epilepticus in Indian children in a tertiary care center. Indian J Pediatr 72: 105–108.
9. Berg AT, Shinnar S, Levy SR, Testa FM, Smith-Rapaport S, et al. (2001) Early development of intractable epilepsy in children: a prospective study. Neurology 56: 1445–1452.
10. Mah JK, Mah MW (1999) Pediatric status epilepticus: a perspective from Saudi Arabia. Pediatr Neurol 20: 364–369.
11. Ozdemir D, Gulez P, Uran N, Yendur G, Kavakli T, et al. (2005) Efficacy of continuous midazolam infusion and mortality in childhood refractory generalized convulsive status epilepticus. Seizure 14: 129–132.
12. Aicardi J, Chevrie JJ (1970) Convulsive status epilepticus in infants and children. A study of 239 cases. Epilepsia 11: 187–197.
13. Dunn DW (1988) Status epilepticus in children: etiology, clinical features, and outcome. J Child Neurol 3: 167–173.
14. DeLorenzo RJ, Towne AR, Pellock JM, Ko D (1992) Status epilepticus in children, adults, and the elderly. Epilepsia 33 Suppl 4: S15–25.
15. Banerjee PN, Hauser WA (2007) Incidence and Prevalence. In: Engel J, Pedley TA, Aicardi J, Dichter MA, Moshé S et al., editors. Epilepsy: A Comprehensive Textbook: Lippincott Williams & Wilkins. pp. 45–56.
16. DeLorenzo RJ, Hauser WA, Towne AR, Boggs JG, Pellock JM, et al. (1996) A prospective, population-based epidemiologic study of status epilepticus in Richmond, Virginia. Neurology 46: 1029–1035.
17. Knake S, Rosenow F, Vescovi M, Oertel WH, Mueller HH, et al. (2001) Incidence of status epilepticus in adults in Germany: a prospective, population-based study. Epilepsia 42: 714–718.
18. Logroscino G, Hesdorffer DC, Cascino G, Hauser WA, Coeytaux A, et al. (2005) Mortality after a first episode of status epilepticus in the United States and Europe. Epilepsia 46 Suppl 11: 46–48.
19. Chevrie JJ, Aicardi J (1979) Convulsive disorders in the first year of life: persistence of epileptic seizures. Epilepsia 20: 643–649.
20. Sharip A, Sorvillo F, Redelings MD, Mascola L, Wise M, et al. (2006) Population-based analysis of meningococcal disease mortality in the United States: 1990–2002. Pediatr Infect Dis J 25: 191–194.
21. Day JF, Shaman J (2009) Severe winter freezes enhance St. Louis encephalitis virus amplification and epidemic transmission in peninsular Florida. J Med Entomol 46: 1498–1506.
22. Barnard C, Wirrell E (1999) Does status epilepticus in children cause developmental deterioration and exacerbation of epilepsy? J Child Neurol 14: 787–794.
23. Kang DC, Lee YM, Lee J, Kim HD, Coe C (2005) Prognostic factors of status epilepticus in children. Yonsei Med J 46: 27–33.

24. Callenbach PM, Westendorp RG, Geerts AT, Arts WF, Peeters EA, et al. (2001) Mortality risk in children with epilepsy: the Dutch study of epilepsy in childhood. Pediatrics 107: 1259–1263.
25. Brevoord JC, Joosten KF, Arts WF, van Rooij RW, de Hoog M (2005) Status epilepticus: clinical analysis of a treatment protocol based on midazolam and phenytoin. J Child Neurol 20: 476–481.
26. Chin RF, Verhulst L, Neville BG, Peters MJ, Scott RC (2004) Inappropriate emergency management of status epilepticus in children contributes to need for intensive care. J Neurol Neurosurg Psychiatry 75: 1584–1588.
27. Molinero MR, Holden KR, Rodriguez LC, Collins JS, Samra JA, et al. (2009) Pediatric convulsive status epilepticus in Honduras, Central America. Epilepsia 50: 2314–2319.
28. Kramer U, Shorer Z, Ben-Zeev B, Lerman-Sagie T, Goldberg-Stern H, et al. (2005) Severe refractory status epilepticus owing to presumed encephalitis. J Child Neurol 20: 184–187.
29. Sadarangani M, Seaton C, Scott JA, Ogutu B, Edwards T, et al. (2008) Incidence and outcome of convulsive status epilepticus in Kenyan children: a cohort study. Lancet Neurol 7: 145–150.
30. Berg AT, Shinnar S, Testa FM, Levy SR, Frobish D, et al. (2004) Status epilepticus after the initial diagnosis of epilepsy in children. Neurology 63: 1027–1034.
31. Ryan CA, Dowling G (1993) Drowning deaths in people with epilepsy. CMAJ 148: 781–784.
32. Wilson FC, Harpur J, Watson T, Morrow JI (2003) Adult survivors of severe cerebral hypoxia–case series survey and comparative analysis. NeuroRehabilitation 18: 291–298.
33. Morrison G, Gibbons E, Whitehouse WP (2006) High-dose midazolam therapy for refractory status epilepticus in children. Intensive Care Med 32: 2070–2076.
34. Waterhouse EJ, Garnett LK, Towne AR, Morton LD, Barnes T, et al. (1999) Prospective population-based study of intermittent and continuous convulsive status epilepticus in Richmond, Virginia. Epilepsia 40: 752–758.
35. Konrad F, Schreiber T, Brecht-Kraus D, Georgieff M (1994) Mucociliary transport in ICU patients. Chest 105: 237–241.
36. Li JM, Chen L, Zhou B, Zhu Y, Zhou D (2009) Convulsive status epilepticus in adults and adolescents of southwest China: mortality, etiology, and predictors of death. Epilepsy Behav 14: 146–149.
37. Prasad K, Krishnan PR, Al-Roomi K, Sequeira R (2007) Anticonvulsant therapy for status epilepticus. Br J Clin Pharmacol 63: 640–647.
38. Lowenstein DH, Bleck T, Macdonald RL (1999) It's time to revise the definition of status epilepticus. Epilepsia 40: 120–122.
39. Logroscino G, Hesdorffer DC, Cascino GD, Annegers JF, Bagiella E, et al. (2002) Long-term mortality after a first episode of status epilepticus. Neurology 58: 537–541.
40. de Pont AC, de Jager CP, van den Bergh WM, Schultz MJ (2011) Recovery from near drowning and postanoxic status epilepticus with controlled hypothermia. Neth J Med 69: 196–197.
41. Maytal J, Shinnar S, Moshe SL, Alvarez LA (1989) Low morbidity and mortality of status epilepticus in children. Pediatrics 83: 323–331.
42. Scholtes FB, Renier WO, Meinardi H (1996) Status epilepticus in children. Seizure 5: 177–184.
43. Kim SJ, Lee DY, Kim JS (2001) Neurologic outcomes of pediatric epileptic patients with pentobarbital coma. Pediatr Neurol 25: 217–220.
44. Tabarki B, Yacoub M, Selmi H, Oubich F, Barsaoui S, et al. (2001) Infantile status epilepticus in Tunisia. Clinical, etiological and prognostic aspects. Seizure 10: 365–369.
45. Ogutu BR, Newton CR, Crawley J, Muchohi SN, Otieno GO, et al. (2002) Pharmacokinetics and anticonvulsant effects of diazepam in children with severe falciparum malaria and convulsions. Br J Clin Pharmacol 53: 49–57.
46. Singhi S, Murthy A, Singhi P, Jayashree M (2002) Continuous midazolam versus diazepam infusion for refractory convulsive status epilepticus. J Child Neurol 17: 106–110.
47. KarasalIhoGlu S, Oner N, CeLtik C, Celik Y, Biner B, et al. (2003) Risk factors of status epilepticus in children. Pediatr Int 45: 429–434.
48. Asadi-Pooya AA, Poordast A (2005) Etiologies and outcomes of status epilepticus in children. Epilepsy Behav 7: 502–505.
49. Maegaki Y, Kurozawa Y, Hanaki K, Ohno K (2005) Risk factors for fatality and neurological sequelae after status epilepticus in children. Neuropediatrics 36: 186–192.
50. Ahmad S, Ellis JC, Kamwendo H, Molyneux E (2006) Efficacy and safety of intranasal lorazepam versus intramuscular paraldehyde for protracted convulsions in children: an open randomised trial. Lancet 367: 1591–1597.
51. Chen L, Zhou B, Li JM, Zhu Y, Wang JH, et al. (2009) Clinical features of convulsive status epilepticus: a study of 220 cases in western China. Eur J Neurol 16: 444–449.
52. Hayashi K, Osawa M, Aihara M, Izumi T, Ohtsuka Y, et al. (2007) Efficacy of intravenous midazolam for status epilepticus in childhood. Pediatr Neurol 36: 366–372.
53. Muchohi SN, Obiero K, Newton CR, Ogutu BR, Edwards G, et al. (2008) Pharmacokinetics and clinical efficacy of lorazepam in children with severe malaria and convulsions. Br J Clin Pharmacol 65: 12–21.
54. Mpimbaza A, Ndeezi G, Staedke S, Rosenthal PJ, Byarugaba J (2008) Comparison of buccal midazolam with rectal diazepam in the treatment of prolonged seizures in Ugandan children: a randomized clinical trial. Pediatrics 121: e58–64.
55. Siddiqui TS, Anis ur R, Jan MA, Wazeer MS, Burki MK (2008) Status epilepticus: aetiology and outcome in children. J Ayub Med Coll Abbottabad 20: 51–53.
56. Lin KL, Lin JJ, Hsia SH, Wu CT, Wang HS (2009) Analysis of convulsive status epilepticus in children of Taiwan. Pediatr Neurol 41: 413–418.

Permissions

All chapters in this book were first published in PLOS ONE, by The Public Library of Science; hereby published with permission under the Creative Commons Attribution License or equivalent. Every chapter published in this book has been scrutinized by our experts. Their significance has been extensively debated. The topics covered herein carry significant findings which will fuel the growth of the discipline. They may even be implemented as practical applications or may be referred to as a beginning point for another development.

The contributors of this book come from diverse backgrounds, making this book a truly international effort. This book will bring forth new frontiers with its revolutionizing research information and detailed analysis of the nascent developments around the world.

We would like to thank all the contributing authors for lending their expertise to make the book truly unique. They have played a crucial role in the development of this book. Without their invaluable contributions this book wouldn't have been possible. They have made vital efforts to compile up to date information on the varied aspects of this subject to make this book a valuable addition to the collection of many professionals and students.

This book was conceptualized with the vision of imparting up-to-date information and advanced data in this field. To ensure the same, a matchless editorial board was set up. Every individual on the board went through rigorous rounds of assessment to prove their worth. After which they invested a large part of their time researching and compiling the most relevant data for our readers.

The editorial board has been involved in producing this book since its inception. They have spent rigorous hours researching and exploring the diverse topics which have resulted in the successful publishing of this book. They have passed on their knowledge of decades through this book. To expedite this challenging task, the publisher supported the team at every step. A small team of assistant editors was also appointed to further simplify the editing procedure and attain best results for the readers.

Apart from the editorial board, the designing team has also invested a significant amount of their time in understanding the subject and creating the most relevant covers. They scrutinized every image to scout for the most suitable representation of the subject and create an appropriate cover for the book.

The publishing team has been an ardent support to the editorial, designing and production team. Their endless efforts to recruit the best for this project, has resulted in the accomplishment of this book. They are a veteran in the field of academics and their pool of knowledge is as vast as their experience in printing. Their expertise and guidance has proved useful at every step. Their uncompromising quality standards have made this book an exceptional effort. Their encouragement from time to time has been an inspiration for everyone.

The publisher and the editorial board hope that this book will prove to be a valuable piece of knowledge for researchers, students, practitioners and scholars across the globe.

List of Contributors

Margarita M. Correa
Grupo de Microbiología Molecular, Escuela de Microbiología, Universidad de Antioquia, Medellín, Colombia

Erika A. Rodríguez and J. Natalia Jiménez
Grupo de Investigación en Microbiología Básica y Aplicada- MICROBA, Escuela de Microbiología Universidad de Antioquia, Medellín, Colombia

Sigifredo Ospina and Santiago L. Atehortúa
Hospital Universitario de San Vicente Fundación, Medellín, Colombia

Xiaoxia Wang and Sherry Towers
Mathematical, Computational and Modeling Sciences Center, School of Human Evolution and Social Change, Arizona State University, Tempe, Arizona, United States of America

Gerardo Chowell
Mathematical, Computational and Modeling Sciences Center, School of Human Evolution and Social Change, Arizona State University, Tempe, Arizona, United States of America
Division of Epidemiology and Population Studies, Fogarty International Center, National Institutes of Health, Bethesda, Maryland, United States of America

Sarada Panchanathan
Department of Pediatrics, Maricopa Integrated Health System, Phoenix, Arizona, United States of America
Department of Biomedical Informatics, Arizona State University, Tempe, Arizona, United States of America

Andrew Copas
University College London, Research Department of Infection and Population Health, London, United Kingdom

Raluca Buzdugan
University College London, Research Department of Infection and Population Health, London, United Kingdom
University of California, Berkeley, School of Public Health, Berkeley, California, United States of America

Frances M. Cowan
University College London, Research Department of Infection and Population Health, London, United Kingdom
University of Zimbabwe, ZAPP-UZ, Community Medicine, Harare, Zimbabwe

Constancia Watadzaushe, Jeffrey Dirawo and Lisa Langhaug
University of Zimbabwe, ZAPP-UZ, Community Medicine, Harare, Zimbabwe

Oscar Mundida
National AIDS Council, Harare, Zimbabwe

Nicola Willis
Africaid, Harare, Zimbabwe

Karin Hatzold
Population Services International, Harare, Zimbabwe

Getrude Ncube and Owen Mugurungi
Ministry of Health and Child Welfare, Harare, Zimbabwe

Clemens Benedikt
UNFPA, Harare, Zimbabwe

Olufunke Fasawe
Master of International Health Management, Economics and Policy Program, SDA Bocconi School of Management, Milan, Italy

Carlos Avila
Senior Health Economist, Principal Associate, Abt Associates, Bethesda, Maryland, United States of America

Nathan Shaffer
PMTCT Technical Lead, HIV Department, World Health Organization, Geneva, Switzerland

Erik Schouten
HIV Advisor, Management Sciences for Health, Lilongwe, Malawi

Frank Chimbwandira
Director of the HIV and AIDS Department, Ministry of Health, Lilongwe, Malawi

David Hoos
Assistant Professor of Clinical Epidemiology, Senior Implementation Director, ICAP, Columbia University, Mailman School of Public Health, New York, New York, United States of America

Olive Nakakeeto
Health Economist, Independent Consultant, Saint-Genis-Poully, France,

Paul De Lay
Deputy Executive Director, Joint United Nations Programme on HIV/AIDS (UNAIDS), Geneva, Switzerland

Ana Julia Velez Rueda and Alicia Susana Mistchenko
Laboratorio de Virología, Hospital de Nin˜ os "Dr. Ricardo Gutiérrez", Ciudad Autónoma de Buenos Aires, Argentina
Comisión de Investigaciones Científicas (CIC), La Plata, Provincia de Buenos Aires, Argentina

Mariana Viegas
Laboratorio de Virología, Hospital de Nin˜ os "Dr. Ricardo Gutiérrez", Ciudad Autónoma de Buenos Aires, Argentina
Consejo Nacional de Investigaciones Científicas y Técnicas (CONICET), Ciudad Autónoma de Buenos Aires, Argentina

Nei-Yuan Hsiao
Division of Virology, University of Cape Town and National Health Laboratory Service, Cape Town, South Africa

Kathryn Stinson and Landon Myer
Centre for Infectious Diseases Epidemiology and Research, School of Public Health and Family Medicine, University of Cape Town, Cape Town, South Africa

Zhuo Zhou, Xin Gao, Yaying Wang, Hongli Zhou, Chao Wu, Li Guo and Jianwei Wang
MOH Key Laboratory of Systems Biology of Pathogens and Christophe Mérieux Laboratory, IPB, CAMS-Fondation Mérieux, Institute of Pathogen Biology (IPB), Chinese Academy of Medical Sciences (CAMS) and Peking Union Medical College (PUMC), Beijing, People's Republic of China

Gláucia Paranhos-Baccalà and Guy Vernet
Fondation Mérieux, Lyon, France

Miguel de Mulder, Gonzalo Yebra and África Holguín
HIV-1 Molecular Epidemiology Laboratory, Microbiology and Parasitology Department, Hospital Universitario Ramón y Cajal, IRYCIS and CIBER-ESP, Madrid, Spain

Adriana Navas
Pediatrics Department, Hospital Universitario Infanta Leonor, Madrid, Spain

María Isabel de José
Pediatrics Department, Hospital Universitario La Paz, Madrid, Spain

María Dolores Gurbindo and Jesús Saavedra-Lozano
Pediatrics Department, Hospital General Universitario Gregorio Marañón, Madrid, Spain

María Isabel González-Tomé
Pediatrics Department, Hospital Universitario Doce de Octubre, Madrid, Spain

María José Mellado
Pediatrics Department, Hospital Carlos III, Madrid, Spain

María Ángeles Munñoz-Fernández and Santiago Jiménez de Ory
Molecular Immunobiology Laboratory, Hospital General Universitario Gregorio Marañón, Madrid, Spain

José Tomás Ramos
Pediatrics Department, Hospital Universitario de Getafe, Madrid, Spain

Chia-Jie Lee
Department of Pediatrics, Chang Gung Memorial Hospital at Linkou, Kweishan, Taoyuan, Taiwan

Yhu-Chering Huang, Chih-Jung Chen, Yu-Chia Hsieh, Cheng-Hsun Chiu and Tzou-Yien Lin
Department of Pediatrics, Chang Gung Memorial Hospital at Linkou, Kweishan, Taoyuan, Taiwan
Chang Gung University College of Medicine, Kweishan, Taoyuan, Taiwan

Shuan Yang and Kuo-Chien Tsao
Chang Gung University College of Medicine, Kweishan, Taoyuan, Taiwan
Department of Laboratory Medicine, Chang Gung Memorial Hospital at Linkou, Kweishan, Taoyuan, Taiwan

Ravi Tandon and Lishomwa C. Ndhlovu
Hawaii Center for AIDS, Department of Tropical Medicine, John A. Burns School of Medicine, University of Hawaii, Honolulu, Hawaii, United States of America

Devi SenGupta, Vanessa A. York and Douglas F. Nixon
Division of Experimental Medicine, University of California San Francisco, San Francisco, California, United States of America

Maria T. M. Giret and Esper G. Kallas
Division of Clinical Immunology and Allergy, University of São Paulo, São Paulo, Brazil

Andrew A. Wiznia and Michael G. Rosenberg
Albert Einstein College of Medicine, Bronx, New York, United States of America

René Geyeregger, Christine Freimüller, Julia Stemberger and Jasmin Dmytrus
Department of Clinical Cell Biology and FACS Core Unit, Children's Cancer Research Institute (CCRI), Vienna, Austria

Gerhard Fritsch
Department of Clinical Cell Biology and FACS Core Unit, Children's Cancer Research Institute (CCRI), Vienna, Austria
Department Pediatrics, Medical University of Vienna, Vienna, Austria

Thomas Lion
Department Pediatrics, Medical University of Vienna, Vienna, Austria
Department of Molecular Microbiology, Children's Cancer Research Institute (CCRI), Vienna, Austria

Anita Lawitschka and Susanne Matthes
Department Pediatrics, Medical University of Vienna, Vienna, Austria
Department of Stem Cell Transplantation, St. Anna Children's Hospital, Vienna, Austria

Stefan Stevanovic, Gabor Mester and Hans-Georg Rammensee
Department of Immunology, Institute for Cell Biology, Eberhard-Karls-Universität Tübingen, Tübingen, Germany

Gottfried Fischer
Department of Blood Group Serology and Transfusion Medicine, Medical University of Vienna, Vienna, Austria

Britta Eiz-Vesper
Institute for Transfusion Medicine, Hannover Medical School, Hannover, Germany

Patrícia Machado, Cláudia Gomes, Cristina Mendes, João Pinto, Virgílio E. do Rosário and Ana Paula Arez
Centro de Malária e outras Doenças Tropicais, Unidade de Parasitologia Médica, Instituto de Higiene e Medicina Tropical, Universidade Nova de Lisboa, Lisboa, Portugal

Licínio Manco
Centro de Investigação em Antropologia e Saúde (CIAS), Universidade de Coimbra, Coimbra, Portugal

Natércia Fernandes, Graça Salomé, Luis Sitoe and Sérgio Chibute
Faculdade de Medicina da Universidade Eduardo Mondlane, Maputo, Mozambique

José Langa
Banco de Sangue do Hospital Central de Maputo, Maputo, Mozambique

Letícia Ribeiro
Departmento de Hematologia, Centro Hospitalar de Coimbra, Coimbra, Portugal

Juliana Miranda
Hospital Pediátrico David Bernardino, Luanda, Angola

Jorge Cano
Centro Nacional de Medicina Tropical, Instituto de Salud Carlos III, Madrid, Spain

António Amorim
Instituto de Patologia e Imunologia Molecular da Universidade do Porto (IPATIMUP), Porto, Portugal
Faculdade de Ciências da Universidade do Porto, Porto, Portugal

Zhiqiang Hu, Lili Liu and Min Chen
Department of Pharmacy, West China Second University Hospital, Sichuan University, Sichuan, China
West China School of Pharmacy, Sichuan University, Sichuan, China

Linan Zeng, Lingli Zhang and Yuan Chen
Department of Pharmacy, West China Second University Hospital, Sichuan University, Sichuan, China
Key Laboratory of Birth Defects and Related Diseases of Women and Children, Sichuan University, Ministry of Education, Sichuan, China
Evidence-Based Pharmacy Centre, West China Second University Hospital, Sichuan University, Sichuan, China

Emily A. Ehle
Department of Pharmacy, The Nebraska Medical Centre, Omaha, Nebraska, United States of America

Emily H. Stewart
Walter Reed National Military Medical Center, Bethesda, Maryland, United States of America

Brian Davis
University of Texas Southwestern Medical Center, Dallas, Texas, United States of America

B. Lee Clemans-Taylor and Robert M. Centor
The University of Alabama at Birmingham, Huntsville Campus, Huntsville, Alabama, United States of America

Benjamin Littenberg
University of Vermont, Burlington, Vermont, United States of America

Carlos A. Estrada
University of Alabama at Birmingham, Birmingham, Alabama, United States of America
Birmingham Veterans Affairs Medical Center and Veterans Affairs Quality Scholar Program, Birmingham, Alabama, United States of America

Solange Ouédraogo, Blaise Traoré, Zah Ange Brice Nene Bi, Firmin Tiandama Yonli, Donatien Kima, Pierre Bonané, Lassané Congo, Rasmata Ouédraogo Traoré and Diarra Yé
Charles de Gaulle Pediatric University Hospital, Ouagadougou, Burkina Faso

Christophe Marguet
Respiratory Diseases, Allergy and CF Unit, Paediatric Department, Rouen University Hospital Charles Nicolle, EA3830, Inserm CIC204, Rouen, France

Jean-Christophe Plantier and Marie Gueudin
Laboratory of Virology, GRAM EA 2656 Rouen University Hospital Charles Nicolle, Rouen, France

Astrid Vabret
Laboratory of Human and Molecular Virology, Caen University Hospital Clemenceau, Caen, France

Malik Coulibaly, Elisabeth Thio and Issa Siribié
Projet MONOD ANRS 12206, Centre de Recherche Internationale pour la Santé, Site ANRS Burkina, Université de Ouagadougou, Ouagadougou, Burkina Faso

Nicolas Meda
Projet MONOD ANRS 12206, Centre de Recherche Internationale pour la Santé, Site ANRS Burkina, Université de Ouagadougou, Ouagadougou, Burkina Faso
Centre Muraz, Bobo Dioulasso, Burkina Faso

Caroline Yonaba and Ludovic Kam
Service de Pédiatrie, CHU Yalgado Ouédraogo, Ouagadougou, Burkina Faso

Sylvie Ouedraogo, Fla Koueta and Diarra Ye
Service de Pédiatrie Médicale, CHU Charles de Gaulle, Ouagadougou, Burkina Faso

Malika Congo
Laboratoire de Bactériologie - Virologie CHU Yalgado Ouédraogo, Ouagadougou, Burkina Faso

Mamoudou Barry
Service de laboratoire, CHU Charles de Gaulle, Ouagadougou, Burkina Faso

Stéphane Blanche
Groupe hospitalier Necker- Enfants malades, Paris, France

Phillipe Van De Perre
Inserm U1058, Université Montpellier 1, Montpellier, France

Valériane Leroy
Inserm, U897, Institut de Santé Publique, Epidémiologie et Développement (ISPED), Université de Bordeaux, Bordeaux, France

Evelien Kerkhof, Henriette A. Moll and Rianne Oostenbrink
Erasmus MC-Sophia Children's Hospital, Department of General Pediatrics, Rotterdam, The Netherlands

Monica Lakhanpaul
Department of General and Adolescent Pediatrics, University College London, Institute of Child Health, London, United Kingdom

Samiran Ray
Pediatric Intensive Care Unit, Great Ormond Street Hospital, London, United Kingdom

Jan Y. Verbakel
Department of General Practice, Katholieke Universiteit Leuven, Leuven, Belgium

Ann Van den Bruel and Matthew Thompson
Department of Primary Care Health Sciences, University of Oxford, Radcliffe Observatory Quarter, Oxford, United Kingdom

Marjolein Y. Berger
Department of General Practice, University Groningen, University Medical Centre Groningen, Groningen, The Netherlands

Narcisse Muganga
Kigali University Teaching Hospital, Department of Pediatrics, Kigali, Rwanda

Philippe R. Mutwa
Kigali University Teaching Hospital, Department of Pediatrics, Kigali, Rwanda

Department of Global Health and Amsterdam Institute for Global Health and Development, Academic Medical Center, Amsterdam, The Netherlands

Brenda Asiimwe-Kateera, Joep M. A. Lange and Peter Reiss
Department of Global Health and Amsterdam Institute for Global Health and Development, Academic Medical Center, Amsterdam, The Netherlands

Sibyl P. M. Geelen
Department of Global Health and Amsterdam Institute for Global Health and Development, Academic Medical Center, Amsterdam, The Netherlands
Wilhelmina Children's Hospital, University Medical Centre Utrecht, Utrecht, The Netherlands

Kimberly R. Boer
Department of Global Health and Amsterdam Institute for Global Health and Development, Academic Medical Center, Amsterdam, The Netherlands
Biomedical Research, Epidemiology Unit, Royal Tropical Institute, Amsterdam, The Netherlands

Janneke van de Wijgert
Department of Global Health and Amsterdam Institute for Global Health and Development, Academic Medical Center, Amsterdam, The Netherlands
Institute of Infection and Global Health, University of Liverpool, Liverpool, United of Kingdom
Rinda Ubuzima, Kigali, Rwanda

Diane Tuyishimire
Outpatients Clinic, Treatment and Research on HIV/AIDS Centre, Kigali, Rwanda

Anita Asiimwe
Ministry of Health of Rwanda, Kigali, Rwanda

Dodi Safari and Miftahuddin Majid Khoeri
Eijkman Institute for Molecular Biology, Jakarta, Indonesia

Nia Kurniati
Department of Child Health, Dr. Cipto Mangunkusumo Hospital/Faculty of Medicine Universitas Indonesia, Jakarta, Indonesia

Lia Waslia
Eijkman Oxford Clinical Research Unit, Jakarta, Indonesia

Tiara Putri
Faculty of Biology, Gajah Mada University, Yogyakarta, Indonesia

Debby Bogaert and Krzysztof Trzciński
Department of Pediatric Immunology and Infectious Diseases, Wilhelmina's Children Hospital, University Medical Center Utrecht, Utrecht, the Netherlands

Elise Martin and Thomas Blanchais
CHU Nantes, Hôpital de la Mére et de l9Enfant, Clinique médicale pédiatrique, Faculté de médecine de Nantes, Nantes, France

Elise Launay
CHU Nantes, Hôpital de la Mére et de l9Enfant, Clinique médicale pédiatrique, Faculté de médecine de Nantes, Nantes, France
Inserm U1153, Obstetrical, Perinatal and Pediatric Epidemiology Research Team, Research Center for Epidemiology and Biostatistics Sorbonne Paris Cité (CRESS), Paris Descartes University, Paris, France

Christéle Gras-Le Guen
CHU Nantes, Hôpital de la Mére et de l9Enfant, Clinique médicale pédiatrique, Faculté de médecine de Nantes, Nantes, France
3 CHU Nantes, Hôpital de la Mére et de l9Enfant, Urgences pe´diatriques, Faculte´ de médecine de Nantes, Nantes, France

Catherine Deneux-Tharaux
Inserm U1153, Obstetrical, Perinatal and Pediatric Epidemiology Research Team, Research Center for Epidemiology and Biostatistics Sorbonne Paris Cité (CRESS), Paris Descartes University, Paris, France

Martin Chalumeau
Inserm U1153, Obstetrical, Perinatal and Pediatric Epidemiology Research Team, Research Center for Epidemiology and Biostatistics Sorbonne Paris Cité (CRESS), Paris Descartes University, Paris, France
Hôpital Necker Enfants Malades, AP-HP, Service de pédiatrie générale, Paris Descartes University, Paris, France

Alain Martinot
CHU de Lille, Hôpital R. Salengro, Unité d'urgences pédiatriques et de maladies infectieuses, Université de Lille-Nord de France, Lille, France

Rémy Assathiany
Association pour le Recherche et l9Enseignement en Pédiatrie Générale (AREPEGE); Association Française de Pédiatrie Ambulatoire (AFPA), Cabinet de Pédiatrie, Issy-les-Moulineaux, France

Jean-Christophe Rozé
CHU Nantes, Hôpital de la Mère et de l9Enfant, Réanimation pédiatrique et néonatale, Faculté de médecine de Nantes, Nantes, France

Alain Moreau and Francis Barin
Université François-Rabelais, Institut National de la Santé et de la Recherche Médicale - Unité 966 et Laboratoire de Virologie, Centre Hopsitalier Universitaire Bretonneau, Tours, France

Antoine Chaillon
Université François-Rabelais, Institut National de la Santé et de la Recherche Médicale - Unité 966 et Laboratoire de Virologie, Centre Hopsitalier Universitaire Bretonneau, Tours, France
University of California San Diego, Department of Pathology, San Diego, California, United States of America

Tanawan Samleerat
Université François-Rabelais, Institut National de la Santé et de la Recherche Médicale - Unité 966 et Laboratoire de Virologie, Centre Hopsitalier Universitaire Bretonneau, Tours, France
Faculty of Associated Medical Sciences, Chiang Mai University, Chiang Mai, Thailand

Sara Gianella
University of California San Diego, Department of Pathology, San Diego, California, United States of America

Faustine Zoveda, Sébastien Ballesteros and Frantz Depaulis
Laboratoire Ecologie et Evolution, Centre National de la Recherche Scientifique - Unité Mixte de Recherche 7625-Ecole Normale Supérieure, Paris, France

Nicole Ngo-Giang-Huong, Gonzague Jourdain and Marc Lallemant
Institut de Recherche pour le Développement, Chiang Mai, Thailand
Harvard School of Public Health, Department of Immunology and Infectious Diseases, Boston, Massachusetts, United States of America

Erica L. Pufall, Jeffrey W. Eaton, Laura Robertson and Simon Gregson
Department of Infectious Disease Epidemiology, Imperial College London, St. Mary's Campus, Norfolk Place, London, United Kingdom

Constance Nyamukapa
Department of Infectious Disease Epidemiology, Imperial College London, St. Mary's Campus, Norfolk Place, London, United Kingdom
Biomedical Research and Training Institute, Avondale, Harare, Zimbabwe

Reggie Mutsindiri, Godwin Chawira and Shungu Munyati
Biomedical Research and Training Institute, Avondale, Harare, Zimbabwe

Gerardo Alvarez-Uria, Raghavakalyan Pakam, Praveen Kumar Naik and Manoranjan Midde
Department of Infectious Diseases, Rural Development Trust Hospital, Bathalapalli, AP, India

Julie A. Cakebread, Hans Michael Haitchi and Yunhe Xu
Academic Unit of Clinical and Experimental Sciences, University of Southampton Faculty of Medicine, University Hospital Southampton, Southampton, United Kingdom

Stephen T. Holgate, Graham Roberts and Donna E. Davies
Academic Unit of Clinical and Experimental Sciences, University of Southampton Faculty of Medicine, University Hospital Southampton, Southampton, United Kingdom
NIHR Respiratory Biomedical Research Unit, University Hospital Southampton, Southampton, United Kingdom

Rong Zhou
State Key Laboratory of Respiratory Diseases, Guangzhou Medical University, Guangzhou, People's Republic of China

Michael A. Pfaller
JMI Laboratories, North Liberty, Iowa, United States of America
Department of Pathology, University of Iowa, Iowa City, Iowa, United States of America

Daniel J. Diekema
Department of Pathology, University of Iowa, Iowa City, Iowa, United States of America

David R. Andes
Department of Medicine, University of Wisconsin, Madison, Wisconsin, United States of America

Amer Alshekhlee
Department of Neurology, St Louis University, St. Louis, Missouri, United States of America

Lin Xu, Xia He, Ding-mei Zhang, Fa-shen Feng, Zhu Wang, Lin-lin Guan, Jueheng Wu, Meng-feng Li and Kai-yuan Cao
Department of Microbiology, Zhongshan School of Medicine, Sun Yat-sen University, Guangzhou, People's Republic of China

Key Laboratory of Tropical Disease Control, Ministry of Education, Sun Yat-Sen University, Guangzhou, People's Republic of China
Sun Yat-sen University - University of Hong Kong Joint Laboratory of Infectious Disease Surveillance, Sun Yat-sen University, Guangzhou, People's Republic of China

Bo-jian Zheng and Kwok-yung Yuen
Sun Yat-sen University - University of Hong Kong Joint Laboratory of Infectious Disease Surveillance, Sun Yat-sen University, Guangzhou, People's Republic of China
Department of Microbiology, University of Hong Kong, Hong Kong SAR, China

Diane S. Lauderdale and Jocelyn Wilder
Department of Health Studies, University of Chicago, Chicago, Illinois, United States of America

Michael Z. David
Department of Health Studies, University of Chicago, Chicago, Illinois, United States of America
Department of Pediatrics, University of Chicago, Chicago, Illinois, United States of America
Department of Medicine, University of Chicago, Chicago, Illinois, United States of America

Robert S. Daum
Department of Pediatrics, University of Chicago, Chicago, Illinois, United States of America

David L. Horn
David Horn LLC, Doylestown, Pennsylvania, United States of America

Annette C. Reboli
Department of Medicine, Cooper Medical School of Rowan University, Camden, New Jersey, United States of America

Coleman Rotstein
Division of Infectious Diseases, Department of Medicine, University of Toronto, Toronto, Ontario, Canada

Billy Franks and Nkechi E. Azie
Astellas Scientific and Medical Affairs, Northbrook, Illinois, United States of America

Vanja M. Dukic
Department of Applied Mathematics, University of Colorado, Boulder, Colorado, United States of America

Tobias Loddenkemper, Sriram Ramgopal and Sanjeev V. Kothare
Department of Neurology, Children's Hospital Boston and Harvard Medical School, Boston, Massachusetts, United States of America

Tanvir U. Syed, Deepak Gulati and Sikawat Thanaviratananich
Department of Neurology, Case Western Reserve University and University Hospitals, Cleveland, Ohio, United States of America

Mohamad Z. Koubeissi
Department of Neurology, Case Western Reserve University and University Hospitals, Cleveland, Ohio, United States of America
Department of Neurology, George Washington University, Washington, D.C., United States of America

Index

www.ingramcontent.com/pod-product-compliance
Lightning Source LLC
Chambersburg PA
CBHW080514200326
41458CB00012B/4204
* 9 7 8 1 6 3 2 4 2 7 7 9 3 *